# Visit our website

to find out about additional books from Baillière Tindall
and other Harcourt Health Sciences imprints

## Register free at
**www.harcourt-international.com**

and you will get

- the latest information on new books, journals and electronic
  products in your chosen subject areas

- the choice of e-mail or post alerts or both, when there are any
  new books in your chosen areas

- news of special offers and promotions

- information about products from all Harcourt Health Sciences
  companies including Baillière Tindall, Churchill Livingstone,
  Mosby and W. B. Saunders

You will also find an easily searchable catalogue, online ordering,
information on our extensive list of journals...and much more!

**Visit the Harcourt Health Sciences website today!**

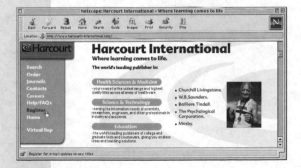

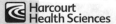

# Baillière's

# Nurses'
# Dictionary

*For Baillière Tindall:*

*Senior Commissioning Editor:* Jacqueline Curthoys
*Project Manager:* Gail Murray
*Project Development Manager:* Karen Gilmour
*Designer:* George Ajayi

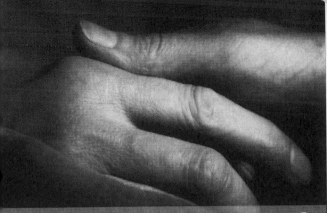
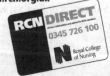

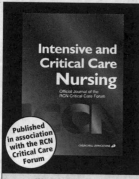

# Complementary Therapies in Nursing & Midwifery

## New larger bound format in 2000

**ISSN 1353 6117, 4 issues**

Editor: Denise Rankin-Box, UK
Deputy Editor: Caroline Stevensen, UK

### Now published in MEDLINE and PubMed

Complementary Therapies in Nursing & Midwifery is the first internationally refereed journal published to meet the specific needs of the nursing profession in the integration of complementary therapies from aromatherapy and massage to acupuncture and herbal medicine into conventional patient care practices.

# European Journal of Oncology Nursing

## The official Journal of the EUROPEAN ONCOLOGY NURSING SOCIETY

**ISSN 1364-9825, 4 issues**

Editor: A Richardson, UK
Associate Editors: L Robinson, UK • C Krcmar, Germany

European Journal of Oncology Nursing seeks to provide a forum for the exchange of knowledge and experience through which nurses can address issues of importance in cancer care.

It aims to inform the practice of cancer nursing through the report of current and ongoing research and relevant developments in practice, policy and education. Nurses involved in the practice, education and research setting are located in a variety of different contexts and the journal aims to reflect both the richness and the diversity of contemporary cancer nursing.

**IDEAL**

# Journal of Orthopaedic Nursing

**ISSN 1361-3111, 4 issues**

Editor-in-Chief: Peter Davis, UK
Associate Editor: Anne Footner, UK

Journal of Orthopaedic Nursing aims to propel orthopaedic nurses into the future. Orthopaedic nursing is changing at an unprecedented pace and will continue to do so at an accelerated rate in the future. It seeks to ensure that orthopaedic nurses, and allied health care professionals, are able to move forward positively and proactively to continually improve their patients' and clients' outcomes at home or in hospital.

# Nurse Education Today

**ISSN 0260 6917, 8 issues**

Editor-in-Chief: Prof Peter Birchenall, UK

Nurse Education Today promotes scholarship and scholarly writing among educators in nursing, midwifery and health visiting. At the same time the journal acts as an interface between the theory and the practice of nurse education, stimulating change and cross-fertilization of ideas. The Network section of the journal focuses on strategic issues pertinent to education within health care.

**IDEAL**

# Midwifery

**ISSN 0266-6138, 4 issues**

Editor-in-Chief: Ann M. Thomson, UK

Midwifery aims to enhance the quality of care for childbearing women and their families and to encourage midwives to explore and develop their knowledge, skills and attitudes.

It also provides an international, interdisciplinary forum for the publication, dissemination and discussion of advances, controversies and current research.

**IDEAL**

# Working for you

## Working well?

The RCN's Working Well initiative has been up and running since 1998. It brings together our work to safeguard the physical and mental well-being of nurses and to encourage employers to provide a safe and supportive working environment.

## Workability: getting disabled and injured nurses back into the workplace

It makes sense to use everybody's skills, even if they have a disability, illness or injury. This campaign encourages employers in all sectors of nursing and education to see that there are ways of employing people who don't fit their idea of the norm. There are lots of ways not to waste talent: for example, a nurse who uses a wheelchair can answer patient enquiries for NHS Direct; and there is already a pioneering deaf midwife in Leeds.

One community nurse in southern England explains how important a supportive environment was to help her back to work:

*'I had been off with stress and depression. My GP and community psychiatric nurse (CPN) felt I could go back to work, but only if I didn't have to return to the same place – I was convinced it was that which had made me so ill. I needed to get back to work as I had run out of sick pay. So I was moved to a different area under a more sympathetic manager in a team where I could be better supported. My CPN even came to meet my new manager with me to explain that I could not take a full caseload for some time. I also had a mentor who was great, and helped me regain my confidence.*

The workability campaign also encourages fast-tracking injured or ill nurses for assessment and treatment, so that they can recover and get back to work (good sense for employers in a time of nursing shortages). A resolution at Congress in 2000, put forward by the RCN UK Safety Reps committee, urged Council to press the four UK health departments to introduce just such fast-track treatment.

- For more information on workability, contact RCN WING (020 8649 9536) or call RCN Direct (0345 726 100) for a workability pack, publication code 001 175.
- The RCN website has full details too — www.rcn.org.uk

## Needlestick injuries

Another new campaign aims at increasing awareness of how to prevent needlestick injuries (NSI) to help reduce the number of injuries and improve methods of dealing with them when they happen.

There will be a programme of educational and research activities, including a new resource pack for RCN safety representatives, infection control nurses and occupational health nurses, and a general information leaflet for all RCN members. New research will collate injury rates, and find out what are the key activities which put nurses and patients at risk.

- Look out for announcements in the *RCN Bulletin* and *Nursing Standard* of when campaign materials are available.

## Latex allergy

RCN safety representatives and staff continue to campaign to raise awareness of the dangers of latex allergy. Many employers have been persuaded to change the gloves they provide. A recent IES survey shows 34% of NHS trusts now provide non-powdered gloves only, but 48% still provide both powdered and powder-free latex gloves, which relies on staff making an informed choice about which gloves to use. We are also lobbying for parliamentary support to pressure NHS Supplies to remove powdered gloves from their catalogue.

We support the cases of individual members who've developed a serious allergy. Often they can't get disability benefit because latex allergy is not on the DSS list of 'prescribed diseases'.

- Ask for information from your local safety representative, or call RCN Direct for a leaflet (publication code 000 948).

## Making time: employee friendly policy campaign

This campaign, launched last autumn, is gathering speed. It recognises that it's important to provide working arrangements which suit the professional and personal commitments of all nurses (not only those with families), and that achieving a balance between work and home is a vital part of working healthily. In Northern Ireland and Wales, we're lobbying for these considerations to be taken into account in the development of health service human resource strategies; in Scotland, we're part of a social partnership team looking at flexible working, and we're working with the NHS Executive regional task forces on employee friendly policies in England.

- *Having a life: an RCN guide to employee friendly policies* gives examples of good practice. Copies are available from RCN Direct (publication code 001 097) or look on our website, http://www.rcn.org.uk

*Working well in brief*

- **Violence against nurses**. Nurses from A&E to nursing homes face aggression and violent attack every day. Recent figures show 11 violent incidents a month for every 1000 NHS nurses in England. The RCN continues to work with employers to try to improve safety, and we support the NHS Zero Tolerance campaign. We are also lobbying to ensure that offenders are properly punished.

- **Stress**. We'll be producing guidance towards the end of 2000 on how employers can analyse what causes of stress have the most damaging effect on nurses' health.

- **Back injury**. A new RCN research project will look at back injury for nurses working in nursing homes, and how better equipment can reduce incidence.

- **Bullying and harassment**. Towards the end of 2000, there will be a new information pack for members on dealing with bullying and harassment, and a programme of training for RCN stewards to help better support members in the workplace.

- For immediate help with bullying, contact your steward, RCN office, or call RCN Direct. RCN Counselling may also be able to help you — call 0345 726 100 for information.

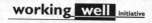

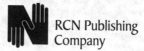

RCN Publishing
Company

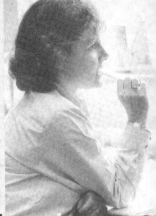
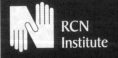

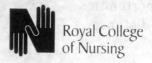Royal College
of Nursing

# CONFERENCES AND EVENTS

The RCN Conference & Events Unit aims to be the leading producer of professionally organised, value for money, innovative events for nurses and about nursing. It brings together the expertise of the RCN to communicate and influence nursing and healthcare policy and practice. The aim is to inform and inspire and the unit is committed to supporting nurses in their personal and professional development to help them deliver the highest quality of patient care.

To receive information on any of the Conference & Events Unit's national and international conferences:

Write:      Conference & Events Unit
            Royal College of Nursing
            20 Cavendish Square
            London
            W1M 0AB
Call:       020 7409 3333
Fax:        020 7647 3435
E-mail:     conference.unit@rcn.org.uk
Click:      www.rcn.org.uk

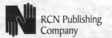

# Ⓝline

If you really want to know what's happening in nursing today, look no further on-line than the world's first weekly nursing journal website.

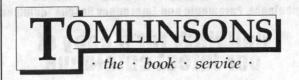

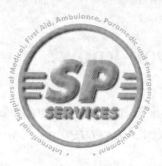
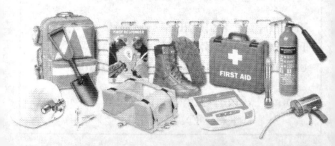

# Baillière's
# NURSES'
# DICTIONARY

EDITED BY
## Barbara F. Weller MSc RGN RSCN RNT

*Independent Nurse Consultant; Honorary Consultant Lecturer, Thames Valley University, London; Editor, Journal of Neonatal Nursing; Formerly Nursing Officer, Department of Health and Chief Nursing Adviser, British Red Cross Society, UK*

FOREWORD BY
## Christine Watson President, Royal College of Nursing, London, UK

*Twenty-third Edition*

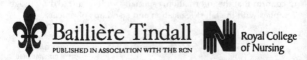

## Baillière Tindall
PUBLISHED IN ASSOCIATION WITH THE RCN

Royal College of Nursing

Edinburgh London New York Philadelphia St Louis Sydney Toronto 2000

BAILLIÈRE TINDALL
An imprint of Harcourt Publishers Limited
© Harcourt Publishers Limited 2001

 is a registered trademark of Harcourt Publishers Limited

First published 1912
Twenty-second edition (PVC and low-price) 1996
Twenty-second edition (PVC and low-price) reprinted 1999
Twenty-third edition (PVC and international) published 2000
Reprinted 2001

ISBN 0 7020 2557 7
International Edition ISBN 0 7020 2549 6

**British Library Cataloguing in Publication Data**
A catalogue record for this book is available from the British Library

**Library of Congress Cataloging in Publication Data**
A catalog record for this book is available from the Library of
Congress

**Note**
Medical knowledge is constantly changing. As new information
becomes available, changes in treatment, procedures, equipment and
the use of drugs become necessary. The editor, contributors and the
publishers have taken care to ensure that the information given in this
text is accurate and up to date. However, readers are strongly advised
to confirm that the information, especially with regard to drug usage,
complies with the latest legislation and standards of practice.

The
publisher's
policy is to use
**paper manufactured
from sustainable forests**

Printed in China

# Contents

# Contributors

**Gary Barrett** BSc(Hons) MBA MEd RGN RSCN ENB 405 Cert Ed FETC
Senior Lecturer, School of Paediatric Nursing and Child Health, Faculty of Health, South Bank University, London, UK

**Dee Beresford** MSc RGN RM ENB 405, 904, 870, 998
Executive Officer, Neonatal Nurses Association, Nottingham, UK

**Robert J. Pratt** BA MSc RN RNT DN(Lond)
Professor of Nursing, Wolfson Institute of Health Sciences, Thames Valley University, London, UK

# Appendices Contributors

**Christine Bishop** BSc(Hons)
Managing Editor, Journal of Neonatal Nursing, Bishop's Stortford, UK

**Helen Caulfield** LLB MA
Solicitor, Royal College of Nursing, London, UK

**Lindsay Creek** RGN ENB 199, 998 ALS(I) PALS(I)
Community Resuscitation Training Officer, East Anglian Ambulance NHS Trust, Newmarket, UK

**Joan M. Datsun**
Retired Medical Secretary

**John Driscoll** BSc(Nursing) DPSN Cert Ed RNT RMN RGN
Director, Transformational Learning Consultants Co Ltd, Sudbury, UK

**Chris Evans** BSc MRPharmS DMS
Principal Pharmacist, St George's Hospital, London, UK

**Gary Frost** PhD SRD
Head of Nutrition and Dietetics, Department of Nutrition and Dietetics, Hammersmith Hospital, London, UK

**Caroline King** BSc SRD
Chief Dietician Paediatrics, Department of Nutrition and Dietetics, Hammersmith Hospital, London, UK

**Hilary Peake** BSc SRD
Senior Dietician, Department of Nutrition and Dietetics, Hammersmith Hospital, London, UK

**Judy Rivett** RGN ONHCert PgDip in Health and Safety
Occupational Health and Safety Consultant, Ketteringham, UK

**Paul Thacker** RGN NDNCert
Clinical Manager, Liaison/OPD, West Suffolk Hospital, Bury St Edmunds, UK

# Foreword

Nursing is both a responsive and a proactive profession. As nurses we are sensitive to the changing needs of those for whom we care. We also pioneer new ways of improving care. The language we use reflects this approach, constantly modifying and embracing new terms to express fresh concepts and aspects of practice.

Since the last edition of this nursing dictionary we have seen yet more rapid change within the health service. Modernization plans cast nursing in a central role with an emphasis on both expanding nursing practice and building on core nursing values. During this period, nursing as a profession continues to develop its own skills and competencies. We are also increasingly receptive to new ideas from other professions and disciplines in order to complement our own practice and knowledge. Given this pace of change, it is inevitable that the scope and variety of our language is growing. Our nursing language is a vibrant, living entity – though it also suffers from its fair share of jargon and mystifying acronyms.

The new edition of this dictionary serves as an essential guide to today's nursing language. Over the years, the content of the dictionary has evolved, moving away from the more obscure medical references to focus more on nursing interventions. The changing policy framework is well served with, for example, a new appendix on clinical supervision and clinical governance, and updated sections on nurse prescribing and community care. The inclusion of information on nursing on the internet is also timely when considering the major implications for nursing of the revolution in information technology.

But though its content must move with the times, other important characteristics of the dictionary remain firmly intact. This is a pocket book which is designed for quick and easy access. It remains uncompromisingly relevant to practice. These constant features have made this dictionary an indispensable ally for generations of nurses, during those early days as a nursing student and throughout nursing careers.

Nurses – and many others – will continue to use *Baillière's Nurses' Dictionary* as a handy source for reliable and accessible information on important nursing issues, as well as a guide to and interpreter of language.

Congratulations must go to editor Barbara Weller, who once again has achieved a marvellous job in keeping up to date a tried and trusted friend.

CHRISTINE WATSON

# Preface

Words, words and more words. This could be one description of a dictionary, or of any other tome for that matter. But the difference for this nurses' dictionary, now in its 23rd edition, is that it provides for the user–reader insight into the meaning of those words that are being used currently in the provision of health care services.

In reading and comparing past editions with this new one, the main impression gained is of the way in which nursing has moved out of the realm of anatomy, drugs and applied treatments into the wider arena of health sciences. This has been a gradually evolving process which the 23rd edition continues to reflect. The issues for care are now even wider, encompassing health maintenance, education, the use and relevance of complementary therapies, and the impact of modern management on the delivery of care, for example clinical governance.

Today's health care professional has a broad remit to deliver a high quality of care in a variety of settings. To help support these objectives this 23rd edition seeks to provide the user with a wide range of definitions that are based on contemporary everyday usage of words used to communicate in professional life.

Communication in the health care services involves team work. The editing of this dictionary too involved several key players. I should like to thank all the contributors for their definitions and ideas, all the appendix writers and the staff of Harcourt Publishers for their support and interest. In addition, I should like to thank Mrs Joan Hunter and colleagues of the Clinical Resources Centre and Library of the West Suffolk Hospitals NHS Trust for their assistance and support; and colleagues at the East Anglian Ambulance NHS Trust for their contributions and advice. Finally, I should like to acknowledge the patience of my husband David Fisher over the burning of the midnight oil to meet deadlines.

Norfolk 2000                                         BARBARA F. WELLER

# Publisher's Acknowledgements

The publishers would like to thank the following for their kind permission to reproduce material in this dictionary: W. B. Saunders for figures in airway, cell, fluid, intussusception, leukocytes, and Trousseau's sign; McGraw-Hill for figure in injection; Resuscitation Council for figures in resuscitation; Royal College of Nursing for information on universal precautions and extending prescribing powers to nurses.

We are also grateful to the following Baillière Tindall authors for their kind permission to use material from their texts: Margaret Adams, for figures in graafian follicle and ectopic gestation (from Tiran D *Baillière's Midwives' Dictionary* 9th edn, 1997); Ann Faulkner, for figure in Maslow's hierarchy of needs (from Faulkner A *Nursing: A Creative Approach* 1985); Sheila Jackson and Penelope Bennett, for figures in bone (compact), ear, endometrium, hair and heart (from Jackson S and Bennett P *Physiology with Anatomy for Nurses* 1988); and Mike Walsh, for figure of a normal electrocardiogram (from Walsh M (ed.) *Watson's Clinical Nursing and Related Sciences* 5th edn, 1997).

# Style Guide

## *Pronunciations*

### Introduction
The pronunciations are transcribed using ordinary English-spelling letters. So that the guide is consistent and unambiguous, these characters have been combined together in precise ways (see below). The avoidance of the use of phonetic symbols (with the exception of the upside-down 'e' or 'schwa' (ə)) ensures that the guide is more or less immediately, and to some extent intuitively, understandable.

### Style of Transcription
All pronunciations are found in parentheses immediately after the bold main entry word (or variant, if one exists). The pronunciations reflect what could be called 'unaccented' or 'neutral' British English. Furthermore, transcriptions reflect *current, spoken usage* of the terms rather than how the term 'should' be pronounced, i.e. the guide does not attempt to be didactic or prescriptive.

#### *Variant Pronunciations and Spellings*
Where alternative pronunciations for a word are given, or where alternative spellings or synonyms are given, pronunciations are separated by commas. For example:

> **medicine** ('medisin, 'medsin)
> **neurone (neuron)** ('nyooə·rohn, 'nyooə·ron)

Alternative pronunciations are often given in a truncated form with the use of hyphens. For example:

> **encephalitis** (en'kefə'lietis, -sef-)

*Entries with Repeated Words*
Note that when a transcription for a particular word has been given at the bold main entry, any other entries that use the same word do not have a repeated transcription.

*Characters and Combinations used to Represent Sound*
In the pronunciation guide, single letters represent single sounds and where two or more characters are combined, as in the following tables, these also represent precise sounds.

**Pronunciation Style Guide**

| *Vowel Sounds* | | *Nearest international phonetic alphabet character* |
|---|---|---|
| **a** | as in **bad** (bad) | æ |
| **ah** | as in **father** ('fahdhə) | ɑ: |
| **air** | as in **hair** (hair) | ɛə or eə |
| **aw** | as in **water** ('wawtə) | ɔ: (cf. or) |
| **ay** | as in **fatal** ('fayt'l) | ɛI |
| **e** | as in **bed** (bed) | ɛ or e |
| **ee** | as in **fetus** ('feetəs) | i: |
| **i** | as in **film** (film) | I |
| **ie** | as in **bite** (biet) | aI |
| **i.ə** | as in **chloropsia** (klor'ropsi.ə) | Iə |
| **iə** | as in **fear** (fiə) | Iə |
| **ieə** | as in **diet** ('dieət) | aIə |
| **o** | as in **body** ('bodee) | ɒ |
| **oh** | as in **choke** (chohk) | əʊ |
| **oo** | as in **boot** (boot) | u: |
| **ooə** | as in **cure** (kyooə) | ʊə |
| **or** | as in **claw** (klor) | ɔ: (cf. aw) |
| **ow** | as in **now** (now) | aʊ |
| **owə** | as in **hour** (owə) | aʊə |
| **oy** | as in **goitre** ('goytə) | ɔI |
| **oyə** | as in **soya** ('soyə) | ɔIə |
| **u** | as in **tongue** (tung) | ʌ |
| **uh** | as in **put** (puht) | ʊ |
| **ə** | as in **mother** ('mudhə) | ə |
| **ər** | as in **bird** (bərd) | ɜ: |
| **y** | as in **yet** (yet) | j (semivowel) |

*Consonant Sounds*

| | | |
|---|---|---|
| b | as in **baby** ('baybee) | b |
| ch | as in **chart** (chaht) | tʃ |
| d | as in **digit** ('dijit) | d |
| dh | as in **they** (dhay) | ð |
| f | as in **fever** ('feevə) | f |
| g | as in **gag** (gag) | g |
| h | as in **heal** (heel) | h |
| j | as in **jump** (jump) | dʒ |
| k | as in **king** (king) | k |
| kh | as in **loch** (lokh) | χ or x |
| l | as in **light** (liet) | l |
| m | as in **man** (man) | m |
| n | as in **need** (need) | n |
| ng | as in **sung** (sung) | ŋ |
| nh | as in **restaurant** ('restəronh) | õ or ā |
| ny | as in **nutrition** (nyoo'trishən) | nj |
| p | as in **pelvis** ('pelvis) | p |
| r | as in **rod** (rod) | r |
| s | as in **sack** (sak) | s |
| sh | as in **fish** (fish) | ʃ |
| t | as in **test** (test) | t |
| th | as in **thirst** (thərst) | θ |
| v | as in **vein** (vayn) | v |
| w | as in **weight** (wayt) | w |
| z | as in **zero** ('ziə‧roh) | z |
| zh | as in **pleasure** ('plezhə) | ʒ |

*Stress Marks*

These are used where the word or term has more than one syllable, with the stress mark placed *before* the syllable to be stressed. The primary stressed syllable is indicated by a superior stress mark (') and secondary stress by an inferior stress mark (ˌ). For example:

> **respiration** (ˌrespi'rayshən)
> **respirator** ('respiˌraytə)
> **respiratory** (ri'spirətə.ree, 'respərətree)

*Syllabic Apostrophe*
Where a consonant is preceded by an apostrophe, this indicates that
the consonant should be pronounced. For example:

**hospital** ('hospit'l)

*Use of the Baseline Dot*
Where two letters occur together that may be mistaken for a different
sound from that intended, a full point is added on the baseline to separate the characters. For example:

**myopia** (mie'ohpi·ə)

## Subentries

The term being sought may be a main entry or a subentry under the
main entry. In subentries, the main entry is represented by its initial
letter if it is singular, and by the addition of an apostrophe and *s* if it is
plural. Subentries are listed alphabetically under the main entry. For
example:

**abdomen** . . .
*Acute a.* . . .
*Pendulous a.* . . .
*Scaphoid (navicular) a.* . . .

## Cross-referencing

Throughout the dictionary, cross-references are given within the text
as SMALL CAPITALS. For example:

**fibrin** ('fiebrin) an insoluble protein that is essential to
CLOTTING of blood, formed from fibrinogen by action of
thrombin.

There are also situations where it is simply more convenient to
define the word in a different location, to which the reader is then
referred.

## Translations

Where a translation of a foreign term occurs, it is indicated in *italic type*
immediately after the abbreviation for the language (which is in
square brackets). For example:

**acus** ('akəs) [L.] *a needle*

**Abbreviations Used in this Dictionary**

| | | | |
|---|---|---|---|
| *b.* born | | L. Latin | |
| Fr. French | | *pl.* plural | |
| Ger. German | | *sing.* singular | |

**Drug Names**

Where possible, only generic names are used; however, some proprietary drug names and names for preparations are included, with information (and sometimes cross-references) about the generic drug(s) involved. Inclusion of a drug in the dictionary does not imply endorsement.

**Alphabetical Order**

Entries in this dictionary are alphabetized as whole words rather than letter by letter, e.g. ABO system precedes abortion, and all-or-none law precedes allantois.

# A

**A** accommodation; adenine; anode (anodal); anterior; axial; symbol for ampere and mass number.

**A-scan** ('ayskan) ultrasonographic display used for measuring the size and thickness of organs and tissues accurately.

**abacterial** (‚aybak'tiə.ri.əl) indicating a condition not caused by bacteria.

**abatement** (ə'baytmənt) a decrease in the severity of a pain or a symptom.

**abdomen** ('abdəmən, ab'doh-) the belly. The cavity between the diaphragm and the pelvis, lined by a serous membrane, the peritoneum, and containing the stomach, intestines, liver, gallbladder, spleen, pancreas, kidneys, suprarenal glands, ureters and bladder. For descriptive purposes, its area can be divided into nine regions (*see* Figure). *Acute a.* any abdominal condition urgently requiring treatment, usually surgical. *Pendulous a.* a condition in which the anterior part of the abdominal wall hangs down over the pubis. *Scaphoid (navicular) a.* a hollowing of the anterior wall commonly seen in grossly emaciated people.

**abdominal** (ab'domin'l) pertaining to the abdomen. *A. aneurysm* a dilatation of the abdominal aorta. *A. aorta* that part of the aorta below the diaphragm. *A. breathing* deep breathing; hyperpnoea. *A. reflex* reflex contraction of abdominal

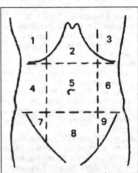

1, Right hypochondriac; 2, epigastric; 3, left hypochondriac; 4, right lumbar; 5, umbilical; 6, left lumbar; 7, right iliac; 8, hypogastric; 9, left iliac.

**REGIONS OF THE ABDOMEN**

wall muscles observed when skin is lightly stroked. *A. section* incision through the abdominal wall. *A. thrust see* HEIMLICH MANOEUVRE.

**abdominopelvic** (ab‚dominoh'pelvik) concerning the abdomen and the pelvic cavity.

**abdominoperineal** (ab‚dominoh'peri'neeəl) pertaining to the abdomen and the perineum. *A. excision* an operation performed through the abdomen and the perineum for the excision of the rectum or bladder.

Often done as a synchronized operation by two surgeons, one working at each approach.

**abdominoposterior** (ab͵dominohpo'stiə.ri.ə) indicating a position of the fetus with its abdomen turned towards the maternal back.

**abduce** (ab'dyoos) to abduct or to draw away.

**abducent** (ab'dyoosənt) leading away from the midline. *A. muscle* the external rectus muscle of the eye, which rotates it outward. *A. nerve* the cranial nerve that supplies this muscle.

**abductor** (ab'duktə) a muscle that draws a limb away from the midline of the body. The opposite of adductor.

**aberrant** (a'berənt) taking an unusual course. Used of blood vessels and nerves.

**aberration** (͵abə'rayshən) deviation from the normal. In optics, failure to focus rays of light. *Mental a.* mental disorder of an unspecified kind.

**ability** (ə'bilitee) the power to perform an act, either mental or physical, with or without training. *Innate a.* the ability with which a person is born.

**ablation** (ab'layshən) removal or destruction, by surgical or radiological means, of neoplasms or other body tissue.

**abnormal** (ab'nawm'l) varying from what is regular or usual.

**ABO system** (͵sistəm) *see* BLOOD GROUP.

**abort** (ə'bawt) 1. to terminate a process or disease before it has run its normal course. 2. To remove or expel from the womb an embryo or fetus before it is capable of independent existence.

**abortifacient** (ə'bawti'fayshənt) an agent or drug that may induce abortion.

**abortion** (ə͵bawshən) 1. premature cessation of a normal process.

2. emptying of the pregnant uterus before the end of the 24th week. 3. the product of such an abortion. *Complete a.* one in which the contents of the uterus are expelled intact. *Criminal a.* the termination of a pregnancy for reasons other than those permitted by law (i.e. danger to mental or physical health of mother or child or family) and without medical approval. *Incomplete a.* one in which some part of the fetus or placenta is retained in the uterus. *Induced a.* the intentional emptying of the uterus. *Inevitable a.* abortion where bleeding is profuse and accompanied by pains, the cervix is dilated and the contents of the uterus can be felt. *Missed a.* one where all signs of pregnancy disappear and later the uterus discharges a blood clot surrounding a shrivelled fetus, i.e. a carneous mole. *Septic a.* abortion associated with infection. *Therapeutic (legal) a.* one induced on medical advice because the continuance of the pregnancy would involve risk to the life of the pregnant woman, or injury to the physical or mental health of the pregnant woman or any existing children of her family, greater than if the pregnancy were terminated; or because there is a substantial risk that if the child were born it would suffer from such physical or mental abnormalities as to be seriously handicapped (1976 Abortion Act, as amended by the Human Fertilization and Embryology Act 1990). *Threatened a.* the appearance of signs of premature expulsion of the fetus; bleeding is slight, the cervix is closed. *Tubal a.* the termination of a tubal pregnancy caused by rupture of the uterine tube.

**abrasion** (ə'brayzhən) a superficial injury, where the skin or mucous membrane is rubbed or torn. *Corneal a.* this can occur when the surface of the cornea has been removed, e.g. by a scratch or other injury.

**abreaction** (ˌabriˈakshən) the reliving of a painful experience, with the release of repressed emotion.

**abruptio placentae** (əˌbrupshioh pləˈsentee) premature detachment of the placenta, causing maternal shock.

**abscess** ('abses) a collection of pus in a cavity. Caused by the disintegration and replacement of tissue damaged by mechanical, chemical or bacterial injury. *Alveolar a.* an abscess in a tooth socket. *Brodie's a.* a bone abscess, usually on the head of the tibia. *Cold a.* the result of chronic tubercular infection and so called because there are few, if any, signs of inflammation. *Psoas a.* a cold abscess that has tracked down the psoas muscle from caries of the lumbar vertebrae. *Subphrenic a.* one situated under the diaphragm.

**absorbent** (əbˈsawbənt, -ˈzaw-) 1. able to take in, or suck up and incorporate. 2. a tissue structure involved in absorption. 3. a substance that absorbs or promotes absorption.

**absorption** (əbˈsawpshən, -ˈzaw-) 1. in physiology, the taking up by suction of fluids or other substances by the tissues of the body. 2. in psychology, great mental concentration on a single object or activity. 3. in radiology, uptake of radiation by body tissues.

**abstinence** ('abstinəns) a refraining from the use of or indulgence in food, stimulants or coitus. *A. syndrome* withdrawal symptoms.

**abuse** (əˈbyoos) misuse, maltreatment or excessive use. *Child a.* the non-accidental use of physical force or the non-accidental act of omission by a parent or other custodian responsible for the care of a child. *Drug a.* use of illegal drugs or misuse of prescribed drugs. *Solvent a.*

the deliberate inhalation of volatile chemicals with the aim of inducing intoxication.

**acapnia** (ayˈkapni.ə) a deficiency of carbon dioxide in the blood.

**acaricide** (aˈkarisied) an agent that destroys mites or ticks.

**Acarus** ('akə.rəs) a genus of small mites. *A. scabiei* (*Sarcoptes scabiei*) the cause of scabies.

**acatalepsy** (ayˈkatəˌlepsee) lack of understanding.

**acataphasia** (ˌayˌkatəˈfaysi.ə) loss of the ability to express connected thought, resulting from a cerebral lesion.

**accessory** (akˈsesə.ri ˌək-) supplementary. *A. nerve* the 11th cranial nerve. It is made up of two portions: the cranial and the spinal.

**accident and emergency** ('aksidənt) sometimes referred to as casualty or trauma medicine. A setting for dealing with problems which require immediate attention and where patients can be directed or referred by a general practitioner or the emergency services.

**accident form** ('aksidənt ˌfawm) a form which provides a record of any accident to any person on NHS trust and other health care premises. Employers require that the form, now used widely, is completed as soon after the accident as possible.

**accommodation** (əˌkoməˈdayshən) adjustment. In ophthalmology, the term refers specifically to adjustment of the ciliary muscle, which controls the shape of the lens. *Negative a.* the ciliary muscle relaxes and the lens becomes less convex, giving long-distance vision. *Positive a.* the ciliary muscle contracts and the lens becomes more convex, giving near vision.

**accountable** (əˈkowntəbˈl) liable to be held responsible for a course of action. A qualified nurse has a duty of care according to law; in nursing, being accountable refers to the responsibility the qualified nurse takes for prescribing and initiating nursing care. Nurses are accountable to their patients, their peers and their employing authority, according to the Code of Professional Conduct. Registered practitioners (nurses, midwives or health visitors) are accountable at all times for their actions, on or off duty and whether engaged in current practice or not.

**accreditation** (ə,kredə'tayshən) a process of evaluation whereby an institution or an individual undergoes regular appraisal against agreed criteria, which, if met, result in the individual or institution being given official recognition by the accrediting organization.

**accretion** (ə'kreeshən) growth. The accumulation of deposits, e.g. of salts to form a calculus in the bladder. In dentistry, the growth of tartar on the teeth.

**ACE inhibitors** (,ays in'hibitəz) a group of drugs used in the treatment of hypertension. Their name, angiotensin converting enzyme inhibitors, explains part of their mode of action, although it is thought that some of their other actions may also be important in reducing blood pressure.

**acet-** combining form denoting acid. From the Latin *acetum*, vinegar.

**acetabuloplasty** (,asi'tabyuhloh,plastee) an operation performed to improve the depth and shape of the hip socket in correcting congenital dislocation of the hip or in treating osteoarthritis of the hip (*see* Figure).

**acetabulum** (,asi'tabyuhləm) the cup-like socket in the innominate bone, in which the head of the femur moves.

**acetate** ('asi,tayt) a salt of acetic acid.

**acetazolamide** (ə,setə'zoləmied) a sulphonamide compound which is

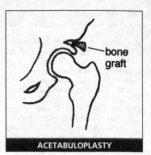

**ACETABULOPLASTY**

an oral diuretic and is used in the treatment of congestive heart failure and of glaucoma.

**acetoacetic acid** (,asithə.ə'seetik, ə,-seetoh.ə'seetik) diacetic acid. A product of fat metabolism. It occurs in excessive amounts in diabetes and starvation, giving rise to acetone bodies in the urine.

**acetonaemia** (,asitə'neemi.ə, ə,see-) the presence of acetone bodies in the blood.

**acetone** ('asi,tohn) a colourless inflammable liquid with a characteristic odour. Traces are found in the blood and in normal urine. *A. bodies* ketones found in the blood and urine of uncontrolled diabetic patients and also in acute starvation as a result of the incomplete breakdown of fatty and amino acids.

**acetonuria** (,asitə'nyooə.ri.ə, ə,see-) the presence of an excess quantity of acetone bodies in the urine, giving it a peculiar sweet smell.

**acetylcholine** (,asitiel'kohleen, ,asi-til-) a chemical transmitter that is released by some nerve endings at the synapse between one neurone and the next or between a nerve ending and the effector organ it supplies. These nerves are said to be cholinergic, e.g. the parasympathetic nerves and the lower motor

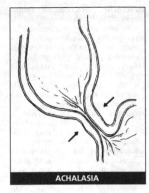

ACHALASIA

neurones to skeletal muscles. Acetylcholine is rapidly destroyed in the body by cholinesterase.

**acetylcoenzyme A** (ˌasitielkoh'enziem, ˌasitil-) active form of acetic acid, to which carbohydrates, fats and amino acids not needed for protein synthesis are converted.

**acetylsalicylic acid** (ˌasitiel'sali'silik, ˌasitil-) aspirin. An analgesic, antipyretic and antirheumatic drug. It is available in its pure form or in combination with other drugs.

**achalasia** (akə'layzi.ə) failure of relaxation of a muscle sphincter causing dilatation of the part above, e.g. of the oesophagus above the cardiac sphincter (*see* Figure).

**ache** (ayk) a dull continuous pain.

**Achilles** (ə'kileez) Greek mythological hero who could be wounded only in the heel. *A. tendon* tendo calcaneus, connecting the soleus and gastrocnemius muscles of the calf to the heel bone (os calcis). Tapping the Achilles tendon normally produces the Achilles reflex or ankle jerk.

**achlorhydria** (ˌayklor'hiedri.ə) the absence of free hydrochloric acid in the stomach. May be found in pernicious anaemia, pellagra and gastric cancer.

**acholia** (ay'kohli.ə) lack of secretion of bile.

**acholuria** (ˌaykə'lyooə.ri.ə) deficiency or lack of bile in the urine.

**acholuric** (ˌaykə'lyooə.rik) pertaining to acholuria. *A. jaundice* jaundice without bile in the urine.

**achondroplasia** (ayˌkondroh'playzi.ə) an inherited condition in which there is early union of the epiphysis and diaphysis of long bones. Growth is arrested resulting in short stature.

**achromasia** (ˌaykroh'mayzi.ə) 1. lack of colour in the skin. 2. absence of normal reaction to staining in a tissue or cell.

**achromatopsia** (ˌaykrohmə'topsi.ə) complete colour blindness caused by disease or trauma. It may be congenital.

**achylia** (ay'kieli.ə) absence of hydrochloric acid and enzymes in the gastric secretions. *A. gastrica* a condition in which gastric secretion is reduced or absent.

**acid** ('asid) 1. sour or sharp in taste. 2. a substance which, when combined with an alkali, will form a salt. Any acid substance will turn blue litmus red. Individual acids are given under their specific names. *A.-alcohol-fast* descriptive of stained bacteria that are resistant to decolorization by both acid and alcohol. *A.-base balance* the normal ratio between the acid ions and the basic or alkaline ions required to maintain the pH of the blood and body fluids.

**acidaemia** (ˌasi'deemi.ə) abnormal acidity of the blood, which contains an excess of hydrogen ions.

**acidity** (ə'siditee) 1. sourness or sharpness of taste. 2. the state of being acid.

**acidosis** (ˌasi'dohsis) a condition in which the relation of alkalinity to acidity of the blood is disturbed, with an increase in the hydrogen ion concentration. It is characterized by vomiting, drowsiness, hyperpnoea, acetone odour of breath (of 'new-mown hay') and acetone bodies in the urine. It may occur in diabetes mellitus owing to incomplete metabolism of fat. *See also* KETOSIS.

**acidotic** (ˌasi'dotik) 1. pertaining to acidosis. 2. a person suffering from acidosis.

**aciduria** (ˌasi'dyooə.ri.ə) a condition in which acid urine is excreted.

**acinus** ('asinəs) a minute saccule or alveolus of a compound gland, lined by secreting cells. The secreting portion of the mammary gland consists of acini.

**acme** ('akmee) 1. the highest point. 2. the crisis of a fever when the symptoms are fully developed.

**acne** ('aknee) an inflammatory condition of the sebaceous glands in which blackheads (comedones) are usually present together with papules and pustules. **A. keratitis** inflammation of the cornea associated with acne rosacea. **A. rosacea** a redness of the forehead, nose and cheeks due to chronic dilatation of the subcutaneous capillaries, which becomes permanent with the formation of pustules in the affected areas. **A. vulgaris** form that occurs commonly in adolescents and young adults, affecting the face, chest and back.

**acneiform** (ak'nee.i.fawm) resembling acne.

**acousma** (ə'koosmə) the hearing of imaginary sounds.

**acoustic** (ə'koostik) relating to sound or the sense of hearing.

**acquired** (ə'kwieəd) pertaining to disease, habits or immunity developed after birth; not inherited.

**acquired immune deficiency syndrome** abbreviated AIDS. *See* AIDS.

**acrid** ('akrid) bitter; pungent; irritating.

**acrocentric** (ˌakroh'sentrik) a chromosome in which the centromere is situated at or very near one end.

**acrocephalia** (ˌakrohke'fayli.ə, -se-) malformation of the head, in which the top is pointed. Oxycephaly.

**acrocyanosis** (ˌakroh.sieə'nohsis) persistent cyanosis, coldness of the hands and feet and profuse sweating of the digits, often associated with a vasomotor defect.

**acrodynia** (ˌakroh'dini.ə) an allergic reaction to mercury in children, causing pain and erythema in the fingers and toes. Pink disease.

**acromegaly** (ˌakroh'megalee) a chronic condition producing gradual enlargement of the hands, feet, and bones of the head and chest. Associated with overactivity of the anterior lobe of the pituitary gland in adults.

**acromioclavicular** (ə.krohmiohklə-'vikyuhlə) pertaining to the joint between the acromion process of the scapula and the lateral aspect of the clavicle.

**acromion** (ə'krohmi.ən) the outward projection of the spine of the scapula, forming the point of the shoulder.

**acroparaesthesia** (ˌakroh.paris'theezi.ə) condition in which pressure on the nerves of the brachial plexus causes numbness, pain and tingling of the hand and forearm.

**acrophobia** (ˌakroh'fohbi.ə) morbid terror of being at a height.

**acrosclerosis** (ˌakrohsklə'rohsis) a type of scleroderma that affects the hands, feet, face or chest.

**acrosome** ('akrə.sohm) part of the head of a spermatozoon containing enzymes which break down the cell membrane of the ovum and allow penetration.

**ACTH** adrenocorticotrophic hormone; corticotrophin.

**actin** ('aktin) the protein of myofibrils responsible for contraction and relaxation of muscles.

**actinodermatitis** (ˌaktinohˌdermə 'tietis) inflammation of the skin due to the action of ultraviolet or X-rays.

*Actinomyces* (ˌaktinoh'mieseez) a genus of branching, spore-forming, vegetable parasites, which may give rise to actinomycosis and from which many antibiotic drugs are produced, e.g. streptomycin.

**actinomycin** (ˌaktinoh'miesin) a group of cytotoxic drugs used in the treatment of malignant disease.

**actinomycosis** (ˌaktinohmie'kohsis) a chronic infective disease of cattle that is also found in humans. Granulated tumours occur, chiefly on the tongue and jaws.

**actinotherapy** (ˌaktinoh'therəpee) treatment of disease by rays of light, e.g. artificial sunlight.

**action** ('akshən) the accomplishment of an effect, whether mechanical or chemical, or the effect so produced. *A. research* a method of undertaking social research that incorporates the researcher's involvement as a direct and deliberate part of the research, i.e. the researcher acts as a change agent. *Cumulative a.* the sudden and markedly increased action of a drug after administration of several doses. *Reflex a.* an involuntary response to a stimulus conveyed to the nervous system and reflected to the periphery, passing below the level of consciousness (*see also* REFLEX).

**activator** (ˌakti'vaytə) a substance, hormone or enzyme that stimulates a chemical change, although it may not take part in the change. In chemistry, a catalyst. For example, yeast is the activator in the process by which sugar is converted into alcohol; the digestive secretions are activated by hormones to carry out normal digestion.

**active** ('aktiv) causing change; energetic. *A. immunity* an immunity in which individuals have been stimulated to produce their own antibodies. *A. movements* movements made by the patient, as distinct from passive movements. *A. principle* the ingredient in a drug that is primarily responsible for its therapeutic action.

**activities of daily living** (ak'tivitiz əv ˌdaylee ˌliving) abbreviated ADL. Those activities usually performed in the course of a person's normal daily routine, such as eating, cleaning teeth, washing and dressing.

**actomysin** (ˌaktoh'miesin) muscle protein complex; the myosin component acts as an enzyme which causes the release of energy.

**acuity** (ə'kyooitee) sharpness. *A. of hearing* an acute perception of sound. *A. of vision* clear focusing ability.

**acupuncture** ('akyuhˌpungkchə) a Chinese medical system which aims to diagnose illness and promote health by stimulating the body's self-healing powers. The insertion of special needles into specific points along the 'meridians' of the body is used for the production of anaesthesia, the relief of pain and the treatment of certain conditions.

**acute** (ə'kyoot) a term applied to a disease in which the attack is sudden, severe and of short duration.

**acute respiratory distress syndrome** (dis'tres) abbreviated ARDS. A severe form of acute lung function failure which occurs after an event such as trauma, inhalation of a toxic substance or septic shock. There is severe breathlessness and a dangerous reduction in the supply of oxygen to the blood.

**acyclic** (ay'sieklik) occurring independently of a natural cycle of events (such as the menstrual cycle).

**acyclovir** (ay'sieklohviə) an antiviral agent used to treat herpes viruses. Uses include the treatment of varicella zoster and herpes simplex. It is only active if started at the onset of the infection. May also be used as prophylaxis in the immunocompromised and for prevention of recurrence.

**Adam's apple** (ˌadəmz ˈapəl) the laryngeal prominence, a protrusion of the front of the neck formed by the thyroid cartilage.

**adamantine** (ˌadəˈmanteen, -tien) pertaining to the enamel of the teeth.

**adaptation** (ˌadapˈtayshən) 1. the process of modification that a living organism undergoes when adjusting itself to new surroundings or circumstances. 2. a function of the stimulus to which the individual is exposed and of the individual's accommodation to the situation. The adaptation response may relate to physiological needs, role, 'self' concept and interdependence. 3. the process of overcoming difficulties and adjusting to changing circumstances. Neuroses and psychoses are often associated with failure of adaptation. 4. used in ophthalmology to mean the adjustment of visual function according to the ambient illumination. *Colour a.* 1. changes in visual perception of colour with prolonged stimulation. 2. adjustment of vision to degree of brightness or colour tone of illumination. *Dark a.* adaptation of the eye to vision in reduced illumination. *Light a.* adaptation of the eye to vision in bright illumination (photopia), with reduction in the concentration of the photosensitive pigments of the eye.

**addict** (ˈadikt) a person exhibiting addiction.

**addiction** (əˈdikshən) the taking of drugs or alcohol leading to physiological and psychological dependence with a tendency to increase use. *See* DEPENDENCE and DRUG (ADDICTION).

**Addison's anaemia** (ˈadisənz) T. *Addison, British physician, 1793–1860.* Pernicious anaemia.

**Addison's disease** deficiency disease of the suprarenal cortex; often tuberculous. There is wasting, brown pigmentation of the skin and extreme debility.

**adducent** (əˈdyoosənt) leading towards the midline. *A. muscle* the medial rectus muscle of the eye, which turns it inwards.

**adductor** (əˈduktə) a muscle that draws a limb towards the midline of the body. The opposite of abductor.

**adenectomy** (ˌadəˈnektəmee) excision of a gland.

**adenine** (ˈadəˌneen) one of the purine bases found in DNA.

**adenitis** (ˌadəˈnietis) inflammation of a gland.

**adenocarcinoma** (ˌadənohˌkahsiˈnohmə) a malignant new growth of glandular epithelial tissue.

**adenofibroma** (ˌadənohfieˈbrohmə) a benign tumour of connective tissue which contains glandular structures.

**adenoid** (ˈadəˌnoyd) resembling a gland. Generally applied to abnormal lymphoid growth in the nasopharynx (*see* Figure).

**adenoidectomy** (ˌadənoyˈdektəmee) the surgical removal of adenoid tissue from the nasopharynx.

**adenoma** (ˌadəˈnohmə) a nonmalignant tumour of glandular tissue.

**adenomatome** (ˌadəˈnohməˌtohm) an instrument for the removal of adenoids.

**adenomyoma** (ˌadənohmieˈohmə) an innocent new growth involving both endometrium and muscle tissue; found in the uterus or uterine ligaments.

**adenopathy** (ˌadəˈnopəthee) enlargement of any gland, especially those of the lymphatic system.

**adenosarcoma** (ˌadənohsahˈkohmə) a malignant tumour of connective

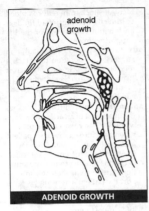

adenoid growth

**ADENOID GROWTH**

and glandular tissue. *Embryonal a.* nephroblastoma.

**adenosclerosis** (,adənohsklə'rohsis) hardening of a gland. Usually the result of calcification.

**adenosine** (a'denoh,seen) a nucleoside consisting of adenine and D-ribose (a pentose sugar). *A. triphosphate* abbreviated ATP. A compound containing three phosphoric acids. It is present in all cells and serves as a store for energy.

**adenovirus** (,adənoh'vierəs) a virus of the Adenoviridae family. Many types have been isolated, some of which cause respiratory tract infections, while others are associated with conjunctivitis, epidemic keratoconjunctivitis or gastrointestinal infection.

**ADH** antidiuretic hormone. Vasopressin.

**adhesion** (ad'heezhən) union between two surfaces normally separated. Usually the result of inflammation when fibrous tissue forms, e.g. peritonitis may cause adhesions between organs. A possible cause of intestinal obstruction.

**adiaphoretic** (ay,dieəfor'retik) an anhidrotic agent. A drug that prevents the secretion of sweat.

**adipocele** ('adipoh,seel) a hernia, with the sac containing fatty tissue.

**adipose** ('adi,pohs, -z) of the nature of fat. Fatty.

**adiposity** (,adi'positee) the state of being too fat. Obesity.

**adiposuria** (,adipoh'syooə.ri.ə) the presence of fat in the urine. Lipuria.

**aditus** ('aditəs) an opening or passageway; often applied to that between the middle ear and the mastoid antrum.

**adjustment** (ə'justmənt) in psychology, the ability of a person to adapt to changing circumstances or environment.

**adjuvant** ('ajəvənt) 1. any treatment used in conjunction with another to enhance its efficacy. 2. a substance administered with a drug to enhance its effect.

**ADL** activities of daily living.

**Adler's theory** ('adləz ,theeəri) *A. Adler, Austrian psychiatrist, 1870–1937.* The theory that neuroses develop as a compensation for feelings of inferiority, either social or physical.

**adnexa** (ad'neksə) appendages. *Uterine a.* the ovaries and tubes.

**adolescence** (,adə'lesəns) the period between puberty and maturity. In the male, 14–25 years. In the female, 12–21 years.

**adrenal** (ə'dreen'l) 1. near the kidneys. 2. a triangular endocrine gland situated above each kidney.

**adrenalectomy** (ə,dreenə'lektəmee) surgical excision of adrenal gland.

**adrenaline** (ə'drenəlin) a hormone secreted by the medulla of the adrenal gland. Has an action similar to normal stimulation of the sympathetic nervous system: (a) causing dilatation of the bronchioles; (b) raising the blood pressure by constriction of surface vessels and stimulation of the cardiac output;

(c) releasing glycogen from the liver. It is therefore used to treat such conditions as asthma, collapse and hypoglycaemia. It acts as a haemostat in local anaesthetics.

**adrenergic** (ˌadrəˈnərjik) pertaining to nerves that release the chemical transmitter noradrenaline in order to stimulate the muscles and glands they supply.

**adrenocorticotrophin** (əˌdreenoh-ˌkawtikohˈtrohfin) adrenocorticotrophic hormone (ACTH); secreted by the anterior lobe of the pituitary body. Stimulates the adrenal cortex to produce cortisol. Corticotrophin.

**adrenogenital** (əˌdreenohˈjenitˈl) relating to both the adrenal glands and the gonads. *A. syndrome* a condition of masculinization caused by overactivity of the adrenal cortex resulting in precocious puberty in the male infant and masculinization in the female. Both sexes are liable to Addisonian crises.

**adrenolytic** (əˈdreenohˈlitik) a drug that inhibits the stimulation of the sympathetic nerves and the activity of adrenaline.

**adsorbent** (ədˈsawbənt, -ˈzawb-) a substance that has the power of attracting gas or fluid to itself.

**adsorption** (ədˈsawpshən, -ˈzawp-) the power of certain substances to attach gases or other substances in solution to their surface and so concentrate them there. This is made use of in chromatography.

**adult** (əˈdult, ˈadult) mature. A mature person.

**adulteration** (əˌdultəˈrayshən) addition of an impure, cheap or unnecessary ingredient to cheat with, cheapen or falsify a preparation.

**advanced trauma life support** (adˈvahnst) a set of protocols recommended for use by doctors and paramedics when dealing with seriously injured people at the scene of an accident. The immediate treatment of shock from reduced blood volume by the infusion of fluids is an integral component of the life support regime.

**advancement** (ədˈvahnsmənt) in surgery, an operation to detach a tendon or muscle and reattach it further forward. Used in the treatment of strabismus and plastic surgery.

**adventitia** (ˌadvenˈtishi.ə, - ˈtishə) the outer coat of an artery or vein.

**advocacy** (ˈadvəkəsee) the process whereby a nurse provides a patient and/or the family with information to enable them to make informed decisions relating to the care situation. The nurse is then able to support the patient's decision vis-à-vis other professionals and also to incorporate the informed decisions into care planning.

**aeration** (airˈrayshən) supplying with air. Used to describe the oxygenation of blood which takes place in the lungs.

**aerobe** (ˈair.rohb) an organism that can live and thrive only in the presence of oxygen.

**aerobic exercise** (airˈrohbik) physical exercises for which the degree of effort is such that it can be maintained for long periods without undue breathlessness. The aim of this form of exercising is to increase the effectiveness of the heart and lungs and the supply of oxygen to the tissues of the body.

**aeropathy** (airˈropəthee) commonly called the bends (decompression sickness).

**aerophagy** (airˈrofajee) the excessive swallowing of air.

**aerosol** (ˈair.rəˌsol) finely divided particles or droplets. *A. sprays* used in medicine to humidify air or oxygen, or for the administration of drugs by inhalation.

**Æsculapius** (ˌeeskyuhˈlaypi.əs, ˈes-) the god of healing in Roman mythology.

**aetas** ('eetas) [L.] *age*; abbreviated aet.

**aetiology** (,eeti'olajee) the science of the cause of disease.

**afebrile** (ay'feebriel, -'feb-) without fever.

**affect** ('afekt, ə'fekt) in psychiatry, the feeling experienced in connection with an emotion or mood.

**affection** (ə'fekshən) 1. a morbid condition or disease state. 2. a warm feeling for someone or something.

**affective** (ə'fektiv) pertaining to the emotions or moods. *A. psychoses* major mental disorders in which there is grave disturbance of the emotions.

**afferent** ('afə,rənt) conveying towards the centre. *A. nerves* the sensory nerve fibres that convey impulses from the periphery towards the brain. *A. paths* or *tracts* the course of the sensory nerves up the spinal cord and through the brain. *A. vessels* arterioles entering the glomerulus of the kidney, or lymphatics entering a lymph gland. See EFFERENT.

**affiliation** (ə,fili'ayshən) the judicial decision about the paternity of a child with a view to the issue of a maintenance order.

**affinity** (ə'finitee) in chemistry, the attraction of two substances to each other, e.g. haemoglobin and oxygen.

**afibrinogenaemia** (ayfie,brinəjə-'neemi.ə) absence of fibrinogen in the blood. The clotting mechanism of the blood is impaired as a result.

**African tick fever** ('afrikən) disease caused by a spirochaete, *Borrelia duttonii*. Transmitted by ticks. See RELAPSING FEVER.

**afterbirth** ('ahftə,bərth) a lay expression used to describe the placenta, cord and membranes expelled after childbirth.

**aftercare** ('ahftə,kair) social, medical or nursing care provided after a period of hospital treatment.

**afterimage** ('ahftə,imij) a visual impression that remains briefly after the cessation of sensory stimulation.

**afterpain** ('ahftə,payn) pain due to uterine contraction after childbirth.

**afunctional** (ay'fungkshən'l) lacking function.

**agammaglobulinaemia** (ay,gamə-,globyuhli'neemi.ə) a condition in which there is no gamma-globulin in the blood. The patients are therefore susceptible to infections because of an inability to form antibodies.

**agar** ('aygah) a gelatinous substance prepared from seaweed. Used as a culture medium for bacteria and as a laxative because it absorbs liquid from the digestive tract and swells, so stimulating peristalsis.

**age** (ayj) 1. the duration, or the measure of time, of the existence of a person or object. 2. to undergo change as a result of the passage of time. *Achievement a.* 1. see DEVELOPMENTAL (MILESTONES). 2. proficiency in study expressed in terms of the chronological age of a normal child showing the same degree of attainment. 3. acquirement of a new skill or interest in old age or a praiseworthy accomplishment by an aged person. *Chronological a.* the actual measure of time elapsed since a person's birth. *Gestational a.* an expression of age of a developing fetus, usually given in weeks. It is measured from the date of the mother's last menstrual period, and so is approximately 2 weeks longer than time from conception. *Mental a.* the age level of mental ability of a person as gauged by standard intelligence tests.

**ageing** ('ayjing) the structural changes that take place with time and are not caused by accident or disease.

**ageism** ('ayjizəm) the systematic discrimination against people on the grounds of age, based on stereotyping of the elderly as helpless, infirm, confused and requiring health care and supportive social services.

**agenesis** (ay'jenəsis) failure of a structure to develop properly.

**agent** ('ayjənt) any substance or force capable of producing a physical, chemical or biological effect. *Alkylating a.* a cytotoxic preparation. *Chelating a.* a chemical compound that binds metal ions. *Wetting a.* a substance that lowers the surface tension of water and promotes wetting.

**agglutination** (ə,glooti'nayshən) collecting into clumps, particularly of cells suspended in a fluid and of bacteria affected by specific immune serum. *A. test* a means of aiding diagnosis and identification of bacteria. If serum containing known agglutinins comes into contact with the specific bacteria, clumping will take place (*see* WIDAL REACTION). *Cross a.* a simple test to decide the group to which blood belongs (*see* BLOOD GROUP).

**agglutinative** (ə'glootinə,tiv) 1. adherent or gluing together. 2. serum that causes clumping of bacteria, e.g. in the Widal reaction.

**agglutinin** (ə'glootinin) any substance causing agglutination (clumping together) of cells, particularly a specific antibody formed in the blood in response to the presence of an invading agent. Agglutinins are proteins (IMMUNOGLOBULIN) and function as part of the immune mechanism of the body. When the invading agents that bring about the production of agglutinins are bacteria, the agglutinins produced bring about agglutination of the bacterial cells.

**agglutinogen** (,agluh'tinəjən) any substance that, when present in the bloodstream, can cause the production of specific antibodies or agglutinins.

**aggregation** (,agri'gayshən) the massing together of materials, as in clumping. *Familial a.* the increased incidence of cases of a disease in a family compared with that in control families. *Platelet a.* the clumping together of platelets, which may be induced by a number of agents, such as thrombin and collagen.

**aggression** (ə'greshən) animosity or hostility shown towards another person or object as a response to opposition or frustration.

**agitation** (,aji'tayshən) 1. shaking. 2. mental distress causing extreme restlessness.

**aglutition** (,aygloo'tishən) difficulty in the act of swallowing. Dysphagia.

**agnosia** (ag'nohziə) an inability to recognize objects because the sensory stimulus cannot be interpreted, in spite of the presence of a normal sense organ.

**agonist** ('agənist) the prime mover. A muscle opposed in action by another (the antagonist).

**agony** ('agənee) extreme suffering, either mental or physical.

**agoraphobia** (,agə.rə'fohbi.ə) a fear of open spaces.

**agranulocyte** (ay'granyuhloh,siet) a white blood cell without granules in its cytoplasm. The term includes monocytes and lymphocytes.

**agranulocytosis** (ay,granyuhlohsie-'tohsis) a condition in which there is a marked decrease or complete absence of granular leukocytes in the blood, leaving the body defenceless against bacterial invasion. May result from: (a) the use of toxic drugs; (b) irradiation. Characterized by a sore throat, ulceration of the mouth and pyrexia. It may result in severe prostration and death.

**agraphia** (ay'grafi.ə) absence of the power of expressing thought in writing. It arises from a lack of muscular coordination or as a result of a cerebral lesion.

**ague** ('aygyoo) malaria.

**AHF** antihaemophilic factor (clotting factor VIII).

**AHG** antihaemophilic globulin (clotting factor VIII).

**AID** artificial insemination of a woman with donor semen.

**AIDS** (aydz) acquired immune deficiency syndrome. It is the extreme end of the spectrum of disease caused by human immuno-deficiency virus (HIV) infection, and impairs the body's cellular immune system. This may result in infection by organisms of normally no or low pathogenicity (opportunistic infections), principally *Pneumocystis carinii* pneumonia (PCP), or the development of unusual tumours, namely Kaposi's sarcoma (*KS*). *A.-related complex* (ARC) recurrent symptoms such as lymphadenopathy, night sweats, diarrhoea, weight loss, malaise and chest infections. Examination of the blood may show abnormally low platelet and neutrophil counts as well as low lymphocyte counts.

**AIH** artificial insemination of a woman by her husband's semen.

**ailment** ('ailmənt) any minor disorder of the body.

**air** (air) a mixture of gases that make up the earth's atmosphere. It consists of: non-active nitrogen 79%; oxygen 21%, which supports life and combustion; traces of neon, argon, hydrogen, etc.; and carbon dioxide 0.03%, except in expired air, when 6% is exhaled as a result of diffusion that has taken place in the lungs. Air has weight and exerts pressure, which aids in syphonage from body cavities. *A.-bed* a rubber mattress inflated with air. *A. embolism* an embolism caused by air entering the circulatory system. *A. encephalography* radiological examination of the brain after the injection of air into the subarachnoid space. *A. hunger* a form of dyspnoea in which there are deep sighing respirations, characteristic of severe haemorrhage or acidosis. *Complemental a.* additional air that can be inhaled with inspiratory effort. *Residual a.* air remaining in the lungs after deep expiration. *Stationary a.* that retained in the lungs after normal expiration. *Supplemental a.* the extra air forced out of the lungs with expiratory effort. *Tidal a.* that which passes in and out of the lungs in normal respiratory action.

**airway** ('airway) 1. the passage by which the air enters and leaves the lungs. 2. a mechanical device (tube) used for securing unobstructed respiration during general anaesthesia or on other occasions when the patient is not ventilating or exchanging gases properly. It may be passed through the mouth or nose. The tube prevents a flaccid tongue from resting against the posterior pharyngeal wall and causing obstruction of the airway (*see* Figure on p. 14).

**akinesia** (ˌayki'neezi.ə) loss of muscle power. This may be the result of a brain or spinal cord lesion or, temporarily, of anaesthesia.

**akinetic** (ˌayki'netik) relating to states or conditions where there is lack of movement.

**alacrima** (ay'lakrimə) a deficiency or absence of secretion of tears.

**alalia** (ə'layli.ə) loss or impairment of the power of speech due to muscle paralysis or a cerebral lesion.

**alanine** ('alə,neen, -,nien) an amino acid formed by the ingestion of dietary protein.

**Albers-Schönberg's disease** (ˌalbairz-'shərnbərg) *H. E. Albers-Schönberg, German radiologist, 1865–1921.* Osteoporosis.

**albinism** ('albi,nizəm) a condition in which there is congenital absence of pigment in the skin, hair and eyes. It may be partial or complete.

**albino** (al'beenoh) a person affected with albinism.

**Albright's syndrome** ('awlbriets) *F. Albright, American physician, 1900–1969.* Condition in which there is abnormal development of bone, excessive pigmentation of the skin and, in females, precocious sexual development.

**albumin** ('albyuhmin) 1. any protein that is soluble in water and moderately concentrated salt solutions and is coagulable by heat, e.g. egg white. 2. serum albumin; a plasma protein, formed principally in the liver and constituting about four-sevenths of the 6–8% protein concentration in the plasma. Albumin is a very important factor in regulating the exchange of water between the plasma and the interstitial compartment (space between the cells). A drop in the amount of albumin in the plasma results in an increase in tissue fluid, which, if severe, becomes apparent as oedema. Albumin serves also as a transport protein.

**albuminuria** (al,byoomi'nyooə.ri.ə) the presence of albumin in the urine, occurring e.g. in renal disease, in most feverish conditions and sometimes in pregnancy. *Orthostatic* or *postural a.* a nonpathological form that affects some individuals after prolonged standing but disappears after bedrest for a few hours.

**albumose** ('albyuh,mohs, -,mohz) a substance, formed during gastric digestion, intermediate between albumin and peptone.

**alcohol** ('alkə,hol) a volatile liquid distilled from fermented saccharine liquids and forming the basis of wines and spirits. The official (British Pharmacopoeia) preparation of

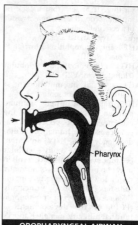

OROPHARYNGEAL AIRWAY

ethyl alcohol (ethanol) contains 95% alcohol and 5% water. Used: (a) as an antiseptic; (b) in the preparation of tinctures; (c) as a perspective for anatomical specimens. Taken internally, it acts as a temporary heart stimulant, and in large quantities as a depressant poison. It has some value as a food, 30 ml brandy producing about 400 J. *Absolute a.* that which contains not more than 1% by weight of water. *A.-fast* pertaining to bacteria that, once having been stained, are resistant to decolorization by alcohol. *A. withdrawal syndrome* a group of symptoms that develop in a person suffering from alcoholism within 6–24 hours of taking the last drink of alcohol. The symptoms include restlessness, tremors, loss of appetite, nausea, vomiting, insomnia, disorientation, seizures and delirium tremens. Treatment involves sedation, improving nutrition, counselling and social support.

**alcoholic** (ˌalkə'holik) 1. pertaining to alcohol. 2. a person addicted to excessive, uncontrolled alcohol consumption. This results in loss of appetite and vitamin B deficiency, leading to peripheral neuritis with eye changes and cirrhosis of the liver and to progressive deterioration in the personality.

**alcoholism** ('alkəˌholizəm) the state of poisoning resulting from alcoholic addiction.

**alcoholuria** (ˌalkəho'lyooə.ri.ə) the presence of alcohol in the urine. This may be estimated when excess blood levels of alcohol are suspected.

**aldosterone** (ˌaldoh'stiə.rohn, al-'dostəˌrohn) a compound, isolated from the adrenal cortex, that aids the retention of sodium and the excretion of potassium in the body, and by so doing aids the maintenance of electrolyte balance.

**aldosteronism** (al'dostə.rəˌnizem) an excess secretion of aldosterone caused by an adrenal neoplasm. The serum potassium is low and the patient has hypertension and severe muscular weakness.

**aleukaemia** (ˌayloo'keemi.ə) an acute condition in which there is an absence or deficiency of white cells in the blood.

**Alexander technique** (alekˌsahndə tek'neek) a process of psychophysical postural re-education. Body posture is believed to affect physical and psychological wellbeing and the postural re-education process aims to assist individuals in monitoring how they consciously use their bodies to promote good health.

**alexia** (ə'leksi.ə, ay-) a form of aphasia in which there is an inability to recognize written or printed words. Word blindness.

**algor** ('algor) chill or rigor; coldness.

**alienation** (ˌayli.ə'nayshən) a feeling of estrangement or separation from others or from self. A symptom of schizophrenia. Sufferers often believe that they are under the control of someone else. Depersonalization.

**alignment** (ə'lienmənt) the state of being arranged in a line, i.e. in the correct anatomical position.

**aliment** ('alimənt) food or nourishment.

**alimentary** (ˌali'mentə.ree, -tree) relating to the system of nutrition. *A. canal* alimentary tract. The passage through which the food passes, from mouth to anus. *A. system* the alimentary tract together with the liver and other organs concerned in digestion and absorption. *A. tract* alimentary canal.

**alimentation** (ˌalimen'tayshən) the giving or receiving of nourishment. The process of supplying the patient's need for nutrition.

**alkalaemia** (ˌalkə'leemi.ə) an increase in the alkali content of the blood. Alkalosis.

**alkali** ('alkəˌlie) a substance capable of uniting with acids to form salts, and with fats and fatty acids to form soaps. Alkaline solutions turn red litmus paper blue. *A. reserve* the ability of the combined buffer systems of the blood to neutralize acid. The pH of the blood is normally slightly on the alkaline side, between 7.35 and 7.45. The principal buffer in the blood is bicarbonate; the alkali reserve is essentially represented by the plasma bicarbonate concentration.

**alkaline** ('alkəˌlien) having the reactions of an alkali. *A. phosphatase* an enzyme localized on cell membranes that hydrolyses phosphate esters, liberating inorganic phosphate, and has an optimal pH of about 10.0. Serum alkaline phosphatase activity is elevated in obstructive jaundice and bone disease.

**alkalinity** (ˌalkə'linitee) 1. the quality of being alkaline. 2. the combining power of a base, expressed as the maximum number of equivalents of acid with which it reacts to form a salt.

**alkaloid** ('alkə,loyd) one of a group of active nitrogenous compounds that are alkaline in solution. They usually have a bitter taste and are characterized by powerful physiological activity. Examples are morphine, cocaine, atropine, quinine, nicotine and caffeine. The term is also applied to synthetic substances that have structures similar to plant alkaloids, such as procaine.

**alkalosis** (,alkə'lohsis) an increase in the alkali reserve in the blood. It may be confirmed by estimation of the blood carbon dioxide content and treated by giving normal saline or ammonium chloride intravenously to encourage the excretion of bicarbonate by the kidneys.

**alkaptonuria** (al,kaptə'nyooə,ri.ə) the excretion of alkapton, an abnormal product of protein metabolism, in the urine. On exposure to air, oxidation takes place, giving a dark-brown colour to the urine.

**alkylating agent** ('alki,layting) a drug that damages the deoxyribonucleic acid (DNA) molecule of the nucleus of the cell. Many are nitrogen mustard preparations and may be termed chromosome poisons; they are used in cancer chemotherapy.

**all-or-none law** (,awlor'nunlor) principle that states that in individual cardiac and skeletal muscle fibres there are only two possible reactions to a stimulus: either there is no reaction at all or there is a full reaction, with no gradation of response according to the strength of the stimulus. Whole muscles can grade their response by increasing or decreasing the *number* of fibres involved.

**allantois** (ə'lantoh.is) a membranous sac projecting from the ventral surface of the fetus in its early stages. It eventually helps to form the placenta.

**allele** (aleel, ə'leel) allelomorph. One of a pair of genes that occupy the same relative positions on homologous chromosomes and produce different effects on the same process of development.

**allelomorph** (ə'leeloh,mawf) allele.

**allergen** ('alə,jen) a substance that can produce an allergy or manifestation of an immune response.

**allergy** ('aləjee) a hypersensitivity to some foreign substances that are normally harmless but which produce a violent reaction in the patient. Asthma, hay fever, angioneurotic oedema, migraine, and some types of urticaria and eczema are allergic states. *See* ANAPHYLAXIS.

**alloaesthesia** (,aloh.is'theezi.ə) allocheiria. A response or sensation felt on (referred to) the opposite side from that to which a stimulus is applied.

**allocate** ('alə,kayt) to assign for a particular purpose.

**allocation** (,alə'kayshən) the act of allocating. *Clinical a.* a period of time spent in ward/department/unit where there are patients/clients. *Patient a.* one nurse is designated as responsible for the care of one patient or a group of patients for a spell of duty. *Task a.* patient care in a ward/unit is provided by a group of nurses. Each nurse is allocated a specific nursing activity (task), e.g. one nurse in the clinical area will be responsible for bed baths while another will be taking and recording vital signs for the same group of patients.

**allograft** ('alloh,grahft) tissue transplanted from one person to another. *Non-viable a.* skin, taken from a cadaver, which cannot regenerate. *Viable a.* living tissue transplanted.

**allopurinol** (,aloh'pyrooə,ri,nol) a drug that reduces the serum and urinary levels of uric acid. Used in the long-term treatment of gout to lessen the frequency and severity of attacks.

**alopecia** (ˌaləˈpeeshi.ə) baldness. Loss of hair. The cause of simple baldness is not yet fully understood, although it is known that the tendency to become bald is limited almost entirely to males, runs in certain families and is more common in certain racial groups than in others. Baldness is often associated with ageing. *A. areata* hair loss in sharply defined areas, usually the scalp or beard. *Cicatricial a., a. cicatrisata* irreversible loss of hair associated with scarring, usually on the scalp. *Male-pattern a.* loss of scalp hair, genetically determined and androgen-dependent, beginning with frontal recession and progressing symmetrically to leave ultimately only a sparse peripheral rim of hair.

**alpha** (ˈalfə) the first letter of the Greek alphabet, α. *A. cells* cells found in the islet of Langerhans in the pancreas. They produce the hormone glucagon. *A. fetoprotein* abbreviated AFP. A plasma protein originating in the fetal liver and gastrointestinal tract. The serum AFP level is used to monitor the effectiveness of cancer treatment; the amniotic fluid AFP level is used in the prenatal diagnosis of neural tube defects. *A. receptors* tissue receptors associated with the stimulation (contraction) of smooth muscle.

**Alport's syndrome** (ˈawlpawts) *A.C. Alport, South African physician, 1880–1959.* A hereditary disorder marked by progressive nerve deafness, progressive pyelonephritis or glomerulonephritis, and occasionally ocular defects.

**alternating current** (ˌawltəˌnaytingˈkurənt) an electrical current that runs alternately from the negative and positive poles.

**alternative medicine** (awlˈternətiv) a form of medicine differing from conventional health care. Consists of a range of treatments essentially based upon a holistic approach to health and wellbeing, including homeopathy, aromatherapy, hypnosis, acupuncture and others. Generally these therapies have not been subject to scientific scrutiny but are often used when conventional treatments have failed. Commonly called complementary therapies (see COMPLEMENTARY).

**altitude sickness** (ˈaltiˌtyood ˌsiknəs) condition caused by hypoxia that occurs as a result of lower oxygen pressure at high altitudes.

**aluminium** (ˌalyəˈmini.əm, ˌalə-) *symbol* Al. A silver-white metal with a low specific gravity, compounds of which are astringent and antiseptic. *A. hydroxide* compound used as an antacid in the treatment of gastric conditions.

**alveolar** (ˌalviˈohlə) concerning an alveolus, or air sac of the lung. *A. air* air found in the alveoli.

**alveolitis** (ˌalviohˈlietis) inflammation of the alveoli. *Extrinsic allergic a.* inflammation of the alveoli caused by inhalation of an antigen, such as pollen.

**Alzheimer's cells** (ˈalts.hiemərz) *A. Alzheimer, German neurologist, 1864–1915.* 1. giant astrocytes with large prominent nuclei found in the brain in hepatolenticular degeneration and hepatic comas. 2. degenerated astrocytes.

**Alzheimer's disease** a progressive form of neuronal degeneration in the brain and the most common cause of dementia in people of all ages. It is more common in older than younger people and is not just a form of presenile dementia, as was originally thought. The degeneration of neurones is accompanied by changes in the brain's biochemistry. At the moment this condition is irreversible and there is no effective treatment.

**amalgam** (ə'malgəm) a compound of mercury and other metals. *Dental a.* used for filling teeth.

**amantadine** (ə'mantə,deen) an antiviral agent used against the influenza A virus; also used as an antidyskinetic in the treatment of Parkinson's disease.

**amaurosis** (,amaw'rohsis) loss of vision, sometimes following excessive blood loss, especially after prolonged bleeding, e.g. haematuria. The visual loss may be partial or complete, temporary or permanent.

**amaurotic** (,amaw'rotik) pertaining to amaurosis. *A. family idiocy* Tay–Sachs disease. A familial metabolic disorder starting in infancy or childhood. Characterized by progressive mental deterioration, blindness and spastic paralysis.

**ambidextrous** (,ambi'dekstrəs) equally skilful with either hand.

**ambivalence** (am'bivələns) the existence of contradictory emotional feelings towards an object, commonly of love and hate for another person. If these feelings occur to a marked degree they lead to psychological disturbance.

**amblyopia** (,ambli'ohpi.ə) dimness of vision without any apparent lesion of the eye. Uncorrectable by optical means.

**ambulant** ('ambyuhlənt) able to walk.

**ambulatory** (,ambyuh'laytə.ree) having the capacity to walk. *A. treatment* or *care* health services provided on an outpatient basis.

**amelioration** (ə,meelyə'rayshən) improvement of symptoms; a lessening of the severity of a disease.

**amenorrhoea** (a,menə'reeə, ay,men-) absence of menstruation. *Primary a.* the non-occurrence of the menses. *Secondary a.* the cessation of the menses, after they have been

| ESSENTIAL AMINO ACIDS | |
|---|---|
| 1 | Threonine |
| 2 | Lysine |
| 3 | Methionine |
| 4 | Valine |
| 5 | Phenylalanine |
| 6 | Leucine |
| 7 | Tryptophan |
| 8 | Isoleucine |
| 9 | Histidine |
| 10 | Arginine |

established, owing to disease or pregnancy.

**amentia** (ay'menshi.ə) mental subnormality. May be due to hereditary factors, failure of development of the embryo or birth trauma.

**amethocaine** ('amethoh,kayn) a local anaesthetic effective when in contact with surfaces as well as when given by injection. *A. pastille* a lozenge that, when dissolved slowly in the mouth, will aid the passage of a bronchoscope or gastroscope.

**ametropia** (,ayme'trohpi.ə) defective vision. A general word applied to incorrect refraction.

**amikacin** (,ami'kaysin) a semisynthetic aminoglycoside antibiotic derived from kanamycin, used in the treatment of a wide range of infections due to susceptible organisms.

**amiloride** (ə'milor.ried) a weak but potassium-retaining diuretic drug.

**amino acid** (ə'meenoh) a chemical compound containing both $NH_2$ and COOH groups. The end-product of protein digestion. *Essential a. a.* one required for replacement and growth but which cannot be synthesized in the body in sufficient amounts and must be obtained in the diet (*see* Table). *Non-essential a. a.* one necessary for proper growth but which can be synthesized in the body and is not specifically required in the diet.

**aminoacidopathy** (ə'meenoh-,asi'dopəthee, ə,mienoh-, ə,minoh-) any inborn error of amino acid metabolism producing a metabolic block that results in accumulation of one or more amino acids in the blood (aminoacidaemia) or excess excretion in the urine (aminoaciduria) or both.

**aminoglutethimide** (ə,meenohgloo-'tethə,mied) a drug which inhibits adrenal hormone synthesis. Its use is sometimes referred to as 'medical adrenalectomy'. The effects are reversible when the drug is discontinued. Used to treat metastatic breast and prostate cancers.

**aminoglycoside** (ə,meenoh'gliekə,sied) any of a group of bacterial antibiotics, derived from various species of *Streptomyces*, that interfere with the function of bacterial ribosomes. The aminoglycosides include gentamicin, netilmicin, streptomycin, tobramycin, amikacin, kanamycin and neomycin. They are used to treat infections caused by Gram-negative organisms and are classified as bactericidal agents because of their interference with bacterial replication. All the aminoglycoside antibiotics are highly toxic, requiring monitoring of blood serum levels and careful observation of the patient for early signs of toxicity, particularly ototoxicity and nephrotoxicity.

**aminophylline** (,ami'nofilin) an alkaloid from camellia, it relaxes plain muscle spasm of the bronchioles and coronary arteries. It may be given by mouth, intravenously or as a suppository, and is useful in treating asthma and heart failure.

**aminosalicylic acid** (,aminoh,sali-'silik) *See* PARA-AMINOSALICYLIC ACID.

**amitosis** (,ami'tohsis) multiplication of cells by simple division or fission.

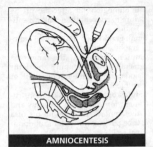

**AMNIOCENTESIS**

**amitriptyline** (,ami'triptə,leen) an antidepressant drug that is chemically related to imipramine. It is useful in relieving tension and anxiety but may cause dizziness and hypotension.

**ammonia** (ə'mohni.ə) $NH_3$. A colourless pungent gas. In solution, used as a cardiac stimulant.

**ammonium** (ə'mohni.əm) $NH_4^+$. A chemical group that combines to form salts similar to those of the alkaline metals. *A. chloride* used as a mild diuretic and to render the urine acid. Widely used in mixtures as an expectorant.

**amnesia** (am'neezi.ə) partial or complete loss of memory. *Anterograde a.* loss of memory of events that have taken place since an injury or illness. *Retrograde a.* loss of memory for events prior to an injury. It often applies to the time immediately preceding an accident.

**amniocentesis** (,amniohsen'teesis) the withdrawal of fluid from the uterus through the abdominal wall by means of a syringe and needle (*see* Figure). It is primarily used in the diagnosis of chromosome disorders in the fetus and in cases of hydramnios. Mothers who are rhesus-negative should be given a reduced dose of anti-D immunoglobulin after the procedure to prevent then making antibodies.

**amniography** (ˌamniˈografee) radiography of the gravid uterus.

**amnion** ('amni.ən) the innermost membrane enveloping the fetus and enclosing the liquor amnii, or amniotic fluid.

**amnioscope** ('amni.əˌskohp) instrument for examining the fetus and the amniotic fluid by means of a tube passing through the abdominal wall.

**amnioscopy** (ˌamniˈoskəpee) inspection of the amniotic sac using an amnioscope.

**amniotic** (ˌamniˈotik) pertaining to the amnion. *A. fluid* the albuminous fluid contained in the amniotic sac. Liquor amnii.

**amoeba** (əˈmeebə) a minute unicellular protozoon. It is able to move by pushing out parts of itself (called pseudopodia). Capable of reproduction by amitotic fission. Infection of the intestines by *Entamoeba histolytica* causes 'amoebic dysentery'.

**amoebiasis** (ˌamiˈbieəsis) infection with amoeba, particularly *Entamoeba histolytica*.

**amoebic** (əˈmeebik) pertaining to, caused by, or of the nature of an amoeba. *A. abscess* an abscess cavity of the liver resulting from liquefaction necrosis due to entrance of *Entamoeba histolytica* into the portal circulation in amoebiasis; amoebic abscesses may affect the lung, brain and spleen. *A. dysentery* a form of dysentery caused by *Entamoeba histolytica* and spread by contaminated food, water and flies; called also amoebiasis. Amoebic dysentery is mainly a tropical disease but many cases occur in temperate countries. Symptoms are diarrhoea, fatigue and intestinal bleeding. Complications include involvement of the liver, liver abscess and pulmonary abscess.

**amoeboid** (əˈmeeboyd) resembling an amoeba in structure or movement.

**amorphous** (əˈmawfəs) without definite shape. The term may be applied to fine powdery particles, as opposed to crystals.

**Amoxil** (əˈmoksil) trade name for a preparation of amoxycillin, an antibiotic.

**amoxycillin** (əˌmoksiˈsilin) a penicillin analogue similar in action to ampicillin but more efficiently absorbed from the gastrointestinal tract and therefore requiring less frequent dosage and not as likely to cause diarrhoea. It also penetrates sputum more readily than ampicillin.

**ampere** ('ampair) *symbol* A. The unit of intensity of an electrical current.

**amphetamine** (amˈfetəˌmeen, -ˌmin) a synthetic drug that stimulates the central nervous system. It is addictive and is now seldom used except in the treatment of narcolepsy.

**amphiarthrosis** (ˌamfiahrˈthrohsis) a form of joint in which the bones are joined together by fibrocartilage, e.g. the junctions of the vertebrae.

**amphoric** (amˈfor.rik) pertaining to a bottle. Used to describe the sound sometimes heard on auscultation over cavities in the lungs, which resembles that produced by blowing across the mouth of a bottle.

**amphotericin** (ˌamfəˈterisin) an antifungal drug which is not absorbed by the gut. The only polyene antibiotic that may be given parenterally. Active against most yeasts and other fungi. Side-effects of fever, nausea and vomiting are common when the drug is given parenterally.

**ampicillin** (ˌampiˈsilin) a broad-spectrum penicillin of synthetic origin, used in treatment of a number of infections. It is active against many of the Gram-negative pathogens, in addition to the usual Gram-positive ones that are sensitive to penicillin.

**ampoule** ('ampyool) a small glass or plastic phial in which sterile drugs of specified dose for injection are sealed.

**ampulla** (am'puhla) the flask-like dilatation of a canal, e.g. of a uterine tube.

**amputation** (,ampyuh'tayshen) surgical removal of a limb or other part of the body, e.g. the breast.

**amputee** (,ampyuh'tee) a person who has had one or more limbs amputated.

**amyl** ('amil) the radical $C_5H_{11}$. *A. nitrite* vasodilator and heart stimulant, prescribed for inhalation in cases of angina pectoris. Capsules can be broken into a handkerchief and the fumes inhaled.

**amylase** ('ami,layz) an enzyme that reduces starch to maltose. Found in saliva (ptyalin) and pancreatic juice (amylopsin).

**amylobarbitone** (ə,mieloh'bahbitohn) one of the barbiturates, used as a short-acting hypnotic and sedative. Effects develop rapidly and the drug is eliminated more quickly than other barbiturates. Regular use may lead to habituation, and overdosage can produce narcosis and death. Classified as a controlled drug.

**amyloid** ('ami,loyd) 1. pertaining to starch. 2. a waxy starch that forms in certain tissues. *A. degeneration* amyloidosis.

**amylopsin** (,ami'lopsin) an enzyme found in the pancrease. Amylase.

**amylum** ('amiləm) [L.] *starch*.

**amyotonia** (ay,mieoh'tohni.ə) atonic condition of the muscles. *A. congenita* any of several rare congenital diseases marked by general hypotonia of the muscles; called also Oppenheim's disease or floppy baby syndrome.

**anabolic** (,anə'bolik) relating to anabolism. *A. compound* a substance that aids in the repair of body tissue, particularly protein. Androgens may be used in this way.

**anabolism** (ə'nabə,lizem) the building up or synthesis of cell structure from digested food materials. *See* METABOLISM.

**anacidity** (,anə'siditee) decrease in normal acidity.

**anaclisis** (,anə'klisis) generally, reclining or leaning; typically, an emotional dependence on others.

**anaclitic** (,anə'klitik) denoting the dependence of the infant on the mother or mother substitute for its sense of wellbeing. *A. choice* a psychoanalytical term for the adult selection of a loved one who closely resembles one's mother (or another adult on whom one depended as a child). *A. depression* severe and progressive depression found in children who have lost their mothers and have not found a suitable substitute.

**anacrotism** (ə'nakrə,tizəm) an abnormal pulse wave tracing embodying a secondary expansion.

**anaemia** (ə'neemi.ə) deficiency in either quality or quantity of red corpuscles in the blood, giving rise especially to symptoms of anoxaemia. There is pallor, breathlessness on exertion, with palpitations, lassitude, headache, giddiness and often a history of poor resistance to infection. Anaemia may be due to many different causes. Increasingly, with the advent of electronic cell counters, anaemia is now classified according to the morphological characteristics of the erythrocytes. *Aplastic a.* the bone marrow is unable to produce red blood corpuscles. A rare condition. *Deficiency a.* any type that is due to the lack of the necessary factors for red cell formation, e.g. hormones or vitamins. *Haemolytic a.* a variety in which there is excessive destruction of red blood corpuscles caused by antibody formation in the blood (*see* RHESUS FACTOR) by drugs or by severe toxaemia, as in extensive burns. *Iron-deficiency a.* the most common type of anaemia, due to a lack of absorbable iron in the diet. It may also be due to excessive or chronic blood loss, or to poor absorption of dietary iron. *Macrocytic a.* a type in which the cells are larger than normal; present in pernicious anaemia. *Microcytic a.* a variety in which the cells are smaller than normal, as in iron deficiency. *Pernicious a.* a variety caused by the inability of the stomach to secrete the intrinsic factor necessary for the absorption of vitamin $B_{12}$ from the diet. *Sickle-cell a.* a hereditary haemolytic anaemia seen most commonly in black people living in or originating from the Caribbean islands, Africa, Asia, the Middle East and the Mediterranean. The red blood cells are sickle-shaped. *Splenic a.* a congenital, familial disease in which the red blood cells are fragile and easily broken down.

**anaerobe** (an'air.rohb, 'anə,rohb) a microorganism that can live and thrive in the absence of free oxygen. These organisms are found in body cavities or wounds where the oxygen tension is very low. Examples are the bacilli of tetanus and gas gangrene.

**anaesthesia** (,anəs'theezi.ə) loss of feeling or sensation in a part or in the whole of the body, usually induced by drugs. *Basal a.* basal narcosis. Loss of consciousness, although supplemental drugs have to be given to ensure complete anaesthesia. *Epidural a.* injection into the extradural space between the vertebral spines and beneath the ligamentum flavum. *General a.* unconsciousness produced by

inhalation or injection of a drug. *Inhalation a.* drugs or gas are administered by a face mask or endotracheal tube to cause general anaesthesia. *Intravenous a.* unconsciousness is produced by the introduction of a drug into a vein. *Local a.* local analgesia. Nerve conduction is blocked by injection of a local anaesthetic, or by freezing with ethyl chloride or by topical application. *Spinal a.* injection of anaesthetic agent into the spinal subarachnoid space.

**anaesthetic** (,anəs'thetik) a drug causing anaesthesia.

**anaesthetist** (ə'neesthətist) a person who is medically qualified to administer an anaesthetic and in the techniques of life support for the critically ill or injured.

**anal** ('ayn'l) pertaining to the anus. *A. eroticism* sexual pleasure derived from anal functions. *A. fissure see* FISSURE. *A. fistula see* FISTULA.

**analeptic** (,anə'leptik) a drug that stimulates the central nervous system.

**analgesia** (,an'l'jeezi.ə) insensibility to pain, especially the relief of pain without causing unconsciousness. *Patient-controlled a.* a preset dose of analgesic, which the patient controls according to need. In-built safety measures prevent accidental overdose.

**analgesic** (,an'l'jeezik, -sik) 1. relating to analgesia. 2. a remedy that relieves pain. *A. cocktail* an individualized mixture of drugs used to control pain.

**analogue** ('anə,log) 1. an organ with a different structure and origin to but the same function as another one. 2. a compound with a similar structure to another but differing in respect of a particular element.

**analysis** (ə'nalisis) 1. the act of determining the component parts of a substance. 2. in psychiatry, a method of trying to understand the complex mental processes, experiences and relationships with other individuals or groups of individuals to determine the reasons for an individual's behaviour.

**anaphase** ('anə,fayz) part of the process of mitosis or meiosis.

**anaphylaxis** (,anəfi'laksis) anaphylactic shock. A severe reaction, often fatal, occurring in response to drugs, e.g. penicillin, but also to bee stings and food allergy, e.g. nuts in sensitive individuals. The symptoms are severe dyspnoea, rapid pulse, profuse sweating and collapse.

**anaplasia** (,anə'playzi.ə) a change in the character of cells, seen in tumour tissue.

**anarthria** (an'ahthri.ə) inability to articulate speech sounds owing to a brain lesion or damage to peripheral nerves innervating articulatory muscles.

**anastomosis** (ə,nastə'mohsis) 1. in surgery, any artificial connection of two hollow structures, e.g. gastroenterostomy. 2. in anatomy, the joining of the branches of two blood vessels.

**anatomy** (ə'natəmee) the science of the structure of the body.

*Ancylostoma* (,ansi'lostəmə) a genus of nematode roundworms which may inhabit the duodenum and cause extreme anaemia. *A. duodenale* a hookworm, very widespread in tropical and subtropical areas.

**androgen** ('andrə,jen) one of a group of hormones secreted by the testes and adrenal cortex. They are steroids which can be synthesized and produce the secondary male characteristics and the building up of protein tissue.

**android** ('androyd) resembling a man. *A. pelvis* a female pelvis shaped like a male pelvis with a wedge-shaped entrance and narrow anterior segment.

**anencephaly** (,anən'kefəlee, -'sef-) congenital absence of the cranial vault, with the cerebral hemispheres completely missing or reduced to small masses.

**anergy** ('anərjee) 1. specific immunological tolerance in which T cells and B cells fail to respond normally. The state can be reversed. 2. tiredness, lethargy, lack of energy.

**aneurine** ('anyuh,reen) thiamine. An essential vitamin involved in carbohydrate metabolism. The main sources are unrefined cereals and pork. Vitamin $B_1$.

**aneurysm** ('anyə,rizəm) a local dilatation of a blood vessel, usually an artery (*see* Figure). Atherosclerosis is responsible for most arterial aneurysms; any injury to the arterial wall can predispose to the formation of a sac. Other diseases that can lead to an aneurysm include syphilis, certain non-specific inflammations, and a congenital defect in the artery. The pressure of blood causes it to increase in size and rupture is likely. Sometimes excision of the aneurysm or ligation of the artery is possible. *Dissecting a.* a condition in which a tear occurs in the aortic lining when the middle coat is necrosed and blood gets between the layers, stripping them apart. *Fusiform a.* a spindle-shaped arterial aneurysm. *Saccular a.* a dilatation of only a part of the circumference of an artery (*see* Figure on p. 24).

**angiitis** (,anji'ietis) inflammation of a blood or lymph vessel.

**angina** (an'jienə, 'anjienə) 1. a tight strangling sensation or pain. 2. an inflammation of the throat causing pain on swallowing. *A. cruris* intermittent claudication. Severe pain in the leg after walking. *A. pectoris* cardiac pain that occurs on exertion owing to insufficient blood supply to the heart muscles. *Vincent's a.* infection and ulceration of the

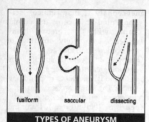

**TYPES OF ANEURYSM**

fusiform    saccular    dissecting

tonsils by a spirochaete, *Borrelia vincentii*, and a bacillus, *Fusiformis fusiformis*.

**angiocardiography** (ˌanjiohˌkahdi'ografee) radiological examination of the heart and large blood vessels by means of cardiac catheterization and an opaque contrast medium.

**angioectasis** (ˌanjioh'ektəsis) abnormal enlargement of capillaries.

**angiography** (ˌanji'ografee) radiological examination of the blood vessels using an opaque contrast medium.

**angioma** (ˌanji'ohmə) a benign tumour composed of dilated blood vessels.

**angioneurosis** (ˌanjiohnyuh'rohsis) a neurosis affecting the blood vessels, which may produce paralysis.

**angioneurotic** (ˌanjiohnyuh'rotik) pertaining to angioneurosis. *A. oedema see* OEDEMA.

**angioplasty** ('anjiohˌplastee) surgery of a narrowed artery to promote the normal flow of blood. A common technique is balloon angioplasty.

**angiosarcoma** (ˌanjiohsah'kohmə) a malignant vascular growth.

**angiospasm** ('anjiospazəm) a spasmodic contraction of an artery, causing cramping of the muscles.

**angiotensin** (ˌanjio'tensin) a substance that raises the blood pressure. It is a polypeptide produced by the action of renin on plasma globulins. Hypertensin.

**anhidrosis** (ˌanhi'drohsis) marked deficiency in the secretion of sweat.

**anhidrotic** (ˌanhi'drotik) an agent that decreases perspiration. An adiaphoretic.

**anhydraemia** (ˌanhie'dreemi.ə) deficiency of water in the blood.

**anhydrous** (an'hiedrəs) containing no water.

**aniline** ('aniˌleen, -ˌlin) a chemical compound derived from coal tar, used for making antiseptic dyes. It is an important cause of serious industrial poisoning associated with bone marrow depression as well as methaemoglobinaemia.

**anima** ('animə) 1. the soul. 2. Jung's term for the unconscious, or inner being, of the individual, as opposed to the personality presented to the world (persona). In Jungian psychoanalysis, the more feminine soul or feminine component of a man's personality.

**anion** ('anˌieən) a negatively charged ion which travels against the current towards the anode, e.g. chloride ($Cl^-$), carbonate ($CO_3^{2-}$). *See* CATION.

**aniridia** (ˌani'ridi.ə) lack of part or the whole of the iris.

**anisocoria** (anˌiesoh'koh.ri.ə) inequality of diameter of the pupils of the two eyes.

**anisocytosis** (anˌiesohsie'tohsis) inequality in the size of the red blood cells.

**anisometropia** (anˌiesohme'trohpi.ə) a marked difference in the refractive power of the two eyes.

**ankle** ('angk'l) the joint between the leg and foot, formed by the tibia and fibula articulating with the talus.

**ankyloblepharon** (ˌangkiloh'blefə.ron) adhesions and scar tissue on the ciliary borders of the eyelids, giving the eye a distorted appearance.

**ankylosis** (ˌangki'lohsis) consolidation, immobility and stiffness of a joint as a result of disease.

**Annelida** (ə'nelidə) a phylum of metazoa, the segmented worms, including the leeches.

**annular** ('anyuhlə) ring-shaped.

**anoci-association** (aˌnohsee.əˌsohsi-'ayshən, -ˌsohshi-) the exclusion of pain, fear and shock in surgical operations, brought about by means of local anaesthesia and basal narcosis.

**anode** ('anohd) the positive pole of an electric battery. *See* CATHODE.

**anodyne** ('anəˌdien) 1. pain-relieving or relaxing. 2. a drug or other treatment that relieves pain.

**anomaly** (ə'nomələee) considerable variation from normal.

**anomie** ('anohmee) a feeling of hopelessness and lack of purpose.

**anonychia** (ˌanə'niki.ə) congenital absence of nails.

*Anopheles* (ə'nofiˌleez) a genus of mosquito. Many are carriers of the malarial parasite and by their bite infect humans. Other species transmit filariasis.

**anophthalmia** (ˌanof'thalmi.ə) congenital absence of a seeing eye. Some portion of the eye, e.g. the conjunctiva, is always present.

**anorexia** (ˌanə'reksi.ə) loss of appetite for food. *A. nervosa* a condition in which there is complete lack of appetite, with extreme emaciation. It is due to psychological causes and usually occurs in young women, leading them to perceive themselves as fat and to take extreme forms of dietary control in order to lose weight.

**anosmia** (an'ozmi.ə) loss of the sense of smell.

**anovular** (an'ohvyuhlə) applied to the absence of ovulation. Usually refers to uterine bleeding when there has been no ovulation, the result of taking contraceptive pills.

**anoxaemia** (ˌanok'seemi.ə) complete lack of oxygen in the blood.

**anoxia** (an'oksi.ə) lack of oxygen to an organ or tissue.

**Antabuse** ('antəˌbyooz) trade name for a preparation of disulfiram, used in the treatment of alcoholism.

**antacid** (ant'asid) a substance neutralizing acidity, particularly of the gastric juices.

**antagonist** (an'tagənist) 1. a muscle that has an opposite action to another, e.g. the biceps to the triceps. 2. in pharmacology, a drug that inhibits the action of another drug or enzyme, e.g. methotrexate is a folic acid antagonist. 3. in dentistry, a tooth in one jaw opposing one in the other jaw.

**anteflexion** (ˌanti'flekshən) a bending forward, as of the body of the uterus. *See* RETROFLEXION.

**antenatal** (ˌanti'nayt'l) before birth. *A. care* care provided by midwives and obstetricians during pregnancy to ensure that the fetal and maternal health are satisfactory. Deviations from normal can be detected and treated early. The mother can be prepared for labour and parenthood and health education offered.

**Antepar** ('antiˌpah) trade name for piperazine.

**antepartum** (ˌanti'pahtəm) shortly before birth, i.e. in the last three months of pregnancy. *A. haemorrhage* bleeding occurring before parturition. *See* PLACENTA PRAEVIA.

**anterior** (an'tiə.ri.ə) situated at or facing towards the front. The opposite of posterior. *A. capsule* the anterior covering of the lens of the eye. *A. chamber of the eye* the space between the cornea in front and the iris and lens behind.

**anterograde** ('antə.rohˌgrayd) extending or moving forwards.

**anteversion** (ˌanti'vərzhən) the forward tilting of an organ, e.g. the normal position of the uterus. *See* RETROVERSION.

**anthelmintic (anthelminthic)** (ˌant.hel'mintik, ˌanthel-) 1. destructive to worms. 2. an agent destructive to worms.

**anthracosis** (ˌanthrə'kohsis) a disease of the lungs, caused by inhalation of coal dust. A form of pneumoconiosis. 'Miner's lung'.

**anthrax** ('anthraks) an acute, notifiable, infectious disease due to *Bacillus anthracis*, acquired through contact with infected animals or their byproducts, such as carcasses, bones or skin, usually by occupational exposure. The incubation period is 2–5 days. A worldwide zoonosis, anthrax is now very uncommon in the UK.

**anthropoid** ('anthrə‚poyd) resembling man. *A. pelvis* female pelvis in which the anteroposterior diameter exceeds the transverse diameter.

**anthropology** (ˌanthrə'poləjee) the study of human beings that focuses on origins, historical and cultural development, and races. *Cultural a.* that branch of anthropology that is concerned with individuals and their relationship to others and to their environment. *Medical a.* biocultural discipline concerned with both the biological and sociocultural aspects of human behaviour, and the ways in which the two interact to influence health and disease. *Physical a.* that branch of anthropology that concerns the physical and evolutionary characteristics of human beings.

**anthropometry** (ˌanthrə'pomətree) the science that deals with the comparative measurement of parts of the human body, such as height, weight, body fat, etc.

**anti-D gamma-globulin** (ˌanti'dee) anti-rhesus antibody which is given to a rhesus-negative woman within 72 hours of delivery of her infant or following termination of her pregnancy, miscarriage or invasive investigations such as amniocente-

sis, to prevent haemolytic disease of the newborn in the next pregnancy. *See* RHESUS FACTOR.

**anti-inflammatory** (ˌanti.inflamə‚tree) a drug that reduces or acts against inflammation. May belong to one of several groups.

**anti-rhesus serum** (ˌanti'reesəs) a substance containing rhesus agglutinins produced in the blood of those who are rhesus-negative if the rhesus-positive antigen obtains access to it, e.g. by blood transfusion. Haemolysis and jaundice are the result. *See* RHESUS FACTOR.

**antibacterial** (ˌantibak'tiə.ri.əl) a substance that destroys or suppresses the growth of bacteria.

**antibiotic** (ˌantibie'otik) substances (e.g. penicillin), produced by certain bacteria and fungi, that prevent the growth of, or destroy, other bacteria. *A. resistance* the evolution and survival, as a result of worldwide antibiotic misuse, of bacteria undergoing the process of natural selection, despite the use of antibiotics to which they were once sensitive.

**antibody** ('anti‚bodee) also known as immunoglobulin, a group of proteins found on the surface of B-lymphocytes (cell-surface antibody) or secreted by B-lymphocytes that have changed into a plasma cell. There are five different types or classes of immunoglobulin (Ig): IgM, IgG, IgD, IgA, IgE. Cell-surface antibody provides a receptor for antigens and secreted antibody combines with antigen to form 'immune complexes'. *See also* IMMUNOGLOBULIN.

**anticholinergic** (ˌanti‚kohli'nəjik) a drug that inhibits the action of acetylcholine.

**anticholinesterase** (ˌanti‚kohli'nestə‚rayz) an enzyme that inhibits the action of the enzyme acetylcholinesterase, thereby potentiating the action of acetylcholine at postsynaptic receptors in the parasympathetic nervous system, thus allowing return of normal muscle contraction.

**anticoagulant** (ˌantikoh'agyuhlənt) a substance that prevents blood from clotting, e.g. heparin.

**anticonvulsant** (ˌantikən'vulsənt) a substance that will arrest or prevent convulsions. Anticonvulsant drugs such as phenytoin are used in the treatment of epilepsy and other conditions in which convulsions occur.

**antidepressant** (ˌantidi'prəs'nt) one of a group of drugs which elevate mood, often diminish anxiety and increase coping behaviour. Tricyclic antidepressants are the most commonly used in treatment of depression. Monoamine oxidase inhibitors (MAOIs) are less commonly used because of the dietary restriction necessary and the toxic side-effects.

**antidiuretic** (ˌanti,dieyuh'retik) a substance that reduces the volume of urine excreted. *A. hormone* abbreviated ADH. A hormone which is secreted by the posterior pituitary gland. Vasopressin.

**antidote** ('anti,doht) an agent that counteracts the effect of a poison.

**antiembolic** (ˌanti,em'bolik) against embolism. Antiembolic hose/stockings are worn to prevent the formation or decrease the risk of deep vein thrombosis, especially in patients after surgery or those confined to bed.

**antiemetic** (ˌanti,i'metik) a drug that prevents or overcomes nausea and vomiting.

**antigen** ('antijen, -jən) any substance, bacterial or otherwise, which in suitable conditions can stimulate the production of an immune response.

**antihaemophilic** (ˌanti,heemoh-'filik) 1. effective against the bleeding tendency in haemophilia. 2. an agent that counteracts the bleeding

tendency in haemophilia. *A. factor* abbreviated AHF. One of the clotting factors, deficiency of which causes classic, sex-linked haemophilia; called also factor VIII and antihaemophilic globulin (AHG). It is available in a preparation for preventive and therapeutic use.

**antihistamine** (ˌanti'histə,meen, -'min) any one of a group of drugs which block the tissue receptors for histamine. They are used to treat allergic conditions, e.g. drug rashes, hay fever and serum sickness, and include promethazine.

**antihypertensive** (ˌanti,hiepə'tensiv) 1. effective against hypertension. 2. an agent that reduces high blood pressure.

**antimetabolite** (ˌantimə'tabəliet) one of a group of chemical compounds which prevent the effective utilization of the corresponding metabolite, and interfere with normal growth or cell mitosis if the process requires that metabolite.

**antimycotic** (ˌantimie'kotik) a preparation effective in treating fungal infections.

**antineoplastic** (ˌanti,neeoh'plastik) effective against the multiplication of malignant cells.

**antiperistalsis** (ˌanti,peri'stalsis) contrary contractions which propel the contents of the intestines backwards and upwards.

**antipruritic** (ˌanti,prooə'ritik) an external application or drug that relieves itching.

**antipyretic** (ˌantipie'retik) an agent that reduces fever.

**antisepsis** (ˌanti'sepsis) the prevention of infection by destroying or arresting the growth of harmful microorganisms.

**antiseptic** (ˌanti'septik) 1. preventing sepsis. 2. any substance that inhibits the growth of bacteria, in contrast to a germicide, which kills bacteria outright.

**antiserum** (ˌanti'siə.rəm) animal or human blood serum which contains antibodies to infective organisms or to their toxins. The serum donor must have previously been infected with the identified organism.

**antisocial** (ˌanti'soshəl) against society. *A. behaviour* in psychiatry, the refusal of an individual to accept the normal obligations and restraints imposed by the community upon its members.

**antispasmodic** (ˌantispaz'modik) any measure used to prevent or relieve the occurrence of muscle spasm.

**antitoxin** (ˌanti'toksin) a substance produced by the body cells as a reaction to invasion by bacteria, which neutralizes their toxins. *See* IMMUNITY.

**antitussive** (ˌanti'tusiv) 1. effective against cough. 2. an agent that suppresses coughing.

**antivenin** (ˌanti'venin) an antitoxic serum to neutralize the poison injected by the bite of a snake or insect.

**antiviral** (ˌanti'vierəl) 1. acting against viruses. 2. a drug that is effective against viruses causing disease, e.g. acyclovir.

**antrectomy** (an'trektəmee) excision of an antrum.

**antrostomy** (an'trostəmee) surgical opening of an antrum, particularly the maxillary antrum, for drainage purposes.

**antrum** ('antrəm) a cavity in bone. *Mastoid a.* the tympanic antrum, which is an air-conditioning cavity in the mastoid portion of the temporal bone. *Maxillary a.* antrum of Highmore. The air sinus in the upper jawbone.

**anuria** (ə'nyooə.ri.ə) cessation of the secretion of urine.

**anus** ('aynəs) the extremity of the alimentary canal, through which the faeces are discharged. *Imper-*

*forate a.* one where there is no opening because of a congenital defect.

**anxiety** (ang'zieətee) a chronic state of tension, which affects both mind and body. *A. neurosis see* NEUROSIS.

**anxiolytic** (ˌangzieoh'litik) a substance, such as diazepam, used for relief of anxiety. Anxiolytics may quickly cause dependence and are not suitable for long-term administration. Also called anti-anxiety agent and minor tranquilliser.

**aorta** (ay'awtə) the large artery rising out of the left ventricle of the heart and supplying blood to all the body. *Abdominal a.* that part of the artery lying in the abdomen. *Arch of the a.* the curve of the artery over the heart. *Thoracic a.* that part which passes through the chest.

**aortic** (ay'awtik) pertaining to the aorta. *A. incompetence* owing to previous inflammation the aortic valve has become fibrosed and is unable to close completely, thus allowing backward flow of blood (*a. regurgitation*) into the left ventricle during diastole. *A. stenosis* a narrowing of the aortic valve. *A. valve* the valve between the left ventricle of the heart and the ascending aorta, which prevents the backward flow of blood through the artery.

**aortitis** (ˌay.aw'tietis) inflammation of the aorta.

**aortography** (ˌay.aw'togrəfee) radiographic examination of the aorta. A radio-opaque contrast medium is injected into the blood to render visible lesions of the aorta or its main branches.

**apathy** ('apəthee) an appearance of indifference, with no response to stimuli or display of emotion.

**aperient** (ə'piəri.ənt) a drug that produces an action of the bowels. A laxative.

**aperistalsis** (ˌayperi'stalsis) lack of peristaltic movement of the intestines.

| APGAR SCORE | | | |
|---|---|---|---|
| **Sign** | | **Score** | |
| | 0 | 1 | 2 |
| Colour | Blue, pale | Body pink, limbs blue | Completely pink |
| Respiratory effort | Absent | Slow, irregular, weak cry | Strong cry |
| Heart rate | Absent | Slow, less than 100 bpm | Over 100 bpm |
| Muscle tone | Limp | Some flexion of limbs | Active movement |
| Reflex response to flicking foot | Absent | Facial grimace | Cry |

**Apert's syndrome** (a'pairz) *E. Apert, French paediatrician, 1868–1940.* A congenital abnormality in which there is fusion at birth of all the cranial sutures, in addition to syndactyly (webbed fingers).

**apex** ('aypeks) the top or pointed end of a cone-shaped structure. *A. beat* the beat of the heart against the chest wall which can be felt during systole. *A. of the heart* the end closing the left ventricle. *A. of the lung* the extreme upper part of the organ.

**Apgar score** ('apgah ˌskor) *V. Apgar, American anaesthetist, 1909–1974.* A system used in the assessment of the newborn: reflex irritability and colour. The Apgar score is assessed 1 min after birth and again at 5 min. Most healthy infants score 9 at birth. A score below 7 would indicate cause for concern (*see* Table).

**APH** antepartum haemorrhage.

**aphagia** (ə'fayji.ə, ay-) loss of the power to swallow.

**aphakia** (ə'fayki.ə, ay-, -'fak-) absence of the lens of the eye. Aphacia.

**aphasia** (ə'fayzi.ə, ay-) a communication disorder due to brain damage; characterized by complete or partial disturbance of language comprehension, formulation or expression. Partial disturbance is also called dysphasia. *Broca's a.* disorder in which verbal output is impaired, and in which verbal communication may be affected as well. Speech is slow and laboured and writing is often impaired. *Developmental a.* a childhood failure to acquire normal language when deafness, learning difficulties, motor disability or severe emotional disturbance are not causes.

**aphonia** (ə'fohni.ə, ay-) inability to produce sound. The cause may be organic disease of the larynx or may be purely functional.

**aphrodisiac** (ˌafrə'diziak) a drug which excites sexual desire.

**aphthae** ('apthee) small ulcers surrounded by erythema on the inside of the mouth (aphthous ulcers).

**apical** ('aypik'l) pertaining to the apex of a structure.

**apicectomy** (ˌaypi'sektəmee) excision of the root of a tooth. Root resection.

**aplasia** (ə'playzi.ə, ay-) incomplete development of an organ or tissue or absence of growth.

**aplastic** (ay'plastik) without power of development. *A. anaemia see* ANAEMIA.

**apnoea** ('apni.ə, ap'neeə) cessation of respiration. *A. mattress* a mattress designed to sound an alarm if the infant lying on it ceases breathing. *A. monitors* designed to give an audible signal when a certain period of apnoea has occurred. *A. of prematurity* apnoeic periods occurring in the respiration of newborn infants in whom the respiratory centre is immature or depressed. *Cardiac a.* the temporary cessation of breathing caused by a reduction of the carbon dioxide tension in the blood, as seen in Cheyne–Stokes respiration. *Sleep a.* transient attacks of failure of autonomic control of respiration, becoming more pronounced during sleep.

**apocrine** ('apǝkrien, -krin) pertaining to modified sweat glands that develop in hair follicles, such as are mainly found in the axillary, pubic and perineal areas.

**apomorphine** (ˌapohˈmawfeen) a derivative of morphine which produces vomiting.

**aponeurosis** (ǝˌponyuhˈrohsis) a sheet of tendon-like tissue which connects some muscles to the parts that they move.

**apophysis** (ǝˈpofisis) a prominence or excrescence, usually of a bone.

**apoplexy** (ˌapǝˈpleksee) a sudden fit of insensibility, usually caused by rupture of a cerebral blood vessel or its occlusion by a blood clot. The symptoms are coma, accompanied by stertorous breathing, and a varying degree of paralysis of the opposite side of the body to the lesion.

**apparition** (ˌapǝˈrishǝn) a hallucinatory vision, usually the phantom appearance of a person. A spectre.

**appendectomy** (ˌapǝnˈdektǝmee) appendicectomy.

**appendicectomy** (ǝˌpendiˈsektǝmee) removal of the vermiform appendix.

**appendicitis** (ǝˌpendiˈsietis) inflammation of the vermiform appendix.

**appendix** (ǝˈpendiks) a supplementary or dependent part. *A. epiploicae* small tag-like structures of peritoneum containing fat, which are scattered over the surface of the large intestine, especially the transverse colon. *Vermiform a.* a wormlike tube with a blind end, projecting from the caecum in the right iliac region. It may be from 2.5 to 15 cm long.

**apperception** (ˌapǝˈsepshǝn) conscious reception and recognition of a sensory stimulus.

**appetite** (ˈapiˌtiet) the desire for food. It is stimulated by the sight, smell or thought of food, and accompanied by the flow of saliva in the mouth and gastric juice in the stomach. The stomach wall also receives an extra blood supply in preparation for its digestive activity. Appetite is psychological, dependent on memory and associations, as compared with hunger, which is physiologically aroused by the body's need for food. Appetite can be discouraged by unattractive food, surroundings or company, and by emotional states such as anxiety, irritation, anger and fear.

**applanation** (ˌaplǝˈnayshǝn) a technique for flattening the cornea to determine the intraocular pressure or detect the presence of glaucoma.

**appliance** (ǝˈplieǝns) a device used for performing a particular function.

**applicator** (ˈapliˌkaytǝ) any device used to apply medication or treatment to a particular part of the body.

**apposition** (ˌapǝˈzishǝn) the bringing into contact of two structures, e.g. fragments of bone in setting a fracture.

**apprehension** (ˌapriˈhenshǝn) a feeling of dread or fear.

**apraxia** (ǝˈpraksi.ǝ) the inability to perform correct movements because of a brain lesion and not because of sensory impairment or loss of muscle power in the limbs. *Oral a.* inability to perform volitional movements of the tongue and lips in the absence of paralysis or paresis. Involuntary movements may, however, be observed, e.g. patients may purse their lips in order to blow out a match.

**aptitude** ('apti,tyood) the natural ability or capacity to acquire mental and physical skills. *A. test* the evaluation of a person's ability for learning certain skills or carrying out specific tasks.

**apyrexia** (,aypie'reksi.ə) the absence of fever.

**aqua** ('akwə) [L.] *water. A. destillata* distilled water. *A. fortis* nitric acid.

**aqueduct** ('akwə,dukt) a canal for the passage of fluid. *A. of Sylvius* the canal connecting the third and fourth ventricles of the brain.

**aqueous** ('akwi.əs, 'ay-) watery. *A. humour* the fluid filling the anterior and posterior chambers of the eye.

*Arachis* ('arəkis) a genus of leguminous plants used in various preparations such as ear wax softeners and skin medications.

**arachnodactyly** (ə,raknoh'daktilee) abnormally long and thin fingers and toes. A congenital condition.

**arachnoid** (ə'raknoyd) 1. resembling a spider's web. 2. a web-like membrane covering the central nervous system between the dura and pia mater.

**arborization** (,ahbərie'zayshən) the branching terminations of many nerve fibres and processes.

**arbovirus** (,ahboh'vierəs) one of a large group of viruses transmitted by insect vectors (anthropodborne), e.g. mosquitoes, sandflies or ticks. The diseases caused include many types of encephalitis, also yellow, dengue, sandfly and Rift Valley fevers.

**arcus** ('ahkəs) [L.] *bow, arch. A. senilis* an opaque circle appearing round the edge of the cornea in old age.

**ARDS** (ahdz) acute respiratory distress syndrome.

**areola** (ə'reeələ) 1. a space in connective tissue. 2. a ring of pigmentation, e.g. that surrounding the nipple.

**argentum** (ah'jentəm) [L.] *silver.*

**arginase** ('ahji,nayz) an enzyme of the liver that splits arginine into urea and ornithine.

**arginine** ('ahji,neen, -,nin) an essential amino acid produced by the digestion of protein. It forms a link in the excretion of nitrogen, being hydrolysed by the enzyme arginase.

**argon** ('ahgon) *symbol* Ar. An inert gaseous element; less than 0.1% in the atmosphere.

**Argyll Robertson pupil** (ah,giel 'robətsən) *D. Argyll Robertson, British ophthalmologist, 1837–1909. See* PUPIL.

**Arnold–Chiari deformity** (,ahn'ld-ki'ahre di,fawmitee) *J. Arnold, German pathologist, 1835–1915; H. Chiari, German pathologist, 1851–1916.* Herniation of the cerebellum and elongation of the medulla oblongata; occurs in hydrocephalus associated with spina bifida.

**aromatherapy** (ə,rohmə'therəpee) the therapeutic use of specially prepared essential or aromatic oils obtained from the different parts of plants, including the flowers, leaves, seeds, wood, roots and bark. The oils may be diluted for use in massage, baths or infusions.

**aromatic** (,arə'matik) 1. having a spicy fragrance. 2. a stimulant spicy medicine.

**arousal** (ə'rowz'l) a state of alertness and increased response to stimuli.

**arrector pili** (ə,rektə 'pielie) a small muscle attached to the hair follicle of the skin. When contracted it causes the hair to become erect, producing the appearance known as gooseflesh.

**arrest** (ə'rest) a cessation or stopping. *Cardiac a.* cessation of ventricular contractions. *Developmental a.* discontinuation of a child's mental or physical development at a certain stage. *Respiratory a.* cessation of breathing.

**arrhenoblastoma** (ə'reenohbla'stomə) a rare ovarian tumour that causes masculinization in women, with male distribution of hair and coarsening of the skin.

**arrhythmia** (ə'ridhmi.ə, ay-) variation from the normal rhythm, e.g. in the heart's action. *Sinus a.* an abnormal pulse rhythm due to disturbance of the sinoatrial node, causing quickening of the heart on inspiration and slowing on expiration.

**arsenic** ('ahsnik) *symbol* As. A metallic element, organic preparations of which were used in medicine in the past.

**art therapy** (aht 'therəpee) the use of art as a medium to encourage patients to express their feelings when unable to do so verbally.

**artefact** ('ahti,fakt) something that is man-made or introduced artificially.

**arteriectomy** (ah,tiə.ri'ektəmee) the removal of a portion of artery wall, usually followed by anastomosis or a replacement graft. *See* ARTERIOPLASTY.

**arteriography** (ah,tiə.ri'ografee) radiography of arteries after the injection of a radio-opaque contrast medium.

**arterioplasty** (ah'tiə.rioh,plastee) the reconstruction of an artery by means of replacement surgery.

**arteriorrhaphy** (ah,tiə.ri'o.rəfee) ligature of an artery.

**arteriosclerosis** (ah,tiə.riohsklə'rohsis) a gradual loss of elasticity in the walls of arteries due to thickening and calcification. It is accompanied by high blood pressure, and precedes the degeneration of internal organs associated with old age or chronic disease.

**arteriotomy** (ah,tiə.ri'otəmee) an incision into an artery.

**arteriovenous** (ah,tiə.rioh'vennəs) both arterial and venous; pertaining to both artery and vein, e.g. an arteriovenous aneurysm, fistula, or shunt for haemodialysis.

**arteritis** (,ahtə'rietis) inflammation of an artery. *Giant cell a.* a variety of polyarteritis resulting in partial or complete occlusion of a number of arteries. The carotid arteries are often involved. *Temporal a.* occlusion of the extracranial arteries, particularly the carotid arteries.

**artery** ('ahtə.ree) a tube of muscle and elastic fibres, lined with endothelium, which distributes blood from the heart to the capillaries throughout the body.

**arthralgia** (ah'thralji.ə) neuralgic pains in a joint.

**arthrectomy** (ah'threktəmee) excision of a joint.

**arthritis** (ah'thrietis) inflammation of one or more joints. Movement in the joint is restricted, with pain and swelling. Arthritis and the rheumatic diseases in general constitute the major cause of chronic disability in the UK, where it is estimated that 20 million persons have a rheumatic disease, of whom between 6 and 8 million are severely affected. *Acute rheumatic a.* rheumatic fever. *Osteo-a.* a degenerative condition attacking the articular cartilage and aggravated by an impaired blood supply, previous injury or overweight, mainly affecting weight-bearing joints and causing pain. *Rheumatoid a.* a chronic inflammation, usually of unknown origin. The disease is progressive and incapacitating, owing to the resulting ankylosis and deformity of the bones. Usually affects the elderly. A juvenile form is known as STILL'S DISEASE.

**arthroclasia** (ˌahthrəˈklayzi.ə) the breaking down of adhesions in a joint to produce freer movement.

**arthrodesis** (ˌahthrəˈdeesis) the fixation of a movable joint by surgical operation.

**arthrodynia** (ˌahthrəˈdini.ə) painful joints. Arthralgia.

**arthrography** (ahˈthrogrəfee) the examination of a joint by means of X-rays. An opaque contrast medium may be used.

**arthrogryposis** (ˌahthrohgrieˈpohsis) 1. a congenital abnormality in which fibrous ankylosis of some or all of the joints in the limbs occurs. 2. a tetanus spasm.

**arthrology** (ahˈthroləjee) scientific study or description of the joints.

**arthroplasty** ('ahthrəˌplastee) plastic surgery for the reorganization of a joint. *Charnley's a. see* McKEE FARRAR A. *Cup a.* reconstruction of the articular surface, which is then covered by a vitallium cup. *Excision a.* excision of the joint surfaces affected, so that the gap thus formed then fills with fibrous tissue or muscle. *Girdlestone a.* an excision arthroplasty of the hip. *McKee Farrar a.* replacement of both the head and the socket of the femur; *Charnley's a.* is similar. *Replacement a.* partial removal of the head of the femur and its replacement by a metal prosthesis.

**arthroscope** ('ahthrəˌskohp) an endoscope for examining the interior of a joint.

**arthrotomy** (ahˈthrotəmee) an incision into a joint.

**articular** (ahˈtikyuhlə) pertaining to a joint.

**articulation** (ahˌtikyuhˈlayshən) 1. a junction of two or more bones. 2. the enunciation of words.

**artificial** (ˌahtiˈfishəl) not natural. *A. feeding* 1. the giving of food other than by placing it directly in the mouth. It may be provided via the mouth, using an oesophageal tube; the food may be introduced into the stomach through a fine tube via the nostril (the nasal route); an opening through the abdominal wall into the stomach (i.e. a gastrostomy) may allow direct introduction; or food may be injected intravenously (*see* PARENTERAL). 2. in reference to the feeding of infants, giving food other than human milk. *A. insemination* the insertion of sperm into the uterus by means of syringe and cannula instead of coitus. The husband's (AIH) or donor (AID) semen may be used. *A. kidney* a dialysis machine to remove unwanted waste materials from the patient with acute or chronic renal failure. *See* HAEMODIALYSIS. *A. respiration* a means of resuscitation from asphyxia. *A. tears* sterile solutions designed to maintain the moisture of the cornea when the latter is abnormally dry due to inadequate tear production. Methylcellulose is a common ingredient.

**arytenoid** (ˌariˈteenoyd) resembling the mouth of a pitcher. *A. cartilages* two cartilages of the larynx; their function is to regulate the tension of the vocal cords attached to them.

**asbestos** (asˈbestos, -təs) a fibrous non-combustible silicate of magnesium and calcium that is a good non-conductor of heat.

**asbestosis** (ˌasbesˈtohsis) a form of pneumoconiosis (chronic lung disease), due to the inhalation of asbestos fibres causing scarring of the lung tissue. It results in breathlessness and may lead to respiratory failure.

**ascariasis** (ˌaskəˈrieəsis) the condition in which roundworms are found in the gastrointestinal tract.

*Ascaris* ('askə.ris) a genus of roundworm. Some types may infest the human intestine.

**Aschoff's nodules** or **bodies** (ashofs bodiz) *K.A.L. Aschoff, German pathologist, 1866–1942.* The nodules present in heart muscle in rheumatic myocarditis.

**ascites** (ə'sieteez) free fluid in the peritoneal cavity. It may be the result of local inflammation or venous obstruction, or be part of a generalized oedema.

**ascorbic acid** (əs'kawbik) vitamin C. This acid is found in many vegetables and fruits and is an essential dietary constituent for humans. Vitamin C is destroyed by heat and deteriorates during storage. It is necessary for connective tissue and collagen fibre synthesis and promotes the healing of wounds. Deficiency causes scurvy.

**asepsis** (ay'sepsis) freedom from pathogenic microorganisms.

**aseptic** (ay'septik) free from sepsis. *A. technique* a method of carrying out sterile procedures so that there is the minimum risk of introducing infection. Achieved by the sterility of equipment and a non-touch technique.

**asexual** (ay'seksyoʊəl, a'sek-) without sex. *A. reproduction* the production of new individuals without sexual union, e.g. by cell division or budding.

**Asilone** ('asilohn) trade name for a proprietary compound antacid mixture.

**asparaginase** (ə'sparəji,nayz) an enzyme that catalyses the deamination of asparagine; used as an antineoplastic agent against cancers, e.g. acute lymphocytic leukaemia, in which the malignant cells require exogenous asparagine for protein synthesis.

**aspartame** (ə,spahtaym) a synthetic compound of two amino acids (L-aspartyl-L-phenylalanine methyl ester) used as a low-calorie sweetener. It is 180 times as sweet as sucrose (table sugar); the amount equal in sweetness to a teaspoon of sugar contains 0.1 calorie (4.2J). Aspartame does not promote the formation of dental caries. The amount of phenylalanine in aspartame must be taken into account in the low-phenylalanine diet for patients with phenylketonuria.

**aspect** ('aspekt) that part of a surface facing in a particular direction. *Dorsal a.* that facing and seen from the back. *Ventral a.* that facing and seen from the front.

**aspergillosis** (,aspərji'lohsis) a bronchopulmonary disease in which the mucous membrane is attacked by the fungus, *Aspergillus.*

*Aspergillus* (,aspərjiləs) a genus of fungi. *A. fumigatus* a common cause of aspergillosis, found in soil and manure.

**aspermia** (ay'spərmi.ə) absence of sperm.

**asphyxia** (as'fiksi.ə) a deficiency of oxygen in the blood and an increase in carbon dioxide in the blood and tissues. Symptoms include irregular and disturbed respirations, or a complete absence of breathing, and pallor or cyanosis. Asphyxia may occur whenever there is an interruption in the normal exchange of oxygen and carbon dioxide between the lungs and the outside air. Common causes are drowning, electric shock, lodging of a foreign body in the air passages, inhalation of smoke and poisonous gases and trauma to or disease of the lungs or air passages. Treatment includes immediate remedy of the situation (*see* RESPIRATION (ARTIFICIAL)) and removal of the underlying cause whenever possible.

**aspiration** (,aspi'rayshən) 1. the act of inhaling. 2. the drawing off of fluid from a cavity by means of suction.

**aspirator** ('aspir,raytə) any apparatus for withdrawing fluid or gases from a cavity of the body by means of suction.

**aspirin** ('asprin) acetylsalicylic acid. It reduces temperature, relieves pain and is an antiplatelet agent to reduce the tendency of the blood to clot within the circulation. *Soluble a.* a combination of aspirin with citric acid and calcium carbonate.

**assay** ('asay, ə'say) a quantitative examination to determine the amount of a particular constituent of a mixture, or of the biological or pharmacological potency of a drug.

**assertiveness** (ə'sərtivnəs) a form of behaviour characterized by a confident declaration or affirmation of a statement without need of proof. To assert oneself is to compel recognition of one's rights or position without either aggressively transgressing the rights of another and assuming a position of dominance, or submissively permitting another to deny one's rights or rightful position. *A. training* instruction and practice in techniques for dealing with interpersonal conflicts and threatening situations in an assertive manner, avoiding the extremes of aggressive and submissive behaviour.

**assessment** (ə'sesmənt) 1. the critical analysis and valuation or judgement of the status or quality of a particular condition, situation or other subject of appraisal. In the nursing process, assessment involves the gathering of information about the health status of the patient/client, analysis and synthesis of the data, and the making of a clinical nursing judgement (*see* NURSING (PROCESS)). The outcome of the nursing assessment is the establishment of the nursing DIAGNOSIS, the identification of the nursing problems. 2. an examination set by an examining authority to test a candidate's nursing skills and knowledge.

**assimilation** (ə,simi'layshən) the process of transforming food so that it can be absorbed and utilized as nourishment by the tissues of the body.

**associate nurse** (ə'sohsi'ət 'nərs) a nurse who, as a member of the primary nursing team, is responsible for effecting a patient's care plans on behalf of the primary nurse. *See* PRIMARY NURSING.

**association** (ə,sohsi'ayshən, -,sohshi-) coordination of function of similar parts. *A. fibres* nerve fibres linking different areas of the brain. *A. of ideas* a mental impression in which a thought or any sensory impulse will call to mind another object or idea connected in some way with the former. *Free a.* a method employed in psychoanalysis in which the patient is encouraged to express freely whatever comes to mind. By this method material that is in the unconscious can be recalled.

**associative play** (ə'sohsi.ətiv) a form of play in which a group of children participate in similar activities without formal organization or direction.

**asthenia** (as'thenia) want of strength. Debility. Loss of tone.

**asthenic** (as'thenik) description of a type of body build: a pale, lean, narrowly built person with poor muscle development.

**asthenopia** (,asthe'nohpi.ə) eye strain giving rise to an aching, burning sensation and headache. Likely to arise in long-sighted people when continual effort of accommodation is required for close work.

**asthma** ('asmə) paroxysmal dyspnoea characterized by wheezing and difficulty in expiration. *Bronchial a.* attacks of dyspnoea in which there is wheezing and difficulty in expiration due to muscular spasm of the bronchi. The attacks may be precipitated by hypersensitivity to foreign substances, air pollution, exertion or infection, or associated with emotional upsets. There is often a family history of asthma or other allergic condition. Treatment is with bronchodilators with or without corticosteroids, usually via an aerosol or a powder inhaler. *Cardiac a.* attacks of dyspnoea and palpitation, arising most often at night, associated with left-sided heart failure and pulmonary congestion. *Renal a.* dyspnoea occurring in kidney disease, which may be a sign of developing uraemia. It is unrelated to true asthma.

**astigmatism** (ə'stigmə,tizəm) inequality of the refractive power of an eye, due to curvature of its corneal meridians. The curve across the front of the eye from side to side is not quite the same as the curve from above downwards. The focus on the retina is then not a point but a diffuse and indistinct area. May be congenital or acquired.

**astringent** (ə'strinjənt) an agent causing contraction of organic tissues, thereby checking secretions, e.g. silver nitrate, tannic acid.

**astrocytoma** (,astrohsie'tohmə) a malignant tumour of the brain or spinal cord. It is slow-growing. A glioma.

**Astrup machine** ('astrup mə,sheen) an apparatus for ascertaining the pH value of arterial blood.

**asymmetry** (ay'simitree, a-) inequality in size or shape of two normally similar structures or of two halves of a structure normally the same.

**asymptomatic** (,aysimptə'matik, a-) without symptoms.

**asynergy** (ay'sinə,jee) lack of coordination of structures which normally act in harmony.

**asystole** (ay'sistəlee) absence of heartbeat. Cardiac arrest.

**at risk** (ət 'risk) whereby an individual or population may be vulnerable to a particular disease, hazard or injury. At risk situations are those involving possible problems that may be preventable with appropriate intervention, or, if they should occur, treatment.

**ataractic** (atə'raktik) 1. pertaining to or characterized by ataraxia. 2. an agent that induces ataraxia; a tranquillizer.

**ataraxia** (,atə'raksi.ə) a state of detached serenity with depression of mental faculties or impairment of consciousness.

**ataxia, ataxy** (ə'taksi) failure of muscle coordination resulting in irregular jerky movements, and unsteadiness in standing and walking from a disorder of the controlling mechanisms in the brain, or from inadequate input to the brain from joints and muscles. *Hereditary a.* Friedreich's ataxia.

**atelectasis** (,atə'lektəsis) a collapsed or airless state of the lung, which may be acute or chronic and may involve all or part of the lung: (a) from imperfect expansion of pulmonary alveoli at birth (*congenital a.*); (b) as the result of disease or injury.

**atheroma** (,athə'rohmə) an abnormal mass of fatty or lipid material with a fibrous covering, existing as a discrete, raised plaque within the intima of an artery.

**atherosclerosis** (,athə.rohsklə'rohsis) a condition in which the fatty degenerative plaques of atheroma are accompanied by arteriosclerosis, a narrowing and hardening of the vessels.

**athetosis** (,athi'tohsis) a recurring series of slow, writhing movements of the hands, usually due to a cerebral lesion.

**athlete's foot** (,athleets) a fungal infection between the toes, easily transmitted to other people. Tinea pedis.

**atlas** ('atləs) the first cervical verte-bra, articulating with the occipital bone of the skull.

**atmosphere** ('atməsˌfiə) 1. the gases that surround the earth, extending to an altitude of 16 km. 2. the air or climate of a particular place, e.g. a smoking atmosphere. 3. mental or moral environment, tone or mood.

**atmospheric pressure** (ˌatməs'ferik) pressure exerted by the air in all directions. At sea level it is about 100 kPa.

**atom** ('atəm) the smallest particle of an element that retains all the prop-erties of that element. It is made up of a central positively charged nu-cleus and, moving around in it in orbit, negatively charged electrons.

**atomizer** ('atəˌmiezə) an instrument by which a liquid is divided to form a fine spray or vapour (nebulizer).

**atony** ('atənee) lack of tone, e.g. in a muscle.

**atopy** ('atəpee) a state of hypersen-sitivity to certain antigens. There is an inherited tendency that includes asthma, eczema and hay fever.

**ATP** adenosine triphosphate.

**atracurium** (ˌatrə'kyooə.ri.əm) a muscle relaxant with a relatively short duration of action used in anaesthesia.

**atresia** (ə'treezi.ə) absence of a nat-ural opening or tubular structure, e.g. of the anus or vagina; usually a congenital malformation.

**atrial** ('aytri.əl) relating to the atri-um. *A. fibrillation* overstimulation of the atrial walls so that many areas of excitation arise and the atrioventricular node is bombarded with impulses, many of which it can-not transmit, resulting in a highly irregular pulse. *A. flutter* rapid regular action of the atria. The atrio-ventricular node transmits alter-native impulses or one in three or four. The atrial rate is usually about 300 beats per minute. *A. septal defect* the non-closure of the fora-

men ovale at the time of birth, giv-ing rise to a congenital heart defect.

**atrioventricular** (ˌaytriohven'trik-yuhlə) pertaining to the atrium and ventricle. *A. bundle see* BUNDLE OF HIS. *A. node* a node of neurogenic tissue situated between the atrium and ventricle and transmitting impulses. *A. valves* the bicuspid and tricuspid valve on the left and right sides of the heart respectively.

**atrium** ('aytri.əm) *pl.* atria. 1. a cavi-ty, entrance or passage. 2. one of the two upper chambers of the heart. Formerly called auricle.

**atrophy** ('atrəfee) wasting of any part of the body, due to degenera-tion of the cells, from disuse, or lack of nourishment or nerve supply. *Acute yellow a.* massive necrosis of liver cells. A rare condition that may follow acute hepatitis or eclampsia or be precipitated by cer-tain drugs. *Progressive muscular a.* (motor neurone disease) degenera-tion of the motor neurones with wasting of muscle tissue.

**atropine** ('atrəˌpeen, -pin) the active principle of belladonna. An alkaloid which inhibits respiratory and gastric secretions, relaxes mus-cle spasm and dilates the pupil.

**attack** (ə'tak) an episode or onset of illness. *A. rate* number of cases of a disease in a particular group, e.g. a school, over a given period, related to the population of that group. *Transient ischaemic a's* brief attacks (a few hours or less) of cerebral dysfunction of vascular origin, without lasting neurological deficit.

**attention deficit syndrome** (ə'ten-shən) a disorder of childhood char-acterized by marked failure of attention, impulsiveness and in-creased motor activity. Affects more boys than girls. Treatment involves medication usually with methyl-phenidate, behaviour therapy and social support.

**attenuation** (ə‚tenyoo'ayshən) a bacteriological process by which organisms are rendered less virulent by culture in artificial media through many generations, exposure to light, air, etc.; it is used for vaccine preparations.

**attitude** ('ati‚tyood) 1. a posture or position of the body; in obstetrics, the relation of the various parts of the fetal body to one another. 2. a pattern of mental views established by cumulative prior experience.

**atypical** (ay'tipik'l) irregular; not conforming to type.

**audiogram** ('awdioh‚gram) a graph produced by an audiometer.

**audiologist** (‚awdi'olǝjist) an allied health professional specializing in audiology, who provides services that include: (a) evaluation of hearing function to detect hearing impairment and, if there is a hearing disorder, to determine the anatomical site involved and the cause of the disorder; (b) selection of appropriate hearing aids; and (c) training in lip reading, hearing aid use and maintenance of normal speech.

**audiology** (‚awdi'olǝjee) the science concerned with the sense of hearing, especially the evaluation and measurement of impaired hearing and the rehabilitation of those with impaired hearing.

**audiometer** (‚awdi'omitə) an instrument for testing hearing, whereby the threshold of the patient's hearing can be measured.

**audit** ('awdit) systematic review and evaluation of records and other data to determine the quality of the services or products provided in a given situation. It is also now a government requirement for the financial review of NHS trusts. *A. Monitor* an adaptation for the UK of the USA Rush Medicus system of assessing quality of nursing care. It consists of 'checklists' for quality, leading to a scoring system. *Medical a.* the systematic critical analysis of the quality of medical treatment and care, including the procedures for diagnosis and treatment, the use of resources, outcomes and the resultant quality of life for the patient. *Nursing a.* an evaluation of structure, process and outcome as a measurement of the quality of nursing care. *Concurrent audits* are conducted at the time the care is being provided to clients/patients. They may be conducted by means of observation and interview of clients/patients, review of open charts, or conferences with groups of consumers and providers of nursing care. *Retrospective audits* are conducted after the patient's discharge. Methods include the study of closed patient's charts and nursing care plans, questionnaires, interviews, and surveys of patients and families.

**Audit Commission** (kǝ'mishǝn) established in 1983 to appoint and regulate external auditors of local authorities in England and Wales. In 1990 its responsibilities were extended to include the NHS. The main duties of the Audit Commission include the promotion of 'best practice' in local government and NHS bodies, encouraging economy, efficiency and effectiveness in both the management and delivery of services.

**aura** ('or.rǝ) the premonition, peculiar to an individual, which often precedes an epileptic fit.

**aural** ('or.rǝl) referring to the ear.

**auricle** ('or.rik'l) 1. the external portion of the ear. 2. obsolete term for the atrium.

**auriscope** ('or.ri‚skohp) an instrument for examining the drum of the ear. An otoscope.

**aurum** ('or.rǝm) [L.] *gold.*

**auscultation** (‚awskǝl'tayshǝn) examining the internal organs by listening to the sounds that they give out. In *direct* or *immediate a.* the ear is placed directly against the body. In *mediate a.* a stethoscope is used.

**Australia antigen** (o'strayli.ə) hepatitis B surface antigen found in the blood of a patient with serum hepatitis or who is a carrier of the virus. Dilute concentrations of the antigen can cause the disease, and health care personnel must take adequate precautions to avoid inoculation accidents. Blood banks routinely screen for the antigen to exclude infected blood donations.

**autism** ('awtizəm) self-absorption. Abnormal dislike of the society of others. *Infantile a.* failure of a child to relate to people and situations, leading to complete withdrawal into a world of private fantasies.

**autistic** (aw'tistik) pertaining to autism.

**autoagglutination** (ˌawtoh.ə.glooti-'nayshən) 1. clumping or agglutination of cells by an individual's own serum, as in autohaemagglutination. Autoagglutination occurring at low temperatures is called cold agglutination. 2. agglutination of particulate antigens, e.g. bacteria, in the absence of specific antigens.

**autoantibody** (ˌawtoh'anti bodee) an antibody formed in response to, and reacting against, an antigenic constituent of the individual's own tissues.

**autoantigen** (ˌawtoh'antijən) a tissue constituent that stimulates production of autoantibodies in the organism in which it occurs.

**autoclave** ('awtə klayv) a steam-heated sterilizing apparatus in which the temperature is raised by reducing the air pressure inside; steam is injected under pressure, bringing about efficient sterilization of instruments and dishes treated in this way.

**autodigestion** (ˌawtohdie'jeschjən, -di-) dissolution of tissue by its own secretions.

**autoeroticism** (ˌawtoh.i'roti sizəm) sexual pleasure derived from self-stimulation of erogenous zones (the mouth, the anus, the genitals and the skin).

**autogenous** (aw'tojənəs) generated within the body and not acquired from external sources.

**autograft** ('awtə grahft) the transfer of skin or other tissue from one part of the body to another to repair some deficiency.

**autoimmune disease** (ˌawtoh.i-'myoon) condition in which the body develops antibodies to its own tissues, e.g. in autoimmune thyroiditis (Hashimoto's disease).

**autoimmunization** (ˌawtoh imyuh-nie'zayshən) the formation of antibodies against the individual's own tissue.

**autoinfection** (ˌawtoh.in'fekshən) self-infection, transferred from one part of the body to another by fingers, towels, etc.

**autoinoculation** (ˌawtoh.i nokyuh-'layshən) inoculation with a microorganism from the body itself.

**autointoxication** (ˌawtoh.in toksi-'kayshən) poisoning by toxins generated within the body itself.

**autologous** (aw'toləgəs) related to self; belonging to the same organism. *A. blood transfusion* abbreviated ABT. The patient donates blood before elective surgery for transfusion postoperatively. ABT may also be obtained as a blood salvage procedure during operation or postoperatively. Avoids cross-matching, compatibility and transfusion infection problems.

**autolysis** (aw'tolisis) a breaking up of living tissues, e.g. as may occur if pancreatic ferments escape into surrounding tissues. It also occurs after death.

**automatic** (ˌawtəˈmatik) performed without the influence of the will.

**automatism** (awˈtoməˌtizəm) performance of non-reflex acts without apparent volition, and of which the patient may have no memory afterwards, as in somnambulism. *Post-epileptic a.* automatic acts following an epileptic fit.

**autonomic** (ˌawtəˈnomik) self-governing. *A. nervous system* the sympathetic and parasympathetic nerves that control involuntary muscles and glandular secretion, over which there is no conscious control.

**autoplasty** ('awtohˌplastee) 1. replacement of missing tissue by grafting a healthy section from another part of the body. 2. in psychoanalysis, instinctive modification within the psychic systems in adaptation to reality.

**autopsy** (awˈtopsee, 'awtəp-) postmortem examination of a body to determine the cause of death.

**autosome** ('awtohˌsohm) any chromosome other than the sex chromosomes. In humans there are 22 pairs of autosomes and 1 pair of sex chromosomes.

**autosuggestion** (ˌawtohsəˈjeschjən) suggestion arising in one's self. Uncritical acceptance of an idea arising in the individual's own mind.

**autotransfusion** (ˌawtohtrans-ˈfyoozhən, -trahns-) reinfusion of a patient's own blood.

**autotransplantation** (ˌawtohˌtransplahnˈtayshən) transfer of tissue from one part of the body to another part.

**avascular** (ayˈvaskyuhlə) not vascular. Bloodless. *A. necrosis* death of bone owing to deficient blood supply, usually following an injury.

**aversion** (əˈvərshən) intense dislike. *A. therapy* a method of treating addictions by associating the craving for what is addictive with painful or unpleasant stimuli. It is rarely used.

**avitaminosis** (ayˌvitəmiˈnohsis) a condition resulting from an insufficiency of vitamins in the diet. A deficiency disease.

**avoidance** (əˈvoydəns) a conscious or unconscious defence mechanism whereby an individual seeks to escape or avoid certain situations, feelings or conflicts.

**avulsion** (əˈvulshən) the tearing away of one part from another. *Phrenic a.* a tearing away of the phrenic nerve. It paralyses the diaphragm on the affected side.

**axilla** (akˈsila) an armpit.

**axis** ('aksis) 1. a line through the centre of a structure. 2. the second cervical vertebra.

**axon** ('akson) the process of a nerve cell along which electrical impulses travel. The nerve fibre.

**axonotmesis** (ˌaksonətˈmeesis) nerve injury characterized by disruption of the axon and myelin sheath but with preservation of the connective tissue fragments, resulting in degeneration of the axon distal to the injury site; regeneration of the axon is spontaneous.

**azathioprine** (ˌazəˈthieəˈpreen) an immunosuppressive drug widely used for transplant recipients and also as treatment for autoimmune conditions.

**azoospermia** (ˌayzoh.ohˈspərmi.ə) absence of spermatozoa in the semen.

**AZT** azidothymidine; *see* ZIDOVUDINE.

**azygos** ('aziˌgos, aˈzie-) something that is unpaired. *A. vein* an unpaired vein that ascends the posterior mediastinum and enters the superior vena cava.

# B

**Ba** symbol for *barium*.

**Babinski's reflex** or **sign** (bə'binskez) *J.F.F. Babinski, French neurologist, 1857–1932.* On stroking the sole of the foot, the great toe bends upwards instead of downwards (dorsal instead of plantar flexion). Present in disease or injury to the upper motor neurone. Babies who have not walked react in the same way, but normal flexion develops later.

**baby** ('baybee) an infant or young child who is not yet walking. *B. blues* the transient feelings of unhappiness and tearfulness that affect many women after the birth of their baby. *B. Friendly Initiative* abbreviated BFI. Part of a global campaign by the World Health Organization and the United Nations Children's Fund to ensure that all mothers are facilitated in breast feeding to enable babies to benefit from the health and social advantages. *Battered b.* one suffering from the result of continued violence; extensive bruising, fractures of limbs, rib and skull, or an internal trauma may be found. *Blue b.* one suffering from cyanosis at birth as a result of atelectasis or congenital heart malformation.

**Bach flower remedies** (baks flowə remədiz) a system of complementary medicine, devised by Dr Edward Bach and based on homeopathic principles. Flower remedies can be used to treat emotional and psychological disorders. There are 38 flower remedies. *See also* HOMEOPATHY.

**bacillaemia** (,basi'leemi.ə) the presence of bacilli in the blood.

**bacilluria** (,basi'lyooə.ri.ə) the presence of bacilli in the blood.

**bacillus** (bə'siləs) loosely, the cause of any bacterial infection by a rod-shaped microorganism, e.g. *Escherichia coli*, the colon bacillus.

**Bacillus** (bə'siləs) a genus of aerobic, spore-bearing Gram-positive bacteria. *B. anthracis* the causative agent of ANTHRAX.

**back** (bak) dorsum. Posterior trunk from neck to pelvis. *B. bone* the vertebral column. *B. slab* plaster or plastic splint in which a limb is supported. *Hunch b.* kyphosis.

**backache** ('bak,ayk) any pain in the back, usually the lower part. The pain is often dull and continuous, but sometimes sharp and throbbing. Backache, or lumbago, is one of the most common ailments and can be caused by a variety of disorders. Nurses are at particular risk and one in six is thought to experience back pain.

**bacteraemia** (,baktə'reemi.ə) the presence of bacteria in the bloodstream.

**bacterial** (bak'tiə.ri.əl) pertaining to bacteria.

**bactericidal** (bak,tiə.ri.si'sied'l) capable of killing bacteria, e.g.

disinfectants, great heat, intense cold or sunlight.

**bactericide** (bak'tiə.ri.sied) an agent that kills bacteria.

**bacteriologist** (bak.tiə.ri'olәjist) one who is qualified in the science of bacteriology.

**bacteriology** (bak.tiə.ri'olәjee) the scientific study of bacteria.

**bacteriolysin** (bak.tiə.ri'olisin, -rioh-'liesin) an antibody produced in the blood to assist in the destruction of bacteria. The action is specific.

**bacteriolysis** (bak.tiə.ri'olisis) the dissolution of bacteria by a bacteriolytic agent.

**bacteriolytic** (bak.tiәrioh'litik) capable of destroying or dissolving bacteria.

**bacteriophage** (bak'tiə.ri.ə.fayj, -.fahzh) a virus that only infects bacteria. Many strains exist, some of which are used for identifying types of staphylococci and salmonellae.

**bacteriostat** (bak'tiə.rioh.stat) an agent that inhibits the growth of bacteria.

**bacteriostatic** (bak.tiə.rioh'static) inhibiting the growth of bacteria.

**bacterium** (bak'tiə.ri.əm) a general name given to a minute vegetable organism which may live on organic matter. There are many varieties, only some of which are pathogenic to man, animals and plants. Each bacterium consists of a single cell and, given favourable conditions, multiplies by subdivision. Bacteria are classified according to their shape (*see* Figure): (a) *bacilli*, rod-shaped; (b) *cocci*, spherical, subdivided into (i) streptococci, in chains; (ii) staphylococci, in groups; (iii) diplococci, in pairs; (c) *spirilla*, *spirochaetes*, spiral. *Pathogenic b.* one whose growth in the body gives rise to disease, either by destruction of tissue or by formation of toxins, which circulate in the blood. Pathogenic bacteria thrive on organic matter in the presence of warmth and moisture.

**bacteriuria** (bak.tiə.ri'yooə.ri.ə) the presence of bacteria in the urine.

**bag** (bag) a sac or pouch. *B. of waters* the membranes enclosing the AMNIOTIC (FLUID) and the developing fetus in utero. *Colostomy b.* a receptacle worn over the stoma by the patient, to receive the faecal discharge. *Douglas b.* a receptacle for the collection of expired air, permitting measurement of respiratory gases. *Ice b.* a rubber or plastic bag half-filled with pieces of ice and applied near or to a part of the body. *Ileostomy b.* any of various plastic or latex pouches attached to the stoma for the collection of faecal material after ILEOSTOMY. *Politizer b.* a soft bag of rubber for inflating the pharyngotympanic tube. *Urine b.* a receptacle used for urine by ambulatory patients with urinary incontinence.

**balanitis** (.balə'nietis) inflammation of the glans penis and of the prepuce, usually associated with phimosis. Balanoposthitis.

**balantidiasis** (.balənti'dieəsis) a rare form of colitis or dysentery caused by intestinal infestation by *Balantidium coli*, a protozoon.

**baldness** ('bawldnəs) absence of hair, especially from the scalp. Alopecia.

**ballottement** (bə'lotmənt) [Fr.] a method of testing for a floating object, e.g. abdominal palpation of the uterus when testing for pregnancy. The uterus is pushed upward by a finger in the vagina, and if a fetus is present it will fall back again like a heavy body in water.

**balsam** ('bawlsəm) an aromatic vegetable juice. *Friar's b.* a compound containing tincture of benzoin. Used for steam inhalations. *Peru b.* used externally as an antiseptic ointment and in *tulle gras*.

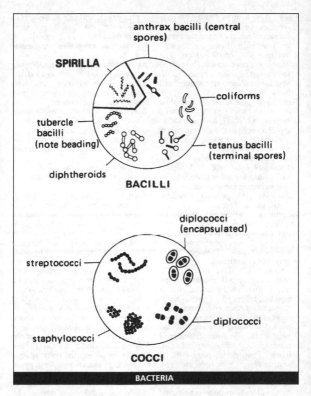

anthrax bacilli (central spores)

**SPIRILLA**

coliforms

tubercle bacilli (note beading)

tetanus bacilli (terminal spores)

diphtheroids

**BACILLI**

diplococci (encapsulated)

streptococci

diplococci

staphylococci

**COCCI**

**BACTERIA**

*Tolu b.* used as an expectorant. A constituent of friar's balsam.

**bandage** ('bandij) 1. a strip or roll of gauze or other material for wrapping or binding any part of the body. 2. to cover by wrapping with such material. Bandages may be used to stop the flow of blood, to provide a safeguard against contamination, or to hold a dressing in place. They may also be used to hold a splint in position or otherwise immobilize an injured part of the body to prevent further injury and to facilitate healing.

**banding** ('banding) placing a band round a vessel to restrict the flow from it. *Pulmonary arterial b.* a palliative operation used in treating infants with ventricular septal defects.

**bank** (bangk) an institution offering services, or a store of donated human tissues for use in the future by other individuals, e.g. *blood b.*, *human milk b.*, *sperm b. Nurse b.* a group of nurses who are known to the employing authority and available for employment on an on-call basis.

**Bankhart's operation** ('bangkhahts) *A.S.B. Bankhart, British orthopaedic surgeon, 1879–1951.* An operation to repair a defect in the glenoid cavity that causes repeated dislocation of the shoulder joint.

**Banti's disease** ('banteez) *G. Banti, Italian pathologist, 1852–1925.* A clinical syndrome characterized by splenomegaly, cirrhosis of the liver, anaemia, leukopenia and gastrointestinal bleeding.

**barbiturates** (bah'bityuh.rəts, - rayts) a large group of sedative and hypnotic drugs derived from barbituric acid, e.g. phenobarbitone, amylobarbitone. Prolonged use may lead to addiction.

**barbotage** (,bahbə'tahzh) [Fr.] a method of spinal anaesthesia by which some of the anaesthetic is injected, followed by partial withdrawal and then reinjection with more of the drug. This process is repeated until the full amount has been given, allowing dilution and mixing with the cerebrospinal fluid.

**barium** ('bair.ri.əm) *symbol* Ba. A soft silvery metallic element. *B. sulphate* a heavy mineral salt that is comparatively impermeable to X-rays and can therefore be used as a contrast medium, given as a meal or as an enema. Used to demonstrate abnormality in the stomach or intestines, and to show peristaltic movement. *B. sulphide* the chief constituent of depilatory preparations, i.e. those which remove hair.

**baroreceptors** (,barohri'septəz) the sensory branches of the glosso-

pharyngeal and vagus nerves that influence the blood pressure. The receptors are situated in the walls of the carotid sinus and aortic arch.

**barotrauma** (,baroh'trawmə) injury due to pressure, such as to structures of the ear, owing to differences between atmospheric and intratympanic pressures.

**Barr body** (bah) *M.L. Barr, Canadian anatomist, b. 1908.* Small, dark-staining area underneath the nuclear membrane of female cells. Represents an inactive X chromosome.

**Barré–Guillain syndrome** (,baray-'giyanh) *see* GUILLAIN–BARRÉ SYNDROME.

**barrier** ('bari.ə) an obstruction. *B. contraceptive* mechanical barrier preventing the sperm from entering the cervical canal, e.g. diaphragm, sheath. *B. nursing* precautions taken by nurses to prevent infection from a patient spreading to other patients and/or staff. This normally involves nursing the patient in a separate room or cubicle. *Blood–brain b.* the selective barrier which separates the circulating blood from the cerebrospinal fluid. *Placental b.* semipermeable membrane between maternal and fetal blood. *Protective b.* radiation-absorbing shield, e.g. lead, concrete, to protect the body against ionizing radiations. *Reverse b. nursing* a technique used by nurses to prevent the transmission of infection to the patient who may be especially vulnerable, e.g. the immunosuppressed patient.

**Bartholin's glands** ('bahtəlinz) *C.T. Bartholin, Danish anatomist, 1655–1738.* Two glands situated in the labia majora, with ducts opening inside the vulva.

**basal** ('bays'l) 1. fundamental. 2. referring to a base. *B. ganglia* the collections of nerve cells or grey matter in the base of the cerebrum. They consist of the caudate nucleus and putamen, forming the corpus striatum, and the globus pallidus. Such cells are concerned with modifying and coordinating voluntary muscle movements. *B. metabolic rate* abbreviated BMR. An indirect method of estimating the rate of metabolism in the body by measuring the oxygen intake and carbon dioxide output on breathing. The age, sex, weight and size of the patient have to be taken into account.

**base** (bays) 1. the lowest part or foundation. 2. the main constituent of a compound. 3. an alkali or other substance that can unite with an acid to form a salt.

**basement membrane** ('baysmənt) a thin layer of modified connective tissue supporting layers of cells, found at the base of the epidermis and underlying mucous membranes.

**basilar** ('basilə) situated at the base. *B. artery* midline artery at the base of the skull, formed by the junction of the vertebral arteries.

**basilic** (bə'silik) prominent. *B. vein* a large vein on the inner side of the arm.

**basophil** ('baysə,fil) adj. *basophilic*. 1. any structure, cell or histological element staining readily with basic dyes. 2. a granular leukocyte with an irregularly shaped, relatively pale-staining nucleus that is partially constricted into two lobes, and with cytoplasm containing coarse bluish-black granules of variable size. 3. a beta cell of the adenohypophysis.

**basophilia** (,baysə'fili.ə) 1. an affinity of cells or tissues for basic dyes. 2. the reaction of relatively immature erythrocytes to basic dyes whereby the stained cells appear blue, grey or greyish-blue, or bluish granules appear.

3. abnormal increase of basophilic leukocytes in the blood. 4. basophilic leukocytosis.

**Batchelor plaster** ('bachələ) *J.S. Batchelor, British surgeon.* A double abduction splint used in the correction of congenital dislocation of the hip.

**bath** (bahth) 1. a medium, e.g. water, vapour, sand or mud, with which the body is washed or in which the body is wholly or partially immersed for therapeutic or cleansing purposes; application of such a medium to the body. 2. the equipment or apparatus in which a body or object may be immersed. *Bed b.* washing a patient in bed. *Emollient b.* a bath in a soothing and softening liquid, used in various skin disorders. It is prepared by adding soothing agents such as gelatin, starch, bran or similar substances to the bath water, for the purpose of relieving skin irritation and pruritus. The patient is dried by patting rather than rubbing the skin. Care must be taken to avoid chilling. *Hot b.* one taken in water at 36–44°C. Care must be taken to avoid faintness. *Sponge b.* one in which the patient's body is not immersed but is wiped with a wet cloth or sponge. Sponge baths are most often employed for reduction of body temperature in the presence of a fever, in which case the water used is tepid and may contain alcohol to increase evaporation of moisture from the skin. *Tepid b.* one taken in water at 30–33°C. *Warm b.* one taken in water at 32–40°C. *Whirlpool b.* (Jacuzzi) one in which the water is kept in constant motion by mechanical means. It has a gentle massaging action that promotes relaxation.

**BCG vaccine** bacille Calmette–Guérin vaccine, a tuberculosis vaccine containing live, attenuated bovine tubercle bacillis (*Myco-bacterium bovis*).

**'bearing down'** (ˌbair.ring 'down) 1. the expulsive pains in the second stage of labour. 2. a feeling of heaviness and downward strain in the pelvis, present with some uterine growths or displacements.

**beat** (beet) pulsation of the heart or an artery. *Apex b.* pulsation of the heart felt over its apex. The beat of the heart is felt against the chest wall. *Dropped b.* the occasional loss of a ventricular beat. *Ectopic b.* one that originates somewhere other than the sino-atrial node.

**Beck inventory of depression** (bek 'invəntari, -tri) abbreviated BID. A self-scoring system used to determine the presence and severity of depression.

**beclomethasone dipropionate** (ˌbek-loh'methəzohn die'prohpianayt) a glucocorticoid administered by aerosol inhalation or Spinhaler to patients who require corticosteroids for control of bronchial asthma or hay fever symptoms.

**becquerel** (be'krel) abbreviated Bq. The SI unit of radioactivity equal to the quantity of material undergoing one disintegration per second; $3.7 \times 10^{10}$ becquerels is equal to 1 curie.

**bed** (bed) 1. a supporting structure or tissue. 2. a couch or support for the body during sleep. *B. cradle* a frame placed over the body of a bed patient. *See* CRADLE. *Capillary b.* the capillaries of a tissue, area or organ considered collectively, and their volume capacity. *Fracture b.* a bed for the use of patients with broken bones. *King's Fund b.* a bed fitted with jointed springs, which may be adjusted to various positions. *See also* KING'S FUND. *Nail b.* the area of modified epidermis beneath the nail over which the nail plate slides as it grows.

**bed-wetting** ('bedˌweting) enuresis; involuntary voiding of urine. *See also* ENURESIS.

**bedboard** ('bedˌbawd) a rigid board placed beneath the mattress of a bed to give firm support to the patient lying upon it.

**bedbug** ('bedˌbug) a bug of the genus *Cimex*, a flattened, oval, reddish insect that inhabits houses, furniture and neglected beds, and feeds on humans, usually at night.

**bedpan** ('bedˌpan) a shallow vessel used for defecation or urination by patients confined to bed.

**bedrest** ('bedˌrest) limiting the patient to staying in bed for a prescribed period for therapeutic reasons.

**bedsore** ('bedˌsor) an ulcer-like sore caused by prolonged pressure of the patient's body. Pressure sore is now the preferred term, as these sores are primarily due to pressure and can also occur in patients who are not confined to bed. A decubitus ulcer.

**bee sting** ('bee sting) injury caused by the venom of a bee. Symptoms of a severe allergic reaction, such as collapse or swelling of the body, indicate ANAPHYLAXIS and require that medical help be sought.

**behaviour** (bi'hayvyə) the way in which an organism reacts to an internal or external stimulus. *B. disorders* may take many forms, such as truancy, stealing, temper tantrums. *B. modification* an approach to correction of undesirable behaviour that focuses on changing observable actions. Modification of the behaviour is accomplished through systematic manipulation of the environmental and behavioural variables related to the specific behaviour to be changed. *B. therapy* a therapeutic approach in which the focus is on the patient's observable behaviour, rather than on conflict and unconscious processes presumed to underlie the maladaptive behaviour. This is accomplished through systematic manipulation of the environmental and behavioural variables related to the specific behaviour to be modified; operant conditioning, systematic desensitization, token economy, aversive control, flooding and implosion are examples of techniques that may be used in behaviour therapy. *Incongruous b.* behaviour that is out of keeping with the person's normal reaction or has the opposite effect to that consciously desired.

**behaviourism** (bi'hayvyə,rizəm) the purely objective study and observation of the behaviour of individuals.

**Behçet's syndrome** ('bayshayz) *H. Behçet, Turkish dermatologist, 1889–1948.* A chronic condition of unknown origin, resulting in painful, recurring mouth and genital ulcers, arthritis, skin lesions and inflammation of the eyes.

**bejel** ('bayjəl) a non-venereal but infectious form of syphilis caused by a treponema indistinguishable from that causing syphilis. Occurs mainly in children of Africa and the Middle East. The primary lesion is on the mouth, spreading to the trunk, arms and legs. Treated with penicillin.

**belching** ('belching) the noisy expulsion of gas from the stomach through the mouth. Eructation.

**beliefs** (bə'leefs) thoughts, ideas and concepts developed by an individual over a period of time from cultural influences, education, religion, parents and family. *Health b.* those beliefs held by an individual regarding the maintenance of his or her state of physical wellbeing, which may be at variance with those beliefs held by the health care practitioner, possibly leading to conflict and non-compliance with prescribed treatment.

**belladonna** (,belə'donə) a drug from the deadly nightshade plant. Used as an antispasmodic in colic, to check secretions and to dilate the pupil of the eye.

**belle indifference** (,bel in'difə,ronhs) [Fr.] an indication of conversion hysteria, in which the patient describes symptoms, appearing not to be distressed by them.

**Bell's palsy** (belz) *Sir C. Bell, British physiologist, 1774–1842.* Facial paralysis due to oedema of the facial nerve.

**bendrofluazide** (,bendroh'flooə,zied) an oral diuretic of the thiazide group. Used primarily to treat mild hypertension and cardiac failure.

**bends** (bendz) a colloquial term for caisson disease. Decompression sickness.

**benign** (bi'nien) 1. the opposite to malignant. 2. describes a non-invasive condition or illness that is not serious even though treatment may be required for health or cosmetic reasons.

**benorylate** (be'nor.rilayt) an ester of paracetamol and aspirin used as an anti-inflammatory and analgesic.

**benzalkonium chloride** (,benzal-'kohni.əm ,klor.ried) a quaternary ammonium compound used as a surface disinfectant and detergent and as a topical antiseptic and antibiotic preservative. Incompatible with soap.

**benzathine penicillin** (,benzə-theen) a long-acting antibiotic. Used in treatment of Gram-positive infections. May be given orally or intramuscularly.

**benzene** ('benzeen) benzol. A coal/tar derivative widely used as a solvent.

**benzhexol** (benz'heksol) an antispasmodic drug that helps to overcome the tremors and ridigity of Parkinson's disease.

**benzocaine** ('benzoh,kayn) a surface anaesthetic used for the relief of pain or to anaesthetize the oropharynx or anus. Available as lozenges or ointment.

**benzyl benzoate** (,benzil 'benzohayt, -ziel) an emulsion used in the treatment of scabies.

**benzylpenicillin** (,benzil,peni'silin, ,benziel-) a widely used soluble penicillin that is quickly absorbed. High blood levels can therefore be obtained.

**bereavement** (bə'reev,mənt) the experience of suffering loss, usually of a loved one by death or separation, but may also include the loss of previous good health, position or wealth. Produces a psychological reaction that has recognized 'stages' that may overlap; these include anger, denial, disbelief and finally acceptance. Collectively recognized as mourning.

**beriberi** (,beri'beri) a deficiency disease due to insufficiency of vitamin $B_1$ in the diet. The disease is more common in areas where refined rice is the main staple in the diet. It is a form of neuritis, with pain, paralysis and oedema of the extremities.

**berylliosis** (bə,rili'ohsis) an industrial lung disease due to the inhaling of the metallic element beryllium. Interstitial fibrosis arises, impairing lung function.

**beta** ('beetə) the second letter in the Greek alphabet, β. *B. blockers* drugs used to block the action of adrenaline on beta-adrenergic receptors in cardiac muscle, thus decreasing the workload of the heart. *B. cells* insulin-producing cells found in the islets of Langerhans in the pancreas. *B. rays* electrons used therapeutically for treatment of lesions of the cornea and iris. *B. receptors* associated with the inhibition (relaxation) of smooth muscle. They also bring an increase in the force of contraction and rate of the heart.

**Betadine** ('betə,deen, -din) trade name for preparations of povidone-iodine, which have a longer antiseptic action than most iodine solutions.

**betamethasone** (,beetə'methə,zohn) a synthetic glucocorticoid which is the most active of the anti-inflammatory steroids.

**bethanechol** (bə'thani,kol) a derivative of choline-like substance, used in the treatment of abdominal distension and urinary retention. Hypotension and dyspnoea may occur as side-effects.

**bethanidine** (bə'thani,deen) an adrenergic blocking agent used in the treatment of hypertension.

**Betnovate** ('betnəvayt) trade name for preparations containing betame-thasone. Used in the treatment of severe inflammatory skin disorders unresponsive to less potent corticosteroids.

**bezoar** ('beezor) a mass of hair, fruit or vegetable fibres sometimes found in the stomach or intestines.

**bhang, bang** (bang) the dried leaves of *Cannabis sativa*, the hemp plant from which marijuana is derived.

**bias** ('bieəs) in research, any tendency for results to differ from the true value in some consistent way.

**bicarbonate** (bie'kaybə,nayt, -nət) any salt containing the $HCO_3$ anion. *Blood b., plasma b.* the bicarbonate of the blood plasma, an important parameter of acid–base balance (*see* ACID) measured in blood gas analysis.

**bicellular** (bie'selyuhlə) composed of two cells.

**biceps** ('bieseps) a muscle with two heads; a flexor of the arm; one of the hamstring muscles of the thigh.

**biconcave** (bie'konkayv) pertaining to a lens or other structure with a

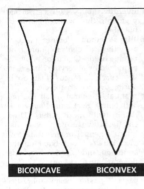

| BICONCAVE | BICONVEX |

hollow or depression on each surface (*see* Figure).

**biconvex** (bie'konvex) pertaining to a lens or other structure that protrudes on both surfaces (*see* Figure).

**bicornuate** (bie'kawnyooayt) having two horns. *B. uterus* a congenital malformation in which there is a partial or complete vertical division into two parts of the body of the uterus (*see* Figure on p. 50).

**bicuspid** (bie'kuspid) having two cusps or projections. *B. teeth* the premolars. *B. valve* the mitral valve of the heart between the left atrium and ventricle.

**bidet** ('beeday) a low narrow basin on a stand for washing the perineum and genitalia.

**bifid** ('biefid) divided or cleft into two parts.

**bifocal** (bie'fohk'l) having two foci, as with spectacles in which the lenses have two different foci.

**bifurcate** (bie'ferkayt) to divide into two branches; arteries bifurcate frequently, thereby getting smaller.

**bifurcation** (,biefə'kayshən) the junction where a vessel divides into two branches, e.g. where the aorta divides into the right and left iliac vessels.

**bigeminal** (bie'jemin'l) double. *B. pulse* two pulse beats which occur together, regular in time and force. A regular irregularity.

**biguanides** (bie'gwahniedz) oral hypoglycaemic agents for treating diabetes. They exert their effect by decreasing gluconeogenesis in muscle tissue. Only effective in those diabetics with functioning islet of Langerhans cells. Most commonly used in non-insulin-dependent diabetics, especially those who are overweight.

**bilateral** (bie'latə.ral) pertaining to both sides.

**bile** (biel) a secretion of the liver, greenish-yellow to brown in colour. It is concentrated in the gallbladder and passes into the small intestine, where it assists digestion by emulsifying fats and stimulates peristalsis. *B. ducts* the canals or passageways that conduct bile. The hepatic and cystic ducts join to form the common bile duct. *B. pigments* bilirubin and biliverdin, produced by haemolysis in the spleen. Normally these colour the faeces only, but in jaundice the skin and urine may also become coloured. *B. salts* sodium taurocholate and sodium glycocholate, which cause the emulsification of fats.

***Bilharzia*** (bil'hahtsi.ə) *T.M. Bilharz, German physician, 1825–1862*. A genus of blood fluke now known as *Schistosoma*.

**bilharziasis** (,bilhah'tsieəsis) schistosomiasis.

**biliary** ('bilyə.ree) pertaining to bile. *B. colic* spasm of muscle walls of the bile duct causing excruciating pain when gallstones are blocking the tube. Pain is in the right upper quadrant of the abdomen and referred to the shoulder. *B. fistula* an abnormal opening

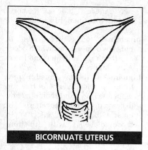

**BICORNUATE UTERUS**

between the gallbladder and the surface of the body.

**biliousness** ('biliəs,nəs) a symptom complex comprising nausea, abdominal discomfort, headache and constipation.

**bilirubin** (,bili'roobin) an orange bile pigment produced by the breakdown of haem and reduction of biliverdin; it normally circulates in plasma and is taken up by liver cells and conjugated to form bilirubin diglucuronide, the water-soluble pigment excreted in the bile. Bilirubin may be classified as indirect ('free' or unconjugated) while en route to the liver from its site of formation by reticulo-endothelial cells, and direct (diglucuronide) after its conjugation in the liver with glucuronic acid. Normally the body produces a total of about 260 mg of bilirubin per day. Almost 99% of this is excreted in the faeces; the remaining 1% is excreted in the urine as UROBILINO-GEN. The typical yellowness of jaundice is caused by the accumulation of bilirubin in the blood and body tissues.

**bilirubinaemia** (,bili,roobi'neemi.ə) the presence of bilirubin in the blood.

**biliuria** (,bili'yooə.ri.ə) bile or bile salts in the urine.

**biliverdin** (,bili'vərdin) a green bile pigment, the oxidized form of bilirubin.

**Billings method** ('bilingz ,methəd) a method of contraception, now rarely used. Ovulation time is estimated by observing changes in the cervical mucus that occur during the menstrual cycle.

**bimanual** (bie'manyooəl) using both hands. *B. examination* examination with both hands. Used chiefly in gynaecology, when the internal genital organs are examined between one hand on the abdomen, and the other hand or a finger within the vagina.

**binary** ('bienə.ree) made up of two parts. *B. fission* the multiplication of cells by division into two equal parts. *B. scale* one used in calculating, in which only two digits, 0 and 1, are used. Digital computers use this scale.

**binaural** (bie'nor.rəl) pertaining to both ears. *B. stethoscope.* See STETHOSCOPE.

**Binet's test** ('beenayz) *A. Binet, French physiologist, 1857–1911.* A method of ascertaining the mental age of children or young persons by using a series of questions standardized on the capacity of normal children at various ages.

**Bing test** (bing) *A. Bing, German otologist, 1844–1922.* A vibrating tuning fork is held to the mastoid process and the auditory meatus is alternately occluded and left open; an increase and decrease in loudness (positive Bing) is perceived by the normal ear and in sensorineural hearing impairment, but in conductive hearing impairment no difference in loudness is perceived (negative Bing).

**binocular** (bi'nokyuhlə, bie-) relating to both eyes.

**binovular** (bi'novyuhlə) derived from two ova. *B. twins* twins, who may or may not be of different sexes.

**bioassay** (ˌbieoh'asay) biological assay. The use of animals or an isolated organ preparation to determine the effect of the active power of a sample of a drug. Comparison is made with the effect of a standard preparation.

**biochemistry** (ˌbieoh'kemistree) the chemistry of living matter.

**biofeedback** (ˌbieoh'feed,bak) visual or auditory evidence provided to an individual of the satisfactory performance of an autonomic body function, e.g. sounding a tone when blood pressure is at a satisfactory level, so that, through conditioning, the patient may assert control over that function.

**biogenesis** (ˌbieoh'jenəsis) 1. the origin of life. 2. the theory that living organisms can originate only from those already living and cannot be artificially produced.

**biohazard** ('bieoh,hazad) any hazard arising from inadvertent human biological processes, e.g. accidental inoculation, needle-stick injury.

**biology** (bie'oləjee) the science of living organisms, dealing with their structure, function and relations with one another.

**biometrics, biometry** (ˌbieə'metriks bie'omətree) 1. anthropometry. 2. the use of statistics in biological science.

**biomicroscopy** (ˌbieohmie'kroskəpee) a microscopic examination of living tissues, e.g. of the structures of the anterior of the eye during life. See SLIT LAMP.

**bionursing** ('bieoh,nərsing) the utilization of knowledge from the life sciences in the theory and practice of nursing.

**biophysical profile** ('bieoh'fizik'l) a non-invasive test of fetal wellbeing using ultrasound to measure fetal heart rate, fetal tone, somatic movements, breathing movements and amniotic fluid volume. Each factor is scored to obtain a total biophysical score, which is an accurate predictor of fetal death in high-risk pregnancies. The score may be affected by gestation, maternal illness, therapeutic medication, substance abuse or fetal abnormality.

**bioplasm** ('bieoh,plazəm) protoplasm. The active principle in matter which produces living organisms.

**biopsy** ('bieopsee) the removal of some tissue or organ from the living body, e.g. a lymph gland, for examination to establish a diagnosis. *Aspiration b.* biopsy in which the tissue is obtained by suction through a needle and syringe. *Cone b.* biopsy in which an inverted cone of tissue is excised, as from the uterine cervix. *Excisional b.* removal of an entire lesion and significant portion of normal-looking tissue for examination. *Needle b.* tissue obtained by the puncture of a lesion with a needle. Rotation of the needle removes tissue within the lumen of the needle. *Punch b.* tissue obtained by a punch.

**biorhythm** ('bieoh,ridhəm) any cyclic biological event, e.g. sleep cycle and menstrual cycle, affecting daily life.

**biosensors** ('bieoh,sensəz) non-invasive instruments that measure the result of biological processes, e.g. body temperature.

**biostatistics** (ˌbieohstə'tistiks) that branch of biometry that deals with the data and laws of human mortality, morbidity, natality and demography; called also vital statistics.

**biosynthesis** (ˌbieoh'sinthəsis) the creation of a compound within a living organism.

**biotin** ('bieətin) formerly termed vitamin H, now part of the vitamin B complex and present in all normal diets.

**biparietal** (biepə'rieət'l) pertaining to both parietal eminences or bones.

**biparous** (bie'parəs) giving birth to two infants at a time.

**bipolar** (bie'pohlə) with two poles. *B. nerve cells* cells having two nerve fibres, e.g. ganglionic cells.

**birth** (bərth) the act of being born. *B. control* limiting the size of the family by abstention from sexual intercourse or the use of contraceptives. *B. mark* a naevus present from birth. *B. notification* a person present, or in attendance, at the birth or up to 6 h afterwards must notify the district medical officer within 36 h (Public Health Act 1936). This responsibility is accepted by the midwife when in attendance. *B. plan* a plan prepared by the expectant mother, usually in conjunction with her partner and midwife, which records her preferences for care during and after labour. *B. rate* the number of births during one year per 1000 total estimated mid-year population (crude birth rate), per 1000 estimated mid-year female population (refined birth rate), or per 1000 estimated mid-year female population of child-bearing age (true birth rate) – that is, between the ages of 15 and 45.

*B. registration* either parent must register the birth within 42 days at the registrar's office in the district in which the birth took place. Failure to do so incurs a fine. The responsibility rests with the midwife if the parents default. *Premature b.* one taking place before term.

**birthing chair** ('bərthing ˌchair) a specially designed chair for use in labour and delivery to promote greater mobility for the mother.

**birthing pool** ('bərthing ˌpool) a specially designed pool allowing mothers to give birth underwater.

**bisacodyl** (ˌbisə'kohdil) a laxative that acts directly on the rectum. Given as tablets or in the form of suppositories.

**bisexual** (bie'seksyooəl) 1. having gonads of both sexes. 2. hermaphrodite. 3. having both active and passive sexual interests or characteristics. 4. capable of the function of both sexes. 5. both heterosexual and homosexual. 6. an individual who is both heterosexual and homosexual. 7. of, relating to or involving both sexes, as in bisexual reproduction.

**bismuth** ('bizməth) *symbol* Bi. A greyish metallic element. Certain of its salts are used as gastric sedatives.

**bistoury** ('bistə.ree) a slender surgical knife, sometimes curved.

**bite** (biet) 1. to seize with the teeth. 2. a wound made by biting. 3. an impression made by the teeth on a thin sheet of malleable material such as wax.

**Bitot's spots** ('beetohz ˌspots) *P.A. Bitot, French physician, 1822–1888.* Collections of dried epithelium, microorganisms, etc., forming shiny, greyish spots on the cornea. A sign of vitamin A deficiency.

**bivalve** ('bie.valv) 1. having two valves, as the shells of molluscs such as oysters. 2. to cut a plaster cast into an anterior and a posterior section. *B. speculum* a vaginal speculum with two blades that can be adjusted for easy insertion.

**blackhead** ('blak.hed) a comedo.

**blackout** ('blakowt) momentary failure of vision and unconsciousness due to cerebral circulatory insufficiency.

**blackwater fever** ('blak ˌwawtə) a form of malignant malaria in which severe haemolysis causes a dark discoloration of the urine.

**bladder** ('bladə) a membranous sac for holding fluid or gas. *Atonic b.* a condition in which there is lack of tone in the bladder wall, which may be the result of incomplete emptying over a long period. *B. worm* a cysticercus. *Irritable b.* a condition in which there is frequent desire to micturate. *Urinary b.* the reservoir for urine.

**Blalock–Taussig operation** (ˌblaylok'tawsig) *A. Blalock, American surgeon, 1899–1964; H.B. Taussig, American paediatrician, 1898–1986.* Operation in which the subclavian artery is anastomosed to the pulmonary artery.

**bland** (bland) non-stimulating. *B. fluids* mild and non-irritating fluids such as barley water and milk.

**blast** (blahst) 1. an immature cell. 2. a wave of high air pressure caused by an explosion.

**blastocyst** ('blastoh,sist) blastula.

**blastoderm** ('blastoh,derm) the germinal cells of the embryo consisting of three layers: the ectoderm, mesoderm and entoderm.

**blastolysis** (bla'stolisis, blastoh'liesis) the destruction of germ substance.

**blastomycosis** (ˌblastohmie'kohsis) a fungal infection, which, after invasion of the skin, may cause granulomatous lesions in the mouth, pharynx and lungs.

**blastula** ('blastyuhlə) blastocyst. An early stage in the development of the fertilized ovum. This stage precedes the gastrula.

**bleb** (bleb) a blister.

**bleeder** ('bleedə) 1. a popular name for one who suffers from haemophilia. 2. a vessel that is difficult to seal at operation.

**bleeding** ('bleeding) 1. escape of blood from an injured vessel. 2. venesection. *B. time* the time taken for oozing to cease from a sharp prick of the finger or ear lobe. The normal value is 1–3 min. *Functional b.* bleeding from the uterus when no organic lesion is present.

**blennorrhagia** (ˌblenə'rayji.ə) 1. an excessive discharge of mucus, e.g. leukorrhoea. 2. gonorrhoea.

**blennorrhoea** (ˌblenə'reeə) blennorrhagia.

**bleomycin** (ˌblio'miesin) an antitumour antibiotic drug especially effective against squamous cell carcinoma.

**blepharitis** (ˌblefə'rietis) inflammation of the eyelids. *Allergic b.* that associated with response to drugs or cosmetics applied to the eye or eyelids. *Squamous b.* that associated with dandruff of the scalp.

**blepharon** ('blefə,ron) the eyelid.

**blepharophimosis** (ˌblefə,rohfie'mohsis) abnormal narrowing of the aperture between the eyelids. Usually congenital but may arise from chronic inflammation.

**blepharospasm** ('blefə,roh,spazəm) prolonged spasm of the orbicular muscles of the eyelids.

**blind** (bliend) without sight. *B. spot* the point where the optic nerve leaves the retina, which is insensitive to light. *Punctum caecum.*

**blind loop syndrome** (bliend 'loop) a condition of stasis in the small intestine, which aids bacterial multiplication, leading to diarrhoea and salt deficiencies. The cause may be intestinal obstruction or surgical anastomosis.

**blindness** ('bliendnəs) lack or loss of ability to see; lack of perception of visual stimuli. Legally, blindness is defined as less than 6/60 vision with glasses (vision of 6/60 is the ability to see only at 6 metres what the normal eye can see at 60 metres).

**blister** (blis'tə) a bleb or vesicle. A collection of serum between the epidermis and the skin. *Blood b.* a blister containing blood, usually caused by a pinch or bruise.

**block** (blok) a stoppage or obstruction. The term is used to describe

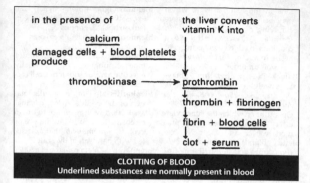

in the presence of
**calcium**
**damaged cells + blood platelets**
produce

thrombokinase ⟶ prothrombin

the liver converts
vitamin K into

thrombin + **fibrinogen**

fibrin + **blood cells**

clot + **serum**

**CLOTTING OF BLOOD**
**Underlined substances are normally present in blood**

(1) various forms of regional anaesthesia, e.g. epidural block; (2) obstruction to the passage of a nervous impulse due to disease, e.g. heart block (*see* HEART); (3) an interruption of mental function.

**blood** (blud) the fluid that circulates through the heart and blood vessels, supplying nutritive material to all parts of the body and carrying away waste products. Blood is a red viscid fluid and consists of plasma in which are suspended erythrocytes (red blood cells), leukocytes (white blood cells) and lymphocytes, and platelets or thrombocytes. (a) The red corpuscles or ERYTHROCYTES contain haemoglobin, which combines with oxygen in passing through the lungs. This oxygen is released into the tissues from the capillaries and oxidation takes place. (b) The white corpuscles or LEUKOCYTES defend against invading microorganisms, which they have power to destroy. (c) Blood platelets or thrombocytes are concerned with the clotting of blood. Plasma also contains many other specialized substances that have important roles to play in immunity and clotting of blood.

**blood bank** 1. a place of storage for blood. 2. an organization that collects, processes, stores and transfuses blood. In most hospitals the blood bank is located in the pathology laboratory.

**blood-borne viruses** (bawn) viruses that are transmitted by blood and some other body fluids (e.g. semen, amniotic fluid), such as hepatitis B virus, hepatitis C virus and human immunodeficiency viruses (HIV-1, HIV-2).

**blood–brain barrier** abbreviated BBB. The membranous barrier separating the blood from the brain. It is permeable to water, oxygen, carbon dioxide, glucose, alcohol, general anaesthetics and some drugs.

**blood casts** casts of coagulated red blood cells formed in the renal tubules and found in the urine.

**blood clotting** coagulation. The formation of a jelly-like substance over the ends or within the walls of a blood vessel, with resultant stoppage of the blood flow. Clotting is one of the natural defence mechanisms of the body when injury

| ABO SYSTEM | | |
|---|---|---|
| Group | Antigen present in red cell | Antibody present in plasma |
| AB | A and B | — |
| A | A | Anti-B (β) |
| B | B | Anti-A (α) |
| O | — | Anti-A and Anti-B (α and β) |

occurs. A clot will usually form within 5 min of a blood vessel being damaged. The exact process of clotting is not known but it is believed that the mechanism is triggered by the platelets, which disintegrate as they pass over rough places in the injured surface. If normal amounts of calcium, platelets and tissue factors are present (*see* Figure on p. 54), prothrombin will be converted to thrombin. Thrombin then acts as a catalyst for the change of fibrinogen into a mesh of insoluble fibrin, in which are embedded erythrocytes and leukocytes and small amounts of fluid (serum). Plasma coagulation factors are:

| I | Fibrinogen |
|---|---|
| II | Prothrombin |
| III | Tissue thromboplastin |
| IV | Calcium ions |
| VII | Factor VII |
| VIII | Antihaemophilic factor (AHF) |
| IX | Christmas factor |
| X | Stuart factor (Power factor) |
| XI | Plasma thromboplastin antecedent (PTA) |
| XII | Hageman factor |
| XIII | Fibrin stabilizing factor |

**blood count** (ˌkownt) the number of blood cells in a given sample of blood, usually expressed as the number of cells per litre of blood (as the red blood cell, white blood cell or platelet count). A differential white cell count determines the number of various types of leuko-

cyte in a sample of blood. For the range of normal values, *see* Appendices.

**blood dyscrasia** any abnormality of the blood cells or of the clotting elements.

**blood group** (ˌgroop) ABO system (*see* Table). In clinical practice there are four main blood types: A, B, O and AB. In addition to this major grouping there is a rhesus (Rh) system that is important in the prevention of haemolytic disease of the newborn resulting from incompatibility of blood groups in mother and fetus. In determining blood group, a sample of blood is taken and mixed with specially prepared sera. One serum, anti-A agglutinin, causes blood of group A to agglutinate; another serum, anti-B agglutinin, causes blood of group B to agglutinate. Thus, if anti-A serum alone causes clumping, the blood is group A; if anti-B serum alone causes clumping, the blood group is B. If both cause clumping, the blood group is AB, and if it is not clumped by either, it is identified as group O. Transfusion with an incompatible ABO group will cause severe haemolytic reaction and death may occur.

**blood pressure** abbreviated BP. The pressure exerted on the artery walls by the blood as it flows through them. It can be measured in milligrams of mercury using a sphygmomanometer. Two readings are made. Arterial pressure fluctuates with each heart beat and one measure records the pressure while the heart is in systole (when the heart is ejecting blood into the arteries) and is the higher, or systolic, pressure. The other records while the heart is in diastole (when the aortic and pulmonary valves are closed and the heart is relaxed) and is the lower, or diastolic, pressure. The range of normal blood pressure recording varies according to age and body size, but in the normal young adult is approximately 100–120/70–80 mmHg.

**blood sugar** the amount of glucose present in the blood. The normal range is 2.5–4.7 mmol/litre. When the amount exceeds 10 mmol/litre, glucose is excreted in the urine, as in diabetes mellitus.

**blood transfusion** introduction of blood from the vein of one person (donor) or from a blood bank into the vein of another (recipient) in cases of severe loss of blood, trauma, septicaemia, etc. It is used to supplement the volume of blood and also to introduce constituents, such as clotting factors or antibodies, that are deficient in the patient. Clotting must be prevented in the transition stage. This is usually done by admixture with sodium citrate (1 g to 459 ml of blood). Too much sodium citrate tends to produce a reaction: rigor and shock may occur.

**blood urea** excretory product of protein present in the blood. The normal range is 3–7 mmol/litre; this increases in renal failure when the kidneys cease to function normally.

**'blue baby'** (bloo) *see* BABY and FALLOT'S TETRALOGY.

**blush** (blush) growing redness of the face, usually a reaction to emotion or heat.

**BMR** basal metabolic rate.

**Bobath technique** ('bohbahht tek‚neek, -bath) an approach to the treatment of neurological conditions developed by Dr and Mrs Bobath. It aims to facilitate movement by inhibiting abnormal tone, abnormal patterns of movement and abnormal balance reactions.

**body** ('bodee) 1. the trunk, or animal frame, with its organs. 2. the largest and most important part of any organ. 3. any mass or collection of material.

**body image** the total concept of the body, including conscious and unconscious feelings, thoughts and perceptions that a person has of it as an object in space, which is dependent and apart from other objects.

**body language** (‚langwij) the expression of thoughts or emotions by means of posture or gestures. Body language may include unintended 'signs' as well as intended communication. Detailed studies of human non-verbal communication have been documented by several observers.

**body mass index** ('mas ‚indeks) abbreviated BMI. The weight (kg) divided by the square of the height (m).

**Body substance isolation** (‚substəns) abbreviated BSI. An INFECTION CONTROL system, developed in 1987, that further elaborated UNIVERSAL PRECAUTIONS and focused on the isolation of all moist and potentially infectious body substances (blood, faeces, urine, sputum, saliva, wound drainage and other body fluids) from all patients, regardless of their presumed infection status, primarily through the use of gloves. This concept has now been further developed and is known by the term STANDARD PRECAUTIONS. *See also* Appendices.

**boil** (boyl) an acute staphylococcal inflammation of the skin and subcutaneous tissues round a hair follicle. It causes a painful swelling with a central core of dead tissue (SLOUGH), which is eventually discharged. A furuncle.

**bolus** ('bohləs) 1. a large pill. 2. a rounded mass of masticated food immediately before being swallowed or one passing through the intestines. 3. a quantity of a drug injected directly to raise its concentration in the blood to a therapeutic level.

**bonding** ('bonding) the attachment process that occurs between an infant and its parents, especially the mother, during the first hours and days following birth. Bonding is a reciprocal process and is a biological need for the future development, both physical and emotional, of the infant.

**bone** (bohn) the dense connective tissue forming the skeleton. It is composed of cartilage or membrane impregnated with mineral salts, chiefly calcium phosphate and calcium carbonate. This is arranged as an outer hard compact tissue and an inner network of cells (CANCELLOUS tissue), in the spaces of which is red bone marrow. In the shaft of long bones is a medullary cavity containing yellow marrow. Microscopically, the bone tissue is perforated with minute HAVERSIAN CANALS containing blood vessels and lymphatics for the maintenance and repair of the cells (*see* Figure). Bone is covered by a fibrous membrane, the PERIOSTEUM, containing blood vessels and by which the bone grows in girth. *D. graft* transplantation of a healthy piece of bone to replace missing or repair defective bone. *B. marrow* substance which fills the marrow cavities of bones. Basically there are two types: yellow and red marrow. The red marrow is responsible for producing the blood cells. The yellow is mostly fatty connective tissue. *B. marrow transplantation* a procedure used

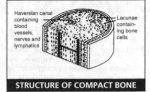

Haversian canal containing blood vessels, nerves and lymphatics — Lacunae containing bone cells

**STRUCTURE OF COMPACT BONE**

to treat aplastic anaemia, acute leukaemia and some rare congenital disorders, with varying success. Healthy bone marrow is taken from the donor and infused into the bloodstream of the recipient; from here it 'homes' in on the bone marrow, where it will grow. Histocompatibility between the donor (usually a sibling) and recipient is essential.

**borborygmus** (ˌbawbə'rigməs) a rumbling sound caused by gas in the intestines.

***Bordetella*** (ˌbawdə'telə) a genus of bacteria. *B. pertussis* the causal agent of whooping cough.

**boric acid** ('bor.rik) a mild antiseptic.

**Bornholm disease** ('bawn,holm) an epidemic myalgia with pleural pain due to Coxsackie virus infection. It is named after the Danish island of Bornholm where there was an outbreak in 1930.

**botulism** ('botyuh,lizəm, 'bochə-) an extremely severe form of food poisoning due to a neurotoxin (botulin) produced by *Clostridium botulinum*, sometimes found in improperly canned or preserved foods. The symptoms include vomiting, abdominal pain, headache, weakness, constipation and nerve paralysis, which causes difficulty in seeing, breathing and swallowing. Death is usually due to paralysis of the respiratory organs.

**bougie** ('boozhee, boo'zhee) a flexible cylindrical instrument used to

dilate a stricture, as in the oesophagus or urethra. *Medicated b.* a
soluble form impregnated with a
medicinal substance. Used for urethral treatment.

**bovine** ('bohvien) relating to the
cow or ox. *B. tuberculosis* that
caused by infection from infected
cows' milk, usually affecting glands
and bones.

**bowel** ('bowəl) the intestine. *B.
sounds* relatively high-pitched
abdominal sounds caused by
the propulsion of the intestinal contents through the lower alimentary
canal.

**bowleg** ('boh,leg) deformity where
there is an outward curvature of
one or both legs near the knee. This
results in a gap between the knees
on standing. Genu varum.

**Bowman's capsule** ('bohmənz) *Sir
W.P. Bowman, British physician,
1816–1892.* The expanded end of
the kidney tubule, which surrounds the glomerulus.

**brace** (brays) 1. a support used in
orthopaedics to hold parts of the
body in their correct positions. 2. an
orthodontic appliance to correct the
alignment of teeth.

**brachial** ('brayki.əl, 'brak-) relating
to the arm. *B. artery* the continuation of the axillary artery along the
inner side of the upper arm. *B.
plexus* a network of nerves at the
root of the neck supplying the
upper limb.

**brachytherapy** (,braki'therəpee)
radiotherapy delivered into or adjacent to a tumour by means of an
intracavitary or interstitial radioactive source.

**bradycardia** (,bradi'kahdi.ə) abnormally low rate of heart contractions
and consequent slow pulse.

**bradykinin** (,bradi'kienin) peptide
formed from the degradation of
protein by enzymes. It is a powerful
vasodilator that also causes contraction of smooth muscle.

**braille** (brayl) a method of printing
developed by *Louis Braille
(1809–1852)* for the blind. Letters of
the alphabet are represented by
patterns of raised dots. These
dots are read by passing the finger-
tips over them.

**brain** (brayn) that part of the central
nervous system contained in the
skull. It consists of the cerebrum,
midbrain, cerebellum, medulla
oblongata and pons varolii.

**bran** (bran) the husk of grain, i.e.
the coarse outer coat of cereals.
High in roughage and vitamins of
the B complex, bran is frequently
recommended as a dietary component both for those with alimentary
disorders and for those in normal
health.

**branchial** ('brangki.əl) relating to
the clefts (branchia) that are present
in the neck and pharynx in the
developing embryo. Normally they
disappear. *B. cyst* a cystic swelling
arising from a branchial remnant in
the neck. *B. sinus* (*lateral cervical
sinus*) a tract leading from the posterior cervical region which opens
in the lower neck in front of the
sternomastoid muscle.

**Braun's frame** ('brawnz ,fraym) *H.F.
W. Braun, German surgeon,
1862–1934.* A metal frame which
incorporates one or more pulleys
and is used to elevate the lower
limb and to apply skeletal traction
for a compound fracture of tibia
and fibula.

**Braxton Hicks contractions**
(,brakstən 'hiks) *J. Braxton Hicks,
British gynaecologist, 1823–1897.*
Painless uterine contractions occurring during pregnancy, becoming
increasingly rhythmic and intense
during the third trimester. Sometimes called 'false labour'.

**breast** (brest) 1. the anterior or front
region of the chest. 2. the mammary
gland. *B. access* formation of pus in
the mammary gland. *B. bone* the

sternum. *B. cancer* the breast is the most common site of malignant tumours in women. In the United Kingdom 13 000 women a year die of this condition and although the survival rates for breast cancer continue to increase, albeit slowly, the incidence of the disease in the Western world is also increasing. Improvement in these survival rates has come from increased public awareness, breast self-examination, breast screening programmes and improved methods of treatment. Women should train themselves to perform a simple self-examination of the breasts, described in the Figure on p. 61. The best time for this is just after menstruation when the breasts are normally soft. If any lump in the breast can be felt, a doctor should be consulted immediately. More than 90% of breast cancers are discovered by the patients themselves. *B. feeding* the method of feeding a baby with milk directly from the mother's breasts. Midwives and paediatricians agree that breast feeding is usually better for the baby and the mother, both physically and emotionally *See* Table on p. 60. *B. pump* an apparatus for removal of milk from the breast. *Pigeon b.* prominent sternum, a deformity resulting from rickets.

**breath** (breth) the air taken in and expelled by the expansion and contraction of the thorax. *B. holding* when a young child cries, holds its breath and goes blue. *B. sounds* the sounds heard when a stethoscope is placed over the lungs during respiration.

**breathing** ('breedhing) the alternate inspiration and expiration of air into and out of the lungs (*see also* RESPIRATION).

**breech** (breech) the buttocks. *B. presentation* a position of the fetus in the uterus such that the buttocks present.

**bregma** ('bregmə) the anterior fontanelle. The membranous junction between the coronal and sagittal sutures.

**bridge** (brij) in dentistry, an irremovable prosthesis carrying false teeth that bridges gaps left when natural teeth are extracted.

**British National Formulary** (ˌbritish ˌnashn'l) abbreviated BNF. A publication produced twice a year by the British Medical Association and the Pharmaceutical Society of Great Britain, containing details of nearly all the drugs currently available on prescription in the United Kingdom. The Nurse Prescribers' formulary is published as an addendum to the BNF. *See also* Appendices.

**British Pharmacopoeia** abbreviated BP. The official publication containing the list of drugs and other medicinal substances in use in the United Kingdom. The book gives details of how these substances are obtained or prepared, and their dosages and methods of administration. It is compiled under the auspices of the General Medical Council and is regularly revised and brought up to date.

**broad ligaments** ('brawd) folds of peritoneum extending from the uterus to the sides of the pelvis, and supporting the blood vessels to the uterus and uterine tubes.

**Broca's area of speech** ('brohkəz ˌair.riə) *P.P. Broca, French surgeon, 1824–1880.* The motor centre for speech, situated in the left cerebral hemisphere. Damage to the nerve cells contained in it can impair speech.

**Brodie's abscess** (ˌbrohdiz) *Sir B.C. Brodie, British surgeon, 1783–1862.* A chronic abscess of bone.

**bromhidrosis** (ˌbromhi'drohsis) offensive and fetid sweat.

**bromide** ('brohmied) a compound of bromide. Bromides are sedatives

---

### TEN STEPS TO SUCCESSFUL BREAST FEEDING

- Breast feeding policy available which is communicated to all staff.
- All health-care staff trained to implement the policy.
- All pregnant mothers informed of the benefits and management of breast feeding.
- Mothers assisted to commence breast feeding within half an hour of delivery.
- Education of mothers re breast feeding and maintenance of lactation even if they are separated from their babies.
- Neonates to be given nothing other than breast milk unless medically necessary.
- 24-hour rooming-in.
- On-demand breast feeding.
- No teats or pacifiers to be given to breast feeding babies.
- Establishment of breast feeding support groups.

Source: UNICEF UK Baby Friendly Initiative.

---

that are strongly depressant and cumulative in action.

**bromocriptine** (ˌbrohmoh'kripteen) a dopamine agonist used in the treatment of Parkinsonism in cases where levodopa is not well tolerated.

**Brompton cocktail** (ˌbromptən 'koktayl) name given to mixtures containing various combinations of morphine, diamorphine and cocaine. These mixtures often contained gin and/or chlorpromazine. They were used in the relief of pain in terminal care. They have now been replaced by a simple solution of morphine in chloroform water.

**bromsulphthalein** (ˌbromsulf'thayleen) a dye used in certain tests for liver function.

**bronchi** ('brongkee) plural of bronchus.

**bronchiectasis** (ˌbrongki'ektəsis) chronic dilatation of the bronchi and bronchioles with secondary infection, usually involving the lower lobes of the lung. The condition may occur as a congenital malformation of the alveoli with resultant dilatation of the terminal bronchi. Most often it is an acquired disease secondary to partial obstruction of the bronchi with necrotizing infection. The symptoms include a chronic cough and purulent sputum.

**bronchiole** ('brongkiˌohl) one of the smallest of the subdivisions of the bronchi.

**bronchiolitis** (ˌbrongkioh'lietis) inflammation of the bronchioles.

**bronchitis** (brong'kietis) inflammation of the bronchi. *Acute b.* a short-lived infection, common in young children and the elderly. It is a descending infection from the common cold, influenza, measles and other upper respiratory conditions. *Chronic b.* a chronic infection, usually associated with infection of the upper respiratory tract. It may in time lead to emphysema.

**bronchoadenitis** (ˌbrongkohˌadə'nietis) inflammation of the bronchial glands.

**bronchodilator** (ˌbrongkohdie'laytə) any agent that causes dilatation of the bronchi.

**bronchography** (brong'kografee) radiography of the bronchial tree after introduction of a radio-opaque medium.

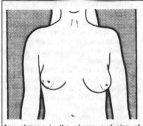

Any change in the shape and size of either breast or nipple should first be noted by looking in the mirror

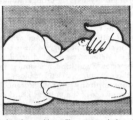

Lying down with a pillow or towel placed under the shoulder helps to spread the breast tissue for easier self-examination

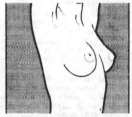

In front of the mirror, and with arms raised, view the breasts from different angles

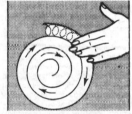

Rotate fingers in small circles and trace a spiral route around the breast to check for any lumps or unusual thickening

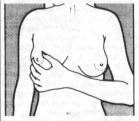

Squeeze each nipple gently, noting any discharge or bleeding

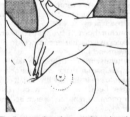

Finally, examine the armpits using the spiral technique and note any unusual findings

**BREAST SELF-EXAMINATION**

**bronchomycosis** (ˌbrongkohmie-'kohsis) an industrial disease chiefly affecting agricultural and stable workers, etc., and due to inhalation of microfungi which infect the air passages. Causes can be *Actinomyces* or *Aspergillus* species. Symptoms are similar to those of pulmonary tuberculosis.

**bronchophony** (brong'kofənee) resonance of the voice as heard in the chest over the bronchi on auscultation.

**bronchopneumonia** (ˌbrongkoh-nyoo'mohni.ə) a descending infection starting around the bronchi and bronchioles; *see also* PNEUMONIA.

**bronchopulmonary** (ˌbrongkoh'pulmə,nə.ree, -'puhl-) relating to the lungs, bronchi and bronchioles. *B. dysplasia* abbreviated BPD. A chronic respiratory condition occurring in babies who have been ventilated for long periods or have needed prolonged oxygen therapy. It results in serious disruption of lung growth. Examination of radiographs and lung specimens reveals patches of collapse and fibrosis. Following ventilation, these babies usually require supplementary oxygen for several weeks or even months to keep the arterial oxygen tension above 55 kPa.

**bronchorrhoea** (ˌbrongkə'reeə) an excessive discharge of mucus from the bronchi.

**bronchoscope** ('brongkohˌskohp) an endoscope that enables the operator to see inside the bronchi. It can also be used to wash out the bronchi, to remove foreign bodies or to take a biopsy.

**bronchoscopy** (brong'koskə,pee) examination of the bronchi by means of a bronchoscope.

**bronchospasm** (ˌbrongkoh'spazəm) difficulty in breathing caused by the sudden constriction of plain muscle in the walls of the bronchi. This may arise in asthma or chronic bronchitis.

**bronchospirometer** (ˌbrongkohspie-'romitə) an instrument used to measure the capacity of one lung or of one lobe of the lung, or of each lung separately.

**bronchotracheal** (ˌbrongkoh'traki.əl, -trə'keeəl) relating to both the trachea and the bronchi. *B. suction* the removal of mucus with the aid of suction.

**bronchus** (ˌbrongkəs) any of the larger passages conveying air to (right or left principal bronchus) and within (lobar and segmental bronchi) the lungs.

**Broviac catheter** ('brohviak) trade name for a special catheter used to provide a central venous line.

**brow** (brow) the forehead. *B. presentation* a position of the fetus such that the forehead appears at the cervix first.

**brown fat** (brown) special type of adipose tissue found in the newborn infant, and which is widely distributed throughout the body. The tissue is highly vascular and owes its colour to the large number of mitochondria found in the cytoplasm of its cells. It allows the infant to increase its metabolic rate and thus its heat production when subjected to cold. At the same time the fat itself is used up.

**Brown-Séquard's syndrome** (brown-'saykahdz) *C.E. Brown-Séquard, French physiologist, 1818–1894.* Paralysis and loss of discriminatory and joint sensation on one side of the body and of pain and temperature sensation on the other, due to a lesion involving one side of the spinal cord.

*Brucella* (broo'selə) a genus of bacteria primarily pathogenic in animals but which may affect humans.

**brucellosis** (ˌbroosi'lohsis) a generalized infection involving primarily the reticuloendothelial system, marked by remittent undulant fever (*see* below), malaise, headache and anaemia. It is caused by various species of *Brucella* and is transmitted to humans from domestic animals such as pigs, goats and cattle, especially through infected milk or contact with the carcass of an infected animal. The disease is also called undulant fever because one of the major symptoms in humans is a fever that fluctuates widely at regular intervals. Prevention is best accomplished by the pasteurization of milk and a programme of testing, vaccination and elimination of infected animals. Also called Malta fever, abortus fever and Mediterranean fever.

**Brudzinski's sign** (broo'jinskiz) *J. Brudzinski, Polish physician, 1874–1917.* 1. passive flexion of one thigh causing spontaneous flexion of the opposite thigh. 2. flexion of the neck causing bilateral flexion of the hips and knees. These signs are indicative of meningeal irritation.

**bruise** (brooz) a superficial injury to tissues produced by sudden impact in which the skin is unbroken. A contusion.

**bruit** ('brooee) [Fr.] an abnormal sound or murmur heard on auscultation of the heart and large vessels.

**bruxism** ('brooksizəm) teeth clenching, particularly during sleep. This occurs in persons under tension and may cause headaches as a result of muscle fatigue.

**bubo** ('byooboh) inflammation of the lymphatic glands of the axilla or groin. Typical of bubonic plague (see PLAGUE) and venereal infections.

**buccal** ('buk'l) pertaining to the cheek or to the mouth.

**Budd–Chiari syndrome** (,budki'ahri) *G. Budd, British physician, 1808–1882; H. Chiari, Austrian pathologist, 1851–1916.* A condition in which thrombosis of the hepatic vein causes vomiting, jaundice, enlargement of the liver and ascites.

**Buerger's disease** ('bərgəz) *L. Buerger, American physician, 1879–1943.* Thromboangiitis obliterans.

**buffer** ('bufə) 1. a physical or physiological system that tends to oppose change within that system, e.g. the reflexes involved in blood pressure homeostasis. 2. a chemical system that acts to prevent change in the concentration of another chemical substance. Sodium bicarbonate is the chief buffer of the blood and tissue fluids. 3. anything that is used to reduce shock or jarring upon contact.

**buggery** ('bugə.ree) anal intercourse, either heterosexual or homosexual. In law the term also includes sexual contact with an animal. Also known as sodomy.

**bulbar** ('bulbə) pertaining to the medulla oblongata. *B. paralysis see* PARALYSIS.

**bulbourethral** (,bulboh.yuh'reethrəl) relating to the bulb of the urethra (bulb of the penis). *B. glands* small glands opening into the male urethra. Cowper's glands.

**bulimia** (byoo'limi.ə) abnormal increase in the sensation of hunger. *B. nervosa* a pattern of 'binge eating', or episodes of uncontrolled and compulsive overeating occurring in response to stress. Bulimic 'binges' often occur in anorexia nervosa.

**bulla** ('buhlə) a large, fluid-containing blister.

**bumetanide** (byoo'metə,nied) a quick-acting diuretic drug which prevents the resorption of urine from Henle's loop in the renal tubule.

**bundle** ('bund'l) a collection of nerve fibres all running in the same direction. *B. branch block* the delay in conduction along either branch of the atrioventricular bundle of the heart. The abnormality is detected by an ECG recording.

**bundle of His** ('his) *L. His Jr, German physiologist, 1863–1934.* The band of neuromuscular fibres which, passing through the spectrum of the heart, divides at the apex into two parts, these being distributed into the walls of the ventricles. The impulse of contraction is conducted through the structure. Atrioventricular bundle.

**bunion** ('bunyən) a prominence of the head of the metatarsal bone at its junction with the great toe, caused by inflammation and swelling of the bursa at that joint. Usually due to shoes that distort the natural shape of the foot.

**buphthalmos** (buf'thalməs) abnormal enlargement of the eyes in congenital GLAUCOMA.

**Burkitt's tumour** ('bərkits) *D.P. Burkitt, Irish surgeon, b. 1911.* African lymphoma. A lymphosarcoma, frequently of the jaw, occurring almost exclusively in children living in low-lying moist areas. Occurs in New Guinea and Central Africa. The Epstein–Barr virus (EB virus), a herpes virus, has been isolated from Burkitt's lymphoma cells in culture, and has been implicated as a causative agent.

**burn** (bərn) an injury to tissues caused by: (a) physical agents, the sun, excess heat or cold, friction, nuclear radiation; (b) chemical agents, acids or caustic alkalis; (c) electrical current. Burns are described as being partial thickness (involving only the epidermis) or full thickness (involving the dermis and underlying structures). Clinically, emphasis is placed on the percentage of the body affected by the burn. The treatment of shock and prevention of infection and malnutrition need special attention.

**burnout** ('bərnowt) a term used to describe the result of chronic stress amongst workers and commonly in members of the helping professions. Burnout is characterized by chronic low energy, defensiveness and emergence of manoeuvres designed to create distance between helper and patient/client. Dissatisfaction and tension may be carried over from the work situation into the personal one and self-esteem and confidence may suffer badly.

**burr** (bər) a bit for a surgical drill, used for cutting bone or teeth. *B. hole* a circular hole drilled in the cranium to permit access to the brain or to release raised intracranial pressure.

**bursa** ('bərsə) a small sac of fibrous tissue, lined with synovial membrane and containing synovial fluid. It is situated between parts that move upon one another at a joint to reduce friction.

**bursitis** (bər'sietis) inflammation of the bursa. It produces pain and may impede movement of the joint. *Pre-patellar b.* housemaid's knee.

**Buscopan** ('buskə,pan) trade name for a preparation of hyoscine butylbromide. An antispasmodic that relaxes smooth muscle in the gastrointestinal tract.

**busulphan** (byoo'sulfan) a cytotoxic drug that depresses the bone marrow and may be used to treat myeloid leukaemia.

**butobarbitone** (,byootoh'bahbi,tohn) an intermediate-acting barbiturate, formerly much used as a sedative. Now used only in severe insomnia.

**buttock** ('butək) either of the two prominences formed by the flesh-covered gluteal muscles at either side of the lower spine.

**butyrophenone** (,byootiroh'feenohn) a chemical class of major tranquillizers, especially useful in the treatment of manic and moderate to severe agitated states and in the control of the vocal utterances and tics of GILLES DE LA TOURETTE'S SYNDROME.

**bypass** ('bie,pahs) diversion of flow. Formation of a shunt. *Aortocoronary b.* diversion of flow from the aorta to the coronary arteries via a saphenous vein or artificial graft. *Femoropopliteal b.* diversion of flow from the femoral to the popliteal artery to overcome an occlusion.

**byssinosis** (,bisi'nohsis) an industrial disease caused by inhalation of cotton or linen dust in factories. A type of pneumoconiosis.

# C

**C** symbol for *carbon; centigrade* or *celsius; cytosine*.

**Ca** symbol for *calcium*.

**cachexia** (kə'keksi.ə) a condition of extreme debility. The patient is emaciated, the skin being loose and wrinkled from rapid wasting, but shiny and tense over bone. The eyes are sunken, the skin yellowish, and there is a grey 'muddy' complexion. The mucous membranes are pale and anaemia is extreme. The condition is typical of the late stages of chronic diseases.

**cadaver** (kə'davə, -'day-) a corpse. The dead body used for dissection.

**caecostomy** (see'kostəmee) the making of a surgical fistula into the caecum by incision through the abdominal wall.

**caecum** ('seekəm) the blind pouch forming the beginning of the large intestine. The vermiform appendix is attached to it.

**caesarean section** (si,zairi.ən 'sekshən) delivery of a fetus by an incision through the abdominal wall and uterus. Performed for the safety of either the mother or the infant. Tradition has it that Julius Caesar was born in this way.

**caesium** ('seezi.əm) *symbol* Cs. A metallic element. *C.-137* radioactive caesium; a fission product from uranium. Sealed in a suitable container it can be used instead of cobalt for beam therapy; sealed in needles, tubes or applicators it can be used for local application.

**café-au-lait spot** (,kafay oh 'lay ,spot) pigmented macules of a distinctive light-brown colour, like coffee with milk, as in neurofibromatosis and Albright's syndrome.

**caffeine** ('kafeen, 'kafi,een) an alkaloid of tea and coffee which acts as a nerve stimulant and diuretic. Mixed with aspirin and codeine it is often used as an analgesic.

**caffeinism** (ka'fee.inizəm) an agitated state due to the excessive ingestion of caffeine.

**caisson disease** ('kays'n) decompression sickness.

**calamine** ('kalə,mien) preparation of zinc carbonate or zinc oxide coloured pink with ferric oxide. It is an astringent and antipruritic used in lotion or ointment form for skin diseases.

**calcaneum** (kal'kayni.əm) the heel bone. Calcaneus.

**calcareous** (kal'kair.ri.əs) chalky. Containing lime.

**calciferol** (kal'sifə.rol) the chemical name for vitamin D.

**calcification** (,kalsifi'kayshən) 1. the deposit of lime in any tissue, e.g. in the formation of callus. 2. the deposit of lime salts in cartilage as part of the normal process of bone formation. *Dystrophic c.* the deposition of calcium in abnormal tissue, such as scar tissue or atheroscler-

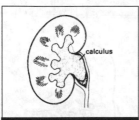

**STAGHORN OR MANY-BRANCHED CALCULUS IN THE RENAL PELVIS**

otic plaques, without abnormalities of blood calcium.

**calcitonin** (ˌkalsiˈtohnin) a polypeptide hormone, produced by the parafollicular or C cells of the thyroid gland, which regulates blood calcium levels.

**calcium** (ˈkalsi.əm) *symbol* Ca. A metallic element necessary for the normal development and functioning of the body. Calcium is the most abundant mineral in the body; it is a constituent of bones and teeth. Deficiency or excess of serum calcium causes nerve and muscle dysfunctions and abnormalities in blood clotting. The correct concentration is regulated by hormones. *C. carbonate* chalk. *C. gluconate* used as an antacid. A compound that is easily absorbed and can be given by intramuscular or intravenous route to raise the blood calcium. *C. lactate* a compound that increases the coagulability of blood; used orally as a calcium supplement.

**calculus** (ˈkalkyuhləs) 1. a stony concretion which may be formed in any of the secreting organs of the body or their ducts (*see* Figure). 2. a calcified deposit that forms on the surface of the teeth leading to tooth decay and gum disease.

**calibrator** (ˈkalibraytə) 1. an instrument for measuring the size of openings. 2. an instrument used

to dilate a tube, e.g. in urethral stricture.

**caliper** (ˈkalipə) a two-pronged instrument that may be used to exert traction on a part. *Walking c.* an appliance fitted to a boot or shoe to give support to the lower limb. It may be used when the muscles are paralysed or in the repair stage of fractures.

**calipers** (ˈkalipəz) compasses for measuring diameters and curved surface. *Skinfold c.* an instrument used in nutritional assessment for determining the amount of body fat. A fold of skin and subcutaneous tissue, usually over the triceps muscle, is pinched away from the underlying muscle using the thumb and forefinger (*see* Figure on p. 68).

**callisthenics** (ˌkalisˈtheniks) mild gymnastics for developing the muscles and producing a graceful carriage.

**callosity** (kəˈlositee) the plaques of thickened skin often seen on the soles of the feet or the palms of the hand, areas subject to friction.

**callous** (ˈkaləs) hard and thickened.

**callus** (ˈkaləs) 1. a callosity. 2. the tissue that grows round fractured ends of bone and develops into new bone to repair the injury.

**Calmette–Guérin bacillus** (ˌkalmet geˌranh) *A.L.C. Calmette, French bacteriologist, 1863–1933; C. Guérin, French bacteriologist, 1872–1961.* A deactivated tuberculosis bacillus from which the antituberculosis vaccine, BCG vaccine, is made.

**calor** (ˈkalə) [L.] *heat*; one of the signs of inflammation.

**caloric** (kaˈlor.rik, ˈkalə.rik) pertaining to heat or calories.

**calorie** (ˈkalə.ree) *symbol* cal. A unit of heat. Used to denote physiological values of various food substances, estimated according to the amount of heat they produce on being oxidized in the body. *See*

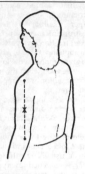

Triceps skinfold is measured at midpoint between acromion and olecranon

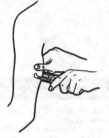

Skin is pinched and calipers are placed over skinfold

**SKINFOLD CALIPERS**

OXIDIZATION. A calorie (or kilocalorie) represents the heat required to raise 1 kg (1000 g) of water by 1°C. A small calorie equals the heat produced in raising 1 g of water by 1°C. In the SI system the calorie is replaced by the joule (1 cal = 4.18 kJ).

**calorific** (ˌkaləˈrifik) heat-producing.

**calorimeter** (ˌkaləˈrimitə) an apparatus for measuring the heat that is produced or lost during a chemical or physical change.

**calx** (kalks) calcium oxide or lime. The basis of slaked lime, bleaching powder and quicklime.

**calyx** ('kayliks, 'kal-) any cup-shaped vessel or part. *C. of kidney* the cup-like terminations of the ureter in the renal pelvis surrounding the pyramids of the kidney.

**camphor** ('kamfə) a crystalline substance prepared from the camphor laurel. It is used internally as a carminative.

**Camphorated oil** (ˌkamfəraytəd oyl) 1 part camphor to 4 parts of oil, prepared for external application as a rubefacient.

*Campylobacter* ('kampilohˌbaktə) a genus of bacteria, family Spirillaceae, made up of Gram-negative, non-spore-forming, motile, spirally curved rods. Causes an acute intestinal illness lasting several days. Usually associated with unpasteurized milk, partially cooked meat and poultry.

**canal** (kəˈnal) a tubular passage. *Alimentary c.* the passage along which the food passes on its way through the body. *C. of Schlemm* that which drains the aqueous humour. *Cervical c.* that through the cervix of the uterus. *Semicircular c.* one of the three canals in the middle ear responsible for maintenance of balance.

**canaliculus** (ˌkanəˈlikyuhləs) a small channel or canal.

**cancellous** ('kansələs) being porous or spongy. Applied to the honeycomb type of bone tissue in the ends of long bones in flat and irregular bones.

**cancer** ('kansə) a general term to describe malignant growths in tissue, of which CARCINOMA is of epithelial and SARCOMA of connective tissue origin, as in bone and muscle. The basic aetiology of cancer remains unknown but many potential causes are now recognized, e.g. cigarette smoking, ionizing radiation, exposure to certain chemicals and overexposure to the sun. Hereditary factors also play an important part in its development. A cancerous growth is one that is not encapsulated, but infiltrates surrounding tissues, the cells of which it replaces by its own. It is spread by the lymph and blood vessels and causes metastases in other parts of the body. Death is caused by destruction of organs to a degree incompatible with life, by extreme debility and anaemia, or by haemorrhage. For early warning signs of cancer, *see* Table. *C. phobia* an irrational fear of cancer.

**cancroid** ('kangkroid) 1. resembling cancer. 2. a skin tumour of moderate degree of malignancy.

**cancrum oris** (ˌkangkrəm 'or.ris) gangrenous stomatitis. An ulceration of the mouth which is a rare complication of measles in debilitated children. Noma.

*Candida* ('kandidə) a genus of small fungi, formerly called *Monilia*. *C. albicans* the variety that causes candidiasis.

**candidiasis** (ˌkandi'dieəsis) infection by the *Candida* fungus. Occurs particularly in moist areas, such as mouth, vagina and skin folds. Popularly known as thrush. Candidiasis can occur as a result of a debilitating illness or immunosuppressive therapy and/or cytotoxic drugs. The infection may also occur as a result of disturbed intestinal flora, and in pregnancy. Oral infection may be due to poor hygiene, carious teeth or badly fitting dentures.

**canine** ('kaynien) 1. pertaining to a dog. 2. an 'eye tooth'. There are two in each jaw between the incisors and the molars.

**cannabis** ('kanəbis) an illegal drug which may be swallowed or smoked. It produces hallucinations

---

### EARLY WARNING SIGNS OF CANCER

- Any lump or thickening, especially in the breast, lip or tongue.
- Any irregular or unexplained bleeding. Blood in the urine or bowel movements. Blood or bloody discharge from the nipple or any body opening. Unexplained vaginal bleeding or discharge, or any bleeding, after the menopause
- A sore that does not heal, particularly around the mouth, tongue or lips, or anywhere on the skin.
- Noticeable changes in the colour or size of a wart, mole or birthmark.
- Loss of appetite or continual indigestion.
- Persistent hoarseness, cough or difficulty in swallowing.
- Persistent change in normal elimination (bowel habits).

*Special note*: Pain is not usually an early warning sign of cancer.

and a temporary sense of well-being, followed by extreme lethargy. Alternative terms for cannabis include marijuana, hashish, blow, draw, hash, grass, pot, the weed, ganja, kaya, kif and bhang.

**cannula** ('kanyuhlə) a hollow tube for insertion into the body by which fluids are introduced or removed. Usually a trocar is fitted into it to facilitate its introduction.

**canthus** ('kanthəs) the angle formed by the junction of the upper and lower eyelids.

**CAPD** continuous ambulatory peritoneal dialysis.

**capeline bandage** ('kayplien) a cap-like covering of two interwoven bandages used for protecting the head or a limb stump.

**capillarity** (,kapi'laritee) the action by which a liquid will rise upwards in a fibrous substance or in a fine tube. Capillary attraction.

**capillary** (kə'pilə.ree) 1. hair-like. 2. a minute vessel connecting an arteriole and a venule. 3. a minute vessel of the lymphatic system.

**capreomycin** (,kaprioh'miesin) a polypeptide antibiotic produced by *Streptomyces capreolus*, which is active against human strains of *Mycobacterium tuberculosis* and has four microbiologically active components.

**capsular** ('kapsyuhlə) relating to a capsule. *C. ligaments* those that completely surround a movable joint, forming a capsule which loosely encloses the bones and is lined with synovial membrane which secretes a fluid for lubrication of the articular surfaces. Also called articular capsule.

**capsule** ('kapsyool) 1. a fibrous or membranous sac enclosing an organ. 2. a small soluble case of gelatin in which a nauseous medicine may be enclosed. 3. the gelatinous envelope which surrounds and protects some bacteria.

**capsulectomy** (,kapsyuh'lektəmee) surgical excision of a capsule.

**capsulitis** (,kapsyuh'lietis) inflammation of the capsule of a joint.

**capsulotomy** (,kapsyuh'lotəmee) the incision of a capsule, particularly that of a joint or of the lens of the eye.

**caput** ('kapuht) head. *C. succedaneum* a transient soft swelling on an infant's head, due to pressure during labour, which disappears within the first few days of life.

**carbachol** ('kahbə,kol) a drug related to and acting like acetylcholine, but more stable. It causes contraction of plain muscle and relaxation of the voluntary sphincter, so relieving postoperative retention of urine. Also occasionally used in the treatment of glaucoma.

**carbamazepine** (,kahbə'mazi,peen) a drug used to control epilepsy and also to relieve pain; used in the treatment of trigeminal neuralgia.

**carbaminohaemoglobin** (kah,baminoh,heemə'glohbin) a compound of carbon dioxide and haemoglobin, present in the blood.

**carbenicillin** (,kahbeni'silin) a synthetic penicillin which is principally used in the treatment of serious infections caused by *Pseudomonas aeruginosa* and other Gram-negative organisms. Large doses, which need to be given intravenously, are required to obtain sufficiently high concentrations in the blood and tissues to be effective.

**carbenoxolone** (,kahbe'noksə,lohn) an anti-inflammatory drug used in the treatment of gastric ulcers.

**carbidopa** (,kahbi'dohpə) an inhibitor of the decarboxylation of levodopa (L-dopa) in peripheral tissues, which does not cross the blood–brain barrier. It is used in combination with levodopa to control the symptoms of PARKINSON'S DISEASE. In the presence of carbidopa, levodopa enters the brain in larger quantities, thus avoiding the need for excessively high doses.

**carbimazole** (kah'bimə,zohl) an antithyroid drug that is used to stabilize a patient with thyrotoxicosis.

**carbohydrate** (,kahboh'hiedrayt) a compound of carbon, hydrogen and oxygen. Carbohydrates are classified into mono-, di-, tri-, poly- and heterosaccharides. In food they are an important and immediate source of energy for the body; 1 g of carbohydrate yields 17 kJ (14 kcal). They are synthesized by all green plants. In the body they are absorbed immediately or stored in the form of glycogen.

**carbolic acid** (kah'bolik) phenol.

**carbon** ('kahbən) *symbol* C. A non-metallic element. *C. dioxide* a gas which, dissolved in water, forms weak carbonic acid. As a product of metabolism by the oxidation of carbon, it leaves the body via the lungs. It can be compressed until it freezes, and then forms a solid (carbon dioxide snow, also known as dry ice) used as an escharotic in various skin conditions. Inhalations of the gas in a 5–7% mixture with oxygen are useful for stimulating the depth of respiration. *C. monoxide* a colourless gas that is very poisonous. It is a major constituent of coal gas and is usually present in the exhaust gases from petrol and diesel engines. In poisoning there is vertigo, flushed face with very red lips, loss of consciousness, and convulsions. The blood is bright red because of the formation of carboxyhaemoglobin. *C. tetrachloride* a powerful anthelmintic used in treating hookworm and whipworm. Also used in cleaning fluids; the inhalation of its vapours in solvent abuse can depress central nervous system activity and cause degeneration of the liver and kidneys.

**carbonic anhydrase** (kah,bonik an-'hiedrayz) an enzyme that catalyses the decomposition of carbonic acid into carbon dioxide and water, facilitating transfer of carbon dioxide from tissues to blood and from blood to alveolar air.

**carboxyhaemoglobin** (kah'boksi-,heemə'glohbin) the combination of carbon monoxide with haemoglobin in the blood in carbon monoxide poisoning.

**carbuncle** ('kahbungk'l) an acute staphylococcal inflammation of subcutaneous tissues, which causes local thrombosis in the veins and death of tissue with several discharging sinuses. In appearance it resembles a collection of boils.

**carcinogen** ('kahsinə,jen, kah'sinə-jən) any substance or agent that can produce a cancer.

**carcinogenic** (,kahsinoh'jenik) pertaining to substances or agents that produce or predispose to cancer.

**carcinoid syndrome** ('kahsi,noyd) a rare condition associated with certain bowel tumours, which spread to other parts of the body. Marked by attacks of severe cyanotic flushing of the skin and by diarrhoea, bronchoconstrictive attacks, pain, serious heart damage, sudden drops in blood pressure, oedema and ascites. Symptoms are caused by serotonin, prostaglandins and other biologically active substances secreted by the tumour.

**carcinoma** (,kahsi'nohmə) a malignant growth of epithelial tissue. Microscopically the cells resemble those of the tissue in which the growth has arisen. *Adenoic c.* adenocarcinoma. *Basal cell c.* a rodent ulcer (*see* ULCER). *Epithelial c.* epithelioma. *Squamous cell c.* one arising from the squamous epithelium of the skin.

**carcinomatosis** (,kahsi,nohmə-'tohsis) the condition in which a carcinoma has given rise to wide-spread metastases.

**cardia** ('kahdiə) the cardiac orifice of the stomach.

**cardiac** ('kahdi,ak) 1. pertaining to the heart. 2. pertaining to the cardia. *C. arrest* the cessation of the heart beat. *C. asthma see* ASTHMA. *C. atrophy* fatty degeneration of the heart muscle. *C. bed* one that can be manipulated to form a chair shape for those who are comfortable only when sitting up. *C. catheterization* a procedure whereby a radio-opaque catheter is passed from an arm vein to the heart. Its passage through the heart can be watched on a screen. Also blood pressure readings and specimens can be taken, thus aiding diagnosis of heart abnormalities. *C. cycle* the sequence of events, lasting about 0.8 s, during which the heart completes one contraction. *C. massage* rhythmic compression of the heart performed in order to re-establish circulation of the blood in cardiac arrest. *C. monitor* (cardiorator) equipment used to monitor and visually record the cardiac cycle. *C. pacemaker* an electrical device that stimulates the heart muscle to maintain myocardial contractions. *See* PACEMAKER. *C. stimulant* a pharmacological agent that increases the action of the heart. Cardiac glycosides, e.g. digoxin and digitalis, increase myocardial contractions and decrease the heart rate and conduction velocity, thus allowing more time for the ventricles to relax and fill with blood.

**cardialgia** (,kahdi'alji.ə) pain in the region of the heart. Cardiodynia.

**cardinal** ('kahdin'l) of first importance. Fundamental. *C. ligaments* deep transverse cervical ligaments. Mackenrodt's ligaments.

**cardiogenic** (,kahdioh'jenik) originating in the heart. *C. shock* shock caused by disease or failure of heart action.

**cardiography** (,kahdi'ografee) the recording of the force and movements of the heart.

**cardiologist** (,kahdi'oləjist) a medically qualified person skilled in the diagnosis of heart disease.

**cardiology** (,kahdi'oləjee) the study of the heart: how it works and its diseases.

**cardiomyopathy** (,kahdiohmie-'opəthee) a chronic disorder of the heart muscle not resulting from atherosclerosis.

**cardiopathy** (,kahdi'opəthee) any disease of the heart.

**cardiopulmonary** (,kahdioh'pulmənə.ree) relating to the heart and lungs. *C. bypass* the use of the heart–lung machine to oxygenate and pump the blood round the body while the surgeon operates on the heart.

**cardioscope** ('kahdioh,skohp) a flexible instrument with a lens and illumination attachment; used for examining the inside of the heart.

**cardiospasm** ('kahdioh,spazəm) spasm of the sphincter muscle at the cardiac end of the stomach. It may result in dilatation of the oesophagus, difficulty in swallowing solids and liquids, and regurgitation of undigested food. Achalasia.

**cardiothoracic** (,kahdiohthor'rasik) pertaining to the heart and thoracic cavity. A specialized branch of surgery.

**cardiotocography** (,kahdiohtə'kografee) the simultaneous recording of the fetal heart rate, fetal movements and uterine contractions in order to discover possible lack of oxygen (hypoxia) to the fetus. Fetal monitoring.

**cardiotomy** (,kahdi'otəmee) surgical incision into the heart or the cardia. *C. syndrome* an inflammatory reaction after heart surgery. There is pyrexia, pericarditis and pleural effusion.

**cardiotoxic** (ˌkahdioh'toksik) anything that has a deleterious or poisonous effect on the heart.

**cardiovascular** (ˌkahdioh'vaskyulə) concerning the heart and blood vessels. *C. system* the heart together with the two chief networks of blood vessels: the systemic circulation and the pulmonary circulation.

**cardioversion** (ˌkahdioh'vərshən) a method of restoring an abnormal heart rhythm to normal (as in atrial fibrillation) by means of an electric shock.

**carditis** (kah'dietis) inflammation of the heart.

**care pathway** ('kair ˌpahthwei) an integrated approach or pathway which determines and utilizes locally agreed multidisciplinary practice based on guidelines and evidence for a specific patient or client group. It may form part of all of the clinical record, it documents the care given and facilitates the evaluation of outcomes.

**care plans** (ˌplanz) *see* NURSING (CARE PLAN).

**carer** ('kairə) a non-professional who provides care for someone in need at home; most commonly a member of the individual's family.

**caries** ('kair.reez) suppuration and subsequent decay of bone, corresponding to ulceration in soft tissues. In caries, the bone dissolves; in necrosis it separates in large pieces and is thrown off. *Dental c.* decay of the teeth due to penetration of bacteria through the enamel to the dentine. *Spinal c.* tuberculosis of the spine. Pott's disease.

**carminative** (kah'minətiv) an aromatic drug that relieves flatulence and associated colic. Cloves, ginger, cardamon and peppermint are examples.

**carneous** ('kahni.əs) fleshy. *C. mole* a tumour of organized blood clot surrounding a dead fetus in the uterus. *See* ABORTION.

**carotene** ('karəˌteen) the colouring matter in carrots, tomatoes and other yellow foods and in fats. It is a provitamin capable of conversion into vitamin A in the liver.

**carotid** (kə'rotid) the principal artery on each side of the neck. *C. bodies* chemoreceptors in the bifurcation of both carotid arteries which monitor the oxygen content of the blood. *C. sinuses* dilated portions of the internal carotids containing the baroreceptors that monitor blood pressure.

**carpal** ('kahp'l) relating to the carpus or wrist. *C. tunnel syndrome* compression of the median nerve at the wrist causing numbing and tingling in the fingers.

**carpopedal** (ˌkahpoh'ped'l) relating to the wrist and foot. *C. spasm* spasm of the hands and feet such as occurs in tetany.

**carpus** ('kahpəs) the eight bones forming the wrist and arranged in two rows: (a) scaphoid, lunate, triquetral, pisiform; (b) trapezium, trapezoid, capitate, hamate (*see* Figure on p. 74).

**carrier** ('kari.ə) 1. a person who harbours the microorganisms of an infectious disease but is not necessarily affected by it, although that person may infect others. 2. one who carries and passes on a hereditary abnormality.

**cartilage** ('kahtilij) a specialized, fibrous connective tissue present in adults and forming most of the temporary skeleton in the embryo. The three most important types are hyaline cartilage, elastic cartilage and fibrocartilage. Also, a general term for a mass of such tissue in a particular site in the body. *Elastic c.* cartilage containing elastic fibres and forming the pinna of the ear, the epiglottis and part of the nasal septum. *Fibro-c.* cartilage in which

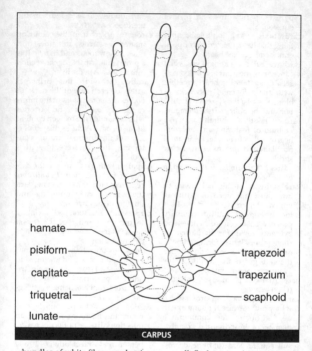

hamate

pisiform

capitate

triquetral

lunate

trapezoid

trapezium

scaphoid

**CARPUS**

bundles of white fibres predominate, forming the intervertebral discs and costal cartilages. *Hyaline c.* flexible, somewhat elastic, semi-transparent cartilage with an opalescent bluish tint, composed of a basophilic fibril-containing substance with cavities in which the chondrocytes occur.

**cartilaginous** (ˌkahti'lajinəs) of the nature of cartilage.

**caruncle** ('karəngk'l) a small fleshy swelling. *Lacrimal c.* a small reddish body situated at the medial junction of the eyelids. *Urethral c.* a small fleshy growth occurring at the urinary orifice in females and giving rise to great pain on micturition.

**cascara** (kas'kahrə) a laxative prepared from the bark of the Californian buckthorn. It may be prepared as an elixir or tablets.

**case** (kays) a particular instance of disease, as in a case of leukaemia; sometimes used incorrectly to designate the patient with the disease. *C. conference* a meeting of professionals involved in the care of a particular person (often a child), to agree patterns of action and to monitor progress. *C.-control study* an epidemiological study in which the characteristics of cases of disease are compared with a matched control group of persons without the disease. Also called retrospective study, case referent study. *C. fatality rate* the number of persons dying of a particular disease expressed as a proportion of the total contracting the disease; usually expressed as a percentage. *C. history* the collected data concerning an individual and that person's family and environment, including the medical history and any other information that may be useful in analysing and diagnosing the health issues or for instructional or research purposes. *C. load* a system of care whereby a nurse, midwife or health visitor is responsible for a group of patients or clients. *C. mix database* computerized record system which combines all the data received from patient administration systems and operational systems to provide a comprehensive set of information about all the treatment and services received by each patient/client during an episode of care. The information helps to develop normal care profiles for different groups, to analyse and compare different treatment regimes, to produce comparative costings for different treatments, etc. It may also be used as part of the medical audit process.

**caseation** (ˌkaysiˈayshən) degeneration of diseased tissue into a cheesy mass.

**casein** (ˈkaysi.in, -seen) the chief protein of milk. It forms a curd from which cheese is made. *C. hydrolysate* a predigested concentrated protein; a useful supplement for a high-protein diet.

**cast** (kahst) 1. a positive copy of an object, e.g. a mould of a hollow organ (a renal tubule, bronchiole, etc.), formed of effused plastic matter and extruded from the body, as in a urinary cast; named, according to constituents, as epithelial, fatty, waxy, etc. 2. a positive copy of the tissues of the jaws, made in an impression, over which denture bases or other restorations may be fabricated. 3. to form an object in a mould. 4. a stiff dressing or casing, usually made of plaster of Paris, used to immobilize body parts. 5. strabismus.

**castor oil** (ˈkahstə oyl) a vegetable oil. Internally it is a purgative. Externally it is protective and soothing and may be used in ointments or in eye drops.

**castration** (kasˈtrayshən) the removal of the testes in the male or the ovaries in the female.

**CAT** (kat) computerized axial tomography.

**cat-scratch disease (fever)** (ˈkat-skratch) a benign, subacute, regional lymphadenitis resulting from a scratch or bite of a cat or a scratch from a surface contaminated by a cat. No specific causative agent has been isolated but a viral aetiology is suspected.

**catabolism** (kəˈtabəˌlizəm) the chemical breakdown of complex substances in the body to form simpler ones, with a release of energy. *See* METABOLISM.

**catalase** (ˈkatəˌlayz) an enzyme found in body cells, including red blood cells and liver cells.

**catalyst** (ˈkatəˌlist) a substance that hastens or brings about a chemical change without itself undergoing alteration; for example, enzymes act as catalysts in the process of digestion.

**cataplasm** (ˈkatəˌplazəm) a poultice. It acts as a counter-irritant. Materials of which it can be made are linseed, bread and bran, but kaolin is more frequently used.

cataplexy ('katə,pleksee) sudden recurrent loss of muscle power without unconsciousness, often associated with narcolepsy. It may be produced by any strong emotion.

cataract ('katə,rakt) opacity of the crystalline lens of the eye causing partial or complete blindness. It may be congenital or may be due to senility, injury or diabetes.

catarrh (kə'tah) chronic inflammation of a mucous membrane accompanied by an excessive discharge of mucus.

catatonia (,katə'tohni.ə) a syndrome of motor abnormalities occurring in schizophrenia, but less commonly in organic cerebral disease, characterized by stupor and the adoption of strange postures, or outbursts of excitement and hyperactivity. The patient may change suddenly from one of these states to the other.

catchment area ('kachmənt ,air.ri.ə) a specific geographical area for which an NHS trust or health centre is responsible for providing the health care services.

catecholamines (,kati'kolə,meenz) a group of compounds that have the effect of sympathetic nerve stimulation. They have an aromatic and an amine portion and include dopamine, adrenaline and noradrenaline.

catgut ('kat,gut) a substance prepared from the intestines of sheep and used in surgery for sutures and ligatures. It is gradually absorbed in the body at a variable rate, according to the preparation.

catharsis (kə'thahsis) 1. a cleansing or purgation. 2. the bringing into consciousness and the emotional reliving of a forgotten (repressed) painful experience as a means of releasing anxiety and tension.

cathartic (kə'thahtik) a purgative drug.

catheter ('kathitə) a tubular, flexible instrument, passed through body channels for withdrawal of fluids from (or introduction of fluids into) a body cavity. Catheters are made of a variety of materials including plastic, metal, rubber and gum-elastic. *Angiographic c.* one through which a contrast medium is injected for visualization of the vascular system of an organ. *Arterial c.* one inserted into an artery and utilized as part of a catheter–transducer–monitor system to continuously observe the BLOOD PRESSURE of critically ill patients. An arterial catheter also may be inserted for radiological studies of the arterial system and for delivery of chemotherapeutic agents directly into the arterial supply of malignant tumours. *Cardiac c.* a long, fine catheter especially designed for passage, usually through a peripheral blood vessel, into the chambers of the heart under fluoroscopic control. *Central venous c.* a long, fine catheter inserted into a vein for the purpose of administering, through a large blood vessel, parenteral fluids (as in parenteral NUTRITION), antibiotics and other therapeutic agents. This type of catheter is also used in the measurement of central venous pressure (*see* CENTRAL (VENOUS PRESSURE)). *Self-retaining c.* a catheter made in such a way that after introduction the blind end expands so that it can remain in the bladder. Useful for continuous or intermittent drainage or where frequent specimens are required. *Ureteric c.* a fine gum-elastic catheter passed up the ureter to the renal pelvis and used to insert a contrast medium in retrograde urography.

catheterization (,kathitə.rie'zay-shən) the insertion of a catheter into a body cavity.

cathode ('kathohd) 1. the negative electrode or pole of an electric current. 2. the negative pole of a battery. *See* ANODE.

**cation** ('katie.ən) a positively charged ion, which moves towards the cathode when an electric current is passed through an electrolytic solution, e.g. hydrogen ($H^+$), sodium ($Na^+$). *See* ANION.

**cauda** ('kawdah) a tail-like appendage. *C. equina* the bundle of coccygeal, sacral and lumbar nerves with which the spinal cord terminates.

**caudal** ('kawd'l) referring to a cauda. *C. block* a local anaesthetic agent injected into the sacral canal so that operations may be carried out in the peritoneal area without a general anaesthetic.

**caul** (kawl) the amnion, which occasionally does not rupture but envelops the infant's head at birth.

**causalgia** (kaw'zalji.ə) an intense burning pain which persists after peripheral nerve injuries.

**caustic** ('kostik, 'kaw-) a substance, usually a strong acid or alkali, capable of burning organic tissue. Silver nitrate (*lunar c.*), carbolic acid and carbon dioxide snow are those most commonly used.

**cauterization** (kawtə.rie'zayshən) the destruction of tissue with cautery.

**cautery** ('kawtə.ree) 1. the application of searing heat by a hot instrument, an electric current or other means such as a laser. 2. an agent so used. *Cold c.* cauterization by carbon dioxide, called also cryocautery.

**cavernous** ('kavənəs, kə'vərnəs) having caverns or hollows. *C. breathing* sounds heard on auscultation over a pulmonary cavity. *C. sinus* a venous channel lying on either side of the body of the sphenoid bone through which pass the internal carotid artery and several nerves. *C. sinus thrombosis* a serious complication of any infection of the face, the veins from the orbit draining into the sinus and carrying the infection into the cranium.

**cavitation** (kavi'tayshən) the formation of cavities, e.g. in the lung in tuberculosis.

**cavity** ('kavitee) a confined space or hollow or potential hollow within the body or one of its organs, e.g. the abdominal cavity or a decayed hollow in a tooth.

**CCU** critical care unit; coronary care unit.

**cefotaxime** (kefoh'takseem) a third generation cephalosporin antibiotic having a broad spectrum of activity, used to treat intra-abdominal infections, bone and joint infections, gonorrhoea, and other infections due to susceptible organisms, including penicillinase-producing strains.

**cefoxitin** (ke'foksitin) a semisynthetic cephalosporin antibiotic, especially effective against Gram-negative organisms, with strong resistance to degradation by β-lactamase.

**Celevac** (sele'vak) trade name for methylcellulose.

**cell** (sel) 1. the basic structural unit of living organisms (*see* Figure on p. 78). A microscopic mass of protoplasm, consisting of a nucleus surrounded by cytoplasm and enclosed in a cell membrane, from which all organic tissues are constructed. Each cell can reproduce itself by mitosis. 2. a small, more or less enclosed, space.

**cellulitis** (selyuh'lietis) a diffuse inflammation of connective tissue, especially of subcutaneous tissue, which causes a typical brawny, oedematous appearance of the part; local abscess formation is not common.

**cellulose** ('selyuh lohs, - lohz) a carbohydrate forming the covering of vegetable cells, i.e. vegetable fibres. Not digestible in the alimentary tract of humans but gives bulk and, as 'roughage', stimulates peristalsis.

**Celsius scale** ('selsi.əs) *A. Celsius, Swedish astronomer, 1701–1744.* A

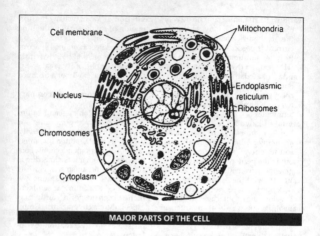

**MAJOR PARTS OF THE CELL**

temperature scale with the melting point of ice set at 0° and the boiling point of water at 100°. The normal temperature of the human body is 36.9°C. Formerly known as the centigrade scale. *See* FAHRENHEIT SCALE.

**cementum** (si'mentəm) cement. Connective tissue with a bone-like structure which covers the root of a tooth and supports it within the socket.

**censor** (ˌsensə) 1. a member of a committee on ethics or for critical examination of a medical or other society. 2. the psychic influence that prevents unconscious thoughts and wishes coming into consciousness.

**censorship** ('sensəˌʃip) in psychiatry, the process of selecting, accepting or rejecting conscious ideas, memories and impulses arising from the individual's subconscious.

**census** ('sensəs) enumeration of a population. The national census was first introduced in England and Wales in 1801 and has since

been repeated every 10 years (except in 1941). It usually records name, address, age, sex, occupation, marital status and other social information.

**Centers for Disease Control** ('sentəz) abbreviated CDC. An agency of the US Department of Health and Human Services, located in Atlanta, Georgia, which serves as a centre for the control, prevention and investigation of diseases. A similar function is performed in England and Wales by the Communicable Diseases Surveillance Centre and in Scotland by the Communicable Diseases (Scotland) Unit.

**centigrade** ('sentiˌgrayd) *see* CELSIUS SCALE.

**centile** ('sentiel) *see* PERCENTILE.

**central** ('sentrəl) pertaining to the centre or midpoint. *C. nervous system* abbreviated CNS. The brain and spinal cord. *C. venous pressure* the pressure recorded by the introduction of a catheter into the right atrium in order to monitor the condition of a patient after a major operative procedure, such as heart surgery.

**centrifugal** (sentri'fyoog'l) conveying away from a centre, such as from the brain to the periphery. Efferent; the reverse of centripetal.

**centrifuge** ('sentri,fyooj) an apparatus that rotates at high speed. If a test tube, for example, is filled with a fluid such as blood or urine and rotated in a centrifuge, any bacteria, cells or other solids in it are precipitated.

**centripetal** (sen'tripit'l, 'sentri-,peet'l) conveying from the periphery to the centre. Afferent; the reverse of centrifugal.

**centromere** ('sentroh,mia) the region(s) of the chromosomes which become(s) allied with the spindle fibres at mitosis and meiosis.

**centrosome** ('sentra,sohm) a body in the cytoplasm of most animal cells, close to the nucleus. It divides during mitosis, one half migrating to each daughter cell.

**centrosphere** ('sentra,sfia) the cell centre, in an area of clear cytoplasm near the nucleus.

**cephalexin** (,kefa'leksin, ,sef-) a cephalosporin antibiotic that may be administered orally.

**cephalhaematoma** (,kefal,heema-'tohma, ,sef-) a swelling beneath the pericranium, containing blood, which may be found on the head of the newborn infant. Caused by pressure during labour. Gradually reabsorbed within the first few days of life.

**cephalocele** ('kefaloh,seel, 'sef-) cerebral hernia. See HERNIA.

**cephalography** (,kefa'lografee, ,sef-) radiographic examination of the contours of the head.

**cephalometry** (,kefa'lomatree, ,sef-) measurement of the dimensions of the head of a living person either

directly or by radiography. See also PELVIMETRY.

**cephaloridine** (,kefa'lor,rideen, ,sef-) an antibiotic that is effective against a wide range of organisms.

**cephalosporin** (,kefaloh'spor,rin, ,sef-) any one of a group of broad-spectrum antibiotics derived from the mould *Cephalosporium*.

**cephradine** ('kefradeen, 'sef-) a cephalosporin antibiotic similar in action to cephaloridine.

**cerclage** (sar'klahzh) [Fr.] encircling of a part with a ring or loop, as for correction of an incompetent cervix uteri or fixation of the adjacent ends of a fractured bone. See SHIRODKAR'S SUTURE.

**cerebellum** (,seri'belam) the portion of the brain below the cerebrum and above the medulla oblongata. Its functions include the coordination of fine voluntary movements and posture.

**cerebral** ('seribral) relating to the cerebrum. *C. cortex* the outer layer of the cerebrum, composed of neurones. *C. haemorrhage* rupture of a cerebral blood vessel. Likely causes are aneurysm and hypertension. See APOPLEXY. *C. hernia see* HERNIA. *C. irritation* a condition of general nervous irritability and abnormality, often with photophobia, which may be an early sign of meningitis, tumour of the brain, etc. It is also associated with trauma. *C. palsy* a condition caused by injury to the brain during or immediately after birth. Coordination of movement is affected, and may cause the child to be flaccid or athetoid, in which condition there is constant random and uncontrolled movement. See SPASTIC.

**cerebration** (,seri'brayshan) mental activity.

**cerebrospinal** (,seribroh'spien'l) relating to the brain and spinal cord. *C. fluid* abbreviated CSF. The fluid made in the choroid plexus of the

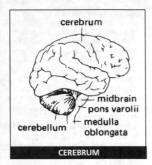

cerebrum

midbrain
pons varolii
medulla
oblongata
cerebellum

**CEREBRUM**

ventricles of the brain and circulating from them into the subarachnoid space around the brain and spinal cord.

**cerebrovascular** (ˌseribroh'vaskyuhlə) pertaining to the arteries and veins of the brain. *C. accident* a disorder arising from an embolus, thrombus or haemorrhage in the cerebrum. *C. disease* any disorder of the blood vessels of the brain and its meninges.

**cerebrum** ('seribrəm) the largest part of the brain, occupying the greater portion of the cranium and consisting of the right and left hemispheres divided by the longitudinal fissure (*see* Figure). Each hemisphere contains a lateral ventricle. The internal substance is white and the convoluted surface is grey. The centre of the higher functions of the brain.

**cerumen** (si'roomən) a waxy substance secreted by the ceruminous glands of the auditory canal. Ear wax.

**cervical** ('sərvik'l, sə'vie-) pertaining to the neck or the constricted part of an organ, e.g. uterine cervix. *C. canal* the passage through the uterine cervix. *C. cancer* cancer of the uterine cervix. *C. collar* a rigid or semirigid immobilizing support

for the neck. *C. rib* a short, extra rib, often bilateral, which sometimes occurs on the seventh cervical vertebra and may cause pressure on an artery or nerve. *C. smear* a test for disorders of the cervical cells; material is scraped from the uterine cervix and examined microscopically. *C. spondylosis* a degenerative disease of the intervertebral joints and discs of the neck. *C. vertebra* one of the seven bones forming the neck portion of the spinal column.

**cervicitis** (ˌsərvi'sietis) inflammation of the neck of the uterus.

**cervix** ('sərviks) a constricted portion or neck. *C. uteri* the neck of the uterus; it is about 2 cm long and projects into the vagina. Capable of wide dilatation during childbirth.

**CESDI** ('kezdee) Confidential Enquiry into Stillbirths and Deaths in Infancy. *See* CONFIDENTIAL ENQUIRY.

**cestode** ('sestohd) tapeworm.

**cetrimide** ('setri,mied) cetyltrimethylammonium bromide (CTAB). A detergent and antiseptic widely used for preoperative skin preparation and the cleansing of wounds.

**chafe** (chayf) irritation of the skin as caused by the friction between skinfolds. Occurs particularly in moist areas.

**chalazion** (kə'lazi.ən) a meibomian or tarsal cyst. A swollen sebaceous gland in the eyelid. A small, hard tumour may develop.

**chancre** ('shangkə) 1. the initial lesion of syphilis developing at the site of inoculation. 2. a papular lesion occurring at the site of infection in tuberculosis or in sporotrichosis.

**chancroid** ('shangkroyd) soft chancre. A venereal ulceration, due to *Haemophilus ducreyi*, accompanied by inflammation and suppuration of the local glands.

**character** ('karəktə) the combination of traits and qualities distinguishing the unique nature of the individual. *C. change* indicates alteration in a person's recognized behaviour to one alien to the person's normal manner of conduct. *C. disorder* a chronic state in which the person exhibits maladaptive and unacceptable forms of behaviour and social response.

**Charcot's disease or joint** (shah'kohz) *J.M. Charcot, French neurologist, 1825–1893.* A chronic progressive, degenerative disease of the stress-bearing portion of one or more joints. The disease is the result of an underlying neurological disorder, e.g. tabes dorsalis from syphilis or diabetic neuropathy or leprosy.

**Charcot's triad** ('triead) nystagmus, intention tremor and scanning speech. A trio of signs of disseminated sclerosis.

**Charnley's arthroplasty** ('chahnliz) *Sir J. Charnley, British orthopaedic surgeon, 1911–1982.* The replacement of the hip joint using a plastic acetabulum and a steel femoral head. *See* ARTHROPLASTY.

**chart** (chaht) a record in graphic or tabular form. *Genealogical c.* a graph showing various descendants of a common ancestor, used to indicate those affected by genetically determined disease. *Reading c.* a chart with material printed in gradually increasing type sizes, used in testing acuity of near vision. *Reuss' c's* charts with coloured letters printed on coloured backgrounds, used in testing colour vision. *Snellen's c.* a chart printed with block letters in gradually decreasing sizes, used in testing visual acuity.

**charting** ('chahting) the keeping of a clinical record of the important facts about a patient and the progress of his or her illness. The patient's chart usually contains a medical history, a nursing history, results of physical examinations, laboratory reports, results of special diagnostic tests, and the observations of the nursing staff. Medical treatments, medications and nursing approaches to problems are recorded on the chart, as are the patient's response to treatment. *See also* PROBLEM-ORIENTED RECORD.

**cheilosis** (kie'lohsis) maceration at the angles of the mouth; fissures may also occur. It may be associated with general debility or riboflavin deficiency.

**cheiropompholyx** (,kieroh'pomfohliks) a skin disease characterized by vesicles on the palms and soles.

**chelate** ('keelayt) a chemical compound in which an atom of a metal is held in a molecular ring.

**chelating agent** (ki'layting) a drug that has the power of combining with certain metals and so aiding excretion, to prevent or overcome poisoning. *See* DIMERCAPROL and PENICILLAMINE.

**chemistry** ('kemistree) the science of dealing with the elements, the atoms which compose them and the compounds that they form.

**chemoreceptor** (,keemohri'septa, ,kem-) a sensory nerve ending or group of cells that is sensitive to chemical stimuli in the blood.

**chemosis** (kee'mohsis) swelling of the conjunctiva due to the presence of fluid; an oedema of the conjunctiva.

**chemosurgery** (,keemoh'sarja,ree, ,kem-) the destruction of tissue by chemical agents for therapeutic purposes, originally applied to chemical fixation of malignant, gangrenous or infected tissue with use of frozen sections to facilitate systematic microscopic control of its excision.

**chemotaxis** (,keemoh'taksis, ,kem-) the reaction of living cells to chemical stimuli. These are either attracted (*positive c.*) or repelled (*negative* *c.*) by acids, alkalis or other substances.

**chemotherapy** (ˌkeemoh'therəpee, ˌkem-) the specific treatment of disease by the administration of chemical compounds.

**chest** (chest) the thorax. *Barrel c.* one more rounded than usual, with raised ribs and, usually, kyphosis. It is often present in emphysema. *C. leads* leads applied to the chest during the course of an electrocardiographic recording. *Flail c.* one where part of the chest wall moves in opposition to respiration as a result of multiple fractures of the ribs. *Pigeon c.* a chest with the sternum protruding forwards.

**Cheyne–Stokes respiration** ('chayn 'stohks) *J. Cheyne, British physician, 1776–1836; W. Stokes, British physician, 1804–1878.* Tidal respiration. A form of irregular but rhythmic breathing with temporary cessations (apnoea). It is likely to be present in cerebral tumour, in narcotic poisoning and in advanced cases of arteriosclerosis and uraemia.

**chiasma** (kie'azmə) a crossing point. *Optic c.* the crossing point of the optic nerves.

**chickenpox** ('chikinˌpoks) varicella.

**chilblain** ('chilˌblayn) a condition resulting from defective circulation when exposure to cold causes localized swelling and inflammation of the hands or feet, with severe itching and burning sensations.

**child** (chield) the human young, from infancy to puberty. *C. abuse* the non-accidental use of physical force or the non-accidental act of omission by a parent or other custodian responsible for the care of a child. Child abuse encompasses malnutrition and other kinds of neglect through ignorance, as well as deliberate withholding from the child of the necessary and basic physical care, including the medical and dental care necessary for

the child to grow. Examples of physical abuse range from burns and exposure to extreme cold, to beating, poisoning, strangulation, and withholding food and water. If a child is seen to be in danger of suffering significant harm, from physical, sexual, emotional or neglectful causes, the child may be registered on the Child Protection Register. If a nurse, health visitor or midwife has reasonable cause to suspect the abuse of a child, appropriate action must be taken in order to protect that child. *See also* CHILDREN ACT 1989. *Deprived c.* a vague term usually implying that the child in question has been raised in a situation lacking in love, affection and consistent parenting responses from adults. Sometimes used to suggest that the child has experienced a generalized deficit of life opportunities, both interpersonal and social. *C. sexual abuse* the subjection of a child to sexual activity likely to cause physical or psychological harm.

**child care** any matter associated with the upbringing and welfare of children, both familial and in relation to welfare and social services. *C. officer* a social worker who has a responsibility to investigate any situation where a child is thought to be at risk of harm due to neglect, injury or desertion, and in those situations where the child is considered 'beyond control' by the parents/guardians or is offending.

**child development** (di'veləpmənt) The stages of physical, psychological and social growth and attainment that occur from birth to adulthood.

**child health clinic** a centre which infants and preschool children attend on a regular basis to ensure normal progress and development. A medical officer and a health visitor are in attendance. Immunizations against infectious diseases, screening and health promotion information are also provided.

**child minder** (ˌmiendə) a person who is registered with the local authority social services department and who is approved by the department to mind an agreed number of children aged from birth to 5 years during the day.

**childbirth** ('chield barth) the act or process of giving birth to a child. Parturition.

**Children Act 1989** ('childrən akt) the main principles of this legislation for the care and welfare of children are as follows. (a) The welfare of children is the prime consideration and wherever possible they should be cared for within their own families. Parents with children in need should be helped and supported by the local authorities, and in partnership with other agencies, to bring up their children themselves. Parents should be informed of their right to complain if they are not satisfied with the services offered. (b) Children should be kept safe and protected by effective intervention if they are in danger but this should be open to parental challenge through the courts. (c) The courts, when dealing with children, should avoid any delays when processing their cases, and should only make an order if to do so is better for the child than making no order at all. (d) Children should be kept informed of any decisions taken in their interests and should participate as far as possible in any decisions or actions taken. (e) Parents continue to have responsibility for their children, even when they are no longer living with them. Parents should be kept informed of and invited to participate in any decisions about their children's future. (f) Local authorities are required to take account of

children's racial origins, culture, linguistic background and religion when making decisions about them.

**Chinese medicine** (chie'neez) a traditional system based on the principles of Yin and Yang, combining acupuncture with a range of medications from herbal and animal sources.

**Chinese restaurant syndrome** ('restəronh) transient arterial dilatation due to ingestion of monosodium glutamate, which is used in seasoning Chinese food; marked by throbbing head, light-headedness, tightness of the jaw, neck and shoulders, and backache.

**chiropody** (ki'ropədee, shi-) the study and care of the feet and the treatment of foot diseases.

**chiropractic** (ˌkierə'praktik) a system of treatment employing manipulation of the spine and other bony structures.

**Chlamydia** (klə'midi.ə) a genus of bacteria comprising two species: *C. trachomatis* which causes lymphogranuloma venereum, trachoma, conjunctivitis and non-gonococcal urethritis; and *C. psittaci*, which causes psittacosis (parrot fever).

**chloasma** (kloh'azmə) a condition in which there is brown, blotchy discoloration of the skin of the face, especially during pregnancy.

**chloral** ('klor.ral) an oily liquid formed by the reaction of chlorine and alcohol. Used in the production of *c. hydrate*, a drug used as a hypnotic; it is well tolerated by children and old people.

**chlorambucil** (klor'rambyuhsil) an alkylating drug used in treating chronic leukaemia. A cytotoxic drug.

**chloramphenicol** (ˌklor.ram'feniˌkol) an antibiotic. It gives rise to agranulocytosis and is used only for serious infectious diseases, such as typhoid fever, and in drops and ointment for eye infections.

**chlorcyclizine** (klor'siekli,zeen) an antihistamine used for travel sickness.

**chlorhexidine** (klor'heksi,deen) an antibacterial compound used for surgical scrub, preoperative skin preparation and cleansing skin wounds.

**chlorine** ('klor.reen, -rin) *symbol* CI. A yellow, irritating poisonous gas. A powerful disinfectant, bleach and deodorizing agent. Used in hypochlorites for sterilization purposes.

**chlormethiazole** (,klorma'thiea,zohl) a hypnotic and sedative drug used to treat insomnia, chiefly in elderly people.

**chloroacetone** (,klor.roh'asi,tohn) chloroacetone. Tear gas.

**chlorocresol** (,klor.roh'kreesol) a coal tar product with a bacterial action more powerful than phenol and with a lower toxicity. Used as an antiseptic and as a preservative in injection fluids.

**chloroform** ('klo.ra,fawm) a colourless volatile liquid administered through inhalation as a general anaesthetic. Now rarely used.

**chloroma** (klor'rohma) a tumour having a greenish colour, usually found in skull bones. It is associated with myeloid leukaemia.

**chlorophyll** ('klo.ra,fil) the green pigment of plants which absorbs solar energy for the synthesis of complex materials from the carbon dioxide and water taken in by the plant.

**chloroquine** ('klor.roh,kween) an antimalarial drug that has a strong suppressant action and is also used in the treatment of amoebic hepatitis, rheumatoid arthritis and lupus erythematosus.

**chlorothiazide** (,klor.roh'thieazied) an oral diuretic used in the treatment of fluid retention and hypertension.

**chlorotrianisene** (,klor.rohtrie-,aniseen) a long-acting oestrogen used in the treatment of menopausal symptoms and in cancer of the prostate.

**chloroxylenol** (,klor.roh'zielanol) an antiseptic that is less irritating to the skin and mucous membranes than cresol and has a powerful disinfectant action.

**chlorpheniramine** (,klorfe'nira,meen) an antihistamine drug used in the treatment of allergies such as hay fever and urticaria.

**chlorpromazine** (,klor'prohma,zeen) a sedative antiemetic drug widely used to treat anxiety, agitation and vomiting, particularly in the elderly, and in the management of psychiatric patients. It is also hypotensive and enhances the effect of analgesics and anaesthetics.

**chlorpropamide** (,klor'prohpa,mied) an oral hypoglycaemic agent used in the treatment of mild diabetes.

**chlorprothixene** (,klorproh'thikseen) a tranquillizer used in the treatment of schizophrenia, psychoneuroses and behaviour disorders.

**chlortetracycline** (,klortetra'siekleen) a broad- spectrum antibiotic effective in treating many bacterial and protozoal infections.

**chlorthalidone** (,klor'thalidohn) a diuretic used in the treatment of oedema, hypertension and diabetes.

**cholangiography** (ka,lanji'ografee) radiography of the hepatic, cystic and bile ducts after the insertion of a radio- opaque contrast medium.

**cholangitis** (,kohlan'jietis) inflammation of the bile ducts.

**cholecystectomy** (,kohlisi'stekt-amee) excision of the gallbladder.

**cholecystitis** (,kohlisi'stietis) inflammation of the gallbladder.

**cholecystoduodenostomy** (,kohli-,sistoh,dyooadi'nostamee) an anastomosis between the gallbladder and the duodenum.

**cholecystoenterostomy** (ˌkohliˌsi-stohˌentəˈrostəmee) the formation of an artificial opening from the gallbladder into the intestine. An operation performed in cases of irremovable obstruction of the bile duct.

**cholecystography** (ˌkohlisiˈstogrə-fee) radiography of the gallbladder after administration of a radio-opaque contrast medium.

**cholecystokinin** (ˌkohliˌsistohˈkienin) a hormone, released by the presence of fats in the duodenum, which causes contraction of the gallbladder.

**cholecystolithiasis** (ˌkohliˌsistolhiˈthiesis) the presence of stones in the gallbladder.

**cholecystotomy** (ˌkohlisiˈtotəmee) an incision into the gallbladder, usually to remove gallstones.

**choledocholithiasis** (ˌkohliˌdohkohliˈthiesis) the presence of stones in the bile duct.

**choledocholithotomy** (ˌkohliˌdoh-kohliˈthotəmee) incision into the bile ducts to remove stones.

**choledochostomy** (ˌkohlidoh-ˈkostəmee) opening and draining the common bile duct.

**cholelithiasis** (ˌkohliliˈthiesis) presence of gallstones in the gallbladder or bile ducts.

**cholera** (ˈkoləˌrə) an acute, notifiable, infectious enteritis endemic and epidemic in Asia and, more recently, also in Africa. Caused by *Vibrio cholerae*, it is marked by profuse diarrhoea, muscle cramp, suppression of urine and severe prostration; it is often fatal. Travellers to areas where cholera is endemic should protect themselves by vaccination, though this only provides partial immunity. The local drinking water should be boiled or sterilized and uncooked foods avoided.

**cholestasis** (ˌkohliˈstaysis) arrest of the flow of bile due to obstruction of the bile ducts.

**cholesteatoma** (ˌkohliˌsteeəˈtohmə) a small tumour containing cholesterol. It may occur in the middle ear or in the meninges, central nervous system or bones of the skull.

**cholesterol** (kəˈlestəˌrol) a sterol found in nervous tissue, red blood corpuscles, animal fat and bile. It is a precursor of bile acids and steroid hormones, and occurs in the most common type of gallstone, in atheroma of the arteries, in various cysts and in carcinomatous tissue. Most of the body's cholesterol is synthesized, but some is obtained in the diet.

**cholesterolosis** (kəˌlestəˌroˈlohsis) a chronic form of cholecystitis when the mucosa of the gallbladder is studded with deposits of cholesterol.

**cholestyramine** (ˌkohliˈstierəmeen) a drug that causes the excretion of bile salts by binding with them. Given to lower blood levels of cholesterol and other fats.

**choline** (ˈkohleen) an essential amine, found in the blood, cerebrospinal fluid and urine, which aids fat metabolism. Formerly classified as a vitamin of the B complex. *C. theophyllinate* an antispasmodic drug used in respiratory conditions.

**cholinergic** (ˌkohliˈnərjik) pertaining to nerves that release acetylcholine, as the chemical stimulator, at their nerve endings. *C. drugs* drugs that inhibit cholinesterase and so prevent the destruction of acetylcholine.

**cholinesterase** (ˌkohliˈnestəˈrayz) an enzyme that rapidly destroys acetylcholine.

**chondroblast** (ˈkondrohˌblast) an embryonic cell that forms cartilage.

**chondroma** (konˈdrohmə) an innocent new growth arising in cartilage.

**chondromalacia** (ˌkondrohmə-ˈlayshi.ə) a condition of abnormal softening of cartilage.

**chondrosarcoma** (ˌkondrohsah-'kohmə) a malignant new growth arising from cartilaginous tissue.

**chorda** ('kawdə) a sinew or cord.

**chordee** (kaw'dee) downward curvature of the penis caused by congenital anomaly (common in hypospadias) or urethral infection.

**chorditis** (kaw'dietis) inflammation of the vocal or spermatic cords.

**chordotomy** (kaw'dotəmee) an operation on the spinal cord to divide the anterolateral nerve pathways for relief of intractable pain. Cordotomy.

**chorea** (ko'reeə) a symptom of disease of the basal ganglia when the individual suffers from spasmodic, involuntary, rapid movements of the face, shoulders and hips. *Huntington's c.* (or Huntington's disease) a rare hereditary disorder which manifests itself in early middle age. The individual also suffers from progressive dementia, which often precedes a premature death. *Sydenham's c.* St Vitus's dance. Occurs in childhood and is associated with rheumatic fever.

**choreiform** (ko'ree.ifawm) resembling chorea.

**choriocarcinoma** (ˌko.riohˌkahsi-'nohmə) formerly known as chorioepithelioma. A highly malignant NEOPLASM usually arising from the trophoblast of a hydatidiform mole (*see* HYDATIDIFORM MOLE). It may develop after an abortion or even the evacuation of a hydatidiform mole or even in normal pregnancy. Metastases usually develop rapidly but the disease normally carries a good prognosis if early treatment is given.

**chorioepithelioma** (ˌko.riohˌepiˌtheeli'ohmə) choriocarcinoma.

**chorion** ('ko.rion, 'kor.ri.ən) the outer membrane enveloping the fetus; the placenta.

**chorionic** (ˌko.ri'onik) pertaining to the chorion. *C. gonadotrophin* human chorionic gonadotrophin (HCG). *C. villi* small protrusions on the chorion from which the placenta is formed. They are in close association with the maternal blood and, by diffusion, interchange of nutriment, oxygen and waste matters is effected between the maternal and the fetal blood. *C. villus biopsy* tissue removed from the gestational sac early in pregnancy so that chromosomal and other inherited disorders can be identified. Can be carried out at an earlier stage than amniocentesis.

**chorioretinitis** (ˌko.riohˌreti'nietis) choroidoretinitis.

**choroid** ('ko.royd) the pigmented and vascular coat of the eyeball, continuous with the iris and situated between the sclera and retina. It reduces the amount of light which falls upon the retina. *C. plexus* specialized cells in the ventricles of the brain which produce cerebrospinal fluids. There is one choroid plexus in each ventricle.

**choroiditis** (ˌko.roy'dietis) inflammation of the choroid.

**choroidoretinitis** (koˌroydohˌreti'nietis) an inflammatory condition of both the choroid and retina of the eye.

**Christmas disease** ('krisməs) a hereditary bleeding disease similar to haemophilia. The name is derived from that of the first patient to be studied.

**chromatography** (ˌkrohmə'togrəfee) a method of chemical analysis by which substances in solution can be separated as they percolate down a column of powdered absorbent or ascend an absorbent paper by capillary traction. A definite pattern is produced and substances may be recognized by the use of appropriate colour reagents. Amino acids can be identified in this way.

**chromatometry** (ˌkrohmə'tomətree) the measurement of colour perception.

**chromic acid** ('krohmik) a strong caustic sometimes used for the removal of warts.

**chromicize** ('krohmiˌsiez) to impregnate with chromic acid, e.g. chromicized catgut, which is particularly strong and durable.

**chromosome** ('krohməˌsohm) in animal cells, a structure in the nucleus, containing a linear thread of DEOXYRIBONUCLEIC ACID (DNA), which transmits genetic information and is associated with RIBONUCLEIC ACID (RNA) and histones. During cell division the material composing the chromosome is compactly coiled. Each organism of a species is normally characterized by the same number of chromosomes in its somatic cells, 46 being the number usually present in humans: 22 pairs of autosomes, and two sex chromosomes (XX or XY), which determine the sex of the organism. In the mature GAMETE (ovum or spermatozoon) the number of chromosomes is halved as a result of MEIOSIS.

**chronic** ('kronik) of long duration; the opposite of acute.

**Chvostek's sign** ('vosteks) *F. Chvostek, Austrian surgeon, 1835–1884.* A spasm of the facial muscles which occurs in tetany. It can be elicited by tapping the facial nerve.

**chyle** (kiel) digested fats which, as a milky fluid, are absorbed into the lymphatic capillaries (lacteals) in the villi of the small intestine.

**chylothorax** (ˌkieloh'thor.raks) the presence of effused chyle in the pleural cavity.

**chyme** (kiem) the semiliquid acid mass of food that passes from the stomach to the intestines.

**chymotrypsin** (ˌkiemoh'tripsin) an enzyme secreted by the pancreas. It is activated by trypsin and aids in the breakdown of proteins.

**Ci** symbol for curie.

**cicatrix** ('sikətriks) the scar of a healed wound (*see* KELOID).

**cilia** ('siliə) 1. the eyelashes. 2. microscopic filaments projecting from some epithelial cells, known as ciliated membranes, as in the bronchi, where cilia wave the secretion upwards.

**ciliary** ('siliə.ree) hair-like. *C. body* a structure just behind the corneoscleral margin, composed of the ciliary muscle and processes. *C. muscle* the circular muscle surrounding the lens of the eye. *C. processes* the fringed part of the choroid coat arranged in a circle in front of the lens.

**cimetidine** (si'metiˌdeen) a histamine H₂ receptor antagonist which reduces gastric acid secretion; used in the treatment of peptic ulcers.

**Cimex** ('siemeks) a genus of bloodsucking bugs. *C. lectularius* the common bedbug.

**cinchocaine** ('sinchohˌkayn) a local anaesthetic agent used mainly as a spinal anaesthetic.

**cineangiocardiography** (ˌsiniˌanjiohˌkahdi'ogrəfee) angiography using a cine camera to show the movements of the heart and blood vessels.

**cineradiography** (ˌsiniˌraydi'ogrəfee) the making of a motion picture record of successive images appearing on a fluoroscopic screen.

**cinnarizine** (si'narizeen) an antihistamine drug which may also be used to treat nausea, vertigo, labyrinthine disorders and motion sickness.

**circadian** (sər'kaydi.ən) denoting a period of 24 h. *C. rhythm* the rhythm of certain biological activities that take place daily.

**circinate** ('sərsiˌnayt) having a circular outline. *Tinea circinata* is ringworm.

**circle of Willis** (ˌsɜːkˈl əv 'wilis) T. Willis, British physician and anatomist, 1621–1675. An anastomosis of arteries at the base of the brain, formed by the branches of the internal carotid and the basilar arteries.

**circulation** (ˌsɜːkjuh'layshən) movement in a circular course, as of the blood. *Collateral c.* enlargement of small vessels establishing adequate blood supply when the main vessel to the part has been occluded. *Coronary c.* the system of vessels that supplies the heart muscle itself. *Extracorporeal c.* 1. removal of the blood by intravenous cannulae, passing it through a machine to oxygenate it, and then pumping it back into circulation. 2. the 'heart–lung' machine or pump respirator, used in cardiac surgery. *Lymph c.* the flow of lymph through lymph vessels and glands. *Portal c.* the passage of blood from the alimentary tract, pancreas and spleen, via the portal vein and its branches through the liver and into the hepatic veins. *Pulmonary c.* passage of the blood from the right ventricle via the pulmonary artery through the lungs and back to the heart by the pulmonary veins. *Systemic c.* the flow of blood throughout the body. The direction of flow is from the left atrium to the left ventricle and through the aorta, with its branches and capillaries. Veins then carry it back to the right atrium, and so into the right ventricle.

**circumcision** (ˌsɜːkəm'sizhən) excision of the prepuce or foreskin of the penis. An operation performed for religious reasons, or sometimes for phimosis or paraphimosis. *Female c.* excision of the labia minora and/or labia majora, and sometimes the clitoris; still performed ritualistically in certain countries, the extent of the surgery varying from one culture to another.

**circumduction** (ˌsɜːkəm'dukshən) moving in a circle, e.g. the circular movement of the upper limb.

**circumoral** (ˌsɜːkəm'or.rəl) around the mouth. *C. pallor* a pale area around the mouth contrasting with the flushed cheeks, e.g. in scarlet fever.

**circumvallate** (ˌsɜːkəm'valayt) surrounded by a wall or raised ring. *C. papilla see* PAPILLA.

**cirrhosis** (si'rohsis) a degenerative change that can occur in any organ, but especially in the liver. May be due to viruses, microorganisms or toxic substances (*portal c.*). Fibrosis results and interferes with the working of the organ. In the liver it causes portal obstruction, with consequent ascites. *Alcoholic c.* the result of chronic alcoholism and nutritional deficiency which affects the liver. *Cardiac c.* cirrhosis of the liver following chronic heart failure. *Posthepatic c.* cirrhosis of the liver following hepatitis. *Pulmonary c.* cirrhosis of the lung tissue.

**cisplatin** ('sisplə.tin, sis'platin) an antineoplastic drug, containing platinum, used in the treatment of ovarian carcinomas and testicular teratomas.

**cisterna** (si'stɜːnə) a space or cavity containing fluid. *C. chyli* the dilated portion of the thoracic duct containing chyle. *C. magna* the subarachnoid space between the cerebellum and medulla oblongata.

**cisternal** (si'stɜːnəl) concerning the cisterna. *C. puncture* insertion of a hollow needle into the cisterna magna to withdraw cerebrospinal fluid.

**citric acid** ('sitrik) acid found in the juice of lemons, limes, etc. An antiscorbutic.

**CJD** Creutzfeldt–Jakob disease.

**Cl** symbol for *chlorine.*

**clamp** (klamp) a metal surgical instrument used to compress any part of the body.

**clapping** ('klaping) in physiotherapy, rhythmic beating with cupped hands. Frequently used over the chest to aid expectoration.

**claudication** (ˌklawdi'kayshən) lameness. *Intermittent c.* limping, accompanied by severe pain in the legs on walking, which disappears with rest. A sign of occlusive arterial disease.

**claustrophobia** (ˌklostrə'fohbi.ə, ˌklaw-) fear of confined spaces, such as small rooms.

**clavicle** ('klavik'l) the collar bone. A long bone, part of the shoulder girdle.

**clavus** ('klayvəs) a corn.

**clawfoot** (ˌklor'fuht) a deformity in which the longitudinal arch is abnormally raised. Pes cavus.

**clawhand** (ˌklor'hand) a deformity in which the fingers are bent and contracted, giving a claw-like appearance.

**cleft** (kleft) a fissure or longitudinal opening. *C. lip* a congenital fissure in the upper lip, often accompanied by cleft palate. *C. palate* a congenital defect in the roof of the mouth due to failure of the medial plates of the palate to meet. Often associated with cleft lip.

**client** ('klieənt) 1. a recipient of a professional service. 2. a recipient of health care, regardless of the person's state of health and where the service is delivered. 3. a patient.

**climacteric** (klie'makto.rik, ˌkliemak-'terik) the period of the menopause in women. Also used to denote the decline in sexual drive in men.

**climax** ('kliemaks) 1. the stage when a disease is at its greatest intensity. 2. the stage in sexual intercourse when orgasm occurs.

**clindamycin** (ˌklində'miesin) an antibiotic active against Grampositive cocci and many anaerobes.

**clinic** ('klinik) 1. instruction of students at the bedside. 2. a department of a hospital devoted to the treatment of a particular type of disease.

**clinical** ('klinik'l) relating to bedside observation and the treatment of patients. *C. governance* a framework through which NHS organizations are accountable for continuously improving the quality of their services and for safeguarding high standards of care by creating an environment in which excellence in care will flourish (see Appendices). *C. nurse specialist* a qualified nurse who has acquired advanced knowledge and skills in a specific area of clinical nursing. *C. risk index for babies* abbreviated CRIB. A professional scoring tool used in assessing the initial neonatal risks for babies, and also for comparing the performance of one neonatal intensive care unit with another. *C. risk management* the means by which adverse events occurring in organizations and usually related to the delivery of patient care are systematically assessed and reviewed in order to seek ways for prevention of future incidents. *C. skills* skills required by clinicians (doctors, nurses, dentists and other clinical professions). Clinical skills vary depending on specialty but core skills remain constant, e.g. communication skills, history-taking skills, record-keeping, basic physical examination, etc. *C. supervision* an exchange between practising professionals to enable the development of professional skills. Has a vital role in sustaining and developing professional practice in nursing, midwifery and health visiting.

**clip** (klip) a metal device for holding the two edges of a wound together or for controlling the flow of liquid through a tube.

**clitoridectomy** (ˌklitə.ri'dektəmee) excision of the clitoris.

**clitoris** ('klitə.ris, 'kliet-) a small organ, formed of erectile tissue, situated at the anterior junction of the labia minora in the female.

**cloaca** (kloh'ayka) 1. the common intestinal and urogenital opening present in many vertebrates. 2. opening through newly formed bone from a diseased area so that pus may escape. *See* INVOLUCRUM.

**clofibrate** (kloh'fiebrayt) a drug which lowers the blood cholesterol.

**clomipramine** (kloh'miprə.meen) an antidepressant drug used to treat patients with obsessional fears.

**clonazepam** (kloh'nazi.pam) an anticonvulsive drug.

**clone** (klohn) cells which are genetically identical to each other and have descended by asexual reproduction from the parent cell, to which they are also genetically identical.

**clonic** ('klonik) having the character of clonus. The second stage of a grand mal fit; also referred to as a tonic–clonic seizure. *See* EPILEPSY.

**clonidine** ('klohni.deen) an antihypertensive drug which is also used to treat migraine.

**clonus** ('klohnəs) muscle rigidity and relaxation which occurs spasmodically. *Ankle c.* spasmodic movements of the calf muscles when the foot is suddenly pushed upwards, the leg being extended.

*Clostridium* (klo'stridi.əm) a genus of anaerobic spore-forming bacteria, found as commensals of the gut of animals and humans and saprophytes of the soil. Pathogenic species include *C. botulinum* (botulism), *C. tetani* (tetanus) and *C. perfringens* (also known as *C. welchii*) (gas gangrene).

**clot** (klot) a semisolid mass formed in a liquid, such as blood or lymph, by coagulation.

**clotrimazole** (kloh'triemə.zohl) an antifungal drug.

**clotting** ('kloting) coagulation. The formation of a clot; *see* BLOOD CLOTTING. *C. time* coagulation time. The length of time taken for shed blood to coagulate.

**cloxacillin** (ˌkloksə'silin) an antibiotic drug effective against penicillin-resistant staphylococci.

**clubbing** ('klubing) broadening and thickening of the tips of the fingers (and toes) due to bad circulation. It occurs in chronic diseases of the heart and respiratory system, such as congenital cardiac defect and tuberculosis.

**clubfoot** (ˌklub'fuht) talipes.

**clumping** ('klumping) the collecting together into clumps. The reaction of bacteria and blood cells when agglutination occurs.

**Co** symbol for *cobalt*.

**co-trimoxazole** (ˌkohtrie'moksə.zohl) an antibiotic drug, taken orally and used mainly to treat urinary infections.

**coagulase** (koh'agyuh.layz) an enzyme formed by pathogenic staphylococci that causes coagulation of plasma. Such bacteria are termed *c. positive*.

**coagulation** (koh.agyuh'layshən) clotting. *See* BLOOD CLOTTING.

**coagulum** (koh'agyuhləm) the mass of fibrin and cells formed when blood clots; the mass formed when other masses coagulate, e.g. milk curd.

**coal tar** ('kohl tah) a byproduct obtained in the destructive distillation of coal; used in ointment or solution in the treatment of eczema and psoriasis.

**coarctation** (ˌkoh.ahk'tayshən) a condition of contraction or stricture. *C. of aorta* a congenital malformation characterized by deformity of the aorta, causing narrowing, usually severe, of the lumen of the vessel. Surgical resection of the stricture may be performed.

**cobalt** ('kohbawlt) *symbol* Co. A metallic element, traces of which are necessary in the diet to prevent anaemia. *Radioactive c.* cobalt-60, used as a source of gamma irradiation in radiotherapy.

**cocaine** (koh'kayn) a colourless alkaloid, obtained from coca leaves, which has a powerful but brief stimulant action. Formerly used as a local anaesthetic, cocaine has been replaced by less addictive preparations like procaine, lignocaine and amethocaine. It is now a major 'recreational' drug, producing euphoria with many undesirable behavioural and social effects. It is addictive and usually taken by snorting. Also known, in its various forms, as 'crack', 'coke', 'snow', 'Charlie' or 'c'.

**cocainism** (koh'kaynizəm) addiction to cocaine. Long-term abuse is associated with a toxic psychosis similar to that caused by amphetamines.

**coccus** ('kokəs) a bacterium of spheroidal shape.

**coccydynia** (,koksi'dini,ə) persistent pain in the region of the coccyx.

**coccygeal** (kok'sijiəl) pertaining to the coccyx.

**coccyx** ('koksiks) the terminal bone of the spinal column, in which four rudimentary vertebrae are fused together to form a triangle.

**cochlea** ('kokli,ə) the spiral canal of the internal ear.

**Cochrane database** ('kokrən) database of systematic reviews of published research. An international multidisciplinary collaboration of health professionals, consumers and researchers who review randomized controlled clinical trials.

**cod liver oil** (kod ,livə 'oyl) purified oil from the liver of the codfish; valuable source of vitamins A and D.

**code** (kohd) 1. a set of rules governing one's conduct. 2. a system by which information can be communicated. *Genetic c.* the arrangement of nucleotides in the polynucleotide chain of a chromosome that governs the transmission of genetic information. *UKCC c.* a code of professional conduct for the nurse, midwife and health visitor. Revised periodically, this code is intended to provide definite standards of practice and conduct that are essential to the ethical discharge of the nurse's responsibility. *See* Appendices.

**codeine** ('kohdeen) an alkaloid of opium. A mild analgesic and antitussive.

**coeliac** ('seeli,ak) relating to the abdomen. *C. disease* gluten enteropathy. A condition of early childhood occurring soon after the child has been weaned on to cereals; characterized by steatorrhoea, distended abdomen and failure to grow. The failure of carbohydrate and fat metabolism appears to be due to the gluten in wheat and rye. The condition may continue into adult life. It is treated by giving a gluten-free diet. *C. plexus* nerve complex that supplies the abdominal organs.

**coenzyme** (koh'enziem) an organic molecule activator to a larger protein enzyme.

**cognition** (kog'nishən) the action of knowing. Cognitive function of the conscious mind in contrast to the effective (feeling) and conative (willing).

**cohort** (,koh'hawt) a group of people possessing a common characteristic, such as being born in the same year or of the same sex, used in research to make generalizations derived from quantitative data. *C. study* concerning a specific group or subpopulation in a research study.

**coitus** ('koytəs, 'koh.itəs) sexual intercourse between male and female. *C. interruptus* a method of birth control in which the erect penis is removed from the vagina before ejaculation occurs.

**colchicine** ('kolchi‚seen) a drug obtained from the seeds of *Colchicum autumnale*. Used in treating gout.

**cold** (kohld) 1. of low temperature. 2. a viral infection affecting the membranes of the nose and throat and the bronchial tubes. *C. sore* herpes simplex. *See* HERPES.

**colectomy** (koh'lektəmee) the excision of a portion or all of the colon.

**colic** ('kolik) acute paroxysmal abdominal pain. *Biliary c.* pain due to the presence of a gallstone in a bile duct. *Infantile c.* excessive crying due to pain and distress. Most common in the first 3 months of life. The infant may pull up its legs and expel gas from the anus or 'belch'. May be due to air swallowing, milk intolerance or natural hyperactivity. *Intestinal c.* severe griping spasmodic abdominal pain which may be a symptom of food poisoning or of intestinal obstruction. *Renal c.* pain due to the presence of a stone in the ureter. *Uterine c.* spasmodic pain originating in the uterus, as in dysmenorrhoea.

**coliform** ('kohli‚fawm) resembling the bacillus *Escherichia coli*.

**colistin** (koh'listin) an antibiotic produced from *Bacillus polymyxa*. Used to treat gastrointestinal and other bacterial infections.

**colitis** (kə'lietis, koh-) inflammation of the colon. It may be due to a specific organism, as in dysentery, but the term *ulcerative c.* denotes a chronic disease, often of unknown cause, in which there are attacks of diarrhoea, with the passage of blood and mucus.

**collagen** ('koləjən) a fibrous structural protein that constitutes the

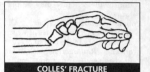

**COLLES' FRACTURE**

protein of the white (collagenous) fibres of skin, tendon, bone, cartilage and all other connective tissues. It also occurs dispersed in a gel to provide stiffening, as in the vitreous humour of the eye. *C. diseases* a group of diseases having in common certain clinical and histological features that are manifestations of involvement of connective tissues (*see* CONNECTIVE (TISSUES)).

**collapse** (kə'laps) 1. a state of extreme prostration due to defective action of the heart, severe shock or haemorrhage. 2. falling in of a structure.

**collar bone** ('kolə ‚bohn) the clavicle.

**collateral** (kə'latə.rəl) accessory to. *C. circulation see* CIRCULATION.

**Colles' fracture** ('koliz) *A. Colles, Irish surgeon, 1773–1843.* Fracture of the lower end of the radius at the wrist following a fall on the outstretched hand. Typically, it produces the 'dinner fork' deformity (*see* Figure).

**collimator** ('koli‚maytə) a shield, shutter or cone device used in radiotherapy machines to help in determining the limits of the treatment field.

**colloid** ('koloyd) 1. glue-like. 2. the translucent, yellowish, gelatinous substance resulting from colloid degeneration. 3. a chemical system composed of a continuous medium of small particles which do not settle out under the influence of gravity and will not pass through a semi-permeable membrane, as in DIALYSIS.

**coloboma** (ˌkoloh'bohmə) a congenital fissure of the eye affecting the choroid coat and the retina.

**colon** ('kohlon) the large intestine, from the caecum to the rectum (*see* Figure). *Ascending c.* that part rising up to the right of the abdomen to in front of the liver. *Descending c.* that part running down from in front of the spleen to the sigmoid colon. *Giant c.* megacolon. *Irritable c. see* IRRITABLE (BOWEL SYNDROME). *Pelvic c., sigmoid c.* that part lying in the pelvis and connecting the descending colon with the rectum. *Transverse c.* that part lying across the upper abdomen connecting the ascending and descending portions.

**colonic** (kə'lonik) pertaining to the colon. *C. irrigation* colonic LAVAGE.

**colonoscope** (koh'lonəˌskohp) a fibreoptic instrument, passed through the anus, for examining the interior of the colon.

**colony** ('kolənee) a mass of bacteria formed by multiplication of cells when bacteria are incubated under favourable conditions.

**colostomy** (kə'lostəmee) an artificial opening (stoma) in the large intestine brought to the surface of the abdomen for the purpose of evacuating the bowel.

**colostrum** (kə'lostrəm) the fluid secreted by the breasts in the last few weeks of pregnancy and for the first 3 or 4 days after delivery, until lactation begins. Colostrum is high in protein and initially low in lactose; its fat content is equivalent to breast milk. It is an important source of passive antibody.

**colour blindness** ('kulə ˌbliendnəs) achromatopsia.

**colour index** (ˌindeks) an index of the amount of haemoglobin in red blood cells. *See* BLOOD.

**colpitis** (kol'pietis) inflammation of the vagina.

**culpocele** ('kolpohˌseel) a hernia of either bladder or rectum into the vagina. Vaginocele.

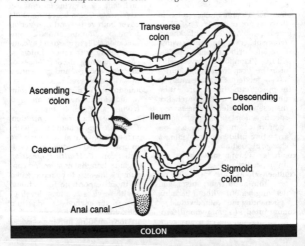

**COLON**

**colpohysterectomy** (ˌkolpohˌhistə-'rektəmee) removal of the uterus through the vagina.

**colpoperineorrhaphy** (ˌkolpohˌperi-ni'orəfee) the repair by suturing of an injured vagina and torn perineum.

**colpopexy** ('kolpohˌpeksee) suture of a prolapsed vagina to the abdominal wall.

**colpoplasty** ('kolpohˌplastee) a plastic operation on the vagina.

**colporrhaphy** (kol'po.rəfee) repair of the vagina. *Anterior c.* repair for cystocele. *Posterior c.* repair for retrocele.

**colposcope** ('kolpəˌskohp) a speculum for examining the vagina and cervix by means of a magnifying lens; used for the early detection of malignant changes.

**coma** ('kohmə) a state of unconsciousness from which the patient cannot be aroused. Characterized by an absence of both spontaneous eye movements and response to painful stimuli. *See* GLASGOW COMA SCALE.

**comatose** ('kohmə.tohs, -ˌtohz) in the condition of coma.

**comedo** (ko'meedoh) a blackhead. A plug of keratin and sebum within the dilated orifice of a hair follicle.

**comfort** ('kumˌfət) to provide relief of or freedom from pain, depression or anxiety. *C. eating* eating at inappropriate times or eating unusual amounts for the relief of distress or anxiety. *C. measure* a specific action taken to promote the comfort of the patient, e.g. re-arranging pillows or providing a change of position.

**comforter** ('kumfəˌtə) a baby's dummy or pacifier.

**commensal** (kə'mensəl) living on or within another organism, and deriving benefit without harming or benefiting the host individual.

**comminuted** ('komiˌnyootid) broken into small pieces, as in a comminuted FRACTURE.

**commissure** ('komisˌyooə) a site of union of corresponding parts, as the angle of the lips or eyelids.

**Committee on Safety of Medicines** (kə'mittee ˌsayftee) abbreviated CSM. An organization responsible for controlling the release of new drugs in the United Kingdom.

**commode** (kə'mohd) a bedside chair with a cutaway seat that allows a receptacle to be fitted underneath for the collection of urine and faeces. Used by a patient who is unable to reach the nearest lavatory.

**communicable disease** (kə'myoon-ikəb'l) a disease, the causative agents of which may pass or be carried from a person, animal or the environment to a susceptible person either directly or indirectly.

**communication skills** (kəˌmyooni-'kayshən skilz) in the broadest sense involve listening, speaking, writing and reading. In the context of health care, they generally focus on listening and giving information to patients. Communication skills cover both verbal and non-verbal forms of communication. Communication skills may extend to communicating with other clinicians, communicating at conferences or formal meetings, and presenting material in class settings.

**community** (kə'myoonitee) a group of individuals living in an area, having a common interest, or belonging to the same organization. *C. care* the care of individuals within the community, as an alternative to institutional or long-stay residential care. *C. Health Council* an organization that enables the consumer's interests to be represented to those responsible for national health services at a local level. *C. nurse* a nurse who is based within the community with a responsibility for providing nursing services within the patient's own home or environment. Community nurses have a strong commitment towards health promotion and the prevention of ill health. *Therapeutic c.* any treatment setting (usually psychiatric) which provides a living–learning situation through group processes emphasizing social, environmental and personal interactions.

**compatibility** (kəmˌpatə'bilitee) mutual suitability. The mixing together of two substances without chemical change or loss of power. *See* BLOOD GROUP.

**compensation** (ˌkompən'sayshən) 1. making good a functional or structural defect. 2. mental mechanism (unconscious) by which a person covers up a weakness by exaggerating a more desirable characteristic.

**competence** ('kompətəns) a set of professionally agreed deliverables, outputs and roles that the health care professional must be able to perform in a particular post.

**competency** ('kompətənsee) a set of behaviour patterns, knowledge and skill that the holder needs to bring to a position in order to perform the required role and functions with competence.

**complement** ('komplimənt) a substance present in normal serum which combines with the antigen–antibody complex (*c. fixation*) to destroy bacteria. *C. fixation test* measurement of the amount of complement with antigen–antibody complex. Complement fixation tests are widely used to detect antibodies for infectious diseases and include the Wassermann test for syphilis.

**complementary** (ˌkompli'mentə.ree) pertaining to that which completes or makes perfect. *C. feed* feed given to infants to supplement breast feeding when the mother has insufficient milk. *C. therapies* a range of treatments, including yoga, reflexology, homeopathy, acupuncture and others, which may be combined with traditional medicine.

**complex** ('kompleks) a grouping of various things, as of signs and symptoms, forming a syndrome. In psychology, a grouping of ideas of emotional origin which are completely or partially represented in the unconscious mind. *Inferiority c.* a compensation by assertiveness or aggression to cover a feeling of inadequacy. *See* ELECTRA COMPLEX and OEDIPUS COMPLEX.

**complication** (ˌkompli'kayshən) an accident or second disease process arising during the course of or following the primary condition; may be fatal.

**compos mentis** (ˌkompəs 'mentis) [L.] *of sound mind.*

**compound** ('kompownd) composed of two or more parts or substances. *C. fracture* a fracture in which a wound through to the skin has also occurred.

**comprehension** (ˌkompri'henshən) mental grasp of the meaning of a situation.

**compress** ('kompres) folded material, e.g. lint (wet or dry), applied to a part of the body for the relief of swelling and pain.

**compression** (kom'preshən) 1. the act of pressing upon or together; the state of being pressed together. 2. in embryology, the shortening or omission of certain developmental stages.

**compulsion** (kəm'pulshən) an overwhelming urge to perform an irrational act or ritual.

**computed axial tomography** (kəm-'pyootid) abbreviated CAT. The utilization of a computerized technique to examine a cross-section of the entire body. The CAT scanner produces an image of tissue density in a complete cross-section of the part of the body being scanned.

**computerized records** (kəm,pyoot-əriezd 'rekordz) many health records are now held on computer systems which are required by law to be secure and to maintain confidentiality, usually achieved by limiting access. Most systems currently also provide a paper printout which is stored as a manual record. *See also* DATA PROTECTION ACT.

**conation** (koh'nayshən) a striving in a certain direction. *See* COGNITION.

**concave** ('konkayv, kon'kayv) hollowed out. The opposite of convex.

**concept** ('konsept) an image or idea held in the mind.

**conception** (kən'sepshən) 1. the act of becoming pregnant, by the fertilization of an ovum. 2. a concept.

**conceptual framework** (kən,septyooəl 'fraymwərk) a group of concepts that are broadly defined and organized to provide a rationale or structure for the interpretation of information.

**concretion** (kən'kreeshən) a calculus or other hardened material present within an organ.

**concussion** (kən'kushən) a violent jarring shock. *C. of the brain* temporary loss of consciousness produced by a fall or a blow on the head. There may be amnesia, slow respiration and a weak pulse.

**conditioned response** (kən,dish-ənd ris'pons) a response that does not occur naturally but may be developed by regular association of some physiological function with an unrelated outside event, such as the ringing of a bell or flashing of a light. Soon the physiological function starts whenever the outside event occurs. Also called conditioned reflex. *Unconditioned r.* an unlearned response, i.e. one that occurs naturally.

**conditioning** (kən'dishəning) a form of learning in which a response is elicited by a neural stimulus that had previously been repeatedly presented in conjunction with the stimulus that originally elicited the response. Also called classical and respondent conditioning.

**condom** ('kondəm) a contraceptive sheath worn during sexual intercourse and affording some protection for both partners against sexually transmitted diseases. Now available for both males and females.

**conductor** (kən'duktə) 1. a substance through which electricity, light, heat or sound can pass. 2. any part of the nervous system that conveys impulses.

**condyle** ('kondiel, -dil) a rounded eminence occurring at the end of some bones, and articulating with another bone.

**condyloma** (,kondi'lohmə) *pl.* condylomata; an elevated wart-like lesion of the skin. *Condyloma acuminata* small, pointed papillomas of viral origin, usually occurring on the skin or mucous surfaces of the external genitalia or perianal region. *Condylomata lata* wide, flat, syphilitic condylomata occurring on most skin, especially about the genitals and anus.

**cone** (kohn) a solid figure with a rounded base, tapering upwards to a point. *C. biopsy* the removal of a cone-shaped section from the cervix of the uterus. It is performed for confirmation of the diagnosis when a cervical smear test result suggests the presence of precancerous cells. *Retinal c.* the cone-shaped end of a light-sensitive cell in the retina, used for acute vision and for distinguishing colours.

**confabulation** (kən,fabyuh'lay-shən) the production of fictitious memories, and the relating of experiences which have no relation to truth, to fill in the gaps due to loss of memory. A symptom of Korsakoff's syndrome.

**confidential enquiry** (ˌkonfiˈden shˈl enˈkwie.ree) a unique form of audit in which case notes are scrutinized by relevant professionals to identify substandard care and make recommendations for future practice. The triennial Confidential Enquiry into Maternal Deaths and the Confidential Enquiry into Stillbirths and Deaths in Infancy (CESDI) are directly related to maternity care, and midwives may be involved in providing appropriate information. The Confidential Enquiry into Perioperative Deaths is also available.

**confidentiality** (ˌkonfiˌdenshiˈali-tee) spoken, written or given in confidence. *See* Appendices, ninth clause of the Professional Code of Conduct published by the United Kingdom Central Council for Nurses, Midwives and Health Visitors.

**conflict** ('konflikt) a mental state arising when two opposing wishes or impulses cause emotional tension and often cannot be resolved without repressing one of the impulses into the unconscious. Conflict situations may be associated with an anxiety neurosis.

**confluent** ('konflooənt) running together.

**confusion** (kənˈfyoozhən) disturbed orientation in regard to time, place or person, sometimes accompanied by disordered consciousness.

**congenital** (kənˈjenitˈl) present at and existing from the time of birth. *C. dislocation of the hip* failure in position of the head of the femur and development of the acetabulum. *C. heart defect* a structural defect of the heart or great vessels or both. *C. infection* an infection which takes place in utero. The most important congenital infections are rubella, cytomegalovirus, herpes simplex, human immuno-deficiency virus (HIV), syphilis and toxoplasmosis.

**congestion** (kənˈjeschən) an abnormal accumulation of blood in any part. *Pulmonary c.* congestion of the lung, as in pneumonia and congestive heart failure.

**conjunctiva** (ˌkonjungkˈtievə) the mucous membrane covering the front of the eyeball and lining the eyelids.

**conjunctivitis** (kənˌjungktiˈvietis) inflammation of the conjunctiva. 'Pink eye' ophthalmia. *Catarrhal c.* a mild form, usually due to cold or irritation. *Granular c.* trachoma. *Phlyctenular c.* marked by small vesicles or ulcers on the membrane. *Purulent c.* caused by virulent organisms, with discharge of pus.

**connective** (kəˈnektiv) joining together. *C. tissues* those that develop from the mesenchyme and are formed of a matrix containing fibres and cells. Areolar tissue, cartilage and bone are examples.

**consanguinity** (ˌkonsangˈgwinitee) blood relationship.

**conscious** ('konshəs) the state of being awake or aware. Levels of consciousness are loosely defined states of awareness of and response to stimuli, essential for the assessment of an individual's neurological status. The level of consciousness is an accurate indicator of the degree of brain (dys)function.

**consent** (kənˈsent) in law, voluntary agreement with an action proposed by another. Consent is an act of reason; the person giving consent must be of sufficient mental capacity and in possession of all essential information in order to give valid and informed consent. *C. forms* in non-emergency situations, written informed consent is generally required before many clinical procedures, such as surgery (including biopsies), endoscopy and radiographic procedures involving catheterization. The doctor must explain to the patient the diagnosis, the nature of the procedure, including the risks involved and the chances of success, and the alternative methods of treatment that are available. It is recommended that consent forms should contain a signed declaration that the doctor has explained the nature of the procedure to the patient in non-technical words. Nurses or other members of the health care team may be involved in filling out the consent form and witnessing the signature of the patient.

**conservative treatment** (kən'sərvətiv) the use of non-radical methods to restore health and preserve function.

**consolidation** (kən‚soli'dayshən) a state of becoming solid. *C. of lung* in pneumonia the infected lobe becomes solid with exudate.

**constipation** (‚konsti'payshən) incomplete or infrequent action of the bowels, with consequent filling of the rectum with hard faeces. *Atonic c.* constipation due to lack of muscle tone in the bowel wall. *Spastic c.* a form of constipation where spasm of part of the bowel wall narrows the canal.

**consumer** (kən'syoomə) in health care, may be the user, client, patient or carer, in terms of the services being provided.

**consumption** (kən'sumpshən) 1. the act of consuming, or the process of being consumed. 2. a wasting away of the body; once applied to pulmonary tuberculosis.

**contact** ('kontakt) 1. a mutual touching of two bodies or persons. 2. an individual known to have been in association with an infected person or animal or a contaminated environment. *C. dermatitis* a skin rash marked by itching, swelling, blistering, oozing and scaling. It is caused by direct contact between the skin and a substance to which the person is allergic or sensitive. *C. lens* a glass or plastic lens worn under the eyelids in the front of the eye. It may be worn for therapeutic or for cosmetic reasons. *C. tracer* a health care worker who visits people known to have an infectious disease, and their partners and family to encourage them to attend a clinic for health care in an attempt to prevent the spread of the infection in the community. *C. tracing* a public health measure taken to limit the spread of infectious disease, e.g. sexually transmitted diseases, tuberculosis.

**contagion** (kən'tayjən) 1. the communication of disease from one person to another by direct contact. 2. an infectious disease.

**containment** (kən'taynmənt) a term used in communicable disease control, meaning prevention of spread of disease from a focus of infection.

**continent** ('kontinənt) 1. able to control urination and defecation. 2. exercising self-restraint, especially abstaining from sexual activity.

**continuing care** (kən'tinyooing) ongoing care of the physically, mentally and emotionally handicapped, and those suffering from chronic incapacitating illness.

**continuing education** (edyoo'kayshən) further study after the attainment of basic qualifications. This is vital for all professional practitioners so that they may keep up to date within their field and is accomplished in the form of organized study days or courses, or by individual reading.

**continuity of care** (‚konti'nyooətee) the concept of a health care provider (general practitioner, health visitor or midwife, etc.) being continually involved with a patient throughout treatment over a period which may extend over years.

**continuous ambulatory peritoneal dialysis** abbreviated CAPD. The patient is ambulant while receiving peritoneal dialysis.

**continuous positive airway pressure** abbreviated CPAP. Medical gas is delivered to the patient at positive pressure to hold open alveoli that would normally close at the end of expiration, thereby increasing oxygenation and reducing the work of breathing.

**contraception** ( ˌkontrə'sepshən) the prevention of conception and pregnancy.

**contraceptive** ( ˌkontrə'septiv) an agent used to prevent conception, e.g. condom, cap that occludes the cervix, spermicidal pessary or cream, intrauterine device (IUD) and oral contraceptives (hormone pills).

**contract** (kən'trakt, 'kontrakt) 1. to make or to enter into an agreement with a person, authority or company to deliver services or goods. 2. In health care, an agreement, usually written between two people with differing interests and concerns, who agree a course of action, behaviour or treatment with defined goals. Consequences or penalties may be included if the contract is not fulfilled.

**contraction** (kən'trakshən) a shortening or drawing together, especially applied to muscle action. *Uterine c's* those occurring during labour.

**contracture** (kən'trakchə) fibrosis causing permanent contraction. *Dupuytren's c.* contraction of the palmar fascia causing permanent bending and fixation of one or more fingers. *Volkmann's ischaemic c.* contraction resulting from impairment of the blood supply. May occur in upper or lower limbs.

**contraindication** ( ˌkontra indi' kayshən) any condition that makes a particular line of treatment impracticable or undesirable.

**contralateral** ( ˌkontrə'latə.rəl) occurring on the opposite side.

**contrast medium** ('kontrahst) a substance used in radiography to make visible or more visible certain organs.

**contrecoup** ( ˌkontrə'koo) [Fr.] an injury occurring on the opposite side or at a distance from the site of the blow, e.g. brain damage on the opposite side of the skull to the blow.

**control** (kən'trohl) 1. restraint or command of objects or events. 2. a standard for testing where the procedure is identical in all respects to the experiment but the factor being studied is absent. *Birth c.* contraception. *C. group* a group of subjects who in the course of an experimental research project do not experience the factor under consideration. This enables the researcher to make a comparison with the effects produced on the experimental group.

**controlled drugs** (kən'trold) preparations subject to the Misuse of Drugs Act (1971), Misuse of Drugs (Notification of and Supply to Addicts) Regulations (1973) and the Misuse of Drugs Regulations (1985), which regulate the prescribing and dispensing of psychoactive drugs, including narcotics, hallucinogens, depressants and stimulants.

**controlled trial** ('trieəl) a research method in which one group of subjects in a trial are not exposed to the experimental treatment or investigation, in an attempt to decrease the possibility of error and increase the possibility that the findings of the study are an accurate reflection of reality.

**contusion** (kən'tyoozhən) a bruise.

**convalescence** ( ˌkonvə'les'ns) period of recovery following illness, injury or operation.

**convection** (kən'vekshən) a method of transmission of heat by the circulation of warmed molecules of a liquid or a gas.

**conversion** (kən'vərshən) 1. the act of changing into something of different form or properties. 2. the transformation of emotions into physical manifestations. 3. manipulative correction of malposition of a fetal part during labour.

**convex** ('konveks, kon'veks) bowing outwards. Having an outline like a segment of a sphere. The opposite of concave.

**convolution** (,konvə'looshən) a fold or coil, e.g. of the cerebrum or renal tubules.

**convulsion** (kən'vulshən) involuntary contractions of the voluntary muscles. Convulsive seizures are symptomatic of some neurological disorders; they are not in themselves a disease entity. *Clonic c.* a convulsion marked by alternative contracting and relaxing of the muscles. *Febrile c.* a convulsion occurring almost exclusively in children aged 6 months to 5 years of age, and associated with a fever of 40°C or higher. *Tonic c.* prolonged contraction of the muscles, as a result of an epileptic discharge. See EPILEPSY.

**Cooley's anaemia** ('kooleez) *T.B. Cooley, American paediatrician, 1871–1945.* Thalassaemia.

**Coombs' test** (koomz) *R.R.A. Coombs, British immunologist, b. 1921.* A test to detect the presence of any antibody on the surface of the red blood cell. Used to detect rhesus incompatibility in maternal or fetal blood and in the diagnosis of haemolytic anaemia.

**coordination** (koh,awdi'nayshən) harmony of movement between several muscles or groups of muscle so that complicated manoeuvres can be made.

**coping** ('kohping) the process of contending with life difficulties in an effort to overcome or work through them. *C. mechanisms* conscious or unconscious strategies or mechanisms that a person uses to cope with stress or anxiety.

**copper** ('kopə) *symbol* Cu. A metallic element, traces of which are present in all human tissues.

**coprolalia** (,koprə'layli.ə) the uncontrolled use of obscene speech.

**coprolith** ('koprəlith) a mass of hard faeces in the rectum or colon.

**copulation** (,kopyu'layshən) coitus. Sexual intercourse between male and female.

**cord** (kawd) a long cylindrical flexible structure. *Spermatic c.* that which suspends the testicle in the scrotum, and contains the spermatic artery and vein and vas deferens. *Spinal c.* the part of the central nervous system enclosed in the spinal column. *Umbilical c.* the connection between the fetus and the placenta, through which the fetus receives nourishment. *Vocal c's* folds of mucous membrane in the larynx, which vibrate to produce the voice.

**corn** (kawn) a local hardening and thickening of the skin from pressure or friction, occurring usually on the feet.

**cornea** ('kawni.ə) the transparent portion of the anterior surface of the eyeball continuous with the sclerotic coat. *Conical c.* keratoconus.

**corneal** ('kawni.əl) pertaining to the cornea. *C. graft* a means of restoring sight by grafting healthy transparent cornea from a donor in place of diseased tissue. Keratoplasty.

**corneoscleral** (,kawnioh'skliə.rəl) relating to both the cornea and sclera. *C. junction* the point where the edge of the cornea joins the sclera. The limbus.

**cornification** (,kawnifi'kayshən) keratinization. The process whereby the skin becomes horny through the deposition of keratin.

**cornu** ('kawnyoo) a horn. *C. of the uterus* one of the two horn-shaped projections where the uterine tubes join the uterus at the upper pole on either side.

**coronal** (ka'rohn'l) relating to the crown of the head. *C. suture* the junction of the frontal and parietal bones.

**coronary** ('ko.rənə.ree) encircling. Crown-like. *C. arteries* the vessels that supply the heart. *C. artery bypass* an operation carried out to bypass a coronary artery narrowed by atheroma using a graft from a healthy saphenous vein or an internal mammary artery. *C. care unit* a ward or unit within a hospital which provides for the monitoring and intensive care by a specialist team of staff of patients who have suffered an attack of coronary thrombosis and of those who are in the immediate postoperative period following heart surgery. *C. circulation* see CIRCULATION. *C. thrombosis* see THROMBOSIS.

**coroner** ('ko.rənə) a public official (e.g. a barrister, solicitor or doctor) who holds inquests concerning sudden, violent or suspicious deaths.

**corpse** (kawps) a dead body; cadaver.

**corpulent** ('kawpyuhlənt) obese.

**corpus** ('korpəs) a body. *C. albicans* the scar tissue on the surface of the ovary which replaces the corpus luteum before the recommencement of menstruation. *C. callosum* the mass of white matter that joins the two cerebral hemispheres together. *C. cavernosum* either of the two columns of the erectile tissue forming the body of the clitoris or the penis. *C. luteum* the yellow body left on the surface of the ovary and formed from the remains of the Graafian follicle after the discharge of the ovum. If it retrogresses, menstruation occurs, but it persists for several months if pregnancy supervenes. *C. striatum* a mass of grey and white matter in the base of each cerebral hemisphere.

**corpuscle** ('kawpəs'l) a small protoplasmic body or cell, as of BLOOD or connective tissue.

**corrosive** (kə'rohsiv, -ziv) a substance that erodes and destroys.

**cortex** ('kawteks) [L.] *an outer layer*, as the bark of the trunk or root of a tree, or the outer layer of an organ or other structure, as distinguished from its inner substance. *Adrenal c.* the tissue surrounding the medulla or core of the adrenal gland. *Cerebral c.* the grey matter covering the two cerebral hemispheres. *Renal c.* the outer covering of the kidney.

**corticospinal** (ˌkawtikoh'spien'l) relating to the cerebral cortex and the spinal cord. *C. tract* the pyramidal tract. The nerve fibres making up the main pathway for rapid voluntary movement.

**corticosteroid** (ˌkawtikoh'stiə.royd) any of the hormones produced by the adrenal cortex or their synthetic substitutes. Glucocorticoids are responsible for carbohydrate, fat and protein metabolism. They have powerful anti-inflammatory properties. Mineralocorticoids, e.g. aldosterone, are responsible for salt and water regulation.

**corticotrophin** (ˌkawtikoh'trohfin) Adrenocorticotrophic hormone (ACTH).

**cortisol** ('kawtiˌsol) the naturally occurring hormone of the adrenal cortex. Hydrocortisone.

**cortisone** ('kawtiˌzohn, -ˌsohn) a naturally occurring corticosteroid. Inactive in humans until converted into cortisol. *C. acetate* a synthetic preparation with anti-inflammatory and antiallergic properties.

**Corynebacterium** (koˌrienibak-'tiə.ri.əm) a genus of slender, rodshaped, Gram-positive and non-motile bacteria. *C. diphtheriae*

Klebs–Löffler bacillus, the causative agent of diphtheria.

**coryza** (kə'riezə) acute infection of the upper respiratory tract, characterized by perfuse discharge from nasal mucous membranes, sneezing and watering of the eyes. The medical name for the common cold.

**cost effectiveness** (ˌkost iˈfektivnəs) a concept which relates cost to the effectiveness of a service and thus provides value for money, e.g. screening programmes to detect cervical cancer, rate of detection, and cost of the service and of treatment.

**costal** ('kost'l) relating to the ribs. *C. cartilages* those that connect the ribs to the sternum directly or indirectly.

**cot death** (kot) *see* SUDDEN INFANT DEATH SYNDROME.

**cotyledon** (ˌkoti'leedən) A cup-shaped depression. Applied to the subdivisions of the placenta.

**cough** (kof) voluntary or reflex explosive expulsion of air from the lungs. Its purpose is usually to expel a foreign body or accumulations of mucus. *Dry c.* one where no expectoration occurs. *Wet c.* one where expectoration of mucus or foreign body occurs. *Whooping c.* infectious disease caused by *Bordetella pertussis*.

**counselling** ('kownsəling) a process of consultation and discussion in which one individual (the counsellor) listens and offers guidance or advice to another who is experiencing difficulties (the client). The counsellor does not direct or make decisions for the client. The general aim is to solve problems and increase awareness. The emphasis is on clients finding their own solutions.

**counterextension** (ˌkowntə.rik'stenshən) 1. the holding back of the upper fragment of a fractured bone while the lower is pulled into posi-

tion. 2. the raising of the foot of the bed in such a way that the weight of the body counteracts the pull of the extension apparatus on the lower part of the limb. Used especially for fracture of the femur.

**counterirritant** (ˌkowntə.iritənt) a substance that produces mild inflammation of the skin when applied to it, but relieves pain and congestion.

**countertraction** (ˌkowntə'trakshən) the reduction of fractures by traction from two opposing directions at once.

**coupling** ('kupling) in cardiology, the frequent occurrence of a normal heart beat followed by an extraventricular one. May be found as a result of digitalis overdose.

**couvade** (koo'vahd) the experiencing of the symptoms of pregnancy and childbirth by the father. This psychosomatic phenomenon is common in many societies.

**coxa** ('koksə) the hip joint. *C. valga* a deformity of the hip in which there is an increase in the angle between the neck and the shaft of the femur. *C. vara* a deformity in which the angle between the neck and the shaft of the femur is smaller than normal.

*Coxiella* (ˌkoksi'elə) a genus of microorganisms of the order Rickettsiales. *C. burnetii* the causative agent of Q fever.

**Coxsackie virus** (kok'sakee) one of a group of enteroviruses that may give rise to a variety of illnesses, including meningitis, pleurodynia, acute myocarditis and acute pericarditis.

**crab louse** ('krab ˌlows) *Phthirus pubis. See* LOUSE.

**crack** (krak) purified form of cocaine, produced by a technique known as 'freebasing'. *See* COCAINE.

**cradle** ('krayd'l) a frame placed over the body or limb of a bed patient for protecting injured parts and preventing them from coming into contact with the bed clothes. 2. infant's bed with protective sides and, in the past, often on rockers. 3. to support, hold, comfort in the arms. *C. cap* an oily crust sometimes seen on the scalp of infants; also called milk crust (crusta lactea). Caused by excessive secretion of the sebaceous glands in the scalp.

**cramp** (kramp) a painful spasmodic muscular contraction which may result from fatigue. *Occupational c.* occurs in miners and stokers; it is associated with intense heat and dehydration.

**cranial** ('krayni.əl) relating to the cranium. *C. nerves* the 12 pairs of nerves arising directly from the brain.

**craniopharingioma** (ˌkrayniohfaˌrinji'ohmə) a cerebral tumour arising in the craniopharyngeal pouch just above the sella turcica.

**craniostenosis** (ˌkrayniohstə'nohsis) premature closure of the suture lines of the skull in an infant. Surgery may be required to relieve raised intracranial pressure.

**craniosynostosis** (ˌkrayniohsi-'nostəsis) premature closure of the cranial sutures.

**craniotabes** (ˌkraynioh'taybeez) a patchy thinning of the bones of the vault of the skull of an infant; associated with rickets.

**craniotomy** (ˌkrayni'otəmee) a surgical opening of the skull made to relieve pressure, arrest haemorrhage or remove a tumour.

**cranium** ('krayni.əm) 1. the skull 2. the bony cavity that contains the brain.

**creatine** ('kreeə teen, - tin) a nitrogenous compound present in muscle. It is also found in the urine in conditions in which muscle is rapidly broken down, e.g. acute fevers and starvation. *C. phosphate* a high-energy phosphate store in muscle.

**creatinine** (kree'atiˌneen) a normal constituent of urine; a product of protein metabolism.

**creatinuria** (kreeˌati'nyooə.ri.ə) increased concentration of creatine in the urine.

**crepitation** (ˌkrepi'tayshən) the grating sound caused by friction of the two ends of a fractured bone.

**crepitus** ('krepitəs) 1. the discharge of flatus from the bowels. 2. crepitation. 3. a crepitant râle.

**cretinism** ('kretiˌnizəm) congenital hypothyroidism. A condition caused by lack of thyroid secretion, characterized by arrested physical and mental development, dull facial expression with dry skin and lack of coordination.

**Creutzfeldt–Jakob disease** (ˌkroytsfelt'yakob) *H.G. Creutzfeldt, German physician, 1885 1961; A. Jakob, German physician, 1884–1931.* Abbreviated CJD. A rapidly progressive disease of the nervous system affecting middle-aged and elderly people. The disease has been reported in younger people treated in the past with human pituitary extract for short stature – now no longer used. It is a spongiform encephalopathy similar to the bovine form (BSE) popularly known as 'mad cow disease', and is known to be associated with an abnormal protein or prion. There is no effective treatment. A new variant of CJD has recently been reported with a shorter incubation period.

**cribriform** ('kribri fawm) perforated like a sieve. *C. plate* part of the ethmoid bone. *See* ETHMOID.

**cricoid** ('kriekoyd) ring-shaped. *C. cartilage* the ring-shaped cartilage at the lower end of the larynx.

**crisis** ('kriesis) 1. a decisive point in acute disease; the turning point towards either recovery or death. *See* LYSIS. 2. a sudden paroxysmal intensification of symptoms in the course of a disease. 3. life crisis; a period of disorganization that occurs when a person meets an obstacle to an important life goal, such as the sudden death of a family member or a difficult family conflict. *Addisonian c., adrenal c.* symptoms of fatigue, nausea and vomiting and collapse accompanying an acute attack of adrenal failure. *Blast c.* a sudden, severe change in the course of chronic myelocytic leukaemia. The clinical picture resembles that seen in acute myelogenous leukaemia, with an increase in the proportion of myeloblasts. *C. intervention* counselling or psychotherapy for patients in a life crisis that is directed at supporting the patient through the crisis and helping the patient to cope with the stressful event that precipitated it. *Identity c.* usually occurring during adolescence, manifested by a loss of the sense of the sameness and historical continuity of one's self, and inability to accept the role the individual perceives as being expected by society.

**criterion** (krie'tiə.riən) the basis on which a decision is made, e.g. for drug dosage, treatment plans, research trials, etc.

**Crohn's disease** (krohnz) *B.B. Crohn, American physician, 1884–1983.* Regional ileitis. See ILEITIS.

**Crosby capsule** ('krozbee) *W.H. Crosby, American physician, b. 1914.* A capsule attached to the end of a flexible tube which is swallowed by the patient. When the capsule reaches the small intestine, as seen on radiological examination, a biopsy of the intestinal mucosa may be taken.

**cross-matching** (ˌkros'maching) a test of the compatibility of donor blood to be transfused to a patient. See BLOOD GROUP.

**croup** (kroop) a condition resulting from acute obstruction of the larynx caused by allergy, foreign body, infection or new growth; occurs chiefly in infants and children. There is spasmodic dyspnoea, a harsh cough and stridor.

**crown** (krown) that part of the tooth that appears above the gum.

**crowning** ('krowning) the stage in labour when the top of the infant's head becomes visible at the vulva.

**cruciate** (ˌkrooshiayt) resembling a cross. *C. ligament see* LIGAMENT.

**crus** (krus) [L.] 1. *the leg*, from knee to foot. 2. a leg-like part.

**'crush' syndrome** (krush) the oedema, oliguria and other symptoms of acute renal failure that follow crushing of a part, especially a large muscle mass, causing the release of myoglobin.

**crutch** (kruch) appliance usually in the form of a light, tubular metal rod with hand grips and plastic loops for the forearms, to aid walking when the patient must not weight-bear (as in fractures of lower limbs) or when a lower limb is missing.

**cryaesthesia** (ˌkrieis'theezi.ə) abnormal sensitivity to cold.

**cryoanalgesia** (ˌkrieoh.anˈljeezi.ə, -si.ə) the relief of pain by application of cold by cryoprobe to peripheral nerves.

**cryobank** ('krieoh.bank) a facility for freezing and preserving semen at low temperatures (usually −196.5 °C) for future use.

**cryoextractor** (ˌkrieoh.ik'straktə) an instrument in which intense cold coagulates the lens of the eye for removal in cataract extraction.

**cryoprecipitate** (ˌkrieohpri'sipitayt) any precipitate that results from cooling. Of particular therapeutic value is the cryoprecipitate from fresh plasma, which is rich in factor VIII and is used to treat haemophilia.

**cryopreservation** (ˌkrieoh preza-'vayshən) maintenance of the viability of excised tissue or organs by storing at very low temperatures.

**cryosurgery** (ˌkrieoh'sərjə.ree) the use of extreme cold to destroy tissue.

**cryotherapy** (ˌkrieoh'therəpee) therapeutic use of cold.

**cryptococcosis** (ˌkriptohkok'ohsis) infection caused by the fungus *Cryptococcus neoformans*, having a predilection for the brain and meninges but also invading the skin, lungs and other parts. It particularly affects persons immunocompromised by disease or therapy.

**cryptorchidism** (krip'tawkiˌdizəm) failure of the testicles to descend into the scrotum; cryptorchism.

**crypts of Lieberkühn** (ˌkripts əv 'leebəˌkoon) *J.N. Lieberkühn, German anatomist, 1711–1756.* Glands, found in the mucous membrane of the small intestine, which secrete intestinal juice.

**CT** *see* COMPUTED AXIAL TOMOGRAPHY.

**Cu** symbol for *copper*.

**cubitus** ('kyoobitəs) 1. the forearm. 2. the elbow. *C. valgus* deformity of the elbow where the palm of the hand is abducted and thus faces outwards. *C. varus* deformity where there is adduction of the forearm.

**culdoscope** ('kuldohˌskohp) an endoscope used in culdoscopy.

**culdoscopy** (kul'doskəpee) direct visual examination of the female viscera through an endoscope introduced into the pelvic cavity through the posterior vaginal fornix.

**culture** ('kulchə) 1. the propagation of microorganisms or of living tissue cells in special media conducive to their growth. 2. a collective noun for the symbolic and acquired aspects of human society, including convention, custom and language. 3. a singular noun for the customs and features of an ethnic (racial, religious or social) group.

**cumulative** ('kyoomyuhlətiv) adding to. *C. action* the toxic effects produced by prolonged use of a drug given in comparatively small doses. Usually occurs as a result of slow excretion of the drug.

**cupping** ('kuping) 1. the formation of a cup-shaped depression with the hand: (a) to produce a skin erythema, thereby improving local circulation; and (b) to loosen excessive secretions from air passages, and perhaps induce coughing. 2. the use of a cupping glass to stimulate skin blood flow.

**curare** (kyoo'rahree) an extract from a South American plant used to poison the tips of arrows. Used in surgery to produce complete muscle relaxation, it is given intravenously as tubocurarine.

**curative** ('kyooə.rətiv) anything which promotes healing by overcoming disease.

**curettage** (ˌkyooə.ri'tahzh, kyuh-'retij) [Fr.] the scraping of a surface with a curette for therapeutic purposes or to obtain biopsy material.

**curette** (kyuh'ret) a spoon-shaped instrument used for the removal of unhealthy tissues by scraping.

**curietron** ('kyooə.riˌtron) an apparatus used for the treatment of cancer of the cervix and body of the uterus. The applicators are placed in the patient and the radioisotope is then moved in and out of the applicators by remote control.

**Curling's ulcer** ('kərlingz) an ulcer of the duodenum seen after severe burns of the body.

**curvature** ('kərvəchə) the curving of a line, whether normal or abnormal. *Spinal c.* abnormal deviation of the vertebral column.

**Cushing's disease** ('kushingz) *H.W. Cushing, American surgeon, 1869–1939.* A condition of over-secretion by the adrenal cortex due to an adenoma of the pituitary gland. Symptoms include obesity, abnormal distribution of hair and atrophy of the genital organs.

**cushingoid** ('kushing.oyd) referring to symptoms resembling those of Cushing's disease, e.g. the side-effects of steroid therapy.

**cusp** (kusp) a pointed or rounded projection, such as on the crown of a tooth, or a segment of a cardiac valve.

**cutaneous** (kyoo'tayni.əs) pertaining to the skin.

**cutdown** ('kut.down) an incision into a vein with insertion of a catheter for intravenous infusion. It is performed when an infusion cannot be started by venepuncture. Also used with hyperalimentation therapy when concentrated solutions need to be given into the superior vena cava.

**cuticle** ('kyootik.l) the narrow band of epidermis extending from the nail wall on to the nail surface; also called eponychium.

**cyanocobalamin** (.sieənohkoh-'baləmin) vitamin $B_{12}$ (anti-anaemic factor) found in liver, eggs and fish. It combines with the intrinsic factor secreted in gastric juice for absorption and is essential for erythrocyte maturation. Administered by injection in the treatment of pernicious anaemia.

**cyanosis** (.sieə'nohsis) a bluish appearance of the skin and mucous membranes, caused by imperfect oxygenation of the blood. It indicates circulatory failure and is common in respiratory diseases. It is also seen in 'blue babies'.

**cyclamate** ('sieklə.mayt, 'siklə.mayt) a non-nutritive sweetener.

**cycle** ('siek'l) a series of recurring events. *Cardiac c.* the events occur-

ring between one heart beat and the next. *Menstrual c.* the changes that occur each month in the female reproductive system.

**cyclic** ('sieklik) pertaining to or occurring in a cycle.

**cyclizine** ('siekli.zeen) an antihistamine.

**cyclobarbitone** (.siekloh'bahbi.tohn) a short-acting barbiturate drug administered orally in cases of insomnia. Prolonged use may lead to dependence.

**cyclodialysis** (.sieklohdie'aləsis) an operation used in glaucoma to improve drainage from the anterior chamber of the eye at the corneo-scleral junction.

**cyclodiathermy** (.siekloh.dieə-'thərmee) a treatment for glaucoma without penetration of the eyeball. Diathermy is applied to the sclera to cause fibrosis around the ciliary body, so allowing the aqueous humour to drain.

**cyclopenthiazide** (.sieklohpen'thiə.zied) an oral diuretic.

**cyclopentolate** (.siekloh'pentə.layt) eye drops that paralyse the ciliary muscles and dilate the pupils.

**cyclophosphamide** (.siekloh'fosfə.mied) a cytotoxic drug used in the treatment of lymphomas and leukaemia.

**cycloplegia** (.siekloh'pleeji.ə) paralysis of the ciliary muscle of the eye.

**cyclopropane** (.siekloh'prohpayn) a gas used for general anaesthesia. It is not irritating to the respiratory tract but is highly inflammable and is therefore potentially dangerous.

**cycloserine** (.siekloh'siə.rien) an antibiotic drug used in the treatment of tuberculosis resistant to first-line therapy.

**cyclosporin** (.siekloh'spo.rin, 'spor.rin) an immunosuppressive agent which does not suppress the production of antibodies. Used as prophylaxis in graft-versus-host (GVH) disease and for the prevention of graft rejection in the field of organ and tissue transplantation.

**cyclothymia** (ˌsiekloh'thiemi.ə) the alteration of mood seen in manic-depressive psychosis.

**cyesis** (sie'eesis) pregnancy. *Pseudo-c.* signs and symptoms suggestive of pregnancy arising when no fertilization has taken place. 'Phantom pregnancy'.

**cyproterone** (sie'prohtə.rohn) an anti-androgen used to treat male hypersexuality and prostatic carcinoma.

**cyst** (sist) 1. a cavity or sac with epithelium, containing liquid or semisolid matter. 2. a stage in the life cycle of certain protozoan parasites when they acquire tough protective coats. *Branchial c.* one formed in the neck from non-closure of the branchial cleft during development. *Chocolate c.* an ovarian cyst occurring in endometriosis. *Daughter c.* a small cyst that develops from a large one. *Dermoid c.* a congenital type containing skin, hair, teeth, etc. It is due to abnormal development of embryonic tissue. *Hydatid c.* the larval cyst stage of the tapeworm, usually found in the liver. *Meibomian c.* a swelling of a Meibomian gland caused by obstruction of its duct. *Multilocular c.* a cyst that is divided into compartments or locules. *Ovarian c.* a cyst of the ovary, usually non-malignant, but sometimes becoming very large and requiring surgical removal. *Retention c.* any cyst caused by blockage of a duct. *Sebaceous c.* a retention cyst caused by the blockage of a duct from a sebaceous gland so that the sebum collects. *Sublingual c.* a ranula. *Thyroglossal c.* one in the thyroglossal tract near the hyoid bone at the base of the tongue.

**cystathioninuria** (ˌsistə.thieohni-'nyooə.ri.ə) a hereditary disorder of cystathionine metabolism, marked by increased concentrations in the urine. May be associated with learning difficulties.

**cystectomy** (si'stektəmee) complete or partial removal of the urinary bladder. The ureters are diverted into an isolated ileal segment (ileal conduit) or into the sigmoid colon.

**cysteine** ('sistiˌeen, sis'tayn) a sulphur-containing amino acid formed by the ingestion of dietary proteins.

**cystic fibrosis** (ˌsistik) generalized hereditary disorder associated with accumulation of excessively thick and tenacious mucus and abnormal secretion of sweat and saliva; called also cystic fibrosis of the pancreas, and mucoviscidosis. The disease is inherited as a recessive trait. The severity of cystic fibrosis varies widely. Although it is congenital, it may not manifest itself during the early weeks of life, or it may cause intestinal obstruction and perforation in the newborn. The chief cause of complications in cystic fibrosis is the extremely thick mucus predisposing to repeated infection, leading to chronic lung disease.

**cysticercosis** (ˌsistisər'kohsis) a disease caused by infestation with the cysticercus of *Taenia solium* (pork tapeworm). Has been eliminated from the UK.

**cysticercus** (ˌsisti'sərkəs) the cystic or larval form of the tapeworm.

**cystine** ('sisteen, -tin) an amino acid closely related to cysteine. Sometimes excreted in urine in the form of minute crystals (cystinuria).

**cystinosis** (ˌsisti'nohsis) an inherited metabolic disorder in which cystine is deposited in the tissues.

**cystitis** (si'stietis) inflammation of the urinary bladder.

**cystocele** ('sistoh.seel) a prolapse of the bladder into the vagina.

**cystodiathermy** (ˌsistoh'dieə.thərmee) the application of a high-frequency electric current to the bladder mucosa, usually for the removal of papillomas.

**cystography** (si'stogrəfee) radiography of the urinary bladder after the introduction of a radio-opaque contrast medium. *Micturating c.* radiographic examination during the act of passing urine.

**cystolithiasis** (ˌsistohli'thieəsis) stone or stones in the urinary bladder.

**cystopexy** ('sistoh,peksee) an operation for stress incontinence in which the bladder neck is fastened to the fascia at the back of the symphysis pubis.

**cystoscope** ('sistə,skohp) an endoscope for examining the interior of the urinary bladder.

**cystostomy** (si'stostəmee) the operation of making a temporary or permanent opening into the urinary bladder.

**cystotomy** (si'stotəmee) incision of the urinary bladder for removal of calculi, etc. *Suprapubic c.* incision above the pubes.

**cystourethrography** (ˌsistoh,yoo.ri-'throgrəfee) radiography of the urinary bladder and urethra.

**cystourethroscope** (ˌsistoh.yoo'ree-thrə,skohp) an instrument for examining the urethra and bladder.

**cytarabine** (si'tarə,been) *see* CYTO-SINE.

**cytogenetics** (ˌsietohjə'netiks) the study of cells during mitosis in order to examine the chromosomes and the relationship between chromosome abnormality and disease.

**cytology** (sie'toləjee) the microscopic study of the form and functions of the cells of the body. *Exfoliative c.* an aid to the early diagnosis of malignant disease. Secretions or surface cells are examined for premalignant changes.

**cytolysin** (sie'tolisin) a substance that causes cytolysis. *See* BACTERIO-LYSIN and HAEMOLYSIN.

**cytolysis** (sie'tolisis) the destruction of cells.

**cytomegalic inclusion disease** (ˌsietoh'megəlik in'kloozhən) an infection due to cytomegalovirus. In the congenital form, there is hepatosplenomegaly with cirrhosis, and microcephaly with learning difficulties and development delay. Acquired disease may cause a clinical state similar to infectious mononucleosis.

**cytomegalovirus** (ˌsietoh,megəloh-'vierəs) a virus belonging to the herpes simplex group.

**cytoplasm** ('sietoh,plazəm) the protoplasmic part of the cell surrounding the nucleus.

**cytosine** ('sietoh,seen) one of the pyrimidine bases found in DEOXY-RIBONUCLEIC ACID (DNA). *C. arabinoside* an antimetabolite used in the treatment of acute leukaemia. Cytarabine.

**cytotoxic** (ˌsietoh'toksik) 1. having a deleterious effect upon cells. 2. an agent or drug that damages or destroys cells. Used to treat various forms of cancer.

**cytotoxin** (ˌsietoh'toksin) a toxin having a specific toxic action on cells of special organs.

# D

**D** symbol for *dioptre*.

**dacryocystorhinostomy** (ˌdakriohˌsistohrie'nostəmee) an operation to create a new opening between the lacrimal sac and the nasal cavity.

**dacryolith** ('dakrioh ˌlith) a calculus in a lacrimal duct.

**dacryoma** (ˌdakri'ohmə) a benign tumour which arises from the lacrimal epithelium.

**dactyl** ('daktil) a finger or toe; a digit.

**dactylology** (ˌdakti'loləjee) communication between individuals by signs made with the fingers and hands.

**daltonism** ('dawltə nizəm) colour blindness; inability to distinguish red from green.

**danazol** ('danə zol) an anterior pituitary suppressant used in the treatment of endometriosis, associated infertility and benign breast disease.

**dander** ('dandə) small scales from the hair or feathers of animals, which may be a cause of allergy in sensitive persons.

**dandruff** ('dandruf) white scales shed from the scalp. If moist from serous exudate they have a greasy appearance.

**dapsone** ('dapsohn) a sulphone drug used in the treatment of leprosy.

**darwinism** ('dahwi nizəm) *C.R. Darwin, British naturalist, 1809–1882*. The theory of the evolution of species through natural selection.

**data** ('daytə) *sing.* datum; a collection of facts. *Continuous d.* data that have a continuous set of values, e.g. for variables such as height, weight and antibody titres in response to vaccination. *D. processing* the storage and analysis of data to produce statistical tabulations, often by computer. *D. Protection Act 1984* this Act gives people the right to know what information is held about them on computers, including health-related data. The Data Protection (Subject Access Modification) (Health) Order 1987 restricted access to health information which might cause serious physical or mental harm to an individual or reveal the identity of another person. The Act did not apply to manual records and in 1990 the Access to Health Records Act was passed to enable people to have access to any computerized or manual health-related records made after 1991. Patients and clients must apply to gain access to their records; the same exceptions to access as in the original Data Protection Act remain. *D. set* a collection of information made on a group and related to certain variables that are being investigated. *Discrete d.* data with a single value or characteristic, e.g. colour of hair.

**database** ('daytəbays) information collected, stored, reviewed and updated, and used for evaluation and audit; e.g. a patient care database, in which information is gained at the initial interview, forms part of the care plan and is available for the evaluation of treatment and care.

**daunomycin** (ˌdawnoh'miesin) a cytotoxic antibiotic; daunorubicin.

**daunorubicin** (ˌdawnoh'roobisin) daunomycin.

**day care** ('day ˌkair) a specialized service for preschool children, either as a substitute for or as an extension to family life. A similar service may be provided for the elderly needing care and support and to provide respite for family carers. *See* DAY CENTRE.

**day centre** (ˌsentə) a specialized facility that offers care, treatment and a respite service for the elderly or the mentally ill.

**day nursery** (ˌnərsəree) a centre for the care, during the daytime, of children up to the age of 5 years. Provided by the social services department or by voluntary agencies. Priority is given to children from 'at risk' families and to those with a handicap.

**day patient care** a service provided either in a specialized ward or in a hospital ward for treatment/investigation/minor surgery. The patient is admitted and discharged on the same day.

**dB** symbol for *decibel*.

**D & C** dilatation and curettage.

**DDT** dichlorodiphenyltrichloroethane; dicophane. A powerful insecticide.

**deafness** ('defnəs) the inability to hear. *Conduction* or *middle ear d.* deafness due to the sound wave failing to reach the cochlea. *Perceptive* or *nerve d.* deafness due to damage to the cochlea or auditory nerve.

**deamination** (deeˌami'nayshən) a process of hydrolysis, taking place in the liver, by which amino acids are broken down and urea is formed.

**death** (deth) the cessation of all physical and chemical processes that occur in all living organisms or their cellular components. *Brain d.* the diagnosis of clinical brain stem death is governed, in the UK, by a set of guidelines ratified by the Medical Royal Colleges and their Faculties. The testing procedure is performed twice by two different doctors to eliminate any observer error. The time interval between testing is not specified. For medicolegal purposes the time of death is that time when the second examination has been completed and the patient fulfils the criteria. Performance of the brain death criteria under the appropriate circumstances allows the patient a dignified death, reduces the agony of the relatives and releases scarce resources for other seriously ill patients. *Clinical d.* the absence of heart beat (no pulse can be felt) and cessation of breathing. *Cot d.* sudden infant death syndrome (SIDS). *D. certificate* certificate issued by the registrar for deaths after receipt of a preliminary certificate completed and signed by an attending doctor, indicating the date and probable cause of death. Only after issue of this certificate, indicating that the death has been registered, can the body be disposed of. *D. instinct* a concept, introduced by Freud, proposing a self-destructive drive opposed by the sexual instinct, which perpetually seeks a renewal of life. May manifest itself as a repetition COMPULSION with the aim of annihilating oneself. *D. rate* the number of deaths per stated number of persons (100 or 10 000 or 100 000) in a certain region in a certain period.

**debility** (dĭ'bĭlĭtee) a condition of weakness and lack of physical tone.

**débridement** (di'breedmonh, day-) [Fr.] the removal of foreign substances and injured tissues from a traumatic wound. Part of the immediate treatment to promote healing.

**Debrisan** ('debrizan) trade name for a preparation of dextranomer beads used to assist wound cleaning and the desloughing of ulcers.

**decalcification** (dee‚kalsifi'kayshən) removal of calcium salts, e.g. from bone in disorders of calcium metabolism.

**decannulation** (dee‚kanyuh'layshən) the removal of a cannula.

**decapsulation** (dee‚kapsyuh'layshən) removal of a fibrous capsule.

**decay** (di'kay) 1. the gradual decomposition of dead organic matter. 2. the process or stage of ageing of living matter. *Radioactive d.* the process by which an unstable atom loses energy by the emission of gamma rays or beta or alpha particles and is transformed to a more stable atom.

**decerebrate** (dee'seri‚brayt) a person with brain damage whose neurological reactions are severely impaired and in whom cerebral functioning has ceased.

**decibel** ('desi‚bel) *symbol* dB. A unit of intensity of sound, used particularly in estimating the degree of deafness.

**decidua** (di'sidyooə) the thickened lining of the uterus for the reception of the fertilized ovum to protect the developing embryo. It is shed when pregnancy terminates.

**deciduoma** (di‚sidyoo'ohmə) an intrauterine tumour containing decidual cells. *D. malignum* chorion epithelioma.

**deciduous** (di'sidyooəs) falling off; subject to being shed, as deciduous teeth.

**decompensation** (‚deekompən'sayshən) failure to compensate. In particular, failure of the heart to overcome disability or increased work load.

**decompression** (‚deekəm'preshən) return to normal environmental pressure after exposure to greatly increased pressure. *Cerebral d.* removal of a flap of the skull and incision of the dura mater for the purpose of relieving intracranial pressure. *D. sickness* a disorder characterized by joint pains, respiratory manifestations, skin lesions and neurological signs, occurring as a result of rapid reduction in air pressure. Aviators flying at high altitudes and persons breathing compressed air in caissons and diving apparatus are particularly susceptible to this disorder.

**decongestant** (‚deekən'jestənt) 1. reducing congestion or swelling. 2. an agent that reduces congestion or swelling, usually of the nasal membranes. Decongestants may be inhaled, taken as spray or nose drops, or used orally in liquid or tablet form.

**decontamination** (‚deekən‚tami'nayshən) the freeing of a person or an object of some contaminating substance such as nerve gas, radioactive material, etc.

**decortication** (dee‚kawti'kayshən) an operation to strip the outer layer of an organ, e.g. the removal of the thickened pleura in the treatment of chronic empyema.

**decrudescence** (‚deekroo'desəns) diminution or abatement of the intensity of symptoms.

**decubitus** (di'kyoobitəs) the position assumed when lying down. *D. ulcer* an ulcer due to interference with the local circulation from prolonged or severe pressure on the surface body tissue resulting in tissue anoxia and cell death; also called bedsore and pressure sore.

**decussation** (deekə'sayshən) a crossing, particularly of nerve fibres. A chiasma. *Pyramidal d.* the crossing of the pyramidal nerve fibres in the medulla oblongata.

**defecation** (ˌdefi'kayshən) elimination of wastes and undigested food, as faeces, from the rectum.

**defence** (di'fens) behaviour directed to protection of the individual from injury. *Character d.* any character trait, e.g. a mannerism, attitude or affectation, which serves as a DEFENCE MECHANISM. *D. mechanism* in psychology, an unconscious mental process or coping pattern that lessens the anxiety associated with a situation or internal conflict and protects the person from mental discomfort. *Insanity d.* a legal concept that a person cannot be convicted of a crime if lacking criminal responsibility by reason of insanity at the time of commission of the crime.

**defervescence** (ˌdeefə'vesəns) the period of abatement of fever.

**defibrillation** (dee,fibri'layshən) the restoration of normal rhythm to the heart in ventricular or atrial fibrillation.

**defibrillator** (di'fibri,laytə) an instrument by which normal rhythm is restored in ventricular or atrial fibrillation by the application of a high-voltage electric current.

**defibrination** (dee,fibri'nayshən) the removal of fibrin from blood plasma to prevent clotting. Used in the preparation of sera.

**deficiency disease** (di'fishənsee) a condition caused by dietary or metabolic deficiency, including all diseases due to an insufficient supply of essential nutrients.

**deficit** ('defəsit) a deficiency or variation from that which is considered to be normal.

**deglutition** (ˌdeegloo'tishən) the act of swallowing.

**dehiscence** (di'hisəns) splitting open, as of a wound.

**dehydration** (ˌdeehie'drayshən) excessive loss of fluid from the body by persistent vomiting, diarrhoea or sweating, or from the lack of intake. Severe dehydration is a serious condition that may lead to fatal SHOCK, ACIDOSIS and the accumulation of waste products in the body, as in URAEMIA.

**deinstitutionalization** (ˌdee,insti-,tyooshənəlie,zayshən) *see* INSTITUTIONALIZATION.

**déjà vu** (ˌdayzhah 'voo) [Fr.] an illusion that a new experience is a repetition of a previous experience.

**deleterious** (ˌdeli'tiə.ri.əs) harmful; injurious.

**delinquency** (di'lingkwənsee) criminal or antisocial conduct, especially among juveniles.

**delirium** (di'liri.əm) mental excitement. A common condition in high fever. It is marked by an irregular expenditure of nervous energy, incoherent talk and delusions. *D. tremens* an acute psychosis common in chronic alcoholism, usually following abstinence from alcohol. *Traumatic d.* a possible occurrence after severe head injury. There is much confusion and disorientation.

**delivery** (di'livə.ree) childbirth; parturition.

**delouse** (dee'lows) to destroy or remove lice.

**Delphi technique** ('delfee tek,neek) a long-range forecasting technique in which qualitative value judgements are made about information. Judgements are made independently and anonymously, pooled and summarized before being fed back to the contributors for another round of opinion.

**deltoid** ('deltoyd) triangular. *D. muscle* the triangular muscle of the shoulder arising from the clavicle and scapula, with insertion into the humerus.

**delusion** (di'loozhən) a false idea or belief held by a person which cannot be corrected by reasoning. *D. of grandeur* erroneous belief in one's own greatness, wealth or position. *D. of persecution* paranoia. *Depressive d.* a sense of unworthiness or sinfulness.

**dementia** (di'menshi.ə) a global and progressive deterioration of the mental faculties which is irreversible and affects memory, intellect, judgement, personality and emotional control. Dementia is the result of an organic brain syndrome. The term 'brain failure' is gradually replacing the term dementia because it conveys the fact that brain failure is a process, while the term dementia simply suggests a state associated with nihilistic views on treatment and prognosis. *Arteriosclerotic d.* dementia due to insufficient blood supply to the brain caused by arteriosclerosis. *Presenile d.* occurring in people aged 40–60 years, it is due to early degeneration of small cerebral blood vessels. *See* ALZHEIMER'S DISEASE and CREUTZFELDT–JAKOB DISEASE. *Senile d.* dementia occurring in old age as the result of cerebral atrophy.

*Demodex* ('deemoh,deks) a genus of mites parasitic in the hair follicles of the host. Species of the genus cause mange in dogs and horses.

**demography** (di'mogrəfee) the social study of people viewed collectively with regard to race, occupation or conditions.

**demulcent** (di'mulsənt) an agent that soothes and allays irritation, especially of sensitive mucous membranes.

**demyelination** (di,mieəli'nayshən) destruction of the medullary or myelin sheaths of nerve fibres, such as occurs in disseminated sclerosis. Demyelinization.

**dendrite** ('dendriet) one of the protoplasmic filaments of a nerve cell by which impulses are transmitted from one neurone to another. Dendron.

**dendritic** (den'dritik) 1. appertaining to a dendrite. 2. branching. *D. ulcer* a corneal ulcer caused by the virus of herpes simplex. It has a branching appearance as it spreads.

**denervation** (,deenər'vayshən) severance or removal of the nerve supply to a part.

**dengue** ('deng.gee) a painful viral disease that occurs in tropical countries throughout the world. The virus that causes the disease, one of four types of a group B arbovirus, is carried by *Aedes* mosquitoes. Because of the intense pain in the bones, dengue is also known as breakbone fever.

**denial** (di'nieəl) a defence mechanism in which the existence of intolerable actions, ideas, changed circumstances, terminal illness, etc. is unconsciously denied.

**dental** ('dent'l) relating to dentistry or to the teeth. *D. hygienist* a trained person carrying out dental procedures such as scaling of the teeth and oral cleansing, who works with the assistance of the dentist in providing preventative dental health care. *D. nurse* assists the dentist at the patient's side in passing instruments, preparing materials and generally assisting the dentist.

**dentine** ('denteen) the calcified substance forming the bulk of a tooth between the pulp and the enamel.

**dentist** ('dentist) a person qualified to practise dentistry.

**dentistry** ('dentistree) the art and science of the teeth, mouth and associated tissues and bone. Dentistry also includes preventative dental care and education concerned with preserving the health of the teeth and gums as well as the supplying and fitting of dentures.

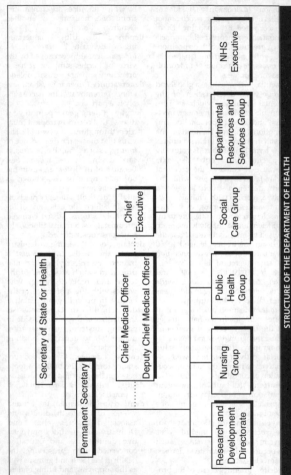

STRUCTURE OF THE DEPARTMENT OF HEALTH

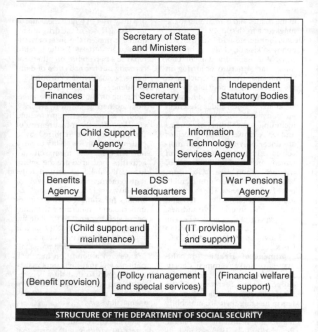

**STRUCTURE OF THE DEPARTMENT OF SOCIAL SECURITY**

**dentition** (den'tishən) the process of teething. *Primary d.* cutting of the temporary or milk teeth, beginning at the age of 6 or 7 months and continuing until the end of the second year. A full set consists of eight incisors, four canines and eight premolars: 20 in all. Deciduous dentition. *Secondary d.* cutting of the permanent teeth, beginning in the 6th or 7th year, and being complete by the 12th to 15th year except for the posterior molars or 'wisdom teeth'. There are 32 permanent teeth—eight incisors, four canines, eight premolars or bicuspids and 12 molars. Permanent dentition.

**dentoid** ('dentoyd) tooth-like.

**denture** ('denchə) a removable dental prosthesis, which may contain one artificial tooth, or several or a full set of teeth.

**deodorant** (di'ohdə.rənt) a substance which destroys or masks an offensive odour.

**deoxycortone** (dee,oksi'kawtohn) a naturally occurring adrenal steroid. *D. acetate* and *d. pivalate* synthetic preparations used in the treatment of adrenocortical insufficiency.

**deoxygenated** (dee'oksijə,naytid) deprived of oxygen. *D. blood* that which has lost much of its oxygen in the tissues and is returning to the lungs for a fresh supply.

**deoxyribonucleic acid** (di͵oksi͵rie-bohnyoo'klee.ik, -'klay-) abbreviated DNA. A nucleic acid of complex molecular structure occurring in cell nuclei as the basic structure of the genes. It is responsible for the control and passing on of hereditary characteristics, and is present in all body cells of every species, including unicellular organisms and DNA viruses. DNA molecules are linear polymers of small molecules called *nucleotides*, each of which consists of one molecule of the five-carbon sugar *deoxyribose*, bonded to a *phosphate* group and to one of the four *bases*. The four bases are two purines, *adenine* (A) and *guanine* (G), and two pyrimidines, *cytosine* (C) and *thymine* (T). The structure of DNA was described in 1953 by J.D. Watson and F.H.C. Crick.

**Department of Health** (də'paht-mənt) a central government department that is responsible for supporting the Secretary of State for Health and other health ministers in meeting their accountability to Parliament for all matters relating to the health of the nation. Reorganized in 1995 so that its structure corresponded with its main responsibilities (*see* Figure on p. 114).

**Department of Social Security** (͵sohshəl sə'kyooəritee) a central government department that is responsible for supporting the Secretary of State for Social Security and other social security ministers in meeting their accountability to Parliament including the national insurance scheme, income support, child support, welfare benefits and social services (*see* Figure on p. 115).

**dependence** (di'pendəns) 1. addiction; the total psychophysical state of a drug user in which the usual or increasing doses of the drug are required to prevent the onset of WITHDRAWAL SYMPTOMS. 2. the level of reliance a person has on others for carrying out the activities of daily living. See DEPENDENCY STUDIES.

**dependency** (di'pendənsee) a state of relying on another for love, affection, mothering, comfort, security, food, warmth, shelter, protection, etc. *D. studies* the measurement of the need for care required by a patient based on the ability to carry out self-care. The main self-care activities measured are the ability to feed, the ability to carry out toilet requirements and the level of mobility, including dressing. *D. studies for staffing ratios* studies undertaken to determine the number of staff required to provide the appropriate skills to care for specific types and numbers of patient.

**depersonalization** (dee͵pərsənəl-ie'zayshən) a condition in which patients feel that their personality has changed so that they become onlookers observing their own actions. It may occur in almost any mental illness.

**depilatory** (di'pilətə͵ree) an agent that will remove hair.

**depressant** (di'presənt) a drug that reduces functional activity of an organ. Anaesthetics, sedatives, tranquillizers and alcohol are depressants.

**depression** (di'preshən) 1. a hollow or depressed area. 2. a lowering or decrease of functional activity. 3. in psychiatry, a morbid sadness, dejection or melancholy, distinguished from grief, which is realistic and proportionate to a personal loss. Profound depression may be symptomatic of a psychiatric disorder or it may constitute the principal manifestation of a neurosis or psychosis. *Endogenous d.* occurs sometimes without obvious cause in the course of manic-depressive psychosis. The mood change is associated with slowing of thought and action and feelings of guilt. *Recessive d.* occurs as a result of some event, such as illness, loss of money, bereavement.

**deprivation** (‚depri'vayshən) loss or absence of parts, organs, powers, or things that are needed. *Emotional d.* deprivation of adequate and appropriate interpersonal or environmental experience in the early developmental years. *Maternal d. syndrome* a group of symptoms, including stunted emotional and physical development, arising in infants who have been deprived of care and love provided by a mother or mothering figure. Deprivation of maternal care during the first 3 years of life is thought to be particularly critical as this is the optimal period for the forming of social attachments. *Sensory d.* deprivation of the usual external stimuli and the opportunity for perception.

**Derbyshire neck** ('dahbishə) *see* GOITRE.

**derealization** (‚deeriəlie'zayshən) loss of a sense of reality. Surroundings and events seem unreal.

**dereism** ('deeri‚izəm) mental activity in which fantasy runs unhampered by logic and experience; describes autistic thinking.

**dermatitis** (‚dərmə'tietis) inflammation of the skin. *Contact d.* that arising from touching a substance to which the person is sensitive. *Exfoliative d.* widespread scaling and itching of the skin, sometimes occurring as a reaction to treatment with certain drugs. *Industrial d., occupational d.* that caused by exposure to chemicals or other substances met with at work. *Sensitization d.* dermatitis due to an allergic reaction. *Traumatic d.* inflammation due to injury.

*Varicose d.* dermatitis, usually of the lower portion of the leg, due to varicosities of the smaller veins. *X-ray d.* radiodermatitis; inflammatory reaction of the skin to radiotherapy.

**dermatoglyphics** (‚dərmətoh'glifiks) study of the patterns of ridges of the skin of the fingers, palms, toes and soles. Of interest in anthropology and law enforcement as a means of establishing identity, and in medicine, both clinically and as a genetic indicator, particularly of chromosomal abnormalities.

**dermatographia** (‚dərmətoh'grafi.ə) a condition in which urticarial weals occur on the skin if a blunt instrument or fingernail is lightly drawn over it.

**dermatology** (‚dərmə'toləjee) the science of skin diseases.

**dermatomycosis** (‚dərmətohmie-'kohsis) a fungal infection of the skin.

**dermatomyositis** (‚dərmətoh‚mieoh-'sietis) a collagen disease producing inflammation of the voluntary muscles with necrosis of the muscle fibres.

**dermatosis** (‚dərmə'tohsis) any skin disease, especially one which does not produce inflammation.

**dermis** ('dərmis) the skin, especially the layer under the epidermis.

**dermoid** ('dərmoyd) pertaining to the skin. *D. cyst see* CYST.

**desensitization** (dee‚sensitie'zayshən) 1. the prevention or reduction of immediate hypersensitivity reactions by the administration of graded doses of allergen; hyposensitization. *See also* IMMUNOTHERAPY. 2. in behaviour therapy, the treatment of phobias and related disorders by intentionally exposing the patient, in imagination or in real life, to emotionally distressing stimuli.

**designer drugs** (di'zienə) drugs illicitly produced to suit the tastes of individuals but now used to describe synthetic variants (drug analogues) of potent controlled drugs (including narcotics and stimulants) but which are not themselves controlled. These substances currently circumvent existing drug legislation and many are relatively easy to synthesize from common industrial chemicals. Many designer drugs are extremely potent (some synthetic analogues of heroin are 1000 times as potent as heroin) and are consequently extremely dangerous.

**desipramine** (de'siprə‚meen) an antidepressant.

**desquamation** (‚deskwə'mayshən) peeling of the superficial layer of the skin, either in flakes or in powdery form.

**detachment** (di'tachmənt) separation from or state of indifference to other people, one's surroundings or environment leading to social isolation. *D. of the retina* separation of the retina, or a part of it, from the choroid.

**detergent** (di'tərjənt) a cleansing and antiseptic agent.

**deterioration** (di‚tiə.ri.ə'rayshən) progressive impairment of function; worsening.

**detoxification** (dee‚toksifi'kayshən) the process of neutralizing toxic substances; detoxication.

**detritus** (di'trietəs) debris; material that has disintegrated.

**detrusor** (di'troozə) muscle of the urinary bladder, the action of which is to push down.

**detumescence** (‚deetyuh'mesəns) 1. the subsidence of a swelling. 2. the subsidence of an erect penis after ejaculation.

**development** (di'veləpmənt) the process of growth and differentiation. *Cognitive d.* the development of intelligence, conscious thought and problem-solving ability that begins in infancy. *Psychosexual d.*

the development of the psychological aspects of sexuality from birth to maturity. *Psychosocial d.* the development of the personality, including the acquisition of social attitudes and skills, from infancy through to maturity.

**developmental** (di‚veləp'ment'l) pertaining to development. *D. anomaly* absence, deformity or excess of body parts as the result of faulty development of the embryo. *D. milestones* significant behaviours used to mark the process of development (*see* AGE (ACHIEVEMENT)). Walking is a developmental milestone in locomotor development, conversation in cognitive development.

**deviance** ('deevi.əns) generally any pattern of behaviour that violates prevailing standards of morality or behaviour within a society. The term is usually qualified to indicate the specific form of deviance.

**deviation** (‚deevi'ayshən) variation from the normal. In ophthalmology, lack of coordination of the two eyes.

**devitalized** (dee'vietə‚liezd) devoid of vitality or life; dead.

**dexamethasone** (‚deksa'methə‚zohn) a powerful anti-inflammatory glucocorticoid.

**dextran** ('dekstran) a plasma volume expander, formed of large glucose molecules, which, given intravenously, increases the osmotic pressure of blood.

**dextrin** ('dekstrin) a soluble carbohydrate that is the first product in the breakdown of starch and glycogen to sugar.

**dextrocardia** (‚dekstroh'kahdi.ə) location of the heart in the right side of the thorax.

**dextromethorphan** (‚dekstrohme-'thorfən) a synthetic morphine derivative used as an antitussive.

**dextromoramide** (‚dekstroh'mo.‚rə‚mied) a narcotic used in the

| DIFFERENCES BETWEEN HYPERGLYCAEMIA AND HYPOGLYCAEMIA IN PATIENTS WITH DIABETES MELLITUS | | |
|---|---|---|
| | Hyperglycaemia | Hypoglycaemia |
| Onset | Slow (2–3 days) | Rapid |
| History | Has not taken insulin/acute infection | Has taken insulin 1/2–4 h previously, but has not eaten/has eaten but had unusual burst of energy |
| Patient reactions | Thirst<br>Nausea<br>Abdominal pain<br>Constipation<br>Vomiting | Irrational<br>Bad-tempered<br>Disorientated (may be mistaken for drunk) |
| Leads to | Ketoacidosis<br>Drowsiness<br>BP↓<br>Pulse weak and rapid<br>Skin dry<br>Tongue dry | Respirations normal<br>No drowsiness<br>BP normal<br>Skin moist<br>Tongue moist |
| Leads to | Coma | Coma |
| Needs | Insulin<br>Restoration of fluid balance | Glucose |
| Avoided by | Recognition of early symptoms and taking appropriate action | |

treatment of chronic pain in terminal disease.

**dextrose** ('dekstrohz, -trohs) an old chemical name for D-glucose, an important energy source for all tissues and the sole energy source for the brain. The term dextrose continues to be used to refer to glucose solutions administered intravenously for fluid or nutrient replacement.

**diabetes** (ˌdiəˈbeetis, -teez) a disease characterized by excessive excretion of urine. *See* POLYURIA. *Bronze d.* haemochromatosis. *D. insipidus* diabetes marked by an increased flow of urine of low specific gravity, accompanied by great thirst. *D. mellitus* a disturbance in the oxidation and utilization of glucose, which is secondary to a malfunction of the beta cells of the pancreas, whose function is the production and release of INSULIN (*see* Table). Because insulin is involved in the metabolism of carbohydrates, proteins and fats, diabetes is not limited to a disturbance of glucose metabolism. Polyuria, thirst and debility are common presenting symptoms. Type I diabetes results from the destruction of the insulin-producing cells of the pancreas occurring most commonly in childhood or adolescence. Type II diabetes or maturity onset diabetes is due to an insufficiency of insulin and usually occurs after the age of

40 years. The goal of treatment is to maintain blood glucose and lipid levels within normal limits and to prevent complications. There is strong support for the concept that microvascular sequelae of the disease from retinopathy and kidney degeneration can be minimized by optimal control. In both types of diabetes treatment is aimed at promoting a sense of health and wellbeing. The diet must be controlled with adequate carbohydrate and the body weight stabilized. Type I is always treated with insulin. Type II may be treated with weight reduction, diet or the use of medications which promote the production of insulin by the pancreas. Insulin therapy has now been standardized at 100 units/ml. Combinations of soluble insulin with slower-acting preparations can be tailored to suit the individual patient in the 24-h control of blood sugar. All insulin has to be given by injection, usually subcutaneously. Pump systems to deliver continuous insulin under the skin are available.

**diabetic** (‚dieə'betik) 1. relating to diabetes. 2. a person affected with diabetes. *D. gangrene*, *d. retinopathy* and *d. cataract* are complications of diabetes mellitus.

**diabetogenic** (‚dieə‚beetoh'jenik) inducing diabetes. Some drugs or physical conditions, such as pregnancy or disease, precipitate the symptoms of diabetes in those prone to the disease.

**diagnosis** (‚dieəg'nohsis) determination of the nature of a disease. *Clinical d.* diagnosis made by the study of signs and symptoms. *Differential d.* the recognition of one disease among several presenting similar symptoms. *Nursing d.* a statement of a health care problem or the potential for one in the health status of the patient/client for which the nurse is competent to intervene and treat.

**dialysate** (di'ali‚sayt) the material passing through the membrane in dialysis.

**dialyser** ('dieə‚liezə) 1. the membrane used in dialysis. 2. the machine or 'artificial kidney' used to remove waste products from the blood in cases of renal failure.

**dialysis** (die'aləsis) the process by which crystalline substances will pass through a semipermeable membrane, whereas colloids will not. In medicine this process is usually employed to remove waste and toxic products from the blood in cases of renal insufficiency. *Peritoneal d.* use of the peritoneum as the semipermeable membrane. A dialysing solution is infused into the abdominal cavity and allowed to run out again when sufficient time has elapsed for dialysis to have occurred. Waste products are thus removed from the blood. *See* HAEMODIALYSIS.

**diameter** (die'amitə) a straight line passing through the centre of a circle to opposite points on the circumference. *Cranial d's* measurement of the skull, usually of the fetal head at term. If these are abnormal, delivery through the vagina may not be possible. *Pelvic d's* measurements between the bones and joints of the pelvis made in women to determine whether the fetus can pass through at the time of childbirth.

**diamorphine hydrochloride** (die‚mawfeen hiedrə'klor‚ried) a morphine derivative similar to heroin; a powerful analgesic and drug of addiction.

**diapedesis** (‚dieəpe'deesis) the passage of white blood cells through the walls of blood capillaries.

**diaphoresis** (‚dieəfə'reesis) perspiration; particularly profuse perspiration.

**diaphoretic** (ˌdiəfor'retik) an agent that increases perspiration, e.g. pilocarpine.

**diaphragm** ('diəˌfram) 1. the muscular dome-shaped partition separating the thorax from the abdomen. 2. any separating membrane or structure. *Contraceptive d.* a rubber cap which occludes the cervix.

**diaphragmatic hernia** (ˌdiəfrag'matik) a protrusion of any or part of an abdominal organ through the diaphragm into the thoracic cavity.

**diaphysis** (di'afisis) the shaft of a long bone.

**diarrhoea** (ˌdiəə'reeə) rapid movement of faecal matter through the intestine resulting in poor absorption of water, nutritive elements and electrolytes, and producing abnormally frequent evacuation of watery stools. *Summer d.* gastroenteritis of infants, probably the result of a virus infection. It is highly contagious. *Tropical d.* sprue.

**diarthrosis** (ˌdieah'throhsis) a freely moving articulation, e.g. ball and socket joint. A synovial joint.

**diastase** ('diəˌstays, -ˌstayz) 1. an enzyme, formed during germination of seeds, which converts starch into sugar. 2. one of the pancreatic enzymes excreted in the urine and the saliva. *D. test* used to estimate the excretion of diastase and therefore pancreatic function.

**diastole** (die'astəlee) the phase of the cardiac cycle in which the heart relaxes between contractions; specifically, the period when the two ventricles are dilated by the blood flowing into them. *See* SYSTOLE.

**diathermy** ('diəˌthərmee) production of heat in a body tissue by a high frequency electric current. *Medical d.* sufficient heat is used to warm the tissues but not to harm them. *Short-wave d.* used in physiotherapy to relieve pain or treat infection *Surgical d.* of very high frequency; used to coagulate blood vessels or to dissect tissues. Cautery.

**diazepam** (die'aziˌpam) a tranquillizer with muscle relaxant and anticonvulsive properties used to relieve anxiety and in the treatment of epilepsy.

**diazoxide** (dieaz'oksied) a vasodilator given by rapid intravenous injection in the treatment of hypertensive emergencies and orally in hypoglycaemia due to a pancreatic tumour.

**DIC** disseminated intravascular coagulation.

**dichloralphenazone** (dieˌklor.ral'fenəˌzohn) a hypnotic drug of the chloral group well suited for children and causing fewer gastrointestinal upsets.

**dichlorphenamide** (ˌdieklor'fenəˌmied) a diuretic used to reduce intraocular pressure in glaucoma.

**dichromatic** (ˌdiekroh'matik) pertaining to colour blindness when there is ability to see only two of the three primary colours.

**dicophane** (di'ekohˌfayn) dichlorodiphenyltrichloroethane; chlorophenothane; DDT. An insecticide.

**dicrotic** (die'krotik) having a double beat. *D. pulse* a small wave of distension following the normal pulse beat; occurring at the closure of the aortic valve.

**dicyclomine** (die'sieklohˌmeen) an anticholinergic drug used in the treatment of peptic ulcer and spastic colon.

**dienoestrol** (ˌdie.en'eestrol) a synthetic oestrogen used to treat symptoms of atrophic vaginitis and kraurosis vulvae.

**diet** ('dieət) the customary amount and kind of food and drink taken by a person from day to day; more narrowly, a diet planned to meet the specific requirements of the individual, including or excluding certain foods. *Bland d.* one that is free from any irritating or stimulating foods. *Elimination d.* one for diagnosis of food allergy, based on omission of foods that might cause symptoms in the patient. *High-calorie d.* one that furnishes more calories than needed to maintain weight, often more than 3500–4000 kcal/day. *High-fibre d.* one relatively high in dietary fibre, which decreases bowel transit time and relieves constipation. *High-protein d.* one containing large amounts of protein, consisting largely of meats, fish, milk, peas, beans and nuts. *Hospital d.* a routine diet plan, provided in a hospital, that includes general, soft and liquid diets and modifications of them to suit the needs of specific patients. *Liquid d.* a diet limited to liquids or to foods that can be changed to a liquid state (*see also* LIQUID (DIET)). *Low-calorie d.* one containing fewer calories than needed to maintain weight, e.g. less than 1200 kcal/day for an adult. *Low-fat d.* one containing limited amounts of fat. *Low-residue d.* one with a minimum of cellulose and fibre and restriction of the connective tissue found in certain cuts of meat. It is prescribed for irritations of the intestinal tract, after surgery of the large intestine, in partial intestinal obstruction, or when limited bowel movements are desirable, as in colostomy patients. Also called low-fibre diet.

**dietetics** (ˌdieə'tetiks) the science of applying the principles of nutrition to the feeding of individuals or groups.

**diethylcarbamazine** (dieˌethilkah-'b+ceməˌzeen) an anthelmintic drug used in the treatment of filariasis.

**diethylpropion** (dieˌethil'prohpi-on) an appetite suppressant in the treatment of obesity, similar in action to an amphetamine drug.

Dependence can occur. Trade names: Apisate and Tenuate Dospan.

**dietitian** (ˌdieə'tishən) one who specializes in dietetics.

**differential** (ˌdifə'renshəl) making a difference. *D. blood count see* BLOOD COUNT. *D. diagnosis see* DIAGNOSIS.

**differentiation** (ˌdifəˌrenshi'ayshən) 1. the distinguishing of one thing from another. 2. the act or process of acquiring completely individual characteristics, such as occurs in the progressive diversification of cells and tissues in the embryo. 3. increase in morphological or chemical heterogeneity.

**diffuse** (di'fyoos, -'fyooz) scattered or widespread, as opposed to localized.

**diffusion** (di'fyoozhən) 1. the spontaneous mixing of molecules of liquid or gas so that they become equally distributed. 2. dialysis.

**diflunisal** (die'flooniˌsal) a salicylic acid derivative that, like aspirin, has analgesic and anti-inflammatory properties. It has fewer side-effects than aspirin, does not affect bleeding time or function, and has a long half-life that permits twice-daily dosage.

**digestion** (die'jeschjən, di-) 1. the act or process of converting food into chemical substances that can be absorbed into the blood and utilized by the body tissues. 2. the subjection of a substance to prolonged heat and moisture, so as to disintegrate and soften it.

**digit** ('dijit) a finger or toe. *Accessory d., supernumerary d.* an additional digit occurring as a congenital abnormality.

**digitalis** (ˌdiji'taylis) a drug used to strengthen the heartbeat and slow down the conducting power of the atrioventricular bundle, thereby enabling the ventricles to beat more effectively. Particularly valuable in treating atrial fibrillation. *Digoxin* is the chief glycoside obtained from the white foxglove. The effects of digitalis are cumulative, indicated by a very slow pulse and coupling of the beats.

**digitalization** (ˌdijitəlieˈzayshən) the administration of digitalis in a dosage schedule designed to produce and then maintain optimal therapeutic concentrations of its cardiotonic glycosides.

**digoxin** (dieˈjoksin) *see* digitalis.

**dihydrocodeine** (dieˌhiedrohˈkohdeen) a synthetic narcotic, analgesic and antitussive drug derived from codeine.

**dihydroergotamine** (dieˌhiedroh.ərˈgotaˌmeen) a drug used in the treatment of migraine. Less effective than ergotamine, but with fewer side-effects.

**dihydrotachysterol** (dieˌhiedrohˌtakiˈstiə.rol) a preparation closely related to vitamin D. Used in cases of vitamin D deficiency and in rickets.

**dilatation, dilation** (ˌdieləˈtayshən; dieˈlayshən) 1. the act of dilating or stretching. 2. the condition, as of an orifice or tubular structure, of being dilated or stretched beyond normal dimensions. *D. and curettage* expanding of the opening of the womb to permit scraping of the walls of the uterus; also called D & C. *D. of the heart* compensatory enlargement of the cavities of the heart, with thinning of the walls.

**dilator** (dieˈlaytə) 1. an instrument used for enlarging an opening or cavity such as the rectum, the male urethra or the cervix. 2. a muscle that causes dilatation. 3. a drug that causes dilatation, e.g. a vasodilator. *Hegar's d's* a series of dilators used to widen the cervical canal before examination of the uterus under anaesthesia.

**diluent** (ˈdilyooənt) 1. diluting. 2. an agent that dilutes or renders less potent or irritant.

**dimenhydrinate** (ˌdiemenˈhiedri.nayt) an antihistamine drug, useful in preventing nausea and vomiting, particularly that associated with motion sickness.

**dimercaprol** (ˌdieməˈkaprol) a drug which combines with heavy metals to form a stable compound, which is rapidly excreted. Used to treat poisoning by antimony, gold, mercury and other metals. Previously called British antilewisite or BAL.

**dimethylphthalate** (dieˌmethilˈthalayt) abbreviated DIMP. An insect repellent in liquid or ointment form that is effective for several hours when applied to the skin.

**diodone** (ˈdieəˌdohn) a contrast medium containing iodine which is similar to iodoxyl. Used in radiology of the urinary tract.

**Diogenes syndrome** (dieˈojiˌneez) gross self-neglect, usually in the elderly.

**dioptre** (dieˈoptə) *symbol* D. The unit used in measuring lenses for spectacles. When parallel light enters a lens and focuses at a distance of 1 m, the refractive power of the lens is 1 dioptre, and from this basis abnormalities are calculated.

**diphtheria** (difˈthiə.ri.ə, dip-) a severe, notifiable, infectious disease, usually of children, characterized by the formation of membranes in the throat and nose and rarely the skin (in an open wound), and toxic neurological and cardiac complications; caused by the bacillus *Corynebacterium diphtheriae*. Primary prevention is provided by the routine immunization of the population in childhood. *See* APPENDICES.

**diphtheroid** (ˈdifthəˌroyd) resembling diphtheria. A general term applied to organisms or membranes similar to true diphtheria types.

*Diphyllobothrium* (dieˌfilohˈbothri.əm) a genus of large tapeworm.

*D. latum*, the broad or fish tapeworm, grows up to 10 m long and may infest humans after the consumption of uncooked infected fish.

**dipipanone** (die'pipə‚nohn) a potent analgesic used for the relief of severe pain.

**diplegia** (die'pleeji.ə) paralysis of similar parts on either side of the body.

**diplococcus** (‚diploh'kokəs) 1. any of the spherical, lanceolate or coffee-bean-shaped bacteria occurring, usually in pairs, as a result of incomplete separation after cell division in a single plane. 2. any organism of the genus *Diplococcus*.

**diploid** ('diployd) 1. having a pair of each chromosome characteristic of a species (in humans, 46). 2. a diploid individual or cell.

**diplopia** (di'plohpi.ə) double vision, in which two images are seen in place of one, due to lack of coordination of the external muscles of the eye.

**diprophylline** (die'prohfileen) a theophylline derivative used in the treatment of bronchospasm or bronchial asthma associated with chronic bronchitis or asthma.

**dipsomania** (‚dipsoh'mayni.ə) a morbid craving for alcohol, which occurs in bouts.

**disability** (‚disə'bilitee) any restriction or lack (resulting from an impairment) of ability to perform an activity in the manner or within the range considered normal for a human being. *Developmental d.* a substantial handicap of indefinite duration, with onset before the age of 18 years, and attributable to mental handicap, autism, cerebral palsy, epilepsy or other neuropathy.

**disaccharide** (die'sakə‚ried) any of a class of sugars, e.g. maltose, lactose, each molecule of which yields two molecules of monosaccharide on hydrolysis. *D. intolerance* the inability to absorb disaccharides owing to an enzyme deficiency.

**disarticulation** (‚disah‚tikyuh'lay-shən) separation; amputation at a joint.

**disc** (disk) a flattened circular structure. *Intervertebral d.* a fibrocartilaginous pad that separates the bodies of two adjacent vertebrae. *Optic d.* a white spot in the retina. It is the point of entrance of the optic nerve.

**discharge** ('dischahj) 1. a setting free, or liberation; used for the release of a patient from hospital, clinic or therapy programme. 2. material or force set free. 3. an excretion or substance evacuated. *D. planning* the preparation required for the return of a patient to the usual life at home. *See* Appendices.

**disclosing solution** (dis'klohzing) a topically applied preparation which reveals plaque and other deposits on teeth by staining them.

**discography** (dis'kogrəfee) radiographic examination after the injection of a radio-opaque contrast medium into an intervertebral disc.

**discrete** (di‚skreet) composed of separate parts that do not become blended.

**disease** (di'zeez) a definite pathological process having a characteristic set of signs and symptoms. It may affect the whole body or any of its parts, and its aetiology, pathology and prognosis may be known or unknown. (For separate diseases, *see* under individual names.)

**disimpaction** (‚disim'pakshən) reduction of an impacted fracture.

**disinfect** (‚disin'fekt) to destroy microorganisms, but not usually bacterial spores, reducing the number of microorganisms to a level which is not harmful to health.

**disinfectant** (‚disin'fektənt) an agent that destroys infection-producing organisms Heat and certain other physical agents, such as steam, can be disinfectants, but in common usage the term is reserved for chemical substances such as glutaraldehyde, sodium hypochlorite or phenol. Disinfectants are usually applied to inanimate objects because they are too strong to be used on living tissues. Chemical disinfectants are not always effective against spore-forming bacteria.

**disinfection** (disin'fekshən) the act of disinfecting. *Terminal d.* disinfection of a sick room and its contents at the termination of a disease.

**disinfestation** (ˌdisinfe'stayshən) destruction of insects, rodents or pests present on the person or the clothes or in the surroundings, and which may transmit disease.

**dislocation** (ˌdislə'kayshən) the displacement of a bone from its natural position upon another at a joint; luxation.

**dismemberment** (dis'membəmənt) the amputation of a limb or a part of it.

**disopyramide** (ˌdiesoh'pirəˌmied) a drug given orally or by slow intravenous injection to treat ventricular arrhythmia.

**disorientation** (disˌor.ri.ent'tayshən) the loss of proper bearings, or a state of mental confusion as to time, place or identity.

**dispensary** (di'spensə.ree) any place where drugs or medicines are actually dispensed.

**displacement** (dis'playsmənt) removal to an abnormal location or position. *D. activity* in psychology, unconscious transference of an emotion from its original object on to a more acceptable substitute.

**disposition** (ˌdispə'zishən) a tendency to suffer from certain diseases.

**dissect** (die'sekt, di-) 1. to cut carefully in the study of anatomy. 2. during operation, to separate

according to natural lines of structure.

**disseminated** (di'semiˌnaytid) widely scattered or dispersed. *D. intravascular coagulation* abbreviated DIC. Widespread formation of thromboses in the capillaries. It is a secondary complication of a diverse group of obstetric, surgical, haemolytic and neoplastic disorders.

**dissociation** (diˌsohsi'ayshən, -ˌsohshi-) separation. 1. the splitting up of molecules of matter into their component parts, e.g. by heat or electrolysis. 2. in psychology, the separation of ideas, emotions or experiences from the rest of the mind, giving rise to a lack of unity of which the patient is not aware.

**distal** ('dist'l) situated away from the centre of the body or point of origin. The opposite of proximal.

**Distalgesic** (ˌdistal'jeezik) a proprietary analgesic composed of dextropropoxyphene and paracetamol.

**distension** (dis'tenshən) enlargement. *Abdominal d.* enlargement of the abdomen by gas in the intestines or fluid in the abdominal cavity.

**distichia, distichiasis** (di'stiki.ə; ˌdisti'kieəsis) the presence of a double row of eyelashes, one or both of which are turned against the eyeball, causing irritation.

**distribution** (distri'byooshən) 1. the sharing out or spreading of an agent, object or population within an area. 2. in research the relative frequencies with which scores of a different size occur.

**disulfiram** (die'sulfiˌram) a drug used in aversion therapy in alcoholism. Antabuse is a proprietary preparation.

**dithranol** ('dithrəˌnol) a synthetic preparation used in the treatment of psoriasis and eczema.

**diuresis** (ˌdieyuh'reesis) increased excretion of urine.

**diuretic** (ˌdieyuh'retik) 1. increasing urine excretion or the amount of urine. 2. an agent that promotes urine secretion. Diuretic drugs are classified by chemical structure and pharmacological action, although a diuretic medication may contain drugs from one or more groups, e.g. loop diuretics, osmotic and potassium-sparing diuretics, and thiazides.

**diurnal** (die'ərnəl) occurring during daytime or period of light. Diurnal animals have one period of rest and one of activity in 24 h.

**diverticulitis** (ˌdievə‚tikyuh'lietis) inflammation of a diverticulum. It is most common in the colon; lower abdominal pain with colic and constipation may occur. Intestinal obstruction or abscesses may develop as a result of collections of bacteria and irritating agents being trapped in small blind pouches formed in the intestinal walls.

**diverticulosis** (ˌdievə‚tikyuh'lohsis) the presence of diverticula in the colon without inflammation.

**diverticulum** (ˌdievə'tikyuləm) a pouch or pocket in the lining of a hollow organ, as in the bladder, oesophagus or large intestine. *Meckel's d.* a small sac occurring in the ileum as a congenital abnormality.

**dizygotic, dizygous** (ˌdiezie'gotik; die'ziegəs) pertaining to or derived from two separate zygotes (fertilized ova); said of twins.

**dizziness** ('dizinəs) a feeling of unsteadiness or haziness, accompanied by anxiety.

**DNA** deoxyribonucleic acid.

**dobutamine** (doh'byootə‚meen) a heart muscle stimulant administered parenterally in short-term treatment of adults with cardiac decompensation either from organic heart disease or from cardiac surgical procedures.

**Döderlein's bacillus** ('dərdə‚lienz) *A.S.G. Döderlein, German obstetrician and gynaecologist, 1860–1941.* A lactobacillus occurring normally in vaginal secretions.

**dolor** ('dolə, 'dohlə) [L.] *pain.*

**domiciliary** (ˌdomi'sil‚yaree) within or at home. *D. midwifery* the confinement of a woman in her own home, attended by a midwife and possibly by the family doctor. *D. services* health and social services provided within the home of the patient/client.

**dominant** ('dominənt) in genetics, capable of expression when carried by only one of a pair of homologous chromosomes. The opposite to recessive. *D. gene* one which will produce its characteristics when it is present in either a hetero- or homozygous state, i.e. it may be inherited from one parent only.

**'domino' booking** ('dominoh ‚buhking) a plan of maternity care whereby a mother has her baby in a consultant unit, cared for by the community midwife. They return home following delivery after an interval of at least 6 h. The name derives from *domiciliary midwife in and out.*

**donor** ('dohnə) 1. an organism that supplies living tissue to be used in another body, such as a person who furnishes blood for transfusion or an organ for transplantation. 2. a substance or compound that contributes part of itself to another substance (acceptor). *Universal d.* a person with group O blood; such blood is sometimes used in emergency transfusion. Transfusion of blood cells rather than whole blood is preferred.

**dopa** ('dohpə) the precursor of dopamine and an intermediate product in the biosynthesis of noradrenaline and adrenaline. It is used in PARKINSON'S DISEASE and manganese poisoning. Also called L-dopa and levodopa.

**dopamine** ('dohpə,meen) a substance allied to noradrenaline and used in the treatment of cardiogenic shock. Also occurs naturally in the adrenal medulla and the brain, where it functions as a transmitter of nervous impulses.

**Doppler effect** ('doplə i,fekt) the relationship of the apparent frequency of waves, as of sound, light and radio waves, to the relative motion of the source of the waves and the observer.

**Doppler ultrasound flowmeter** a device for measuring blood flow that transmits sound at a frequency of several megahertz along a blood vessel. Rapid pulsatile changes in flow as well as steady flow can be recorded, hence, it is helpful in assessing intermittent claudication, thrombus obstruction of deep veins and other abnormalities of blood flow in the major arteries and veins.

**dorsal** ('daws'l) relating to the back or posterior part of an organ.

**dorsiflexion** (,dawsi'flekshən) bending backwards of the fingers or toes, i.e. upwards.

**dorsum** ('dawsəm) 1. the back. 2. the upper or posterior surface.

**dosimeter** (doh'simitə) one of various devices used to detect and measure exposure to radiation; worn by personnel near to radiation sources.

**dothiepin** (doh'thieəpin) a tricyclic antidepressant and sedative drug.

**double-blind trial** (dub'l 'bliend trieəl) a test for the real effect of a new drug or treatment in clinical practice. Neither the patient nor the staff administering the treatment knows which of two apparently identical treatments is the new one being tested.

**douche** (doosh) a stream of fluid directed to flush out a cavity of the body.

**Douglas's pouch** ('dugləsəz) J. Douglas, British anatomist, 1675–1742. Rectouterine pouch.

**Down's syndrome** (downz) J.L.H. Down, British physician, 1828–1896. A congenital condition characterized by physical malformations and some degree of mental handicap. The disorder was formerly known as mongolism. It is also called trisomy 21 syndrome because the disorder is concerned with a defect in CHROMOSOME 21. There is a relatively high incidence in children of mothers who are in the older childbearing age. A particular type of Down's syndrome that occurs in children of younger mothers tends to occur in certain families. The term trisomy refers to the presence of three representative chromosomes in a cell instead of the usual pair. In Down's syndrome the 21st chromosome pair fails to separate when the germ cell (usually the ovum) is being formed. Thus the ovum contains 24 chromosomes, and when it is fertilized by a normal sperm carrying 23 chromosomes, the child is born with an extra chromosome (or total of 47) per cell.

**doxapram** ('doksə,pram) a respiratory stimulant used in carbon monoxide poisoning.

**doxepin** ('doksipin) a tricyclic ANTIDEPRESSANT.

**dracontiasis** (,drakon'tieəsis) a tropical disease caused by infestation with the guinea-worm; acquired by drinking contaminated water.

*Dracunculus* (dra'kungkyuhləs) a genus of roundworms; includes the guinea-worm.

**drain** (drayn) 1. to withdraw liquid generally. 2. any device by which a channel or open area may be established for exit of fluids or purulent material from a cavity, wound or infected area.

**dramatherapy** (ˌdrahmə'therəpee) the therapeutic use of drama, in which clients are encouraged to act out their feelings in order to overcome problems.

**dressing** ('dresing) material applied to cover a wound or a diseased surface of the body.

**drip** (drip) a colloquial term used to denote intravenous infusion of fluid (blood, saline, glucose) into the body.

**drive** (driev) in psychology, an urge or motivating force.

**droperidol** (droh'peri‚dol) a major tranquillizer used to control behavioural disturbances.

**droplet infection** ('droplət) infection due to inhalation of respiratory pathogens suspended in liquid particles exhaled from someone already infected.

**dropsy** ('dropsee) an old-fashioned term used to describe excess fluid in the tissues (oedema).

**drug** (drug) 1. any medicinal substance. 2. a narcotic. 3. to administer a drug. *D. abuse* the use of drugs for purposes other than those for which they are prescribed or recommended. The major groups of drugs and medicines generally considered to be most commonly misused are stimulants ('uppers'), depressants ('downers'), psychedelics and narcotics. *D. addiction* a state of periodic or chronic intoxication produced by the repeated consumption of a drug, characterized by (a) an overwhelming desire or need (compulsion) to continue use of the drug and to obtain it by any means; (b) a tendency to increase the dosage; (c) a psychological and usually a physical dependence on its effects; and (d) a detrimental effect on the individual and on society. *D. idiosyncrasy* an individual response to a drug that is unique to that person and quite different from what is expected. *D. interaction*

modification of the potency of one drug by another (or others) taken concurrently or sequentially. Some drug interactions are harmful and some may have therapeutic benefits. Present knowledge of drug interactions is limited. Drugs may also interact with various foods. In general, these interactions fall into three categories: (a) food malabsorption; (b) nutritional status; and (c) alteration of drug response by nutrients. In teaching patients self-care in the taking of prescribed medications, one should explain the need for meticulously following directions related to the intake of food and drink while the medication regimen is being followed. *D. tolerance* a progressive reduction in the effect of a drug following repeated use. To achieve the desired effect increasingly larger doses of the medication are needed.

**Dubowitz score** ('dyoobohvits ‚skor) a method used to assess gestational age in a low-birth-weight infant.

**Duchenne dystrophy** (doo‚shen) G. *B.A. Duchenne, French neurologist, 1806–1875*. Progressive muscular dystrophy occurring in childhood. *See* DYSTROPHY.

**duct** (dukt) a tube or channel for the passage of fluid, particularly one conveying the secretion of a gland.

**ductless** ('duktləs) without an excretory duct. *D. glands* ENDOCRINE glands.

**ductus** ('duktəs) a duct. *D. arteriosus* a passage connecting the pulmonary artery and aorta in intrauterine life, which normally closes at birth (*see* Figure). When it remains open it is called persistent ductus arteriosus. *See also* PATENT (DUCTUS ARTERIOSUS).

**dumping** ('dumping) the rapid evacuation of the contents of an organ. *D. syndrome* a feeling of fullness,

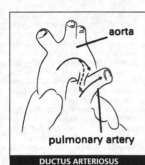

DUCTUS ARTERIOSUS

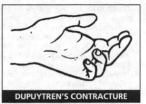

DUPUYTREN'S CONTRACTURE

weakness, sweating and dizziness which may occur after meals following a partial gastrectomy.

**duodenal** (ˌdyooəˈdeenəl) pertaining to the duodenum. *D. intubation* the use of a special tube which is passed via the mouth and stomach into the duodenum. Used for withdrawal of duodenal contents for pathological examination. *D. ulcer* a peptic ulcer occurring in the duodenum near the pylorus.

**duodenostomy** (ˌdyooəˈdiˈnostə-mee) the formation of an artificial opening into the duodenum, through the abdominal wall, for purposes of feeding in cases of gastric disease.

**duodenum** (ˌdyooəˈdeenəm) the first 20–25 cm of the small intestine, from the pyloric opening of the stomach to the jejunum. The pancreatic and common bile ducts open into it.

**Dupuytren's contraction** or **contracture** (ˌduhpwiˈtrenz) *Baron G. Dupuytren, French surgeon, 1777–1835.* Contracture of the palmar fascia, causing permanent bending and fixation of one or more fingers (*see* Figure).

**dura mater** ('dyooə.rə ˌmahtə, ˌmaytə) a strong fibrous membrane forming the outer covering of the brain and spinal cord.

**dwarfism** ('dwawfizəm) the state of being short in stature. Arrest of growth and development, e.g. due to renal rickets, cretinism or deficient pituitary function.

**dynamometer** (ˌdienəˈmomitə) an instrument for measuring the force of muscular contracture.

**dysarthrosis** (ˌdisahˈthrohsis) a deformed, dislocated or false joint.

**dyschondroplasia** (ˌdiskondroh-ˈplayzi.ə) a condition in which cartilage is deposited in the shaft of some bones. The affected bones become shortened and deformed.

**dyscrasia** (disˈkrayzi.ə) a morbid condition, usually referring to an imbalance of component elements. *See also* BLOOD DYSCRASIA.

**dysdiadochokinesis** (ˌdisdie.adə-kohkiˈneesis) a sign of cerebellar disease in which the ability to perform rapid alternating movements, such as rotating the hands, is lost.

**dysentery** ('disˈntree) inflammation of the intestine, especially of the colon, with abdominal pain, tenesmus and frequent stools, often containing blood and mucus. The causative agent may be chemical irritants, bacteria, protozoa, viruses or parasitic worms. *Amoebic d.* common in tropical countries; caused by the protozoon *Entamoeba histolytica*. Spread is decreased in places with high standards of hygiene and sanitation. A notifiable disease in the UK. Also called amoebiasis. *Bacillary d.* the most common and acute form of the disease, caused by bacteria of the genus *Shigella; S. sonnei* is the most frequent cause in the UK. A notifiable disease. Also called shigellosis.

**dysfunction** (dis'fungkshən) impairment of function.

**dysgammaglobulinaemia** (dis-‚gamə‚globyuhli'neemi.ə) an immunological deficiency state marked by selective deficiencies of one or more, but not all, classes of immunoglobulin, resulting in heightened susceptibility to infectious diseases.

**dysgenesis** (dis'jenəsis) defective development.

**dysgerminoma** (‚disjərmi'nohmə) a malignant tumour derived from germinal cells that have not been differentiated to either sex, occurring in either the ovary or the testicle.

**dyshidrosis** (dis.hi'drohsis) a disturbance of the sweat mechanism in which an itching vesicular rash may be present.

**dyskinesia** (‚diski'neezi.ə) impairment of voluntary movement.

**dyslalia** (dis'layli.ə) impairment of speech, caused by a physical disorder.

**dyslexia** (dis'leksi.ə) difficulty in reading or learning to read; accompanied by difficulty in writing and spelling correctly.

**dysmaturity** (‚dismə'tyooə.ritee) the condition of being small or immature for gestational age; said of fetuses that are the product of a pregnancy involving placental insufficiency or dysfunction. Also called small for dates, or light for gestational age.

**dysmenorrhoea** (dis‚menə'reeə) painful menstruation. *Primary (spasmodic) d.* painful menstruation occurring without apparent cause. The onset is usually shortly after puberty and occurs with each subsequent period. May be helped by hormonal therapy. *Secondary (congestive) d.* painful menstruation occurring in a woman who has previously had normal periods for some years. Often due to endometritis. The condition tends to worsen as the local congestion increases.

**dysostosis** (‚diso'stohsis) abnormal development of bone.

**dyspareunia** (‚dispa'rooni.ə) painful or difficult coitus in women.

**dyspepsia** (dis'pepsi.ə) indigestion. There may be abdominal discomfort, flatulence, nausea and sometimes vomiting. *Nervous d.* dyspepsia in which anxiety and tension aggravate the symptoms.

**dysphagia** (dis'fayji.ə) difficulty in swallowing.

**dysphasia** (dis'fayzi.ə) difficulty in speaking as the result of a brain lesion. There is a lack of coordination and an inability to arrange words in their correct order.

**dysplasia** (dis'playzi.ə) abnormal development of tissue.

**dyspnoea** (disp'neeə) difficult or laboured breathing. *Expiratory d.* difficulty in expelling air. *Inspiratory d.* difficulty in taking in air.

**dyspraxia** (dis'praksi.ə) partial loss of ability to perform coordinated movements.

**dysrhythmia** (dis'ridhmi.ə) disturbance of a regularly occurring pattern. Often applied to an abnormality of rhythm of the brain waves, as shown in an electroencephalogram.

**dystaxia** (dis'taksi.ə) difficulty in controlling voluntary movements.

**dystonia** (dis'tohni.ə) a lack of tonicity in a tissue, often referring to the muscles.

**dystrophia** (dis'trohfi.ə) dystrophy. *D. myotonica* a rare hereditary disease of early adult life in which there is progressive muscle wasting and gonadal atrophy.

**dystrophy** ('distrəfee) a disorder of an organ or tissue caused by faulty nutrition of the affected part.

Dystrophia. *Muscular d.* a group of hereditary diseases in which there is progressive muscular weakness and wasting.

**dysuria** (dis'yooə.ri.ə) difficult or painful micturition.

# E

**ear** (iə) the organ of hearing and of equilibrium (*see* Figure). It consists of three parts: (a) the *external e.*, made up of the expanded portion, or pinna, and the auditory canal, separated from the middle ear by the drum, or tympanum; (b) the *middle e.*, an irregular cavity containing three small bones (incus, malleus and stapes) that link the tympanic membrane to the internal ear; it also communicates with the pharyngotympanic tube and the mastoid cells; (c) the *internal e.*, which consists of a bony and a membranous labyrinth (the cochlea and semicircular canals).

**EB virus** Epstein–Barr virus.

**EBM** expressed breast milk. *See* EXPRESSION.

**Ebola virus disease** (eeˈbohlə) a central African viral haemorrhagic fever with acute onset and characteristic morbilliform rash. The incubation period is 2–21 days. Outbreaks have been reported in Sudan and Zaire. It has no known source, although it is probably a

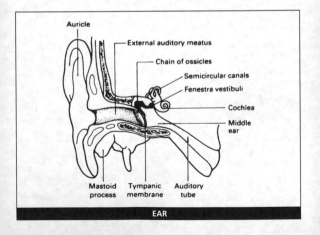

EAR

zoonosis. Person-to-person spread in hospitals and laboratories by accidental inoculation of blood and tissue fluids has occurred.

**ecchymosis** (ˌeki'mohsis) a bruise; an effusion of blood under the skin causing discoloration.

**eccrine** ('ekrien, -rin) secreting externally. Applied particularly to the sweat glands, which are generally distributed over the body. *See* APOCRINE.

**ECG** electrocardiogram.

*Echinococcus* (eˌkienoh'kokəs) a genus of tapeworm. *E. granulosus* infests dogs and may also infect humans. The larval form develops into cysts (hydatids), which occur in the liver, lung, brain and other organs.

**echocardiography** (ˌekoh kahdi'ogrəfee) a method of studying the movements of the heart by the use of ultrasound.

**echoencephalography** (ˌekoh.enˌkefə'logrəfee, - sef-) a method of brain investigation by ultrasonic echoes.

**echolalia** (ˌekoh'layli.ə) the pathological involuntary repetition of phrases or words spoken by another person.

**echopraxia** (ˌekoh'praksi.ə) the automatic repetition of the movements of others.

**echovirus** (ˌekoh'vierəs) a group of viruses (enteroviruses), the name of which was derived from the first letters of the description 'enteric cytopathogenic human orphan'. At the time of the isolation of the viruses the diseases they caused were not known, hence the term 'orphan'. It is now known that these viruses produce many types of human disease, especially aseptic meningitis, diarrhoea and respiratory diseases.

**eclampsia** (i'klampsi.ə) a severe condition in which convulsions may occur as a result of an acute toxaemia of pregnancy.

**ccmnesia** (ek'neezi.ə) forgetfulness of recent events with remembrance of more remote ones.

**ecology** (iˌkolǝjee, ee-) the study of the relationship between living organisms and the environment.

**economy** (i'konǝmee) the management of money or domestic affairs. *Token e.* in behaviour therapy, a programme of treatment in which the patient earns tokens, exchangeable for tangible rewards, by engaging in appropriate personal and social behaviour, and loses tokens for antisocial behaviour.

**ecstasy** ('ekstǝ see) 1. a feeling of exaltation. It may be accompanied by sensory impairment and lack of activity but with an expression of rapture. 2. an illegal drug that has become extremely popular since the late 1980s. It is particularly widely used as an accompaniment to modern dance music. Has resulted in several fatalities in young people. Causes intense thirst leading to the drinking of large quantities of water resulting in fatal damage of the body's fluid balance, kidney failure and coma. Also known as 'MDMA', 'E' or 'ecky'.

**ECT** electroconvulsive therapy.

**ectoderm** ('ektoh dǝrm) the outer germinal layer of the developing embryo from which the skin and nervous system are derived.

**ectogenous** (ek'tojǝnǝs) produced outside an organism. *See* ENDOGENOUS.

**ectoparasite** (ˌektoh'parǝ slet) a parasite that spends all or part of its life on the external surface of its host, e.g. a louse.

**ectopia** (ek'tohpi.ə) displacement or abnormal position of any part. *E. cordis* congenital malposition of the heart outside the thoracic cavity. *E. vesicae* a defect of the abdominal wall in which the bladder is exposed.

**ectopic** (ek'topik) 1. pertaining to or characterized by ectopy. 2. located away from the normal position. 3. arising or produced at an abnormal site or in a tissue where it is not normally found. *E. pregnancy* pregnancy in which the fertilized ovum becomes implanted outside the uterus instead of in the wall of the uterus. Also called extrauterine pregnancy.

**ectopy** ('ektə,pee) displacement or malposition, especially if congenital.

**ectropion** (ek'trohpi.ən) eversion of an eyelid, often due to contraction of the skin or to paralysis. It causes a persistent overflow of tears and hypertrophy of exposed conjunctiva.

**eczema** ('eksimə, 'eksmə) 1. a general term for any superficial inflammatory process involving primarily the epidermis, marked early by redness, itching, minute papules and vesicles, weeping, oozing and crusting, and later by scaling, lichenification and often pigmentation. 2. atopic dermatitis. Eczema is a common allergic reaction in children but it also occurs in adults. Childhood eczema often begins in infancy, the rash appearing on the face, neck and folds of elbows and knees. It may disappear by itself when an offending food is removed from the diet, or it may become more extensive and in some instances cover the entire surface of the body. Severe eczema can be complicated by skin infections. The cause of eczema can be either exogenous (due to external or traumatic factors) or endogenous (due to internal or constitutional factors).

**edentulous** (ee'dentyuhləs, -'dench-) without natural teeth.

**EDTA** ethylenediaminetetra-acetic acid.

**EEG** electroencephalogram.

**effacement** (i'faysmənt) taking up of the cervix. The process by which the internal os dilates, so opening out the cervical canal and leaving only a circular orifice, the external os. This process precedes cervical dilatation, particularly in a primigravida, while both occur simultaneously in a multigravida during labour.

**effector** (i'fektor) a motor or sensory nerve ending in a muscle, gland or organ.

**efferent** ('efə.rənt) conveying from the centre to the periphery. *See also* AFFERENT. *E. nerves* nerves coming from the brain to supply the muscles and glands.

**effleurage** (,eflə'rahzh) [Fr.] stroking movement in massage. In NATURAL CHILDBIRTH, a light circular stroke of the lower abdomen, done in rhythm to control breathing, to aid in relaxation of the abdominal muscles, and to increase concentration during a uterine contraction. The stroking is accomplished by moving the wrist only.

**effort syndrome** ('efət) a condition characterized by breathlessness, palpitations, chest pain and fatigue, caused by an abnormal anxiety; often found in soldiers but may also occur in other individuals.

**effusion** (i'fyoozhən) the escape of blood, serum or other fluid into surrounding tissues or cavities.

**ego** ('eegoh, 'eg-) in psychoanalytical theory, that part of the mind which the individual experiences as 'self'. The ego is concerned with satisfying the unconscious primitive demands of the 'id' in a socially acceptable form.

**eidetic** (ie'detik) having the ability to visualize exactly objects or events which have previously been seen. Having a photographic memory.

**Eisenmenger's complex** ('iez'n,mengəz) *V. Eisenmenger, German* *physician, 1864–1932.* A congenital heart defect in which a ventricular septal defect is associated with increased pulmonary vascular resistance.

**ejaculation** (i,jakyuh'layshən) the act of ejecting semen, a reflex action that occurs as the result of sexual stimulation.

**elastic** (i'lastik) capable of stretching. *E. bandage* one that will stretch and will exert continuous pressure on the part bandaged. *E. stocking* a woven rubber stocking sometimes worn for varicose veins. *E. tissue* connective tissue containing yellow elastic fibres.

**elation** (i'layshən) in psychiatry, a feeling of wellbeing or a state of excitement. It occurs to a marked degree in hypomania and to an intense degree in mania. *See* EUPHORIA.

**elbow** ('elboh) the joint between the upper arm and the forearm. It is formed by the humerus above and the radius and ulna below.

**elective** (i'lektiv) usually pertaining to a surgical procedure that is performed by choice, as opposed to an emergency life-saving procedure. Timing of the procedure may also be arranged to be mutually convenient for the patient and surgeon.

**Electra complex** (i'lektrə) libidinous fixation of a daughter towards her father. The female version of the Oedipus complex.

**electro-oculography** (i,lektroh,-okyuhlogrəfee) *see* ELECTRORETINOGRAPHY.

**electrocardiogram** (i,lektroh'kahdioh,gram) abbreviated ECG. A tracing made of the various phases of the heart's action by means of an electrocardiograph. The normal electrocardiogram is composed of a P wave, Q, R and S waves (known as the QRS COMPLEX, or QRS wave), and a T wave. The P wave occurs at the beginning of each contraction of the atria. The QRS wave occurs at the beginning of each contraction of the ventricles. The T wave seen in a normal electrocardiogram occurs as the ventricles recover electrically and prepare for the next contraction. There is a refractory period between these waves.

**electrocardiograph** (i,lektroh'kahdioh,grahf, -,graf) a machine that records the electrical potential of the heart from electrodes on the chest and limbs.

**electrocautery** (i,lektroh'kawtə,ree) an instrument for the destruction of tissue by means of an electrically heated needle or wire loop.

**electrocoagulation** (i,lektrohkoh,agyuh'layshən) a method of coagulation using a high-frequency current. A form of surgical diathermy.

**electroconvulsive therapy** (i,lektrohkən'vulsiv) abbreviated ECT. Electroplexy. The passage of an electric current through the frontal lobes of the brain, which causes a convulsion. It is used in the treatment of depression and sometimes of schizophrenia. A general anaesthetic and muscle relaxant are given before treatment.

**electrocorticography** (i,lektroh,-kawti'kogrəfee) electroencephalography with the electrodes applied directly to the cortex of the brain during surgery to locate a small lesion, e.g. a scar.

**electrode** (i'lektrohd) the terminal of a conducting system or cell of a battery, through which electricity enters or leaves the body.

**electroencephalogram** (i,lektroh,-en'kafələ,gram, -'sef-) abbreviated EEG. A tracing of the electrical activity of the brain. Abnormal rhythm is an aid to diagnosis in epilepsy and cerebral tumour.

**electroencephalograph** (i,lektroh,en-'kefələ,grahf, -,graf,-'sef-) a machine for recording the electrical activity of the cortex of the brain. The electrodes are applied to the scalp.

**electrolysis** (ˌilek'trolisis, ˌelek-) 1. chemical decomposition by means of electricity, e.g. an electric current passed through water decomposes it into oxygen and hydrogen. 2. the destruction of tissue by means of electricity, e.g. the removal of surplus hair.

**electrolyte** (i'lektrəˌliet) a compound which, when dissolved in a solution, will dissociate into ions. These ions are electrically charged particles and will thus conduct electricity. *E. balance* the maintenance of the correct balance between the different elements in the body tissues and fluids.

**electron** (i'lektron) a negatively charged particle revolving round the nucleus of an ATOM. *E. microscope* a type of microscope employing a beam of electrons rather than a beam of light, which allows very small particles such as viruses to be identified.

**electrophoresis** (iˌlektrohfə'reesis) a method of analysing the different proteins in blood serum by passing an electric current through the serum to separate the electrically charged particles. The particles gradually separate into bands as a result of the difference in rate of movement according to the electrical charge on the particles.

**electroplexy** (iˌlektroh'plekse) electroconvulsive therapy.

**electroretinography** (iˌlektroh.-reti'nogrəfee) a method of examining the retina of the eye by means of electrodes and light stimulation for assessment of retinal damage.

**element** ('elimənt) 1. any of the primary parts or constituents of a compound. 2. in chemistry, a simple substance that cannot be decomposed by ordinary chemical means; the basic 'stuff' of which all matter is composed.

**elephantiasis** (ˌelefən'tieəsis) a chronic disease of the lymphatics producing excessive thickening of the skin and swelling of the parts affected, usually the lower limbs. It may be due to filariasis in tropical and subtropical climates.

**elevator** ('eliˌvaytə) an instrument used as a lever for raising bone, etc. *Periosteal e.* instrument that strips the periosteum in bone surgery.

**elimination** (iˌlimi'nayshən) the removal of waste matter, particularly from the body. Excretion.

**ELISA** (e'liezə) abbreviation for enzyme-linked immunosorbent assay, a blood test first used for the detection of antibodies to the human immunodeficiency virus (HIV) but which may be used to detect the presence of other antibodies in the blood. It may give a false-negative or false-positive result: a follow-up test should always be offered after a positive result.

**elixir** (i'liksə) a sweetened spirituous liquid, used largely as a flavouring agent to hide the unpleasant taste of some drugs.

**emaciation** (iˌmaysi'ayshən) excessive wasting of body tissues. Extreme thinness.

**emasculation** (iˌmaskyuh'layshən) the removal of the penis or testicles; castration.

**embolectomy** (ˌembə'lektəmee) surgical removal of an embolus, frequently arterial emboli that are cutting off the blood supply to the limbs.

**embolism** ('embəˌlizəm) obstruction of a blood vessel by a travelling blood clot or particle of matter. *Air e.* the presence of gas or air bubbles, usually sucked into the large veins from a wound in the neck or chest. *Cerebral e.* obstruction of a vessel in the brain. *Coronary e.* the blockage of a coronary vessel with a clot. *Fat e.* globules of fat released into the blood from a fractured bone. *Infective e.* detached particles of infected blood clot from an area of inflammation which, obstructing small vessels, result in abscess formation, i.e. pyaemia. *Pulmonary e.* blocking of the pulmonary artery or one of its branches by a detached clot, usually due to thrombosis in the femoral or iliac veins. *Retinal e.* blockage, due to air or a blood clot, of the central retinal artery, resulting in loss of vision.

**embolus** ('embələs) a substance carried by the bloodstream until it causes obstruction by blocking a blood vessel. *See* EMBOLISM.

**embrocation** (,embroh'kayshən) a liquid applied to the body by rubbing to treat strains. A liniment.

**embryo** ('embri,oh) the fertilized ovum in its earliest stages, i.e. until it shows human characteristics during the second month. After this it is termed a fetus.

**embryology** (,embri'olajee) the study of the growth and development of the embryo from the unicellular stage until birth.

**emergency** (i'mərjənsee) a sudden crisis requiring urgent intervention. *E. obstetric unit* an emergency team from a consultant obstetric unit which goes out to obstetric emergencies in the community or, in general practitioner units, taking the appropriate equipment, including O-negative blood for transfusion. *E. protection order* a court order whereby a child is arbitrarily removed from the care of the parents in the interests of the child's safety.

**emesis** ('emasis) vomiting.

**emetic** (i'metik) an agent that can induce vomiting.

**eminence** ('eminans) a projection, usually rounded, from a surface, e.g. of a bone.

**emission** (i'mishən) involuntary ejection (of semen).

**EMLA** ('emlə) a cream for local application to a skin site, containing a mixture of local anaesthetics. Particularly useful for children as it allows for painful tests and biopsies to be performed with minimal pain and discomfort.

**emollient** (i'moli,ənt, -'moh-) any substance used to soothe or soften the skin.

**emotion** (i'mohshən) feeling or affect; a state of arousal characterized by alteration of feeling tone and by physiological behavioural changes. The physical form of emotion may be outward and evident to others, as in crying, laughing, blushing or a variety of facial expressions; however, emotion is not always reflected in the appearance and actions even though psychic changes are taking place. Joy, grief, fear and anger are examples of emotions.

**empathy** ('empəthee) the power of projecting oneself into the feelings of another person or into a situation.

**emphysema** (,emfi'seemə, -fie-) the abnormal presence of air in tissues or cavities of the body. *Pulmonary e.* a chronic disease of the lungs. Distension of alveoli causes intervening walls to be broken down and bullae to form on the lung surface. It also causes distension of the bronchioles and eventual loss of elasticity so that inspired air cannot be expired, making breathing difficult. *Surgical e.* the presence of air or any other gas in the subcutaneous tissues, introduced through a wound and evidenced by crepitation on pressure.

**empirical** (em'pirik'l) based on experience and not on scientific reasoning.

**empowerment** (em'powəmənt) the capacity to empower, to give power or authority, e.g. to patients through the mechanism of the

'Patient's Charter' or the 'Changing Childbirth Report' for pregnant women, to take control over their own care and to work in partnership with care providers.

**empyema** (ˌempie'eemə) a collection of pus in a cavity, most commonly referring to the pleural cavity.

**emulsion** (i'mulshən) a mixture in which an oil is suspended in water by the addition of an emulsifying agent.

**en face** (ˌohn 'fas) [Fr.] a position in which the mother's face and that of her infant are on the same plane and approximately 20 cm apart; a position usually held during breastfeeding.

**enamel** (i'naməl) the hard outer covering of the crown of a tooth.

**enarthrosis** (ˌenah'throhsis) a freely moving joint, e.g. ball and socket joint.

**ENB** English National Board for Nursing, Midwifery and Health Visiting. *See* NATIONAL BOARDS.

**encanthis** (en'kanthis) a small fleshy growth at the inner canthus of the eye, which may form an abscess.

**encapsulated** (en'kapsyuh‚laytid) enclosed in a capsule.

**encephalin (enkephalin)** (en'kefəlin, -'sef-) an opiate-like substance produced by the pituitary which has analgesic effects. This substance may also be produced synthetically. *See* ENDORPHIN.

**encephalitis** (en‚kefə'lietis, -‚sef-) inflammation of the brain. There are many types of encephalitis, depending on the causative agent and the structures involved. The symptoms may be mild, with headache, general malaise and muscle ache similar to that associated with influenza. The more acute and serious symptoms may include fever, delirium, convulsions and coma, and in a significant number of patients result in death.

**encephalocele** (en'kefəloh‚seel, -'sef-) herniation of the brain through the skull.

**encephalography** (en‚kefə'logrəfee, -‚sef-) radiographic examination of the ventricles of the brain after the insertion of air or a gas through a lumbar or cisternal puncture.

**encephalomalacia** (en‚kefəlohmə-'layshi.ə, -‚sef-) softening of the brain.

**encephalomyelitis** (en‚kefəloh‚mieə'lietis, -‚sef-) inflammation of the brain and spinal cord.

**encephalomyelopathy** (en‚kefəloh‚mieə'lopəthee, -‚sef-) any disease condition of the brain and spinal cord.

**encephalon** (en'kefəlon, -'sef-) the brain with the spinal cord, constituting the central nervous system.

**encephalopathy** (en‚kefə'lopəthee, -‚sef-) cerebral dysfunction with diffuse disease or damage of the brain. *Dialysis e.* associated with long-term use of haemodialysis; marked by speech disorders and myoclonic fits progressing to global dementia. *Hepatic e.* a condition caused by liver failure, leading to dementia and then coma. *Hypertensive e.* a transient disturbance of function associated with hypertension. Disorientation, excitability and abnormal behaviour occur, which may be reversed if the pressure is reduced. *Wernicke's e.* a complication associated with chronic alcoholism; characterized by paralysis of the eye muscles, diplopia, nystagmus, ataxia and mental changes.

**encopresis** (ˌenkə'preesis) incontinence of faeces not due to organic defect or illness.

**endarterectomy** (ˌendahtə'rektəmee) the surgical removal of the lining of an artery, usually because of narrowing of the vessel by atheromatous plaques. *Thrombo-e.* removal of a clot with the lining.

**endarteritis** (ˌendahtəˈrletis) inflammation of the innermost coat of an artery. *E. obliterans* a type that causes collapse and obstruction in small arteries.

**endemic** (en'demik) pertaining to a disease prevalent in a particular locality.

**endemiology** (enˌdeemi'oləjee) the study of all the factors pertaining to endemic disease.

**endocarditis** (ˌendohkah'dietis) inflammation of the endocardium characterized by vegetations on the endocardium and heart valves. Due to infection by microorganisms, fungi or *Rickettsia*, or to rheumatic fever.

**endocardium** (ˌendoh'kahdi.əm) the membrane lining the heart.

**endocervicitis** (ˌendohˌsərvi'sietis) inflammation of the membrane lining the uterine cervix.

**endocrine** (ˈendohˌkrin, -ˌkrien) secreting within. Applied to those glands whose secretions (hormones) flow directly into the blood and not outwards through a duct. The chief endocrine glands are the thyroid, parathyroids, suprarenals and pituitary. The pancreas, stomach, liver, ovaries and testes also produce internal secretions. *See* EXOCRINE.

**endocrinology** (ˌendohkri'nolajee) the science of the endocrine glands and their secretions.

**endoderm** ('endoh dərm) entoderm.

**endogenous** (en'dojənəs) produced within the organism; *see* EXOGENOUS. *E. depression* one in which the disease derives from internal causes.

**endolymph** ('endoh limf) the fluid inside the membranous labyrinth of the ear.

**endometriosis** (ˌendoh meetri'ohsis) the presence of endometrium in an abnormal situation, e.g. in the ovaries, the intestines or the urinary bladder. The ectopic tissue undergoes the same hormonal changes as normal endometrium (*see* Figure on p. 140). As there is no outlet for bleeding when menstruation occurs, the woman suffers severe pain.

**endometritis** (ˌendohmi'trietis) inflammation of the endometrium.

**endometrium** (ˌendoh'meetri.əm) the mucous membrane lining the uterus.

**endomyocarditis** (ˌendoh mieohkah'dietis) inflammation of the lining membrane and muscles of the heart.

**endoparasite** (ˌendoh'parə siet) a parasite that lives within the body of its host.

**endophthalmitis** (ˌendofthal'mietis) inflammation of the ocular cavity and adjacent structures.

**endorphin** (en'dawfin) one of a group of opiate-like peptides produced naturally by the body at neural synapses at various points in the central nervous system, where they modulate the transmission of pain perceptions. Endorphins raise the pain threshold and produce sedation and euphoria; the effects are blocked by naloxone, a narcotic antagonist.

**endoscope** ('endə skohp) an instrument used for direct visual inspection of a hollow organ or cavity.

**endosteitis** (ˌendosti'ietis) inflammation of the endosteum.

**endosteoma** (en dosti'ohmə) a neoplasm in the medullary cavity of a bone.

**endosteum** (en'dosti.əm) the lining membrane of bone cavities.

**endothelioma** (ˌendoh theeli'ohmə) a malignant growth originating in the endothelium.

**endothelium** (ˌendoh'theeli.əm) the membranous lining of serous, synovial and other internal surfaces.

**endotoxin** (ˌendoh'toksin) a poison produced by and retained within a bacterium, which is released only

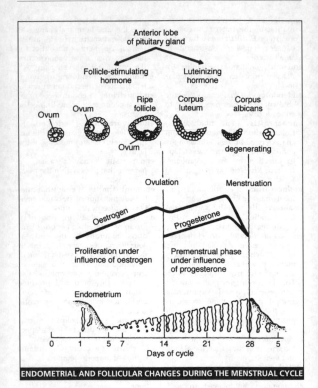

**ENDOMETRIAL AND FOLLICULAR CHANGES DURING THE MENSTRUAL CYCLE**

after the destruction of the bacterial cell. *See* EXOTOXIN.

**endotracheal** (ˌendohtrəˈkeeəl) within the trachea. *E. tube* an airway catheter which is inserted into the trachea when a patient requires ventilatory support. It also allows for the removal of secretions by suction.

**enema** ('enimə) 1. introduction of fluid into the rectum. 2. a solution introduced into the rectum to promote evacuation of faeces or as a means of administering nutrient or medicinal substances. 3. introduction of a radio-opaque material in a radiological examination of the colon (*barium e.*), or via a tube inserted into the jejunum in a radiological examination of the small bowel (*small bowel e.*).

**enervation** (ˌenəˈvayshən) 1. general weakness and loss of strength. 2. removal of a nerve.

**engagement** (inˈgayjmənt) the entry of the presenting part of the fetus, normally the head, into the true pelvis. Occurs in the last stage of pregnancy.

**English National Board for Nursing, Midwifery and Health Visiting** ('inglish) *see* NATIONAL BOARDS.

**enophthalmos** (ˌenofˈthalmos) a condition in which the eyeball is abnormally sunken into its socket.

**ensiform** ('ensiˌfawm) xiphoid; sword-shaped. *E. cartilage* the lowest portion of the sternum.

*Entamoeba* (ˌentəˈmeebə) a genus of protozoa, some of which are parasitic in man. *E. histolytica* the cause of amoebic dysentery.

**enteral** ('entəˌral) within the gastrointestinal tract. *E. diets* or *e. feeding* diets taken by mouth or through a nasogastric tube.

**enterectomy** (ˌentəˈrektəmee) excision of a portion of the intestine.

**enteric** (enˈterik) pertaining to the intestine. *E.-coated* a special coating applied to tablets or capsules which prevents release and absorption of their contents until they reach the intestine.

**enteritis** (ˌentəˈrietis) inflammation of the small intestine.

*Enterobacteriaceae* (ˌentəˌrohbakˌtiəˌriˈaysiˌee) a family of Gramnegative, rod-shaped bacteria, many of which are normally found in the human intestine.

**enterobiasis** (ˌentəˌrohˈbieəsis) infestation by threadworms.

*Enterobius* (ˌentəˈrohbiˌəs) a genus of nematode worms. *E. vermicularis* the threadworm or pinworm, a small white worm parasitic in the upper part of the large intestine. Gravid females migrate to the anal region to deposit their eggs, sometimes causing severe itching. Infection is frequent in children.

**enterococcus** (ˌentəˌrohˈkokəs) any streptococcus of the human intestine. An example is *Streptococcus faecalis*, only harmful out of its normal habitat, when it may cause a urinary infection or endocarditis.

**enterocolitis** (ˌentəˌrohkəˈlietis, -koh) inflammation of both the large and the small intestine.

**enterokinase** (ˌentəˌrohˈkienayz) an intestinal enzyme that converts trypsinogen into trypsin; enteropeptidase.

**enterostomy** (ˌentəˈrostəmee) the formation of an external opening into the small intestine. It may be (a) temporary, to relieve obstruction, or (b) permanent, in the form of an ileostomy in cases of total colectomy.

**enterotomy** (ˌentəˈrotəmee) any incision of the intestine.

**enterotoxin** (ˌentəˌrohˈtoksin) a toxin that is produced by one of the many organisms that cause food poisoning. Such toxins frequently prove more resistant to destruction than the bacteria themselves.

**enterovirus** (ˌentəˌrohˈvierəs) a virus that infects the gastrointestinal tract and then attacks the central nervous system. This subgroup includes Coxsackie, polio and echoviruses, and are now known, together with rhinoviruses, as picornaviruses.

**enterozoon** (ˌentəˌrohˈzoh.on) an animal parasite infesting the intestines.

**entoderm** ('entohˌderm) the innermost of the three germ layers of the embryo along with the mesoderm (intermediate) and ectoderm (outer) layers. It gives rise to the lining of most of the respiratory tract and to the intestinal tract and its glands.

**Entonox** ('entəˌnoks) trade name for a mixture of nitrous oxide and oxygen, 50% of each, premixed in one cylinder and used as an analgesic.

**entropion** (en'trohpi.ən) inversion of an eyelid, so that the lashes rub against the eyeball.

**enucleation** (i.nyookli'ayshən) removal of an organ or other mass intact from its supporting tissues, as of the eyeball from the orbit.

**enuresis** (.enyuh'reesis) involuntary passing of urine, usually during sleep at night (bed-wetting).

**environment** (in'vierənmənt) the surroundings of an organism which influence its development and behaviour.

**Environmental Health Officer** (en.vieə.rən'ment'l 'helth .ofisə) the person employed by the local authority to improve and to regulate the environment and to enforce statutory regulations. Responsibilities include housing, food hygiene, refuse collection, infestation, and air and noise pollution, etc.

**enzyme** ('enziem) a protein that will catalyse a biological reaction. *See* CATALYST.

**enzyme-linked immunosorbent assay** (.enziem.linkt .imyuhno-'zorbənt) *see* ELISA.

**eosin** ('eeohsin) a red dye used to stain biological specimens. A derivative of bromine and fluorescein.

**eosinophil** (eeə'sinəfil) cell having an affinity for eosin. A type of white blood cell containing eosin-staining granules.

**eosinophilia** (.eeə.sinə'fili.ə) excessive numbers of eosinophils present in the blood.

**ependyma** (e'pendimə) the membrane lining the cerebral ventricles and the central canal of the spinal cord.

**ependymoma** (e.pendi'mohmə) a neoplasm arising from the lining cells of the ventricles or central canal of the spinal cord. It gives rise to signs of hydrocephalus and is treated by surgery and radiotherapy.

**ephedrine** ('efi.dreen, -drin) a drug that relieves spasm of the bronchi; it has a similar action to adrenaline but can be taken orally. Widely used in asthma and chronic bronchitis.

**ephidrosis** (.efi'drohsis) profuse sweating; hyperhidrosis.

**epiblepharon** (.epi'blefə.ron) a congenital condition in which an excess of skin of the eyelid folds over the lid margin so that the eyelashes are pressed against the eyeball.

**epicanthus** (.epi'kanthəs) a vertical fold of skin on either side of the nose, sometimes covering the inner canthus; a normal characteristic in persons of certain races, but anomalous in others.

**epicardium** (.epi'kahdi.əm) the visceral layer of the pericardium.

**epicondyle** (.epi'kondiel) a protuberance on a long bone above its condyle.

**epicritic** (.epi'kritik) pertaining to sensory nerve fibres in the skin which give the appreciation of touch and temperature.

**epidemic** (.epi'demik) the presence in a population of disease or infection in excess of that usually expected.

**epidemiology** (.epi.deemi'oləjee) the study of the distribution of diseases in populations. It includes the attack rate (incidence) and the numbers affected at any one time (prevalence).

**epidermis** (.epi'dərmis) the nonvascular outer layer or cuticle of the skin. It consists of layers of cells which protect the dermis.

**epidermoid** (.epi'dərmoyd) pertaining to certain tumours which have the appearance of epidermal tissue.

*Epidermophyton* (epi.dərmoh'fieton) a genus of fungi that attack skin and nails, but not hair. The cause of ringworm and athlete's foot.

**epididymis** (ˌepiˈdidimis) [Gr.] an elongated, cord-like structure along the posterior border of the testis, whose coiled duct provides for the storage, transport and maturation of spermatozoa.

**epididymitis** (ˌepiˌdidiˈmietis) inflammation of the epididymis.

**epididymo-orchitis** (ˌepiˌdidimoh.-awˈkietis) inflammation of the epididymis and the testis.

**epidural** (ˌepiˈdyooəral) outside the dura mater. *E. analgesia* also known as extradural or peridural anaesthesia. A form of pain relief for childbirth and chronic pain, obtained by the injection of a local analgesic into the epidural space in order to block the spinal nerves. It may be approached by two routes: (1) caudal, through the sacro-coccygeal membrane covering the sacral hiatus; or (2) lumbar, through the intervertebral space and ligamentum flavum.

**epigastrium** (ˌepiˈgastri.əm) that region of the abdomen situated over the stomach.

**epiglottis** (ˌepiˈglotis) a cartilaginous structure which covers the opening from the pharynx into the larynx during swallowing and prevents food from passing into the trachea.

**epilation** (ˌepiˈlayshən) removal of hairs with their roots. It may be effected by pulling out the hairs or by electrolysis.

**epilatory** (eˈpilatə.ree) an agent that produces epilation.

**epilepsy** (ˈepiˌlepsee) convulsive attacks due to disordered electrical activity of the brain cells. In a major attack of 'grand mal' the patient falls to the ground unconscious, following an aura or unpleasant sensation. There are first tonic and then clonic contractions, from which stage the patient passes into a deep sleep. A minor attack of 'petit mal' is a momentary loss of consciousness

only. Both these types of epilepsy are idiopathic and are not caused by any damage to the brain. *Focal* or *Jacksonian e.* a symptom of a cerebral lesion. The convulsive movements are often localized and close observation of the onset and course of the attack may greatly assist diagnosis. *Temporal lobe e.* characterized by hallucinations of sight, hearing, taste and smell, paroxysmal disorders of memory and automatism. Caused by temporal or parietal lobe disease.

**epileptiform** (ˌepiˈleptiˌfawm) resembling an epileptic fit.

**epiloia** (ˌepiˈloyə) tuberous sclerosis. A congenital disorder with areas of hardening in the cerebral cortex and other organs, characterized clinically by mental handicap and epilepsy.

**epinephrine** (ˌepiˈnefrin) adrenaline.

**epineurium** (ˌepiˈnyooə.ri.əm) the sheath of tissue surrounding a nerve.

**epiphora** (iˈpifə.rə) persistent overflow of tears, often due to obstruction in the lacrimal passages or to ectropion.

**epiphysis** (iˈpifisis) the end of a long bone, developed separately from but attached by cartilage to the diaphysis (the shaft), with which it eventually unites. Growth in length takes place from the line of junction.

**episcleritis** (ˌepi.sklə'rietis) inflammation of the outer coat of the eyeball. It is seen as a slightly raised bluish nodule under the conjunctiva.

**episiotomy** (əˌpeeziˈotəmee) an incision made in the perineum when it will not stretch sufficiently during the second stage of labour (*see* Figure on p. 144).

**epispadias** (ˌepiˈspaydi.əs) a malformation in which there is an abnormal opening of the urethra on to the

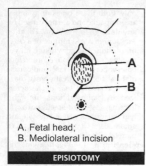

A. Fetal head;
B. Mediolateral incision

**EPISIOTOMY**

dorsal surface of the penis. *See* HYPOSPADIAS.

**epistaxis** (ˌepiˈstaksis) bleeding from the nose.

**epithelioma** (ˌepiˌtheeliˈohmə) any tumour originating in the epithelium.

**epithelium** (ˌepiˈtheeli.əm) the surface layer of cells of the skin or lining tissues.

**epithelization** (ˌepiˌtheelieˈzayshən) development of epithelium. The final stage in the healing of a surface wound. Epithelialization.

**epizoon** (ˌepiˈzoh.on) any external animal parasite.

**Epstein–Barr virus** (ˌepstienˈbah) *M. A. Epstein, British pathologist, b. 1921; Y. Barr, Canadian pathologist, b. 1932.* A herpes virus that causes infectious mononucleosis. It has been isolated from cells cultured from Burkitt's lymphoma, and has been found in certain cases of nasopharyngeal cancer. Also called EB virus.

**Erb's palsy** (airps) *W.H. Erb, German physician, 1840–1921.* Paralysis of the arm, often due to birth injury causing pressure on the brachial plexus or lower cervical nerve roots.

**erectile** (iˈrektiel) having the power of becoming erect. *E. tissue* vascular tissue which, under stimulus, becomes congested and swollen, causing erection of that part. The penis consists largely of erectile tissue.

**erection** (iˈrekshən) the enlarged and rigid state of the sexually aroused penis. Erection can also occur in the clitoris and the nipples of the female.

**erepsin** (iˈrepsin) the enzyme of succus entericus, secreted by the intestinal glands, which splits peptones into amino acids.

**ergometrine** (ˌərgohˈmetreen) an alkaloid of ergot which stimulates contraction of the uterine muscle.

**ergonomics** (ˌərgəˈnomiks) the scientific study of human beings in relation to their work and the effective use of human energy.

**ergosterol** (ərˈgostəˌrol) a sterol occurring in animal and plant tissues which, on ultraviolet irradiation, becomes a potent antirachitic substance, vitamin $D_2$ (ergocalciferol).

**ergot** (ˈərgot) a drug from a fungus that grows on rye. Used chiefly to contract the uterus and check haemorrhage at childbirth.

**ergotamine** (ərˈgotəˌmeen) an alkaloid of ergot used in the treatment of migraine.

**ergotism** (ˈərgəˌtizəm) the effects of poisoning from ergot, which may lead to gangrene of the fingers and toes.

**erogenous** (iˈrojənəs) arousing erotic feelings. *E. zones* areas of the body, stimulation of which produces erotic desire, e.g. the oral, anal and genital orifices and the nipples.

**erosion** (iˈrohzhən) the breaking down of tissue, usually by ulceration. *Cervical e.* a covering of columnar epithelium on the vaginal part of the uterine cervix, arising from erosion of the squamous epithelium, which normally covers it.

**erotic** (i'rotik) pertaining to sexual love or lust.

**eroticism, erotism** (i'roti,sizəm; 'erə,tizəm) a sexual instinct or desire; the expression of one's instinctual energy or drive, especially the sex drive.

**eructation** (,iruk'tayshən) belching; the escape of gas from the stomach through the mouth.

**eruption** (i'rupshən) a breaking out, e.g. of a skin lesion, or the cutting of teeth.

**erysipelas** (,eri'sipələs) a febrile disease characterized by inflammation and redness of the skin and subcutaneous tissues, and caused by group A haemolytic streptococci.

**erysipeloid** (,eri'sipə,loyd) an infective dermatitis or cellulitis due to infection with *Erysipelothrix insidiosa*; it usually begins in a wound (often the result of a prick by a fish bone) and remains localized, rarely becoming generalized and septicaemic.

**erythema** (,eri'theemə) redness of the skin caused by congestion of the capillaries in its lower layers. It occurs with any skin injury, infection or inflammation. *E. induratum* a manifestation of vasculitis. *E. multiforme* an acute eruption of the skin, which may be due to an allergy or to drug sensitivity. *E. nodosum* a painful disease in which bright red, tender nodes occur below the knee or on the forearm; it may be associated with tuberculosis.

**erythematous** (,eri'theemətəs) characterized by erythema.

**erythrasma** (,eri'thrazmə) a skin disease due to infection by *Corynebacterium minutissimum*, attacking the armpits or groins. It causes no irritation but is contagious.

**erythroblast** (i'rithroh,blast) originally, any nucleated erythrocyte, but now more generally used to designate the nucleated precursor from which an erythrocyte develops.

**erythroblastosis** (i,rithrohbla'stohsis) the presence of erythroblasts in the blood. *E. fetalis* a severe haemolytic anaemia with an excess of erythroblasts in the newly born. Due to rhesus incompatibility between the child's and the mother's blood.

**erythrocyanosis** (i,rithroh,sieə'nohsis) swelling and blueness of the legs and thighs occurring mainly in young women and during cold weather.

**erythrocyte** (i'rithrə,siet) a mature red blood cell. The cells contain haemoglobin and serve to transport oxygen. They are developed in the red bone marrow found in the cancellous tissue of all bones (*see* Figure on p. 146). The haemopoietic factor vitamin $B_{12}$ is essential for the change from proerythroblast to normoblast, and iron, thyroxine and vitamin C are also necessary for its perfect structure. *E. sedimentation rate* abbreviated ESR. The rate at which the cells of citrated blood form a deposit in a graduated 200 mm tube (Westergren method). The normal is less than 10 mm of clear plasma in 1 h. This is much increased in severe infection and acute rheumatism.

**erythrocythaemia** (i,rithrohsie'theemi.ə) increase in numbers of red blood cells due to overactivity of the bone marrow; Vaquez' disease; polycythaemia vera.

**erythrocytopenia** (i,rithroh,sietoh'peeni.ə) erythropenia; deficiency in numbers of red blood cells.

**erythrocytosis** (i,rithrohsie'tohsis) erythrocythaemia.

**erythroderma** (i,rithrə'dərmə) abnormal redness of the skin, usually over a large area.

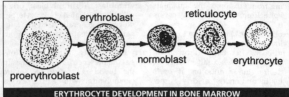

proerythroblast → erythroblast → normoblast → reticulocyte → erythrocyte

**ERYTHROCYTE DEVELOPMENT IN BONE MARROW**

**erythroedema polyneuropathy** (i,rithri'deemə ,polinyooə'ropəthee) a disease of infancy and early childhood. Marked by pain, swelling and ink coloration of the fingers and toes, and by listlessness, irritability, failure to thrive, profuse perspiration and sometimes scarlet coloration of the cheeks and tip of the nose. Called also acrodynia, pink disease.

**erythromycin** (i,rithroh'miesin) a broad-spectrum antibiotic produced by a strain of *Streptomyces erythreus*. It is effective against a wide variety of organisms, including Gram-negative and Gram-positive bacteria.

**erythropoiesis** (i,rithrohpoy'eesis) the manufacture of red blood corpuscles.

**erythropoietin** (i,rithroh'poyitin, -poy'ee-) a hormone, produced by the kidney, which stimulates the production of red blood cells in the bone marrow. *e. therapy* the use of erythropoietin to promote new blood formation as an alternative to blood transfusion.

**erythropsia** (,eri'thropsi.ə) a defect of vision in which all objects appear red. Often occurs after a cataract operation.

**eschar** ('eskar) a slough or scab which forms after the destruction of living tissue by gangrene, infection or burning.

*Escherichia* (,esh.ə'riki.ə) a genus of Enterobacteriaceae. *E. coli* an organism normally present in the intestines of humans and other vertebrates. Although not generally pathogenic, it may set up infections of the gallbladder, bile ducts, and urinary and intestinal tracts. Strain O157, normally found in the gut of cattle, occasionally has been responsible for serious outbreaks of food poisoning in humans.

**Esmarch's tourniquet** ('ezmahks) *J.F. A. von Esmarch, German surgeon, 1823–1908.* A rubber bandage used in surgery to express blood from a limb and render it less vascular.

**esophoria** (,eesoh'for.ri.ə) latent convergent strabismus. The eyes turn inwards only when one is covered up.

**esotropia** (,eesoh'trohpi.ə) convergent strabismus. One or other eye turns inwards, resulting in double vision.

**ESP** extrasensory perception.

**ESR** erythrocyte sedimentation rate.

**ESRD** end-stage renal disease. *See* RENAL.

**essence** ('esəns) 1. an indispensable part of anything. 2. a volatile oil dissolved in alcohol.

**essential** (i'senshəl) indispensable. *E. amino acids* those amino acids that must be obtained in the diet and are necessary for the maintenance of tissue growth and repair. *See* AMINO ACID. *E. fatty acids* unsaturated fatty acids that are necessary for body growth. *E. oils* specially prepared aromatic oils which are obtained from the different parts of plants including flowers, leaves, seeds, wood, roots and bark. Used in aromatherapy.

**ester** ('estə) a compound formed by the combination of an acid and an alcohol, with the elimination of water.

**esterase** ('estə,rayz) an enzyme that causes the hydrolysis of esters into acids and alcohol.

**ethambutol** (e'thambyuh,tol) a drug used in combination with other drugs in the treatment of tuberculosis.

**ethanol** ('ethə,nol, 'eethə-) alcohol.

**ethanolamine** (,ethə'nolə,meen) an intravenous sclerosing agent used to inject varicose veins.

**ether** ('eethə) a volatile inflammable liquid formerly used as a general anaesthetic agent.

**ethics** ('ethiks) a code of moral principles. *Nursing e.* the code governing a nurse's behaviour with patients and their relatives, and with colleagues. *See* Appendices.

**ethmoid** ('ethmoyd) a sieve-like bone separating the cavity of the nose from the cranium. The olfactory nerves pass through its perforations.

**ethmoidectomy** (,ethmoy'dektə-mee) surgical removal of a portion of the ethmoid bone.

**ethnic** ('ethnik) pertaining to a social group, members of which share cultural bonds or physical (racial) characteristics. *E. minority* a social grouping of people who share cultural or racial factors but who constitute a minority within the greater culture or society.

**ethnocentrism** (,ethno'sentriz'm) the belief that one's own group, community, society or even way of doing things is superior to those of others, leading to mistrust or doubt about others' values and beliefs.

**ethnography** (eth'nogrəfee) a qualitative research approach developed by anthropologists with the purpose of describing an aspect of a culture, but also aimed at learning about the culture or factor being studied.

**ethnology** (eth'nolajee) the science dealing with the human races, their descent, relationship, etc.

**ethoheptazine** (,ethoh'heptəzeen) an analgesic related to pethidine. It relieves pain and muscle spasm.

**ethosuximide** (,ethoh'suksi,mied) an anticonvulsant used in the treatment of 'petit mal' epilepsy.

**ethyl chloride** (,ethil 'klor.ried) a volatile liquid used as a local anaesthetic. When sprayed on intact skin it causes local insensitivity, through freezing.

**ethylene oxide** (,ethileen 'oksied) a gas which is sporicidal and viricidal and capable of penetrating relatively inaccessible parts of an apparatus during sterilization. It is used for equipment which is too delicate to be sterilized by other methods.

**ethylenediaminetetra-acetic acid** (,ethileen,dieəmeen,tetra.ə'seetik) abbreviated EDTA. A chelating agent used in the treatment of lead poisoning.

**ethyloestrenol** (,ethil'eestrə,nol) an anabolic steroid that may be used to treat severe weight loss, debility and osteoporosis.

**etiolation** (,eeti.ə'layshən) paleness of the skin due to lack of exposure to sunlight.

**etiology** (,eeti'olajee) *see* AETIOLOGY.

**eucalyptus oil** (,yookə'liptəs ,oyl) an oil derived from the leaves of the eucalyptus tree; it has mild antiseptic properties and is used in the treatment of nasal catarrh.

**eugenics** (yoo'jeniks) the study of measures that may be taken to improve future generations, both physically and mentally.

**eugenol** ('yooji,nol) a local anaesthetic and antiseptic, derived from oil of cloves and cinnamon, used in dentistry.

**eugeria** (yoo'je.riə) the state of a high quality of life in old age. Eugeria should be the normal state for the elderly but may be affected by physical or mental illness.

**Eugynon** (yoo'gienon) *E. 30, E. 50* proprietary preparations of contraceptive tablets containing oestrogen and progesterone.

**eunuch** ('yoonək) a castrated male.

**euphoria** (yoo'for.ri.ə) an exaggerated feeling of wellbeing, often not justified by circumstances. Less than ELATION.

**euplastic** (yoo'plastik) capable of being transformed into healthy tissue. The term may be applied to a wound that is healing well.

**eurhythmics** (yoo'ridhmiks) gentle body exercises performed to music.

**eustachian tube** (yoo stayshən 'tyoob) *B. Eustachio, Italian anatomist, 1520–1574.* The pharyngotympanic tube.

**euthanasia** (,yoothə'nayzi.ə, -zhə) 1. an easy or good death. 2. the deliberate ending of life of a person suffering from an incurable disease; this can be voluntary or involuntary.

**euthyroid** (yoo'thieroyd) having a normally functioning thyroid gland.

**evacuant** (i'vakyooənt) 1. promoting evacuation. 2. an agent that promotes evacuation.

**evacuation** (i,vakyoo'ayshən) 1. an emptying or removal, especially the removal of any material from the body by discharge through a natural or artificial passage. 2. material discharged from the body, especialy the discharge from the bowels.

**evacuator** (i'vakyoo,aytə) an instrument that produces evacuation, e.g. one designed to wash out small particles of stone from the bladder after lithotripsy.

**evaluation** (i,valyoo'ayshən) a critical appraisal or assessment; a judgement of the value, worth, character or effectiveness of that which is being assessed. In the health-care field this includes assessment of the patient's position on the health/illness continuum, and of the effectiveness of patient care activities in bringing about a change in the patient's position. Accepted as the fourth phase of the nursing process.

**eventration** (,eeven'trayshən) 1. the protrusion of the intestines through the abdominal wall. 2. removal of abdominal viscera.

**eversion** (i'vərshən) turning outwards. *E. of the eyelid* ectropion. The upper eyelid may be everted for examination of the eye or for the removal of a foreign body.

**evidence-based practice** ('evidəns,bayst) systematically appraising clinical situations and then using up-to-date research findings as a basis for the nursing or medical decisions. An approach to clinical practice first developed at McMaster University (Canada) which is based on the following four principles: (a) clinical and other health-care decisions should be *based on the best evidence* available from patients and populations as well as from the laboratory; (b) the patient's problem determines the nature and source of evidence to be sought, rather than habit, protocol or tradition; (c) identifying the best evidence calls for the integration of epidemiological and biostatistical ways of thinking with those derived from pathophysiology and clinical experience; (d) the conclusions of this search and critical appraisal of evidence are worthwhile only if they are translated into actions that affect patients.

**evisceration** (i,visə'rayshən) removal of internal organs. *E. of the eye* removal of the contents of the eyeball, but not the sclera.

**evolution** (,eevə'looshən) the development of living organisms which change their characteristics during succeeding generations.

**evulsion** (i'vulshən) extraction by force.

**Ewing's tumour** ('yooingz) J. Ewing, American pathologist, 1866–1943. A form of sarcoma usually affecting the shaft of a long bone in young adults.

**exacerbation** (ek,sasə'bayshən, ig,zasə-) an increase in the severity of the symptoms of a disease.

**exanthem** (eg'zanthəm, ek's-) an infectious disease characterized by a skin rash.

**exanthematous** (,egzan'themətəs, ,eks-) pertaining to any disease associated with a skin eruption.

**excavation** (,ekskə'vayshən) scooping out. *Dental e.* the removal of decay from a tooth before inserting a filling.

**exception** (ek'sepshən) in health care the justification for clinical variance made by a practitioner and usually peer-reviewed by others.

**excision** (ek'sizhən) the cutting out of a part.

**excitation** (,eksie'tayshən) the act of stimulating.

**excitement** (ek'sietmənt) a physiological and emotional response to a stimulus.

**excoriation** (ek,skor.ri'ayshən) an abrasion of the skin.

**excrement** ('ekskrəmənt) faecal matter; waste from the body.

**excrescence** (ek,skresəns) abnormal outgrowth of tissue, e.g. a wart.

**excreta** (ek'skreetə) the natural discharges of the excretory system: faeces, urine and sweat.

**excretion** (ek'skreeshən) the discharge of waste from the body.

**exercise** ('eksə,siez) performance of physical exertion for improvement of health or correction of physical deformity. *Active e.* motion imparted to a part by voluntary contraction and relaxation of its controlling muscles. *Isometric e.* active exercise performed against stable resistance, without change in the length of the muscle. No movement occurs at any joints over which the muscle passes. *Passive e.* motion imparted to a segment of the body by another individual, or a machine or other outside force, or produced by voluntary effort of another segment of the patient's own body. *Range of movement (ROM) e's* exercises that move each joint through its full range of movement, that is, to the highest degree of movement of which each joint is normally capable.

**exfoliation** (eks,fohli'ayshən) the splitting off from the surface of dead tissue in thin flaky layers.

**exhalation** (,eks.hə'layshən) 1. the giving out of a vapour. 2. the act of breathing out.

**exhibitionism** (,eksi'bishə,nizəm) 1. showing off; a desire to attract attention. 2. exposing the genitals to persons of the opposite sex in socially unacceptable circumstances.

**exocrine** ('eksoh,krin, -,krien) pertaining to those glands that discharge their secretion by means of a duct, e.g. salivary glands. *See* ENDOCRINE.

**exogenous** (ek'sojənəs) of external origin.

**exomphalos** (ek'somfələs) 1. hernia of the abdominal viscera into the umbilical cord. 2. congenital umbilical hernia.

**exophthalmometer** (,eksofthal'momitə) an instrument for measuring the extent of protrusion of the eyeball.

**exophthalmos** (,eksof'thalmos) abnormal protrusion of the eyeball which results in a marked stare. May be due to injury or disease and is often associated with thyrotoxicosis.

**exostosis** (ˌekso'stohsis) a bony outgrowth from the surface of a bone.

**exotoxin** (ˌeksoh'toksin) a poison produced by a bacterial cell and released into the tissues surrounding it. *See* ENDOTOXIN.

**exotropia** (ˌeksoh'trohpi.ə) divergent strabismus; the eyes turn outwards.

**expanded role** (ˌeks'pandid) the opportunity for nurses, midwifes and health visitors to undertake an expanded role in relation to patient care beyond that traditionally recognized. The professional framework for nurses, midwives and health visitors in relation to the expanded role is contained within the United Kingdom Central Council for Nursing, Midwifery and Health Visiting's (UKCC's) guidance 'The Scope of Professional Practice' (1992).

**expected outcome** (eks,pektid 'owt-kom) in a nursing care plan the rationale for a statement regarding a nursing intervention and what it is expected to achieve.

**expectorant** (ek'spektə.rənt) a remedy that promotes and facilitates expectoration.

**expectoration** (ek,spektə'rayshən) sputum; secretions coughed up from the air passages. Its characteristics are a valuable aid in diagnosis and note should be taken of the quantity ejected, its colour and the amount of effort required. Frothiness denotes that it comes from an air-containing cavity; fluidity indicates oedema of the lung.

**expiration** (ˌekspi'rayshən) 1. the act of breathing out. 2. termination or death.

**exploration** (ˌeksplə'rayshən) the operation of surgically investigating any part of the body.

**expression** (ek'spreshən) 1. the aspect or appearance of the face as determined by the physical or emotional state. 2. the act of squeezing out or evacuating by pressure, e.g. the removal of breast milk by hand or breast pump. 3. the manifestation of a heritable trait in an individual carrying the gene or genes that determine it.

**exsanguination** (ek,sang.gwi'nayshən) extensive blood loss due to internal or external haemorrhage.

**extension** (ek'stenshən) 1. the straightening out of a flexed joint, such as the knee or elbow. 2. the application of traction to a fractured or dislocated limb by means of a weight.

**extensor** (ek'stensə, -sor) a muscle that extends or straightens a limb.

**exterior** (ek'stiə.ri.ə) on the outside.

**exteriorize** (ek'stiə.ri.ə,riez) 1. to bring an organ or part of one to the outside of the body by surgery. 2. in psychiatry, to turn one's interests outwards.

**extra-** ('ekstrə) prefix denoting outside, additional or beyond.

**extracapsular** (ˌekstrə'kapsyuhlə) outside the capsule. May refer to a fracture occurring at the end of the bone but outside the joint capsule, or to cataract extraction.

**extracellular** (ˌekstrə'selyuhlə) outside the cell. *E. fluid* tissue fluid that surrounds the cells.

**extract** ('ekstrakt) a concentrated preparation of a drug made by extracting its soluble principles by steeping in water or alcohol and then evaporating the fluid.

**extraction** (ek'strakshən) 1. the process or act of pulling or drawing out. 2. the preparation of an extract. *Breech e.* extraction of an infant from the uterus in cases of breech presentation. *Vacuum e.* removal of the uterine contents by application of a vacuum. An alternative to the forceps method of delivering a baby.

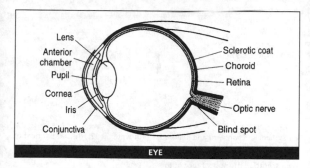

Lens
Anterior chamber
Pupil
Cornea
Iris
Conjunctiva
Sclerotic coat
Choroid
Retina
Optic nerve
Blind spot

**EYE**

**extrapyramidal** (ˌekstrəpi'ramid'l) outside the pyramidal (cerebrospinal) tract. *E. system* the nerve tracts and pathways which are not within the pyramidal tracts.

**extrasensory** (ˌekstrə'sensə.ree) outside or beyond any of the known senses. *E. perception* abbreviated ESP. Appreciation of the thoughts of others or of current or future events without any normal means of communication.

**extrasystole** (ˌekstrə'sistəlee) premature contraction of the atria or ventricles. *See* SYSTOLE.

**extrauterine** (ˌekstrə'yootə,rien) occurring outside the uterus. *E. pregnancy* ectopic gestation; development of a fetus outside the uterus.

**extravasation** (ik,stravə'sayshən) effusion or escape of fluid from its normal course into surrounding tissues. *E. of blood* a bruise.

**extremity** (ek'stremitee) distal part; a hand or foot.

**extrinsic** (ek'strinsik, -zik) originating externally. *E. factor* a substance present in meat and other foodstuffs. Also called cyanocobalamin (vitamin $B_{12}$), it is necessary for the manufacture of red blood cells. The intrinsic factor produced in the stomach is necessary for the absorption of vitamin $B_{12}$. *E. muscle* a muscle originating away from the part that it controls, such as those controlling the movements of the eye.

**extroversion** (ˌekstrə'vorshən) turning inside out, e.g. of the uterus, as sometimes occurs after labour.

**extrovert** ('ekstrə,vərt) a person who is sociable, a good mixer, outgoing and interested in what is going on in the social enviroment. A personality type first described by Jung. *See* INTROVERT.

**extubation** (,ekstyuh'bayshən) removal of a tube used in intubation.

**exudation** (,eksyuh'dayshən) the slow discharge of serous fluid through the walls of the blood cells and its deposition in or on the tissues.

**eye** (ie) the organ of sight. A globular structure with three coats. The nerve tissue of the retina receives impressions of images via the pupil and lens. From this the optic nerve conveys the impressions to the visual area of the cerebrum (*see* Figure).

**eyelid** ('ie,lid) a protective covering of the eye, composed of muscle and dense connective tissue covered with skin, lined with conjunctiva and fringed with eyelashes. Eyelids contain the Meibomian glands.

**eyetooth** (ie'tooth) an upper canine tooth.

# F

**F** symbol for *Fahrenheit* and *fluorine*.

**face** (fays) the front of the head from the forehead to the chin. *F. presentation* the appearance of the face of the fetus first at the cervix during labour.

**facet** ('fasit) a small flat area on the surface of a bone. *F. syndrome* a slight dislocation of the small facet joints of the vertebrae giving rise to pain and muscle spasm.

**facial** ('fayshəl) pertaining to the face or lower anterior portion of the head. *F. nerve* the seventh cranial nerve, which supplies the salivary glands and superficial face muscles. *F. paralysis see* PARALYSIS.

**facies** ('faysi,eez, 'fayshi-) facial expression; it often gives some indication of the patient's condition. *Adenoid f.* the open mouth and vacant expression associated with mouth breathing and nasal obstruction. *Parkinson f.* fixed expression, due to paucity of movement of facial muscles, characteristic of Parkinsonism.

**faecalith** ('feekəlith) a hard stony mass of faecal material. A coprolith.

**faeces** ('feeseez) waste matter excreted by the bowel, consisting of indigestible cellulose, food which has escaped digestion, bacteria (living and dead) and water.

**Fahrenheit scale** ('faran,hiet) *G.D. Fahrenheit, German physicist, 1686–1736.* A scale of heat measurement. It registers the freezing point of water at 32°, the normal heat of the human body at 98.4°, and the boiling point of water at 212°. *See* CELSIUS.

**failure** ('faylyə) inability to perform or to function properly. *F. to thrive* retardation of normal growth and development in an infant. Causes are numerous but malnutrition or difficulty in absorbing essential nutrients is a main factor, as well as those that are psychosocial in origin, e.g. maternal deprivation syndrome. *Heart f.* inability of the heart to maintain a circulation sufficient to meet the body's needs. *Kidney f., renal f.* inability of the kidney to excrete metabolites at normal plasma levels under normal loading, or inability to retain electrolytes when intake is normal; in the acute form, marked by uraemia and usually by oliguria, with hyperkalaemia and pulmonary oedema. *Respiratory f., ventilatory f.* a life-threatening condition in which respiratory function is inadequate to maintain the body's needs for oxygen supply and carbon dioxide removal while at rest.

**fainting** ('faynting) *see* SYNCOPE.

**faith healing** ('fayth) an attempt to cure disease or disability with the use of spiritual powers or by the influence of the personality of the healer.

**falciform** ('falsi,fawm) sickle-shaped. *F. ligament* a fold of peri-

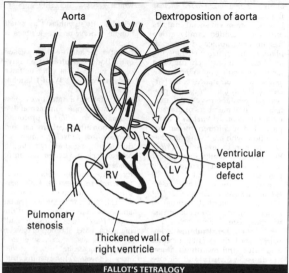

Aorta

Dextroposition of aorta

RA

Ventricular septal defect

RV

LV

Pulmonary stenosis

Thickened wall of right ventricle

**FALLOT'S TETRALOGY**

toneum which separates the two main lobes of the liver and connects it with the anterior abdominal wall and the diaphragm.

**fallopian tube** (fə.lohpi.ən tyoob) *G. Fallopius, Italian anatomist, 1523–1563.* Uterine tube. One of a pair of tubes, about 10–14 cm long, arising out of the upper part of the uterus. The distal end of each tube is fimbriated and lies near an ovary. The tubes' function is to conduct the ova from the ovaries to the interior of the uterus. An oviduct.

**Fallot's tetralogy** (ˌfaloh te'traləjee) *E.L.A. Fallot, French physician, 1850–1911.* A congenital heart disease with four characteristic defects: (a) pulmonary stenosis; (b) interventricular defect of the septum; (c) overriding of the aorta, i.e.

opening into both right and left ventricles; (d) hypertrophy of the right ventricle. *See* Figure.

**falx** (falks) a sickle-shaped structure. *F. cerebri* the fold of dura mater that separates the two cerebral hemispheres.

**familial** (fə'mili.əl) occurring in or affecting members of a family more than would be expected by chance.

**family** ('familee) 1. a group of people related by blood or marriage, especially a husband, wife and their children. 2. a taxonomic category below an order and above a genus. *Blended f.* a family unit composed of a married couple and their offspring, including some from previous marriages. *Extended f.* a nuclear family and their close relatives, such as the children's grandparents, aunts and uncles. *Extended nuclear f.* a nuclear family who nevertheless make frequent social contacts with the extended family group despite geographical distance. *F. planning* the arrangement, spacing and limitation of the children in a family, depending upon the wishes and social circumstances of the parents. *F. therapy* a therapeutic process whereby the psychotherapist treats several members of the family simultaneously. *Nuclear f.* a couple and their children, by birth or adoption, who are living together and are more or less isolated from their extended family. *Single parent f.* a lone parent and offspring living together as a family unit.

**Fanconi's syndrome** (fan'kohneez) *F. Fanconi, Swiss paediatrician, 1892–1979.* A rare inherited disorder of metabolism in which reabsorption of phosphate, amino acids and sugar by the renal tubules is impaired. The kidneys fail to produce acid urine, and resulting features are thirst, polyuria and rickets, leading to chronic renal failure.

**fang** (fang) the root of a tooth.

**fantasy** ('fantəsee) an imagined sequence of events or mental images that serves to satisfy unconscious wishes or to express unconscious conflicts.

**farinaceous** (ˌfari'nayshəs) starchy or containing starch. Refers to foods such as wheat, oats, barley and rice.

**farmer's lung** (ˌfahməz) a disease occurring in those in contact with mouldy hay. It is thought to be due to a hypersensitivity, with widespread reaction in the lung tissue. It causes excessive breathlessness.

**FAS** fetal alcohol syndrome.

**fascia** ('fashi.ə) a sheath of connective tissue enclosing muscles or other organs.

**fasciculation** (fəˌsikyuh'layshən) isolated fine muscle twitching

which gives a flickering appearance.

**fasciculus** (fə'sikyuhləs) a small bundle of nerve or muscle fibres; a fascicle.

**fat** (fat) 1. the adipose or fatty tissue of the body. 2. neutral fat; a triglyceride which is an ester of fatty acids and glycerol. *Wool-f.* lanolin. *See also* BROWN FAT.

**fatigue** (fə'teeg) a state of weariness which may range from mental disinclination for effort to profound exhaustion after great physical and mental effort. *Muscle f.* may occur during prolonged effort owing to oxygen lack and accumulation of waste products.

**fatty** ('fatee) containing or similar to fat. *F. acid see* ESSENTIAL. *F. degeneration* a degenerative change in tissue cells due to the invasion of fat and consequent weakening of the organ. The change occurs as a result of incorrect diet, shortage of oxygen in the tissues or excessive consumption of alcohol.

**fauces** ('fawseez) the opening from the mouth into the pharynx. *Pillars of the f.* the two folds of muscle covered with mucous membrane that pass from the soft palate on either side of the fauces. One fold passes into the tongue, the other into the pharynx, and between them is situated the tonsil.

**favism** ('fayvizəm) an acute haemolytic anaemia caused by ingestion of fava beans or inhalation of the pollen of the plant, usually occurring in certain individuals as a result of a genetic abnormality with a deficiency in an enzyme, glucose-6-phosphate dehydrogenase, in the erythrocytes. Called also fabism.

**favus** ('fayvəs) a type of ringworm infection rare in the UK, with formation of scabs, in appearance like a honeycomb. It usually affects the scalp and is due to a fungus infection (*Trichophyton schoenleinii*).

**Fe** symbol for *iron* (L. *ferrum*).

**fear** (fiə) a normal emotional response, in contrast to anxiety and phobia, to consciously recognized external sources of danger; it is manifested by alarm, apprehension or disquiet. *Obsessional f.* a recurring irrational fear that is not amenable to ordinary reassurance; a phobia.

**febrile** ('feebriel, 'feb-) characterized by or relating to fever. *F. convulsion* a convulsion which occurs in childhood and is associated with pyrexia.

**fecundation** (,fekən'dayshən, ,fee-) fertilization.

**fecundity** (fi'kunditee) the ability to produce offspring frequently and in large numbers. In demography, the physiological ability to reproduce, as opposed to fertility.

**feedback** ('feed,bak) a method of control where some of the output is returned as input for monitoring purposes. Feedback mechanisms are important in the regulation of such physiological processes as hormone and enzyme reactions. *Negative f.* a rise in the output of a substance is detected and further output is thus inhibited. *Positive f.* a rise in output causes either a direct or indirect rise in the output of another substance.

**felon** ('felən) an abscess of the distal phalanx of a finger; a whitlow.

**Felty's syndrome** ('feltiz) *A.R. Felty, American physician, 1895–1963.* The triad of rheumatoid arthritis, splenomegaly and leukopenia. Often associated with anaemia, lymphadenopathy and vasculitic cutaneous ulceration.

**female genital mutilation** (,feemayl ,jenit'l) female circumcision involving excision of the labia majora, labia minora and clitoris and in some cases, partial closure of the introitus. It is prevalent in African countries such as Sudan. Prior to pregnancy it may cause problems with micturition and intercourse. Special care will be required during labour and delivery, and excision and separation of the tissues may be carried out; caesarean section may be necessary.

**feminization** (,feminie'zayshən) 1. the normal induction or development of female sexual characteristics. 2. the induction or development of female secondary sexual characteristics in the male. *Testicular f.* a condition in which the subject is phenotypically female, but lacks nuclear sex chromatin and is of XY chromosomal sex.

**femoral** ('femə,rəl) pertaining to the femur. *F. artery* that of the thigh from groin to knee. *F. canal* the opening below the inguinal ligament through which the femoral artery passes from the abdomen to the thigh.

**femur** ('feemə) the thigh bone.

**fenbufen** (fen'byoofen) a nonsteroidal anti-inflammatory drug (NSAID) that acts as a prodrug. It is associated with a lower incidence of gastrointestinal haemorrhage but a higher incidence of skin rashes than other NSAIDs.

**fenestra** (fə'nestra) a window-like opening. *F. ovalis* the oval opening between the middle and the internal ear.

**fenoprofen** (,feenoh'prohfən) an anti-inflammatory drug used in the treatment of arthritic conditions.

**fentanyl** ('fentə,nil) a short-acting narcotic analgesic, widely used during anaesthesia, especially for children and the elderly.

**ferritin** ('feritin) a complex formed of an iron and protein molecule; one of the forms in which iron is stored in the body.

**ferrous** ('ferəs) containing iron. *F. fumarate, f. gluconate, f. succinate* and *f. sulphate* are iron salts which are given orally to treat iron-deficiency anaemia.

**ferrule** ('ferool, -rel) a rubber cap used on the end of walking sticks, frames and crutches to prevent slipping.

**fertilization** (,fərtilie'zayshən) the impregnation of the female sex cell, the ovum, by a male sex cell, a spermatozoon. *In vitro f.* artificial fertilization of the ovum in laboratory conditions. The timing and conditions for implantation into a uterus have to be perfect if successful pregnancy is to ensue.

**fester** ('festə) to become superficially inflamed and to suppurate.

**festination** (,festi'nayshən) an involuntary tendency to take short accelerating steps in walking; seen in conditions such as Parkinson's disease.

**fetal** ('feet'l) pertaining to the fetus. *F. alcohol syndrome* abbreviated FAS. Physical and mental abnormalities due to maternal alcohol intake during pregnancy. Abnormalities may include microcephaly, growth deficiencies, mental handicap, hyperactivity, heart murmurs and skeletal malformation. The exact amount of alcohol consumption that will produce fetal damage is unknown, but the periods of gestation during which the alcohol is most likely to result in fetal damage are 3–4.5 months after conception and during the last trimester. *F. assessment* determination of the wellbeing of the fetus. Assessment techniques and procedures include: (a) medical and family histories and physical examination of the mother; (b) ULTRASONOGRAPHY; (c) assessment of fetal activity using the Cardiff kick chart; (d) chemical assessment of placental function; (e) assays of amniotic fluid obtained by AMNIOCENTESIS; and (f) electronic and ultrasonic fetal heart rate monitor-

ing. *F. distress* the clinical manifestation of fetal hypoxia which may be due to maternal or fetal causes. *F. position* a position resembling that of the fetus in the womb, sometimes adopted by a child or adult in a state of distress or depression.

**fetishism** ('feti,shizm) a state in which an object is regarded with an irrational fear, or an erotic attraction which may be so strong that the object is necessary for achieving sexual excitement.

**fetor** ('feetə, -tor) an offensive smell.

**fetoscope** ('feetə,skohp) an endoscope for viewing the fetus in utero.

**fetus** ('feetəs) the developing baby between the eighth week and the end of pregnancy.

**fever** ('feevə) 1. an abnormally high body temperature; pyrexia. 2. any disease characterized by marked increase of body temperature.

**fibre** ('fiebə) a thread-like structure.

**fibreoptics** (,fiebə'roptiks) the transmission of light rays along flexible tubes by means of very fine glass or plastic fibres. Use is made of this in endoscopic instruments such as the gastroscope.

**fibrescope** ('fiebə,skohp) an endoscope in which fibreoptics are used.

**fibrillation** (,fibri'layshən, ,fie-) a quivering, vibratory movement of muscle fibres. *Atrial f.* rapid contractions of the atrium causing irregular contraction of the ventricles in both rhythm and force. *Ventricular f.* fine rapid twitchings of the ventricles leading to circulatory arrest. Rapidly fatal unless it can be controlled.

**fibrin** ('fiebrin) an insoluble protein that is essential to CLOTTING of blood, formed from fibrinogen by action of thrombin.

**fibrinogen** (fie'brinəjən) a soluble protein which is present in blood plasma and is converted into fibrin by the action of thrombin when the blood clots.

**fibrinolysin** (ˌfiebriˈnolisin) a pro teolytic enzyme that dissolves fibrin.

**fibrinolysis** (ˌfiebriˈnolisis) the dissolution of fibrin by the action of fibrinolysin. The process by which clots are removed from the circulation after healing has taken place.

**fibrinopenia** (ˌfiebrinohˈpeeni.ə) a deficiency of fibrinogen in the blood. There is a tendency to bleed as the coagulation time is increased.

**fibroadenoma** (ˌfiebrohˌadəˈnohmə) a benign tumour of glandular and fibrous tissue. *See* ADENOMA.

**fibroangioma** (ˌfiebrohˌanjiˈohmə) a benign tumour containing both fibrous and vascular tissue.

**fibroblast** ('fiebrohˌblast) a connective tissue cell.

**fibrocartilage** (ˌfiebrohˈkahtilij) cartilage with fibrous tissue in it.

**fibrochondritis** (ˌfiebrohkonˈdrietis) inflammation of fibrocartilage.

**fibrocystic** (ˌfiebrohˈsistik) fibrous and cystic. *F. disease of the pancreas* an inherited disease affecting the mucus-secreting glands, the sweat glands and the pancreas. It is characterized by fatty stools and repeated lung infections. Mucoviscidosis; cystic fibrosis.

**fibroid** ('fiebroyd) 1. having a fibrous structure. 2. a fibroma or a fibromyoma, usually one occurring in the uterus.

**fibroma** (fieˈbrohmə) a benign tumour of connective tissue.

**fibromyoma** (ˌfiebrohmieˈohmə) a tumour consisting of fibrous and muscle tissue; frequently found in or on the uterus (*see* Figure).

**fibroplasia** (ˌfiebrohˈplayzi.ə) the formation of fibrous tissue when a wound heals. *Retrolental f.* a condition characterized by the presence of fibrous tissue behind the lens, leading to detachment of the retina and blindness, attributed to use of excessively high concentra

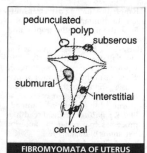

**FIBROMYOMATA OF UTERUS**

tions of oxygen in the care of preterm infants.

**fibrosarcoma** (ˌfiebrohsahˈkohmə) a malignant tumour arising in fibrous tissue.

**fibrosis** (fieˈbrohsis) fibrous tissue formation, such as occurs in scar tissue or as the result of inflammation. It is the cause of adhesions of the peritoneum or other serous membranes. *F. of the lung* condition that may precede bronchiectasis and emphysema.

**fibrositis** (ˌfiebrəˈsietis) inflammation of fibrous tissue. The term is loosely applied to pain and stiffness, particularly of the back muscles, for which no other cause can be found.

**fibula** ('fibyuhlə) the slender bone from knee to ankle, on the outer side of the leg.

**field of vision** (ˌfeeld) the area within view, as for the fixed eye or a camera, or in an operation.

**fight or flight response** (ˌfiet or 'fliet ˌrispons) activation of the sympathetic nervous system in response to danger or stress.

**filament** ('filəmənt) a small threadlike structure.

*Filaria* (fiˈlair.ri.ə) a genus of nematode worms which may be found in the connective tissues and lymphatics, having been transmitted to humans by mosquitoes. Found mainly in the tropics and subtropics.

**filariasis** ( filə'rieəsis) an infection by filaria, particularly by *Wuchereria bancrofti*, resulting in blockage of the lymphatics, which causes swelling of the surrounding tissues. Elephantiasis may occur.

**filiform** ('fili fawm, 'fie-) thread-like. *F. papillae* the fine thread-like processes that cover the anterior two-thirds of the tongue.

**filter** ('filtə) a device for eliminating certain elements, such as (a) particles of certain size from a solution, or (b) rays of a certain wavelength from a stream of radiant energy. *Millipore f.* trade name for a device used to filter nutrient solutions as they are administered intravenously.

**filtrate** ('filtrayt) the fluid that passes through a filter.

**filtration** (fil'trayshən) 1. the removal of precipitate from a liquid by means of a filter. 2. the removal of rays of a certain wavelength from an electromagnetic beam. *F. angle* the angle of the anterior chamber of the eye through which the aqueous humour drains; blockage of this channel gives rise to glaucoma.

**fimbria** ('fimbri.ə) a fringe. *F. of the uterine tube* the thread-like projections that surround the pelvic opening of the uterine tube.

**finger** ('fing.gə) a digit of the hand. *Clubbed f.* one with enlargement of the terminal phalanx with constant osseous changes; occurs in many heart and lung diseases. *Hammer f., mallet f.* permanent flexion of the distal phalanx of a finger due to avulsion of the extensor tendon. *Trigger f.* temporary flexion of a finger which is overcome in a sudden jerk by active or passive extension of the finger. It is caused by thicken-

ing of the flexor tendon in a narrowed tendon sheath. *Webbed f's* fingers more or less united by strands of tissue; syndactyly.

**firm** (fərm) a medical or surgical hospital team, usually comprising two house officers, a senior house officer (SHO), a registrar and a senior registrar, directed by a consultant physician or surgeon.

**first aid** ( fərst 'ayd) emergency care and treatment of an injured person before complete medical and surgical treatment can be secured.

**fission** ('fishən) a form of asexual reproduction by dividing into two equal parts, as in bacteria. *Binary f.* the splitting in two of the nucleus and the protoplasm of a cell, as in protozoa. *Nuclear f.* the splitting of the nucleus of an atom, with the release of a great quantity of energy.

**fissure** ('fishə) a narrow slit or cleft. *Anal f.* a painful crack in the mucous membrane of the anus. *F. of Rolando* a furrow in the cortex of each cerebral hemisphere, dividing the sensory from the motor area; the central sulcus.

**fistula** ('fistyuhlə) an abnormal passage between two epithelial surfaces, usually connecting the cavity of one organ with another or a cavity with the surface of the body. *Anal f.* the result of an ischiorectal abscess where the channel is from the anus to the skin. *Biliary f.* a leakage of bile to the exterior, following operation on the gallbladder or ducts. *Blind f.* one which is open at only one end. *Faecal f.* one in which the channel is from the intestine through the wound caused by an operation on the intestines when sepsis is present. *Rectovaginal f.* fistula from the rectum to the vagina which may result from a severe perineal tear during childbirth. *Tracheo-oesophageal f.* an opening from the trachea into the oesophagus; a congenital deformity. *Vesicovaginal f.* an opening from the bladder to the vagina, either from error during operation or from ulceration, as may occur in carcinoma of the cervix.

**fit** (fit) a commonly used term for paroxysmal motor discharges leading to sudden convulsive movements, as in epilepsy, eclampsia and hysteria. The term is sometimes applied to apoplexy.

**fitness** ('fitnəs) associated with a sense of wellbeing, and the ability to undertake sustained physical exertion without undue breathlessness. Fitness needs to be maintained on a regular basis by the person taking regular physical exertion or exercise.

**fixation** (fik'sayshən) 1. the process of rendering something immovable, such as a joint or a fractured bone. 2. in psychology, a term used to describe a failure to progress wholly or in part through the normal stages of psychological development to a fully developed personality. 3. in ophthalmology, directing the sight straight at an object.

**flaccid** ('flaksid, 'flasid) soft, flabby. *F. paralysis see* PARALYSIS.

**Flagyl** ('flagil) trade name for a preparation of metronidazole, an antibacterial and antiprotozoal.

**flail** (flayl) exhibiting abnormal or pathological mobility, as in flail chest or flail joint. *F. chest* a loss of stability of the chest wall due to multiple rib fractures or detachment of the sternum from the ribs as a result of a severe crushing chest injury. The loose chest segment moves in a direction that is the reverse of normal. *F. joint* an unusually movable joint.

**flap** (flap) a mass of tissue, used for grafting in plastic surgery, which is left attached to its blood supply and used to repair defects either adjacent to it or at some distance from it.

**flare** (flair) the response of the skin to an allergic or hypersensitivity reaction. Reddening of the skin that spreads outwards.

**flatfoot** ('flat,fuht) a condition due to absence or sinking of the medial longitudinal arch of the foot, caused by weakening of the ligaments and tendons. Pes planus.

**flatulence** ('flatyuhləns) excessive formation of gases in the stomach or intestine.

**flatulent** ('flatyuhlənt) suffering from flatulence. *F. distension* swelling due to gas in the stomach or intestines. It is a common complication after abdominal operations and is caused by intestinal stasis.

**flatus** ('flaytəs) gas in the stomach or intestine.

**flea** (flee) a small, wingless bloodsucking insect parasite. The common human flea, *Pulex irritans*, rarely transmits disease. Cat and dog fleas, *Ctenocephalides*, are also relatively harmless. The rat fleas *Xenopsylla* and *Nosopsyllus* are the vectors of bubonic plague.

**flexibilitas cerea** ( fleksi,bilitəs 'seeə.ri.ə) waxy flexibility; a cataleptic state in which the limbs retain any position in which they are placed. A symptom of some forms of schizophrenia; also occurs occasionally in hysteria.

**flexion** ('flekshən) bending; moving a joint so that the two or more bones forming it draw towards each other. *Plantar f.* bending the fingers or toes downwards.

**Flexner's bacillus** ('fleksnəz) *S. Flexner, American bacteriologist, 1863–1946.* One of the group of pathogenic bacteria which cause bacillary dysentery; *Shigella flexneri.*

**flexor** ('fleksə) any muscle causing flexion of a limb or other part of the body.

**flexure** ('flekshə) a bend or curve.

**flight of ideas** (ˌfliet əv ie'diəz) the rapid movement of ideas and speech from one fragmentary topic to another that occurs in mania.

**floaters** ('flohtəz) wisps or strands within the eye that are visible to the patient. Usually caused by detachment and collapse of the vitreous humour and the normal ageing process.

**flooding** ('fluding) 1. excessive loss of blood from the uterus. 2. a form of desensitization for the treatment of phobias and related disorders. The patient is repeatedly exposed, in imagination or real life, to emotionally distressing aversive stimuli of high intensity. Also called implosion.

**florid** ('flo.rid) having a flushed facial appearance.

**flowmeter** ('floh.meetə) an instrument used to measure the flow of liquids or gases.

**flucloxacillin** (ˌflookloksə'silin) an antibiotic drug used in the treatment of infection by penicillin-resistant bacteria.

**fluctuation** (ˌfluktyoo'ayshən, -chyoo-) a wave-like motion felt on palpation of the abdomen.

**fludrocortisone** (ˌfloodroh'kawti-ˌsohn, -ˌzohn) a synthetic corticosteroid used in the treatment of adrenal disorders.

**fluid** ('flooid) 1. a liquid or gas; any liquid of the body. 2. composed of molecules which freely change their relative positions without separation of the mass. *Amniotic f.* the fluid within the amnion that bathes the developing fetus and protects it from mechanical injury. *Body f's* the fluids within the body, composed of water, electrolytes and nonelectrolytes. The volume and distribution of body fluids vary with age, sex and amount of adipose tissue (*see* Figure). *Cerebrospinal f.* the fluid contained within the ventri-cles of the brain, the subarachnoid space and the central canal of the spinal cord. *Interstitial f.* the extracellular fluid bathing most tissues, excluding the fluid within the lymph and blood vessels.

**fluid balance** (ˌbaləns) a state in which the volume of body water and its solutes (electrolytes and nonelectrolytes) is within normal limits and there is normal distribution of fluids within the intracellular and extracellular compartments. The total volume of body fluids should be about 60% of the body weight.

**fluke** (flook) one of a group of parasitic flatworms (Trematoda). Different varieties may affect the blood, the intestines, the liver or the lungs.

**fluorescein** (ˌflooə'resee.in) a dye used to detect corneal ulceration. When it is dropped on the eye the ulcer stains green.

**fluorescence** (ˌflooə'res'ns) the property of reflecting back light waves, usually of a lower frequency than those absorbed so that invisible light (e.g. ultraviolet) may become visible.

**fluorescent** (ˌflooə'res'nt) capable of producing fluorescence. *F. screen* a screen that becomes fluorescent when exposed to X-rays. *F. treponemal antibody test* a serological test for syphilis; the first to become positive after infection.

**fluoridation** (ˌflooə.ri'dayshən) the adding of fluorine to water, in those areas where it is lacking, in order to reduce the incidence of dental caries.

**fluorine** ('flooə.reen) *symbol* F. Any binary compound of fluorine.

**fluoroscope** (ˌflooə.rəskohp) an instrument for the study of moving internal organs and contrast medium using X-rays.

**fluorouracil** (ˌflooə.roh'yooə.rəsil) an antimetabolite cytotoxic drug used particularly in the treatment of solid tumours.

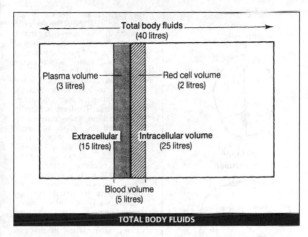

**fluphenazine** (floo'fenə zeen) a major tranquillizer.

**flurandrenolone** (,flooə.ran'drenə lohn) a topical steroid used for eczema and other inflammatory skin conditions that have not responded to weaker steroids.

**flurbiprofen** (,flərbi'prohfen) a non-steroidal anti-inflammatory drug.

**flush** (flush) a redness of the face and neck. *Hectic f.* one occurring in conditions such as septic poisoning and pulmonary tuberculosis. *Hot f.* one occurring during the menopause, accompanied by a feeling of heat.

**flutter** ('flutə) an irregularity of the heartbeat.

**focus** ('fohkəs) 1. the point of convergence of light or sound waves. 2. the local seat of a disease.

**focusing** ('fohkəsing) the ability of the eye to alter its lens power to focus correctly at different distances.

**folic acid** ('fohlik) one of the VITA-MINS of the B complex. Folic acid is involved in the synthesis of amino acids and DNA; its deficiency causes megaloblastic anaemia. Green vegetables, liver and yeast are major sources. *F. a. antagonist* any antimetabolite cytotoxic drug that inhibits the action of the folic acid enzyme.

**folie à deux** (fo'lee a dər) [Fr.] the occurrence of identical psychoses simultaneously in two closely associated persons.

**follicle** ('folik'l) a very small sac or gland. *Hair f.* the sheath in which a hair grows. *F.-stimulating hormone* abbreviated FSH. A hormone, produced by the anterior pituitary gland, which controls the maturation of the GRAAFIAN FOLLICLES in the ovary.

**follicular** (fo'likyuhlə) pertaining to a follicle. *F. conjunctivitis* inflammation occurring in the lower conjunctival fornix. *F. tonsillitis* tonsillitis arising from infection of the tonsillar follicles.

**folliculosis** (fo,likyuh'lohsis) an abnormal increase in the number of

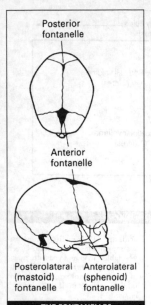

Posterior
fontanelle

Anterior
fontanelle

Posterolateral   Anterolateral
(mastoid)        (sphenoid)
fontanelle       fontanelle

**THE FONTANELLES**

lymph follicles. *Conjunctival f.* a benign non-inflammatory overgrowth of follicles of the conjunctiva of the eyelids.

**fomentation** (ˌfohmenˈtayshən) treatment by warm, moist applications; also, the substance thus applied.

**fomes** (ˈfohmeez) *see* FOMITES.

**fomites** (fəˈmieteez, ˈfohmə-) [L.] *sing.* fomes; inanimate objects or material on which disease-producing agents may be conveyed.

**fontanelle** (ˌfontəˈnel) a soft membranous space between the cranial bones of an infant (*see* Figure). *Anterior f.* that between the parietal and frontal bones, which closes at about the age of 18 months. Rickets causes delay in this process. *Posterior f.* the junction of the occipital and parietal bones, at the sagittal suture, which closes within 3 months of birth.

**food** (food) anything which, when taken into the body, serves to nourish or build up the tissues or to supply body heat. *F. allergy* sensitivity to one or more of the components of a normal diet, e.g. peanut allergy, which is rare but may be dangerous. *F. poisoning* a group of notifiable acute illnesses caused by ingestion of contaminated food. It may result from toxaemia from foods, such as those inherently poisonous or those contaminated by poisons, foods containing poisons formed by bacteria, or food-borne infections. Food poisoning usually causes inflammation of the gastrointestinal tract (gastroenteritis). This may occur quite suddenly, soon after the food has been eaten. The symptoms are acute, and include tenderness, pain or cramps in the abdomen, nausea, vomiting, diarrhoea, weakness and dizziness. *See* BOTULISM.

**foot** (fuht) the terminal part of the lower limb. *Athlete's f.* ringworm of the foot; tinea pedis. *F. drop* inability to keep the foot at the correct angle owing to paralysis of the flexors of the ankle. *F. presentation* the presentation of one or both legs instead of the head during labour.

**foramen** (foˈraymən) an opening or hole, especially in a bone. *F. magnum* the hole in the occipital bone through which the spinal cord passes. *F. ovale* the hole between the left and right atria in the fetus. *Obturator f.* the large hole in the innominate bone. *Optic f.* the opening in the posterior part of the orbit through which the optic nerve and the ophthalmic artery pass.

**forceps** ('forseps) surgical instruments used for lifting or compressing an object. *Artery f. (Spencer Wells f.)* compress bleeding points during an operation. *Cheatle f.* long forceps for lifting utensils. *Obstetric f.* various patterns are used in difficult labour to facilitate delivery. *Vulsellum f.* have clawlike ends for exerting traction.

**forensic** (fə'renzik, -sik) pertaining to or applied in legal proceedings. *F. medicine* the branch that is concerned with the law and has a bearing on legal problems. It includes the investigation of unexplained death or injury.

**foreskin** ('for‚skin) the prepuce.

**formaldehyde** (faw'maldi‚hied) a gaseous compound with strongly disinfectant properties. It is used in solution for disinfection of excreta and utensils and also in the preparation of toxoids from toxins.

**formula** ('fawmyuhlə) [L.] 1. an expression, using numbers or symbols, of the composition of, or of directions for preparing, a compound, such as a medicine; or of a procedure to follow to obtain a desired result; or of a single concept. 2. a mixture for feeding an infant, composed of milk and/or other ingredients.

**formulary** ('fawmyuhlə‚ree) a prescriber's handbook of drugs. *See* BRITISH NATIONAL FORMULARY.

**fornix** ('forniks) an arch. *Conjunctival f.* the reflection of the conjunctiva from the eyelids on to the eyeball. *F. cerebri* an arched structure at the back and base of the brain. *F. of the vagina* the recesses at the top of the vagina in front (*anterior f.*), back (*posterior f.*) and sides (*lateral f.*) of the cervix uteri.

**fossa** ('fosə) a small depression or pit. Usually applied to fossae in bones. *Cubital f.* the triangular depression at the front of the elbow. *Iliac f.* the depression on the inner surface of the iliac bone. *Pituitary f.* the depression in the sphenoid bone. *See* SELLA TURCICA.

**foster children** ('fostə) children under the care of foster parents.

**foster parents** (pair‚rənts) persons who undertake for reward the care of children who are not related to them within the meaning of the Children Act (1989).

**Fothergill's operation** ('fodhə‚gilz) *W.E. Fothergill, British gynaecologist, 1865–1926.* Amputation of the cervix, with anterior and posterior colporrhaphy for prolapse of the uterus.

**fourchette** (fooə'shet) [Fr.] the fold of membrane at the perineal end of the vulva.

**fovea** ('fohvi.ə) a fossa; a small depression, particularly that of the retina that contains a large number of cones, giving form and colour, and is therefore the area of most accurate vision.

**fracture** ('frakchə) 1. to break a part, especially a bone. 2. a break in the continuity of bone. The signs and symptoms are pain, swelling, deformity, shortening of the limb, loss of power, abnormal mobility, and crepitus Fractures are generally caused by trauma, by either a direct or an indirect force on the bone. Fractures may also be caused by muscle spasm or by disease that results in decalcification of the bone. The different types and classification of fractures are shown in the Figure on p. 164. *March f.* a hairline crack in the long bone of the foot caused by repeated trauma associated with long marches and with jogging. *Pathological f.* one due to weakening of the bone structure by pathological processes, such as neoplasia, osteomalacia or osteomyelitis. *Pott's f.* a fracture dislocation of the ankle involving the lower end of the fibula and sometimes the internal malleolus of the tibia. *Spontaneous f.* one that

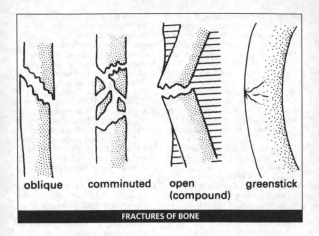

oblique    comminuted    open    greenstick
(compound)

**FRACTURES OF BONE**

occurs as a result of little or no violence, usually of a bone weakened by disease.

**frame** (fraym) a rigid supporting structure or a structure for immobilizing a part. *Braun f.* a metal frame used to elevate the lower limb in fractures of the tibia and fibula. *Quadriplegic standing f.* a device for supporting in the upright position a patient whose four limbs are paralysed. *Stryker f.* one consisting of canvas stretched on anterior and posterior frames, on which the patient can be rotated around the longitudinal axis. *Walking f.* a walking aid with three or four legs.

**framycetin** (,frami'seetin) an aminoglycoside antibiotic, very similar to neomycin. Used for topical application.

**freckle** ('frek'l) a brown pigmented spot on the skin. *Hutchinson's melanotic f.* a non-invasive malignant melanoma which occurs mainly on the face of middle-aged women.

**free association** (free ə,sohsi'ay-shən) in psychoanalysis a spontaneous mental process whereby words used in a non-logical chain suggest ideas, thoughts or feelings without selection or repression.

**Frei's test** (friez) *W.S. Frei, German dermatologist, 1885–1943.* An intradermal test to aid the diagnosis of lymphogranuloma venereum.

**Freiberg's disease** ('friebərgz) *A.H. Freiberg, American surgeon, 1868–1940.* Osteochondritis of the second metatarsal bone, in which there is pain on walking and standing.

**fremitus** ('fremitəs) a thrill or vibration, e.g. that produced in the chest by speaking and felt on palpation.

**frenotomy** (fri'notəmee) the cutting of the frenulum of the tongue to cure tongue-tie.

**frenulum** ('frenyuhləm) frenum; a fold of mucous membrane which limits the movement of an organ. *F. of the tongue* the fold under the tongue.

**Freudian** ('froydi.ən) *S. Freud, Austrian psychiatrist, 1856–1939.* Relating to the theories of Freud, who was the originator of psychoanalysis and the psychoanalytical theory of the cause of neurosis.

**friable** ('friəb'l) easily crumbled or torn.

**friction** ('frikshən) the act of rubbing one object against another. *F. massage* a circular or transverse pressure applied by fingertip or thumb to a localized area. Used for the relief of pain. *F. murmur* the grating sound heard in auscultation when two rough surfaces rub together, as in dry pleurisy.

**Friedländer's bacillus** ('freedlendəz) *K. Friedländer, German pathologist, 1847–1887.* The cause of a rare form of pneumonia. *Klebsiella friedländeri.*

**Friedreich's ataxia** or **disease** ('freedrieks) *N. Friedreich, German physician, 1825–1882.* A rare form of hereditary ataxia.

**frigidity** (fri'jiditee) an absence of normal sexual desire; usually refers to women.

**Frölich's syndrome** ('frɜrliks) *A. Frölich, Austrian neurologist, 1871–1953.* A group of symptoms associated with disease of the pituitary body: increased adiposity, atrophy of the genital organs, and development of feminine characteristics.

**frontal** ('frunt'l) 1. relating to the forehead. 2. relating to the front or anterior aspect of a structure.

**frostbite** ('frost.biet) impairment of circulation, chiefly affecting the fingers, the toes, the nose and the ears, due to exposure to severe cold. The first stage is represented by chilblains. Advanced cases show thrombosis and dry gangrene.

**frottage** (fro'tahzh) [Fr.] 1. a rubbing movement in massage. 2. sexual gratification by rubbing against another person's body.

**frozen shoulder** ('frohzən) a stiff and painful shoulder; capsulitis. Treatment may include stretching under anaesthesia, combined with exercises. The cause is unknown.

**fructose** ('fruktohs, -tohz, 'fruhk-) fruit sugar, a monosaccharide.

**frusemide** ('froozəmied) a diuretic with a rapid and powerful action used in the treatment of oedema and of acute renal failure.

**FSH** follicle-stimulating hormone.

**fugue** (fyoog) a period of altered awareness during which a person may wander for hours or days and perform purposive actions although memory for the period may be lost. It may follow an epileptic fit or occur in hysteria or schizophrenia.

**fulguration** (.fulgyuh'rayshən) the destruction by diathermy of papillomata (warts), particularly inside the urinary bladder.

**fulminating** ('fuhlmi.nayting, 'ful-) sudden in onset and rapid in course.

**fumigation** (.fyoomi'gayshən) disinfection by exposure to the fumes of a vaporized germicide.

**function** ('fungk.shən) 1. the natural action or intended purpose of a person, organ or structure. 2. to perform special work or an action.

**fundus** ('fundəs) the base of an organ or the part farthest removed from the opening. *F. of the eye* the posterior part of the inside of the eye as shown by the ophthalmoscope. *F. of the stomach* that part above the cardiac orifice. *F. of the uterus* the top of the uterus; that part farthest from the cervix.

**fungate** ('fung.gayt) to grow rapidly and produce fungus-like growths. Often occurs in the late stages of malignant tumours.

**fungicide** ('funji.sied) a preparation that destroys fungal infection.

**fungiform** ('funji.fawm) shaped like a fungus or mushroom.

**fungus** ('fung.gəs) a low form of vegetable life which includes mushrooms and moulds. Some varieties cause disease, such as actinomycosis and ringworm.

**funis** ('fyoonis) the umbilical cord.

**funnel chest** ('fun'l) a developmental deformity in which there is a depression in the sternum and an inward curvature of the ribs and costal cartilages.

**furor** ('fyooə.raw) a state of intense excitement during which violent acts may be performed. This may occur after an epileptic fit.

**furuncle** ('fyooə.rungk'l) a boil.

**furunculosis** (fyuh.rungkyuh'loh-sis) a staphylococcal infection represented by many, or crops of, boils.

**furunculus** (fyuh'rungkyuhləs) a furuncle. *F. orientalis* a protozoal infection, mainly of the tropics, which causes a chronic ulceration. Cutaneous leishmaniasis.

**fusidic acid** (fyoo'sidik) an antibiotic used to treat penicillin-resistant staphylococci. It is usually used in combination with another antibiotic effective against staphylococci.

**fusiform** ('fyoozi.fawm) shaped like a spindle.

**fusion** ('fyoozhən) 1. the union between two adjacent structures. 2. the coordination of separate images of the same object in the two eyes into one image.

*Fusobacterium* (.fyoozohbak'tiə.ri.əm) a genus of anaerobic Gram-negative bacteria found as normal flora in the mouth and large bowel, and often in necrotic tissue, probably as secondary invaders.

**Fybogel** ('fiebojel) trade name for preparations of ispaghula husk, a laxative.

# G

**g** symbol for *gram*.

**G** symbol for *guanine*.

**Ga** symbol for *gallium*.

**gag** (gag) 1. an instrument placed between the teeth to keep the mouth open. 2. the reflex action that occurs when the back of the throat is stimulated.

**gait** (gayt) manner of walking. *Ataxic g.* the foot is raised high, descends suddenly, and the whole sole strikes the ground. *Cerebellar g.* a staggering walk indicative of cerebellar disease. *Four-point g.* a method which may be adopted when using sticks or crutches, which allows maximum stability. *Spastic g.* stiff, shuffling walk, the legs being kept together.

**galactorrhoea** (ˌgaləktə'reeə) 1. an excessive flow of milk. 2. secretion of milk after breast feeding has ceased.

**galactosaemia** (gəˌlaktə'seemi.ə) an inborn error of metabolism in which there is inability to convert galactose to glucose. The disorder becomes manifest soon after birth and is characterized by feeding problems, vomiting, diarrhoea, abdominal distension, enlargement of the liver and mental handicap. Treatment consists of exclusion from the diet of milk and all foods containing galactose or lactose.

**galactose** (gə'laktohz, -ohs) a monosaccharide derived from lactose. D-Galactose is found in lactose or milk sugar and cerebrosides of the brain. *G. tolerance test* a laboratory test to determine the liver's ability to convert the sugar galactose into glycogen.

**gall** (gawl) bile, a digestive fluid secreted by the liver and stored in the gallbladder.

**gallamine** ('galəˌmeen) a synthetic muscle relaxant, chemically related to curare but less potent and shorter-acting.

**gallbladder** ('gawlˌbladə) the sac under the lower surface of the liver, which acts as a reservoir for bile.

**gallipot** ('galiˌpot) a small receptacle for lotions.

**gallium** ('gali.əm) *symbol* Ga. A radioisotope used in detecting some soft-tissue disorders.

**gallop rhythm** ('galəp) heart rhythm that may occur when there is ventricular overload.

**gallstone** ('gawlˌstohn) a concretion formed in the gallbladder or bile ducts. Gallstones are often multiple and faceted. *G. colic see* BILIARY (COLIC).

**galvanometer** (ˌgalvə'nomitə) an instrument for detecting or measuring the strength of a current of electricity.

**gamete** ('gameet) a sex cell which combines with another to form a zygote, from which a complete organism develops. A spermatozoon or an ovum.

**gametocyte** (gə'meetoh,siet) a cell that is undergoing gametogenesis.

**gametogenesis** (,gamitoh'jenəsis) the production of the gametes by the gonads.

**gamma** ('gamə) the third letter in the Greek alphabet, γ. *G.-benzene hexachloride* a drug used as a cream, lotion or as a shampoo to treat head lice. *G. camera* an apparatus for depicting a part of the body into which radioactive isotopes emitting gamma rays have been introduced. *G. encephalography* a method of localizing a brain tumour by using radioactive isotopes emitting gamma rays. *G.-globulin* a class of plasma proteins composed almost entirely of IgG, an IMMUNOGLOBULIN protein that contains most antibody activity. *G. rays* electromagnetic rays, of shorter wavelength and with greater penetration than X-rays, which are given off by certain radioactive substances and which are used in radiotherapy. Also used in the sterilization of articles that would be destroyed by the heat and moisture required in autoclaving.

**ganglion** ('gang.gli.ən) 1. a collection of nerve cells and fibres, forming an independent nerve centre, as is found in the sympathetic nervous system. 2. a cystic swelling or a tendon.

**ganglionectomy** (,gang.gli.ə'nektəmee) excision of a ganglion.

**gangrene** ('gang.green) death of body tissue, generally in considerable mass, due either to loss of blood supply or to the effects of certain infections. *Dry g.* occurs gradually and results from slow reduction of the blood flow in the arteries. There is no subsequent bacterial decomposition; the tissues become dry and shrivelled. It occurs only in the extremities, and can occur with ARTERIOSCLEROSIS and DIABETES (MELLITUS). *Gas g.*

results from dirty lacerated wounds infected by anaerobic bacteria, especially species of *Clostridium*. It is an acute, severe, painful condition in which muscles and subcutaneous tissues become filled with gas and a serosanguineous exudate. *Moist g.* caused by sudden stoppage of blood, resulting from burning by heat or acid, severe freezing, physical accident that destroys the tissue, or a clot or other embolism. At first, tissue affected by moist gangrene has the colour of a bad bruise, and is swollen and often blistered. The gangrene is likely to spread with great speed. Toxins are formed in the affected tissues and absorbed.

**Ganser's syndrome (state)** ('ganzəz (stayt)) *S.J.M. Ganser, German psychiatrist, 1853–1931.* Amnesia, disturbance of consciousness and hallucinations, associated with senseless answers to questions, and absurd acts. Usually a transient response to a troublesome situation, e.g. prisoners on remand (prison psychosis).

**gargle** ('gahg'l) 1. a solution for rinsing the mouth and throat. 2. to rinse the mouth and throat by holding a solution in the open mouth and agitating it by expulsion of air from the lungs.

**gargoylism** ('gahgoy.lizəm) *see* HURLER'S SYNDROME.

**gas** (gas) molecules of a substance very loosely combined; a vapour. *G. and air analgesia* an authorized form of analgesia using nitrous oxide and air, by which the pains of labour are lessened without affecting uterine contractions. *Laughing g.* nitrous oxide. *Marsh g.* methane. *Sternutatory g.* one which causes sneezing. *Tear g.* one that is irritating to the eyes and causes excessive lacrimation.

**Gasser's ganglion** ('gasəz) *J.L. Gasser, Austrian anatomist, 1723–*

1765. The trigeminal ganglion. The ganglion of the sensory root of the fifth cranial nerve.

**gastrectomy** (ga'strektəmee) excision of part or whole of the stomach. *Billroth g.* removal of most of the lesser curvature and pyloric portion and joining of the duodenum to the refashioned stomach. This cuts down the production of secretin and acid. *Partial g.* removal of a part, usually the distal portion, of the stomach. Commonly performed in the surgical treatment of peptic ulcer. *Polya g.* removal of the first part of the duodenum and the greater part of the stomach, and anastomosis of the stomach to the jejunum. The blind portion of the duodenum supplies the bile and pancreatic and duodenal secretions.

**gastric** ('gastrik) pertaining to the stomach. *G. analysis* analysis of the stomach contents by microscopy and tests to determine the amount of acid present. *G. bypass* surgical creation of a small gastric pouch that empties directly into the jejunum through a gastrojejunostomy, thereby causing food to bypass the duodenum; performed for the treatment of gross OBESITY. *G. flu* a popular term for what may be any of several disorders of the stomach and intestinal tract. The symptoms are nausea, diarrhoea, abdominal cramps and fever. *G. juice* the clear fluid secreted by the glands of the stomach to assist digestion. It contains an enzyme called pepsin, which acts upon proteins in the presence of weak hydrochloric acid. *G. lavage* a treatment for some types of poisoning where the stomach contents are washed out through a stomach tube. *G. ulcer* ulceration of the gastric mucosa, associated with hyperacidity and often precipitated by HELICOBACTER PYLORI organisms. The condition is often aggravated by stress.

**gastrin** ('gastrin) a hormone, secreted by the walls of the stomach, which excites continued secretion of digestive juice while food is in the stomach.

**gastritis** (ga'strietis) inflammation of the lining of the stomach.

**gastro-oesophagostomy** (,gastroh-.i,sofə'gostəmee) a surgical anastomosis between the stomach and the oesophagus.

**gastrocnemius** (,gastrok'neemi.əs) the principal muscle of the calf of the leg. It flexes both the ankle and the knee.

**gastrocolic** (,gastroh'kolik) pertaining to the stomach and colon. *G. reflex* after a meal, increased peristalsis causes the colon to empty into the rectum. This gives rise to a desire to defecate.

**gastroduodenostomy** (,gastroh-,dyooədi'nostəmee) a surgical anastomosis between the stomach and the duodenum.

**gastroenteritis** (,gastroh,entə'rietis) inflammation of the lining of the stomach and intestine. Psychological causes of gastroenteritis include fear, anger and other forms of emotional upset. Allergic reactions to certain foods can cause gastroenteritis, as can irritation by excessive use of alcohol. Severe gastroenteritis, with such symptoms as headache, nausea, vomiting, weakness, diarrhoea and gas pains, may result from various viral and bacterial infections, such as INFLUENZA.

**gastroenterology** (,gastroh,entə-'roləjee) the study of diseases of the gastrointestinal tract.

**gastroenterostomy** (,gastroh,entə-'rostəmee) a surgical anastomosis between the stomach and small intestine.

**Gastrografin** (,gastroh'grafin) a proprietary oral diagnostic radio-opaque contrast medium.

**gastroileac** (,gastroh'iliak) pertaining to the stomach and ileum.

*G. reflex* food entering the stomach sets up powerful peristalsis in the ileum and opening of the ileocaecal valve.

**gastrointestinal** (,gastroh.in'tes-tin'l) pertaining to the stomach and intestine. *G. tract* the alimentary tract.

**gastrojejunostomy** (,gastroh.jejuh-'nostəmee) a surgical anastomosis between the stomach and the jejunum.

**gastroscope** ('gastrə,skohp) an endoscope especially designed for passage into the stomach to permit examination of its interior. The gastroscope is a hollow, cylindrical tube, fitted with special lenses and lights, which acts by reflecting light and creating a mirror effect, making it possible to 'go around corners', and facilitating visualization of the curvature of the stomach.

**gastrostomy** (ga'strostəmee) the creation of an opening into the stomach. This procedure is done to provide for the administration of food and liquids when stricture of the oesophagus or other conditions make swallowing impossible. *See* ARTIFICIAL (FEEDING).

**gastrotomy** (ga'strotəmee) a surgical incision of the stomach.

**gastrula** ('gastruhlə) an early stage in the development of the fertilized ovum.

**gatekeepers** ('gayt,keepəz) the individuals or groups in an organization who regulate access to goods and services, e.g. the family doctor's receptionist.

**Gaucher's disease** (goh'shayz) *P.C.E. Gaucher, French physician, 1854–1918.* A rare familial disease in which fat is deposited in the reticuloendothelial cells, causing an enlarged spleen and anaemia.

**gauze** (gawz) a thin open-meshed material used for dressing wounds.

**gavage** ('gavahzh) [Fr.] forced feeding; the giving of fluids and nourishment by oesophageal or other type of tube directly into the stomach.

**gay** (gay) popular term for a homosexual, usually male. *G. bowel syndrome* the damaging effects of male homosexual practices on the lower bowel; also includes anal fissures, anal fistulas, haemorrhoids and ulcers.

**Geiger counter** ('giegə ,kowntə) *H. Geiger, German physicist, 1882–1945.* An instrument for detecting and registering radioactivity. The apparatus is sensitive to the rays emitted.

**gelatin** ('jelətin) an albuminoid, obtained from connective tissue or bone. Used in pharmacy for suppositories and capsules, and in bacteriology as a culture medium. In absorbable film and sponge, it is used in surgical procedures.

**gender** ('jendə) sex; the category to which an individual is assigned on the basis of sex. *G. identity disorder* a psychiatric label for those disorders marked by a sense of inappropriateness and attendant discomfort concerning one's sexual anatomy and sex role. This category usually includes transvestism, transsexualism and gender identity disorders in childhood.

**gene** (jeen) one of the biological units of heredity, self-reproducing and located at a definite position (locus) on a particular chromosome. *Dominant g.* one that is capable of transmitting its characteristics irrespective of the genes from the other parent. *G. therapy* the use of 'healthy' genes to cure or treat a hereditary disease. *Recessive g.* one that can pass on its characteristics only if it is present with a similar recessive gene from the other parent. *See* MENDEL'S THEORY.

**General Household Survey (GHS)** (,jenrəl hows'hold) started in 1971, now under the auspices of the Office for National Statistics; initially for use by all government departments but also provides a secondary data source for the social sciences. It is a continuous survey and includes five main areas of investigation: family data, employment, housing, education and health.

**general practitioner (GP)** the role of the general practitioner or primary care physician in the United Kingdom is unique. Besides being the first point of contact for most patients, GPs must offer the first treatment or referral for all problems which are presented to them. In addition, GPs give personal and continuing care to their patients, often over the course of many years.

**genetic** (jə'netik) 1. pertaining to reproduction or to birth or origin. 2. inherited. *G. code* the arrangement of genetic material stored in the DNA molecule of the chromosome. *G. counselling* supportive service for prospective parents who can receive advice as to the likelihood of their children being born with a genetically transmitted disorder.

**genetics** (jə'netiks) the study of heredity and natural development.

**genitalia** (,jeni'tayli.ə) the organs of reproduction.

**genitourinary** (,jenitoh'yooə.rinə.ree) referring to both the reproductive organs and the urinary tract.

**genotype** ('jenoh,tiep,    'jeenoh-) the genetic characteristics of an individual.

**gentamicin** (,jentə'miesin) an antibiotic effective against many Gramnegative bacteria, especially *Pseudomonas* species, as well as certain Gram-positive bacteria, especially *Staphylococcus aureus*.

**genu** ('jenyoo) [L.] *the knee*. *G. valgum* knock-knee. *G. varum* bowleg.

**genupectoral** (,jenyoo'pektə.rəl) relating to the knee and chest. *G. position* the knee–chest position. *See* POSITION.

**geriatrics** (,jeri'atriks) the branch of medicine covering old age and the disorders arising from it.

**germ** (jərm) 1. a microbe. 2. that from which something may develop; a seed.

**German measles** (,jərmən) *see* RUBELLA.

**germicide** ('jərmi,sied) an agent capable of destroying pathogenic microorganisms.

**germinoma** (,jərmi'nohmə) a neoplasm of the testis or ovum.

**gerontology** (,jeron'toləjee) the study of old age and the ageing processes.

**Gessel's developmental chart** ('ges'lz) *A. Gessell, American psychologist, 1880–1961.* A chart which shows the expected motor, social and psychological development of children.

**gestaltism** (gə'shtaltizəm) a theory of holism in psychology which claims that ideas come as a whole and are not subdivisible.

**gestation** (je'stayshən) the period of development of the young in mammals, from the time of fertilization of the ovum to birth. *See also* PREGNANCY. *Ectopic g.* fetal development in some part other than the uterus, usually the uterine tube (*see* Figure on p. 172). *G. period* the duration of pregnancy; in the human female about 280 days when measured from the first day of the last menstrual period.

**Ghon focus** (gon) *A. Ghon, Czechoslovakian pathologist, 1866–1936.* The primary lesion of pulmonary tuberculosis, as seen on chest radiograph, after it has healed by fibrosis and calcification.

**giardiasis** (,jiah'dieəsis) *A. Giard, French biologist, 1846–1908.* An infection with *Giardia lamblia*, a

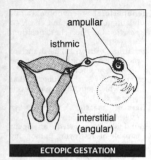

ampullar

isthmic

interstitial
(angular)

**ECTOPIC GESTATION**

pear-shaped protozoon that causes a persistent protracted diarrhoea, often resulting in intestinal malabsorption.

**gigantism** ('jiegan‚tizəm, jie'gantizəm) abnormal growth of the body, often due to overactivity of the anterior lobe of the pituitary gland.

**Gilles de la Tourette's syndrome (disease)** (‚zheel də lah tooə'rets) *G.E.A.B. Gilles de la Tourette, French neurologist, 1857–1904.* Multiple tics, especially of the face and upper part of the body, often associated with involuntary obscene utterances. The condition usually has its onset in childhood and often becomes chronic. The cause is unknown.

**Gilliam's operation** ('gili.əmz) *D.T. Gilliam, American gynaecologist, 1844–1923.* The correction of retroversion of the uterus by shortening the round ligaments; ventrosuspension.

**gingiva** ('jinjivə, jin'jievə) the gum; connective tissue surrounding the necks of the teeth.

**gingivectomy** (‚jinji'vektəmee) the surgical removal of the gum margins to get rid of pockets and improve the shape of the gums.

**gingivitis** (‚jinji'vietis) inflammation of the gums.

**ginseng** ('jinseng) used widely in Chinese medicine; reputed to have the power to cure many diseases and to have properties to improve sexual health and impotence.

**gland** (gland) an organ composed of cells which secrete fluid prepared from the blood, either for use in the body, or for excretion as waste material. *Ductless (endocrine) g.* one that produces an internal secretion but has no canal (duct) to carry the secretion away, e.g. the thyroid gland. *Exocrine g.* one that discharges its secretion through a duct, e.g. the parotid gland. *Lymph g. see* LYMPH (NODES). *Mucous g.* one that secretes mucus.

**glanders** ('glandəz) a disease of horses communicable to humans, and caused by the glanders bacillus, *Pseudomonas mallei*.

**glandular** ('glandyuhlə) pertaining to a gland. *G. fever see* INFECTIOUS (MONONUCLEOSIS).

**glans** (glanz) an acorn-shaped body, such as the rounded end of the penis or the clitoris.

**Glasgow coma scale** (‚glazgoh) a standardized system for quickly evaluating the level of consciousness in the critically ill. Measures include: eye opening according to four criteria, verbal response against five criteria, and motor response using six criteria. Scores of 7 or less qualify as 'coma'. Coma is defined as no response and no eye opening.

**glaucoma** (glaw'kohmə) raised intraocular pressure. *Closed-angle g.* one that occurs when there is a mechanical defect in the drainage angle; may be primary or secondary. It may be acute, when there is pain and blurring of vision, or chronic, when there may be no pain, but a gradual loss of vision. *Open-angle g.* chronic primary glaucoma in which the angle remains open but drainage becomes gradually diminished. *Primary g.* one that occurs without any previous disease. It is a common cause of blindness, partial or complete, in the elderly. *Secondary g.* one that occurs when some ocular disease is complicated by an increase in intraocular pressure.

**gleet** (gleet) chronic gonococcal urethritis marked by a transparent mucous discharge.

**glenoid** ('gleenoyd) resembling a hollow. *G. cavity* the socket of the shoulder joint.

**glia** ('gliea) neuroglia; the connective tissue of the brain and spinal cord.

**glibenclamide** (glie'benklə,mied) an oral hypoglycaemic agent of the sulphonylurea group used in the treatment of maturity onset diabetes mellitus (Type II).

**glioblastoma** (,glieohbla'stohmə) a malignant glioma arising in the cerebral hemispheres.

**glioma** (glie'ohmə) a malignant tumour composed of neuroglial cells affecting the brain and spinal cord; seldom metastasizes.

**globin** ('glohbin) a protein used in the formation of haemoglobin.

**globulins** ('globyuhlinz) a protein group, forming constituents of the blood (*serum g.*) and cerebrospinal fluid.

**globus** ('globəs) a ball or globe. *G. hystericus* a symptom of hysteria when a patient feels unable to swallow because there is a lump in the throat. *G. pallidus* the pale medial part of the lentiform nucleus of the brain.

**glomerulitis** (glo,meryuh'lietis) inflammation of the glomeruli of the kidney.

**glomerulonephritis** (glo,meryuh-lohnə'frietis) a bilateral, non-infectious inflammation of the kidneys. The cause is unknown but the condition is associated with immunological disturbance. It may

be acute, presenting rapidly but reversibly, or it may be chronic, presenting slowly and irreversibly.

**glomerulosclerosis** (glo,meryuh-lohsklə'rohsis) degenerative changes in the glomerular capillaries of the renal tubule, leading to renal failure.

**glomerulus** (glo'meryuhlas) the tuft of capillaries within the nephron, which filters urine from the blood.

**glossal** ('glos'l) relating to the tongue.

*Glossina* (glo'siena) a genus of biting flies, the tsetse flies.

**glossitis** (glo'sietis) inflammation of the tongue.

**glossolalia** (,glosə'layli.ə) 'speaking in tongues'; unintelligible speech. The patient speaks in an imaginary language.

**glossopharyngeal** (,glosoh,fə'rinji.əl, -,farin'jeeəl) pertaining to the tongue and pharynx. *G. nerve* the ninth cranial nerve.

**glossoplegia** (,glosoh'pleeji.ə) paralysis of the tongue.

**glottis** ('glotis) the space between the vocal cords. The term is sometimes used for that part of the larynx which is associated with voice production.

**glucagon** ('glookə,gon) a polypeptide produced by the pancreas. It aids glycogen breakdown in the liver and raises the blood sugar level.

**glucocorticoid** (,glookoh'kawti,koyd) any corticoid substance that raises the concentration of liver glycogen and blood sugar, i.e. cortisol (hydrocortisone), cortisone and corticosterone.

**gluconeogenesis** (,glookoh,neeoh-'jenəsis) the production of glucose from the non-nitrogen portion of the amino acids after deamination. It occurs in the liver and kidneys.

**glucose** ('glookohs, -kohz) dextrose or grape-sugar; a simple sugar, a

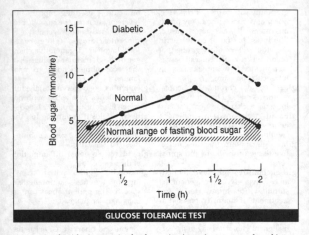

**GLUCOSE TOLERANCE TEST**

monosaccharide in certain foodstuffs, especially fruit, and in normal blood; the chief source of energy for living organisms. *See also* DEXTROSE. *G.-6-phosphate dehydrogenase* a red-cell enzyme. Inherited deficiency causes a tendency to haemolytic anaemia. *See* FAVISM. *G. tolerance test* test in which a quantity of glucose is given and the concentration of glucose in the blood is estimated at intervals afterwards (*see* Figure). Used mainly when diabetes mellitus is suspected.

**glue ear** (ˌgloo iə) the accumulation of sticky material in the middle ear resulting in impaired hearing, most common in young schoolchildren.

**glue sniffing** ('gloo ˌsnifing) solvent abuse.

**glutamic acid** (gloo'tamik) one of the 22 amino acids formed by the digestion of dietary protein.

**glutamic–oxaloacetic transaminase** (glooˌtamikˌoksəloh.əˈseetik tranz-ˈamiˌnayz) an enzyme found in cardiac muscle and the liver. Raised serum levels (SGOT) may indicate an acute myocardial infarction or the presence of liver disease.

**glutamic–pyruvic transaminase** (glooˌtamikpie'roovik tranz'amiˌnayz) an enzyme found in the liver. Measurement of serum levels (SGPT) is used in the study and diagnosis of liver diseases.

**glutaraldehyde** (ˌglootə'raldiˌhied) a disinfectant active against all viruses, fungi, vegetative bacteria and spores. Used in aqueous solution for sterilization of non-heat-resistant equipment.

**gluteal** ('glooti.əl, gloo'ti.əl) relating to the buttocks. *G. muscles* three muscles which form the fleshy part of the buttocks.

**gluten** ('glootən) the protein of wheat and other grains. *G.-induced enteropathy* coeliac disease.

**glycerin** ('glisəˌrin) a colourless syrupy substance obtained from fats and fixed oils. It has a hygroscopic action. As an emollient it is an ingredient of many skin preparations. *G. suppository* one composed of glycerin and gelatin, used as an evacuant. *G. of thymol* an antiseptic mouthwash and gargle.

**glyceryl trinitrate** (ˌglisə.ril trieˈnie-trayt) nitroglycerin. Glyceryl trinitrate is a vasodilator used to relieve certain types of pain, especially in the prophylaxis and treatment of ANGINA (PECTORIS). It is administered sublingually or by transdermal patch or gel.

**glycine** ('glieseen) a non-essential amino acid.

**glycogen** ('gliekəjən) the form in which carbohydrate is stored in the liver and muscles. Animal starch. *G. storage disease* inherited disease in which there is a deficiency in the synthesis of glycogen. This accumulates in the liver, causing enlargement.

**glycogenesis** (ˌgliekoh'jenəsis) the process of glycogen formation from the blood glucose.

**glycogenolysis** (ˌgliekəjə'nolisis) the breakdown of glycogen in the body so that it may be utilized.

**glycoside** ('gliekə.sied) a crystalline body in plants which, when acted on by acids or ferments, produces sugar. If the sugar is glucose it may be termed a glucoside. *See* DIGITALIS.

**glycosuria** (ˌgliekoh'syooə.ri.ə) an excess of glucose in the urine, a symptom of diabetes mellitus. *Renal g.* sugar in the urine, in an otherwise healthy person, due to an inherited inability to reabsorb glucose normally.

**glymidine** ('gliemi.deen) a drug of the sulphonylurea group used in the treatment of diabetes mellitus.

**gnathic** ('nathik) pertaining to the jaw.

**gnathoplasty** ('nathoh.plastee) a plastic operation on the jaw.

**goblet cell** ('goblit ˌsel) a goblet-shaped cell, found in the intestinal epithelium, which produces mucus.

**goitre** ('goytə) enlargement of the thyroid gland, causing a swelling in the front part of the neck. Simple endemic goitre, sometimes referred to as Derbyshire neck, is usually caused by lack of iodine in the diet. *Colloid g.* an enlarged but soft thyroid gland with no signs of hyperthyroidism. *Exophthalmic g.* hyperthyroidism with marked protrusion of the eyeballs (exophthalmos). Graves' disease. *Intrathoracic g.* enlargement of the gland mainly in the thorax, so the swelling may not be easily visible. *Sporadic g.* a simple non-toxic enlargement. *Substernal g.* enlargement of the gland behind the sternum so that swelling in the neck may not be apparent. *Toxic g.* signs of excess of thyroxine in the blood, where the gland has not been previously enlarged. The patient complains of weight loss and is generally nervous. Exophthalmos may be present.

**gold** (gohld) *symbol* Au. A metallic element used in treating rheumatoid arthritis. Gold salts are among the most toxic of therapeutic agents. Toxic reactions may vary from mild to severe kidney or liver damage and blood dyscrasias. *Radioactive g.* an isotope which gives off beta and gamma rays. Used in the form of small grains or seeds, it may be implanted into malignant tissues. In colloidal form it may be instilled into a serous cavity to treat malignant effusions.

**Golgi apparatus** ('goljee apə.raytəs, 'golgee) *C. Golgi, Italian histologist, 1844–1926.* Specialized structures seen near the nucleus of a cell during microscopic examination.

**Golgi's organ** the sensory end-organs in muscle tendons that are sensitive to stretch.

**gonad** ('gohnad, 'gonad) a reproductive gland; the testicle or ovary.

**gonadotrophic** (ˌgonədoh'trohfik) having influence on the gonads. *G. hormones* gonadotrophin.

**gonadotrophin** (ˌgonədoh'trohfin) any hormone having a stimulating effect on the gonads. Two such hormones are secreted by the anterior pituitary: follicle-stimulating hormone (FSH) and luteinizing hormone (LH), both of which are active, but with differing effects, in the two sexes. *Chorionic g.* a gonad-stimulating hormone produced by cytotrophoblastic cells of the placenta; used in the treatment of underdevelopment of the gonads and to induce ovulation in infertile women.

**gonion** ('gohni.ən) [Gr.] the midpoint of the mandible (lower jaw).

**gonioscope** ('gohnioh,skohp) an apparatus for examining the angle of the anterior chamber of the eye.

**goniotomy** (ˌgohni'otəmee) an operation for glaucoma; it consists in opening Schlemm's canal under direct vision.

**gonococcus** (ˌgonoh'kokəs) *Neisseria gonorrhoeae*, a diplococcus which causes gonorrhoea.

**gonorrhoea** (ˌgonə'reeə) a common venereal disease caused by *Neisseria gonorrhoeae* infecting the genital tract of either sex, causing a discharge and pain on micturition, although the disease is often asymptomatic in females. Spread by the bloodstream, it may give rise to iritis or arthritis. Scar tissue formation may bring about urethral stricture or infertility owing to occlusion of the uterine tubes. The eyes of babies may be infected at birth during passage through the birth canal of an infected mother. The condition is called OPHTHALMIA (NEONATORUM) (notifiable disease). In the past it was a major cause of blindness in babies.

**gonorrhoeal** (ˌgonə'reeəl) relating to gonorrhoea. *G. arthritis* intractable infection of joints, causing great pain and disability.

**gouge** (gowj) a curved chisel used for scooping out diseased bone or other hard substances.

**gout** (gowt) a hereditary form of arthritis with an excess of uric acid in the blood. It is characterized by painful inflammation and swelling of the smaller joints, especially those of the big toe and thumb. Inflammation is accompanied by the deposit of urates around the joints.

**GPI** general paralysis of the insane; dementia paralytica. *See* PARALYSIS.

**Graafian follicle** ('grahfi.ən) *R. de Graaf, Dutch physician and anatomist, 1641–1673.* A follicle which is formed in the ovary and contains an ovum (*see* Figure). A follicle matures during each menstrual cycle, ruptures and releases the ovum (ovulation), which is then picked up by the fimbriated end of the uterine tube.

**graft** (grahft) 1. any tissue or organ for implantation or transplantation. 2. to implant or transplant such tissue. *Autogenous g.* a graft taken from and given to the same individual. *Bone g.* a portion of bone transplanted to repair another bone. *Corneal g.* a portion of cornea, usually from a recently dead person, used to repair a diseased cornea. *Homologous g.* tissue obtained from the body of another animal of the same species but with a genotype differing from that of the recipient; a homograft or allograft. *Pedicle g.* a skin graft, one end of which remains attached to its original site until the grafting has become established.

**graft-versus-host disease (reaction)** (ˌgrahftvərsiz'hohst) abbreviated GVH disease. A condition that occurs when immunologically competent cells or their precursors are

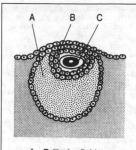

A  Follicular fluid
B  Granulosa cells
C  Ovum

**GRAAFIAN FOLLICLE**

transplanted into an immunologically incompetent recipient (host) that is not histocompatible with the donor. Characteristic signs include skin lesions, ulceration, alopecia, painful joints and haemolytic anaemia. GVH disease is a frequent complication of bone marrow transplants. Human leukocyte antigen (HLA) matching of the donor and recipient reduces the possibility of GVH disease.

**gram** (gram) *symbol* g. The fundamental SI unit of weight, equal to one thousandth of a kilogram.

**Gram's stain** ('gramz ˌstayn) *H. Gram, Danish physician, 1853–1938.* A method of staining bacteria which is used to classify them into Gram-negative and Gram-positive.

**grand mal** (ˌgronh 'mal) [Fr.] major epilepsy. *See* EPILEPSY.

**granular** ('granyuhlə) containing small particles. *G. casts* the degenerated cells from the lining of renal tubules excreted in the urine in certain kidney disorders.

**granulation** (ˌgranyuh'layshən) 1. the division of a hard solid substance into small particles. 2. the growth of new tissue by which ulcers and wounds heal when the edges are not in apposition. It consists of new capillaries and fibroblasts which fill in the space and later form fibrous tissue. The resulting scar is often unsightly.

**granule** ('granyool) 1. a small particle or grain. 2. a small pill made of sucrose.

**granulocyte** ('granyuhlə ˌsiet) any cell containing granules in its cytoplasm, especially polymorphonuclear leukocytes which contain neutrophilic, basophilic and eosinophilic granules in their cytoplasm.

**granulocytopenia** (ˌgranyuhlohˌsietə'peeni.ə) a marked reduction in the number of granulocytes in the blood. The condition may precede agranulocytosis.

**granuloma** (ˌgranyuh'lohmə) a tumour composed of granulation tissue, usually due to chronic infection or invasion by a foreign body.

**granulomatosis** (ˌgranyuhˌlohmə'tohsis) an infection producing granulomata. *Lipoid g.* xanthomatosis; Hand–Schüller Christian disease; *Malignant g.* lymphadenoma; Hodgkin's disease.

**gravel** ('grav'l) small 'sandy' calculi formed in the kidneys and bladder, and sometimes excreted with the urine. They can also form in the gallbladder where they can accumulate or cause low-grade cholecystitis.

**Graves' disease** ('grayvz) *R.J. Graves, Irish physician, 1796–1853.* Exophthalmic goitre; thyrotoxicosis.

**gravid** ('gravid) pregnant.

**gravity** ('gravətee) weight. *Specific g.* the weight of a substance compared with that of an equal volume of water.

**gray** (gray) *symbol* Gy. The SI unit used to denote the absorbed dose in radiation therapy.

**grey-scale display** ('gray,skayl dis-,play) a method to show the texture of tissue on ULTRASOUND display. The amplitude of each echo is represented by varying shades of grey. A bright white outline is seen from specular surfaces, a mottled grey from various tissue areas, and black from collections of fluid, such as the bladder and amniotic sac.

**grief** (greef) *see* BEREAVEMENT.

**griseofulvin** (,grizioh'fuhlvin) an oral antifungal antibiotic that is used in the treatment of infections of the skin, hair and nails.

**groin** (groyn) the junction of the upper thigh with the abdomen. The groins slope outwards and upwards from the pubic region.

**group therapy** (groop) a form of psychotherapy in which a group of patients meets regularly with the therapist in order to discuss and share problems, anxieties and fears in a psychotherapeutic setting. The group also provides emotional support for self-revelation and a structured environment for trying out new ways of relating to people.

**growing pains** ('groh.ing) recurrent quasi-rheumatic limb pains peculiar to early youth, once believed to be caused by the growing process. It is now recognized that growth does not cause pain and that these pains can be a symptom of many different disorders.

**growth** (grohth) 1. the progressive development of a living thing, especially the process by which the body reaches its point of complete physical development. 2. an abnormal formation of tissue, such as a tumour. *G. hormone* a substance that stimulates growth, especially a secretion of the anterior lobe of the PITUITARY gland that directly influences protein, carbohydrate and lipid metabolism, and controls the rate of skeletal and visceral growth. *See* CREUTZFELDT–JAKOB DISEASE (CJD).

**guanethidine** (gwah'nethi,deen) a drug used in the treatment of hypertension. It is an adrenergic blocking agent.

**guanine** ('gwahneen) a purine base, one of the constituents of all nucleic acids.

**guardian** *ad litem* (,gahdi.ən ad 'lietem) a person usually from the local authority social service department, who is appointed by a court to look after the interests of a child before its full Adoption Order is granted. Meanwhile the prospective adoptive parents have continuous possession of the child, and are visited and interviewed by the guardian *ad litem* to ensure that the home will be satisfactory.

**guardian Caldicott** ('kawldi,kot) a named member of an NHS Trust who is responsible for agreeing and reviewing internal protocols governing the protection and use of patient identified information by staff within the health-care system. This nominated person is also responsible for ensuring that these protocols meet the requirements of relevant national guidance and/or policies and that all systems in place are regularly monitored.

**Guillain–Barré syndrome** (,giyanh-'baray) *G. Guillain, French neurologist, 1876–1961; A. Barré, French neurologist, 1880–1967.* Acute infective polyneuritis. After an infection, usually respiratory, there is a general weakness or paralysis which frequently affects the respiratory muscles as well as the peripheral ones.

**guillotine** ('gilə,teen) a surgical instrument used for excising tonsils.

**guinea-worm** ('gini,wərm) a nematode worm, *Dracunculus medinensis*, which burrows into human tissues, particularly into the legs or feet.

**gumboil** ('gum,boyl) the opening on the gum of an abscess at the root of a tooth.

gumma ('gumə) a soft, degenerating tumour characteristic of the tertiary stage of syphilis. It may occur in any organ or tissue.

gustatory (gu'staytə.ree) relating to taste.

gut (gut) the intestine.

Guthrie test ('guthri) a blood test carried out on a neonate between the 6th and 14th days of life to diagnose PHENYLKETONURIA.

gutta ('gutə) a drop. *G. percha* the juice of a tropical tree which, when dried, forms an elastic semisolid substance. Used in dentistry as a root filler.

GVH disease graft-versus-host disease.

Gy symbol for *gray*.

gynaecologist (.gienə'kolə jist) one who specializes in the diseases of the female genital tract.

gynaecology (.gienə'koləjee) the science of those diseases that are peculiar to the female genital tract.

gynaecomastia (.gienəkoh'masti.ə) excessive growth of the male breast.

gypsum ('jipsəm) plaster of Paris (calcium sulphate).

gyrus ('jierəs) a convolution, as of the cerebral cortex.

# H

**H** symbol for *hydrogen*.

**habit** ('habit) automatic response to a specific situation acquired as a result of repetition and learning. *Drug h.* drug addiction. *H. training* a method used in psychiatric nursing whereby deteriorated patients can be rehabilitated and taught personal hygiene by constant repetition and encouragement.

**habituation** (ha,bityuh'ayshən, -,bichuh-) the gradual adaptation to a stimulus or to the environment. The acquisition of a habit, e.g. a condition resulting from the repeated consumption of a drug, but with little or no tendency to increase the dose; there may be psychic but no physical dependence on the drug.

**haemangioblastoma** (hee,manjiohbla'stohmə) a tumour of the brain or spinal cord consisting of proliferated blood vessel cells.

**haemangioma** (,heemanji'ohmə) a benign tumour formed by dilated blood vessels. *Strawberry h.* a birthmark, which may become very large, but frequently disappears in a few years.

**haemarthrosis** (,heemah'throsis) an effusion of blood into a joint.

**haematemesis** (,heemə'teməsis) vomiting of blood. If it has been in the stomach for some time and become partially digested by gastric juice, it is of a dark colour and contains particles resembling coffee grounds.

**haematin** ('heemətin) the iron-containing part of haemoglobin.

**haematocele** ('heemətoh,seel) a swelling produced by effusion of blood, e.g. in the sheath surrounding a testicle or a broad ligament.

**haematocolpos** (,heemətoh'kolpos) an accumulation of blood or menstrual fluid in the vagina.

**haematocrit** ('heemətoh,krit, hi'mətə) the volume of red cells in the blood. Usually expressed as a percentage of the total blood volume.

**haematology** (,heemə'toləjee) the science dealing with the nature, functions and diseases of blood.

**haematoma** (,heemə'tohmə) a swelling containing clotted blood.

**haematometra** (,heemətoh'meetrə) an accumulation of blood or menstrual fluid in the uterus.

**haematomyelia** (,heemətohmie-'eeli.ə) an effusion of blood into the spinal cord.

**haematosalpinx** (,heemətoh'salpingks) an accumulation of blood in the uterine tubes; haemosalpinx.

**haematuria** (,heemə'tyooə,ri.ə) the presence of blood in the urine, due to injury or disease of any of the urinary organs.

**haemochromatosis** (,heemoh,krohmə'tohsis) a condition in which there is high absorption and deposition of iron leading to a high serum level, pigmentation of the skin and liver failure. Bronze diabetes.

**haemoconcentration** (ˌheemoh-konsənˈtrayshən) a loss of circulating fluid from the blood resulting in an increase in the proportion of red blood cells to plasma. The viscosity of the blood is increased.

**haemocytology** (ˌheemohsie'toləjee) the study of the cellular contents of blood.

**haemocytometer** (ˌheemohsie'tomitə) an apparatus for counting the blood corpuscles in a specific volume of blood.

**haemodialysis** (ˌheemohdie'aləsis) the removal of waste material from the blood of a patient with acute or chronic renal failure by means of a dialyser or artificial kidney. The apparatus is coupled to an artery and dialysis is achieved by the blood and rinsing fluid (DIALYSATE) passing through a semipermeable membrane. Blood is returned through a vein.

**haemoglobin** (ˌheemə'glohbin) the complex protein molecule contained within the red blood cells which gives them their colour and by which oxygen is transported.

**haemoglobinaemia** (ˌheeməˌglohbi-'neemi.ə) the presence of haemoglobin in the blood plasma.

**haemoglobinometer** (ˌheeməˌglohbi'nomitə) an instrument for estimating the haemoglobin content of the blood.

**haemoglobinopathy** (ˌheeməˌglohbi'nopəthee) any one of a group of hereditary disorders, including sickle-cell anaemia and thalassaemia, in which there is an abnormality in the production of haemoglobin.

**haemolysin** (hee'molisin) a substance that destroys red blood cells. It may be an antibody, a bacterial toxin or a component of a virus.

**haemolysis** (hee'molisis) the disintegration of red blood cells. Excessive haemolysis, which may produce anaemia, may be caused by poisoning or by bacterial infection.

**haemolytic** (ˌheemə'litik) having the power to destroy red blood cells. *H. disease of the newborn* a condition associated with rhesus incompatibility. *See* RHESUS FACTOR.

**haemophilia** (ˌheemoh'fili.ə) a condition characterized by impaired coagulability of the blood, and a strong tendency to bleed. Over 80% of all patients with haemophilia have haemophilia A (classic haemophilia), which is characterized by a deficiency of clotting factor VIII. Haemophilia B (Christmas disease), which affects about 15% of all haemophiliac patients, results from a deficiency of factor IX. Inherited as an X-linked recessive trait, it is transmitted by females only, to their male offspring. In order to avoid the debilitating and crippling effects of haemophilia, treatment must raise the level of the deficient clotting factor and maintain it in order to stop local bleeding. The patient must learn to avoid trauma and to obtain prompt treatment for bleeding episodes. Before surgery or dental treatment the patient must be given an infusion of the appropriate clotting factor.

*Haemophilus* (hee'mofiləs) a genus of Gram-negative rod-like bacteria. *H. ducreyi* the cause of soft chancre. *H. influenzae* a species once thought to be the cause of epidemic influenza; it produces a highly fatal form of meningitis, especially in infants. *H. pertussis* the cause of whooping cough; Bordet–Gengou bacillus.

**haemophthalmia** (ˌheemof'thalmi.ə) bleeding into the vitreous of the eye, usually the result of trauma; haemophthalmos.

**haemopneumothorax** (ˌheemohˌnyoomoh'thor.raks) the presence of blood and air in the pleural cavity, usually the result of injury.

**haemopoiesis** (ˌheemohpoy'eesis) the formation of red blood cells, which normally takes place in the bone marrow and continues throughout life. *Extramedullary h.* the formation of blood cells other than in the bone marrow, e.g. in the liver or spleen.

**haemopoietic** (ˌheemohpoy'etik) relating to red blood cell formation. *H. factors* those necessary for the development of red blood cells, e.g. vitamin $B_{12}$ and folic acid.

**haemoptysis** (hee'moptisis) the coughing up of blood from the lungs or bronchi. Being aerated, it is bright-red and frothy.

**haemorrhage** ('hemə.rij) an escape of blood from a ruptured blood vessel, externally or internally. Arterial haemorrhage involves bright-red blood which escapes in rhythmic spurts, corresponding to the beats of the heart. Venous haemorrhage involves dark-red blood which escapes in an even flow. Haemorrhage may also be: primary, at the time of operation or injury; reactionary or recurrent, occurring later when the blood pressure rises and a ligature slips or a vessel opens up; secondary, as a rule about 10 days after injury, and usually due to sepsis. Special types are as follows. *Antepartum h.* that which occurs before labour starts. See PLACENTA (PRAEVIA). *Cerebral h.* an episode of bleeding into the cerebrum; one of the three main forms of STROKE. *Concealed h.* collection of the blood in a cavity of the body. *Intracranial h.* bleeding within the cranium, which may be extradural, subdural, subarachnoid or cerebral. *Intradural h.* bleeding beneath the dura mater. It may be due to injury and causes signs of compression. The cerebrospinal fluid will be bloodstained. *Postpartum h.* that which occurs within 12–24 h of delivery, from the genital tract, and

which either measures 500 ml or more, or which adversely affects the woman's condition. Secondary postpartum haemorrhage is excessive bleeding more than 24 h after delivery.

**haemorrhagic** (ˌhemə'rajik) pertaining to or characterized by haemorrhage. *H. disease of the newborn* a self-limited haemorrhagic disorder of the first days of life, caused by deficiency of vitamin K-dependent blood clotting factors II, VII, IX and X. It should be prevented by the prophylactic administration of vitamin K to all newborn babies. *Viral h. fevers* a group of notifiable virus diseases of diverse aetiology but with similar characteristics of fever, headache, myalgia, prostration and haemorrhagic symptoms. They include dengue haemorrhagic fever, Marburg disease, Ebola virus disease, Lassa fever and yellow fever.

**haemorrhoid** ('hemə.royd) a 'pile' or locally dilated rectal vein. Piles may be either external or internal to the anal sphincter. Pain is caused on defecation, and bleeding may occur.

**haemorrhoidectomy** (ˌhemə.roy-'dektəmee) the surgical removal of haemorrhoids.

**haemosiderosis** (ˌheemoh.sidə'rohsis) iron deposits in the tissues resulting from excessive haemolysis of red blood cells.

**haemostasis** (ˌheemoh'staysis, hee-'mostəsis) the arrest of bleeding or the slowing up of blood flow in a vessel.

**haemostatic** (ˌheemoh'statik) a drug or remedy for arresting haemorrhage; a styptic.

**haemothorax** (ˌheemoh'thor.raks) blood in the thoracic cavity, e.g. from injury to soft tissues as a result of fracture of a rib.

**HAI** hospital-acquired infection.

**hair** (hair) a delicate keratinized epidermal filament growing out of

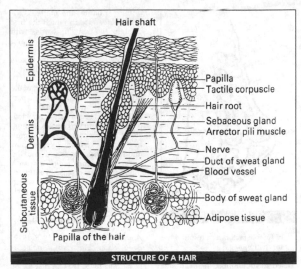

**STRUCTURE OF A HAIR**

the skin. The root of the hair is enclosed beneath the skin in a tubular follicle (*see* Figure). *H. ball see* BEZOAR.

**Haldol** ('haldol) trade name for a preparation of haloperidol, an antipsychotic agent.

**halibut oil** ('halibət ,oyl) a vitamin (A and D)-rich oil derived from the liver of halibut.

**halitosis** (,hali'tohsis) foul-smelling breath.

**hallucination** (hə,loosi'nayshən) a sensory impression (sight, touch, sound, smell or taste) that has no basis in external stimulation. Hallucinations can have psychological causes, as in mental illness, or they can result from drugs, alcohol, organic illnesses, such as brain tumour or senility, or exhaustion.

**hallucinogen** (hə'loosinə,jen) an agent that causes hallucinations, e.g. LSD and cannabis.

**hallux** ('haləks) the big toe. *H. valgus* a deformity in which the big toe is bent towards the other toes (*see* Figure on p. 184). *H. varus* a deformity in which the big toe is bent outwards away from the other toes.

**halo** ('hayloh) a circular structure, such as a luminous circle seen surrounding an object or light. *Glaucomatous h., h. glaucomatosus* a narrow light zone surrounding the optic disc in glaucoma.

**halo effect** (i,fekt) a beneficial effect noted after a health-care intervention, visit or research project. The halo effect cannot be attributed to the content of the interview, visit or project but is the outcome of

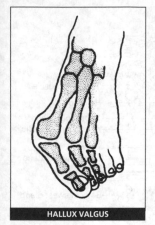

**HALLUX VALGUS**

indefinable factors as a result of the intervention.

**halo splint** an orthopaedic device used to immobilize the head and neck to assist in the healing of cervical injuries and postoperatively after cervical surgery.

**halogen** ('halə‚jen, -lə‚jən) one of the non-metallic elements (others are chlorine, iodine, bromine and fluorine).

**haloperidol** (‚haloh'peri‚dol) a sedative and tranquillizer used in the treatment of schizophrenia and other psychiatric disorders, particularly mania.

**halothane** ('haloh‚thayn) a widely used anaesthetic; used as an inhalation to induce and maintain anaesthesia.

**hamamelis** (‚hamə'meelis) a soothing agent prepared from witch-hazel and used in suppository form in the treatment of haemorrhoids.

**hamartoma** (‚hamah'tohmə) a benign nodule which is an overgrowth of mature tissue.

**hammer** ('hamə) the malleus. **H.-toe** a deformity in which the first phalanx is bent upwards, with plantar flexion of the second and third phalanx.

**hamstring** ('ham‚string) the flexors of the knee joint that are situated at the back of the thigh.

**hand** (hand) the terminal part of the arm below the wrist. **Claw h.** a paralytic condition in which the hand is flexed and the fingers contracted, caused by injury to nerves or muscles. **Cleft h.** a congenital deformity in which the cleft between the third and fourth fingers extends into the palm. **H., foot and mouth disease** a mild infectious disease in children, caused by Coxsackie virus, which results in vesicle formation on all three sites. Not the same as foot and mouth disease.

**Hand–Schüller–Christian disease** (‚hand‚shoolə'krischən) A. Hand, American paediatrician, 1868–1949; A. Schüller, Austrian neurologist, 1874–1958; H.A. Christian, American physician, 1876–1951. A disease of the reticuloendothelial system in which granulomata containing cholesterol are formed, chiefly in the skull.

**handicap** ('handi‚kap) a disadvantage for a given individual, resulting from an impairment or a disability that limits or prevents the fulfilment of a role that is normal (depending on age, sex, and social and cultural factors) for that individual.

**Hansen's disease** ('hansənz) G.H.A. Hansen, Norwegian physician, 1841–1912. Leprosy, caused by Hansen's bacillus, Mycobacterium leprae.

**haploid** ('haemployd) having one set of chromosomes after division instead of two.

**Harrison's groove** or **sulcus** ('haris-‚nz ‚groov) E. Harrison, British physician, 1789–1838. A horizontal groove along the lower border of the thorax corresponding to the

costal insertion of the diaphragm;
seen in rickets.

**Hartnup disease** ('hahtnup) a hereditary defect in amino acid metabolism which may produce learning difficulties (named after the first person found to suffer from it).

**Hashimoto's disease** (ˌhashi'mohtohz) *H. Hashimoto, Japanese surgeon, 1881–1934.* A lymphoadenoid goitre caused by the formation of anti-bodies to thyroglobulin. It is an autoimmune condition giving rise to hypothyroidism.

**hashish** ('hasheesh,-ish) Indian hemp. *See* CANNABIS.

**haustration** (haw'strayshən) a haustrum, or the process of forming one.

**haustrum** ('hawstrəm) any one of the pouches formed by the sacculations of the colon.

**Haversian canal** (hə'varsi.ɔn, -shən) *C. Havers, British physician and anatomist, 1650–1702.* One of the minute canals that permeate compact bone, containing blood and lymph vessels to maintain its nutrition. *See* BONE.

**Hawthorne effect** ('hawthawn i.fekt) the term given to the usual beneficial effect of a study on the persons participating in the study. It was named after an industrial management study in the USA, where the effect was first identified.

**hay fever** (hay) an atopic ALLERGY characterized by sneezing, itching and watery eyes, running nose and a burning sensation of the palate and throat. It is a localized anaphylactic reaction to an extrinsic allergen, most commonly pollens and the spores of moulds. When the allergen comes in contact with mast cell-bound IgE immunoglobulin in the tissues of the conjunctiva, nasal mucosa and bronchial tree, the cells release mediators of ANAPHYLAXIS and produce the characteristic symptoms of hay fever. Atopy.

**HCG** human chorionic gonadotrophin. *See* GONADOTROPHIN.

**HCl** hydrochloric acid.

**He** symbol for *helium*.

**HEA** Health Education Authority. A special health authority responsible for giving authoritative advice both nationally and locally on a wide range of health education issues through campaigns and publications (formerly the Health Education Council). Now an integral part of the health service and thus participates with other health authorities in planning health service policies and priorities.

**head** (hed) the anterior or superior part of a structure or organism, in vertebrates containing the brain and the organs of special sense. *H. injury* traumatic injury to the head resulting from a fall or violent blow. Such an injury may be open or closed and may involve a brain CONCUSSION, skull fracture, or contusions of the brain. All head injuries are potentially dangerous because there may be a slow leakage of blood from damaged blood vessels into the brain, or the formation of a blood clot which gradually increases pressure against brain tissue. Long-term effects of head injury may include chronic headache, disturbances in mental and motor function, and a host of other symptoms that may or may not be psychogenic. Organic brain damage and post-traumatic epilepsy resulting from scar formation are possible sequels to head injury.

**headache** ('hed.ayk) a pain or ache in the head. A symptom rather than a disorder. It accompanies many diseases and conditions, including emotional distress. *See also* MIGRAINE.

**Heaf test** (heef) *F.G.R. Heaf, British physician, 1894–1973.* A form of tuberculin testing. A drop of tuberculin solution on the skin is injected by means of a number of very short needles mounted on a spring-loaded device (Heaf's gun).

**healing** ('heeling) the process of return to normal function after a period of disease or injury. *H. by first intention* union of the edges of a clean incised wound without visible granulations, and leaving only a faint linear scar. *H. by second intention* union of the edges of an open wound by the formation of granulations from the bottom and sides. *H. by third intention* union of a wound that is closed surgically several days after the injury.

**health** (helth) the World Health Organization (WHO) states that 'Health is a state of complete physical, mental and social wellbeing and not merely the absence of disease or infirmity.' *H. assessment* an evaluation made by a health-care professional of an individual's health status, which takes account of the health history and lifestyle together with the findings of a physical examination. *H. authority* a body through which the National Health Service is administered at district level. Established in 1996 as a merger between District Health Authorities and Family Health Services Authorities. *H. centre* a community health organization for providing ambulatory health care and coordinating the efforts of all health agencies, commonly focused around the general practitioner's services. *H. culture* a system that attempts to explain and treat health problems and illness and to maintain health. Part of the wider culture to which people belong, it may be a traditional or a biomedical system. *H. education officer* an officer appointed to make health education resources available to the community. *H. services* the term is usually employed to connote the system or programme by which health care is made available to the population and financed by government or private enterprise, or both. *H. statistics* summated data on any aspect of the health of populations; for example, mortality, morbidity, use of health services, treatment outcome, costs of health care. *Holistic h.* a system of preventive medicine that takes into account the whole individual, and that person's own responsibility for well-being, with the total influences (social, psychological, environmental) that affect health, including nutrition, exercise and mental relaxation. *Public h.* the field of medicine that is concerned with safeguarding and improving the health of the community as a whole.

**health care system** ('sistəm) an organized plan of health services. The term is usually employed to denote the system or programme by which health care is made available to the population and financed by government or private enterprise or both.

**health education** (edyoo'kayshən) various methods of education aimed at the prevention of disease. All nurses, midwives and health visitors have particular responsibilities and opportunities to promote good health.

**Health Improvement Programme** (im'proovmənt ˌprohgram) abbreviated HImP. A 3-year local strategy for improving health within a community, which is updated each year. Developed and led by a health authority it must result in coordinated and shared strategy involving the health authority, local NHS trusts, local authorities, primary care groups, dentists, voluntary organizations and local people. It is designed to cover the main health needs and health care requirements of the local people within the

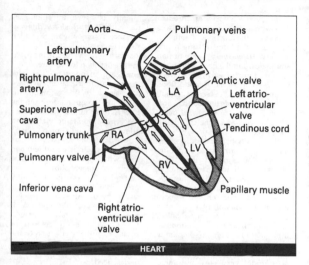

Aorta

Pulmonary veins

Left pulmonary artery

Right pulmonary artery

Superior vena cava

Pulmonary trunk

Pulmonary valve

Inferior vena cava

Right atrioventricular valve

LA

RA

LV

RV

Aortic valve

Left atrioventricular valve

Tendinous cord

Papillary muscle

**HEART**

defined area, together with the investment required in local health services to meet these needs. Also includes the health targets set by central government from 'Our Healthier Nation', etc.

**Health Service Commissioner (Health Service Ombudsman UK)** (ˌsɜrvis kəˈmiʃnə) appointed to protect the interests of patients in relation to the administration and provision of health care delivered in the National Health Service. The Commissioner is responsible to Parliament and can investigate complaints and allegations of maladministration by a health authority, NHS trusts and the clinical practice of medical practitioners.

**health visitor** (ˌvizitə) a registered nurse who may also be a midwife and who has completed a 52-week full-time course in social and preventative medicine leading to a health visiting certificate. The main area of responsibility of health visitors is health education and preventative care of mothers and children under 5 years old, although some specialize in school health and preventative care of the elderly.

**hearing** (ˈhiə.ring) the reception of sound waves and their transmission onwards to the brain in the form of nerve impulses. *H. aid* an apparatus, usually electronic, to amplify sounds before they reach the inner ear.

**heart** (haht) a hollow, muscular organ which pumps the blood throughout the body, situated behind the sternum slightly towards the left side of the thorax (*see* Figure). *H. attack* myocardial infarction. *H. block* impairment of conduction in heart excitation; often applied specifically to atrioventricular heart block. *H. failure* may be acute, as in coronary thrombosis, or chronic. *H.–lung machine* an apparatus used to perform the functions of both the heart and the lungs during heart surgery. *H. murmur* an abnormal sound heard in the heart, frequently caused by disease of the valves. Occurs when the blood flow through the heart exceeds a certain velocity. *H. sounds* the sound heard when listening to the heart beat. They are caused by the closure of the valves.

**heartburn** ('haht,bərn) indigestion marked by a burning sensation in the oesophagus, often with regurgitation of acid fluid. Pyrosis.

**heat** (heet) warmth. A form of energy, which may cause an increase in temperature or a change of state, e.g. the conversion of water into steam. *H. exhaustion* a rapid pulse, anorexia, dizziness, and cramps in arms, legs or abdomen, sometimes followed by sudden collapse, caused by loss of body fluids and salts under very hot conditions. *Prickly h.* miliaria; heat rash. Acute itching caused by blocking of the ducts of the sweat glands following profuse sweating. *H. stroke* a severe life-threatening condition resulting from prolonged exposure to heat. *See* SUNSTROKE.

**hebephrenia** (,hebi'freeni.ə) a form of schizophrenia characterized by thought disorder and emotional incongruity. Delusions and hallucinations are common.

**Heberden's nodes** ('hebə,dənz) *W. Heberden, British physician, 1710–1801.* Bony or cartilaginous outgrowths causing deformity of the terminal finger joints in osteoarthritis.

**hebetude** ('hebityood) emotional dullness. A common symptom in dementia and schizophrenia.

**hectic** ('hektik) occurring regularly. *H. fever* a regularly occurring increase in temperature; it is frequently observed in pulmonary tuberculosis. *H. flush* a redness of the face accompanying a sudden rise in temperature.

**hedonism** ('heedə,nizəm, 'hed-) excessive devotion to pleasure.

**Heimlich manoeuvre** ('hiemlik mə,noovə) *H.J. Heimlich, American physician, b. 1920.* A technique for removing foreign matter from the trachea of a choking person. Wrap the arms around the victim and allow that person's torso to hang forwards. Make a fist with one hand and grasp it with the other, then with both hands against the victim's abdomen (above the navel and below the rib cage), forcefully press into the abdomen with a sharp upward thrust. The manoeuvre may be repeated several times if necessary to clear the air passages. If the victim is unconscious or prone, turn that person on to the back, kneel astride the torso and with both hands use the manoeuvre as described.

*Helicobacter* (,helikoh'baktə) a genus of spiral and flagellated Gram-negative bacteria. *H. pylori* a species found in the stomach. May cause damage to the prostaglandins protecting the mucosal cells in the stomach wall, leading to progressive gastritis and ulceration.

**heliotherapy** (,heelioh'therəpee) treatment of disease by exposure of the body to sunlight.

**helium** ('heeli.əm) *symbol* He. An inert gas sometimes used in conjunction with oxygen to facilitate respiration in obstructional types of dyspnoea and for decompressing deep-sea divers.

**helix** ('heeliks) 1. a spiral twist. Used to describe the configuration of certain molecules, e.g. deoxyribonucleic acid (DNA). 2. the outer rim of the auricle of the ear.

**Hellin's law** ('helinz lor) one in about 89 pregnancies ends in the

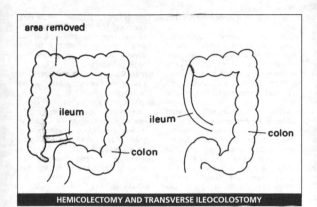

**area removed**

ileum

ileum

colon

colon

**HEMICOLECTOMY AND TRANSVERSE ILEOCOLOSTOMY**

birth of twins; one in $89^2$, or 7921, in the birth of triplets; one in $89^3$, or 704 969, in the birth of quadruplets. Infertility treatments have raised the rate of multiple pregnancies.

**helminthiasis** (ˌhelminˈthieəsis) an infestation with worms.

**hemeralopia** (ˌheməˌraˈlohpi.ə) day blindness. The vision is poor in a bright light but is comparatively good when the light is dim. *See* NYCTALOPIA.

**hemianopia** (ˌhemi.əˈnohpi.ə) partial blindness, in which the patient can see only half of the normal field of vision. It arises from disorders of the optic tract and of the occipital lobe.

**hemiballismus** (ˌhemibəˈlizməs) involuntary chorea-like movements on one side of the body only.

**hemicolectomy** (ˌhemikohˈlektəmee) the removal of the ascending and part of the transverse colon with an ileotransverse colostomy (*see* Figure).

**hemiparesis** (ˌhemipəˈreesis) paralysis on one side of the body; hemiplegia.

**hemiplegia** (ˌhemiˈpleeji.ə, jə) paralysis of one half of the body, usually due to cerebral disease or injury. The lesion is on the side of the brain opposite to the side paralysed.

**hemisphere** ('hemiˌsfiə) a half sphere. In anatomy, one of the two halves of the cerebrum or cerebellum.

**hemp** (hemp) *see* CANNABIS.

**Henle's loop** ('henleez ˌloop) *F.G.J. Henle, German anatomist, 1809–1885.* The U-shaped loop of the uriniferous tubule of the kidney.

**Henoch's purpura** ('henokhs) *E.H. Henoch, German paediatrician, 1820–1910.* Allergic PURPURA.

**heparin** ('hepə.rin) an anticoagulant formed in the liver and circulated in the blood. Injected intravenously it prevents the conversion of prothrombin into thrombin, and is used in the treatment of thrombosis.

**hepatectomy** (ˌhepəˈtektəmee) excision of a part or the whole of the liver.

**hepatic** (hiˈpatik) relating to the liver. *H. flexure* the angle of the colon that is situated under the liver.

**hepaticojejunostomy** (hi,patikoh-,jejuh'nostəmee) the anastomosis of the hepatic duct to the jejunum, usually created after extensive excision for carcinoma of the pancreas.

**hepaticostomy** (hi,pati'kostəmee) a surgical opening into the hepatic duct.

**hepatitis** (,hepə'tietis) inflammation of the liver. *Amoebic h.* inflammation that may arise during amoebic dysentery and lead to liver abscesses. *Anicteric h.* viral hepatitis without jaundice, tending to occur chiefly in infants and young children; symptoms include mild anorexia and gastrointestinal disturbances, slight fever, and enlargement and tenderness of the liver. *Fulminant h.* (acute hepatitis with coma) an acute fulminating form of hepatitis resulting from extensive hepatic necrosis. It may be due to: (a) toxic liver injury, as in carbon tetrachloride poisoning or paracetamol overdose; (b) a hypersensitivity reaction to a drug, such as halothane; or (c) viral hepatitis. Death is usually caused by acute yellow atrophy of the liver. *Viral h.* an acute, notifiable, infectious hepatitis caused by one of several different viruses that infect human liver cells, e.g. hepatitis A virus (HAV), hepatitis B virus (HBV), hepatitis C virus (HCV) and hepatitis E virus (HEV).

**hepatization** (,hepətie'zayshən) the alteration of lung tissue into a solid mass resembling liver, which occurs in acute lobar pneumonia.

**hepatogenous** (,hepə'tojənəs) arising in the liver. Applied to jaundice in which the disease arises in the parenchymal cells of the liver.

**hepatolenticular** (,hepətohlen'ti-kyuhlə) pertaining to the liver and the lentiform nucleus. *H. degeneration* Wilson's disease; a progressive

condition, usually occurring between the ages of 10 and 25 years. There are tremors of the head and limbs, pigmentation of the cornea and sometimes defective twilight vision.

**hepatoma** (,hepə'tohmə) a primary malignant tumour arising in the liver cells.

**hepatomegaly** (,hepətoh'megəlee) an enlargement of the liver.

**hepatosplenomegaly** (,hepətoh-,spleenoh'megəlee) enlargement of the liver and spleen, such as may be found in kala-azar.

**hepatotoxic** (,hepətoh'toksik) applied to drugs and substances that cause destruction of liver cells.

**herbal medicine** ('herb'l) a form of complementary or alternative medicine in which plants are used for their therapeutic properties. Also called phytotherapy.

**herd immunity** (hərd) the immunity of a population. When there is a high enough number of persons in a population immune to a particular infection, the infection fails to spread because of the absence of enough susceptibles. For example, in measles this could probably be achieved by vaccination of 90–95% of the population.

**hereditary** (hi'reditə,ree) derived from ancestry; inherited.

**heredity** (hi'reditee) the transmission of both physical and mental characteristics to the offspring from the parents. Recessive characteristics may miss one or two generations and reappear later.

**hermaphrodite** (hər'mafrə,diet) an individual whose gonads contain both testicular and ovarian tissue. These may be combined as an ovotestis or there may be a testis on one side and an ovary on the other. The external genitalia may be indeterminate of either sex. *Pseudo-h.* one whose gonads are histologically of one sex but in whom the geni-

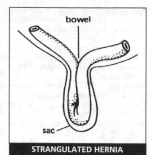

bowel

sac

**STRANGULATED HERNIA**

talia have the appearance of the opposite sex. *True h.* one who possesses both male and female gonads.

**hernia** ('həɪni.ə) a protrusion of any part of the internal organs through the structures enclosing them. *Cerebral h.* a protrusion of brain through the skull. *Diaphragmatic h.* and *hiatus h.* a protrusion of a part of the stomach through the oesophageal opening in the diaphragm. *Femoral h.* a loop of intestine protruding into the femoral canal. More common in females. *Hiatus h.* see DIAPHRAGMATIC H. *Incisional h.* a hernia occurring at the site of an old wound. *Inguinal h.* protrusion of the intestine through the inguinal canal. This may be congenital or acquired, and is commoner in males. A rupture. *Irreducible h.* a hernia that cannot be replaced by manipulation. *Reducible h.* a hernia that can be returned to its normal position by manipulative measures. *Strangulated h.* a hernia of the bowel in which the neck of the sac containing the bowel is so constricted that the venous circulation is impeded, and gangrene will result if not treated promptly (see Figure). *Umbilical h.* protrusion of bowel through the

umbilical ring. This may be congenital or acquired. *Vaginal h.* rectocele or cystocele.

**hernioplasty** ('hərnioh,plastee) a plastic repair of the abdominal wall performed after reduction of a hernia.

**herniorrhaphy** (,hərni'o.rəfee) removal of a hernial sac and repair of the abdominal wall.

**herniotomy** (,hərni'otəmee) an operation to removal a hernial sac.

**heroin** ('heroh.in) a diacetate of morphine used as an analgesic and abused illicitly for its euphoriant effects. The drug readily induces physical dependence and may be sniffed, smoked ('chasing the dragon') or injected subcutaneously or intravenously ('shooting up' or 'mainlining'). Slang terms for heroin include 'smack', 'H' and 'brown sugar'. *H. babies* babies who have received regular heroin (morphine) via the placenta before birth and who show signs of withdrawal after birth. Withdrawal symptoms may persist for 1–4 weeks and include vomiting, diarrhoea, sweating, breathing difficulties and hyperactivity.

**herpes** ('hərpeez) an inflammatory skin eruption showing small vesicles caused by a herpes virus. *H. simplex* a viral infection which gives rise to localized vesicles in the skin and mucous membranes and is characterized by latency and subsequent recurrence. It is caused by herpes simplex viruses types 1 and 2. Type 1 infection is common in children and is often symptomless. Type 2 infection is common in older age groups and is associated with sexual activity. Lesions appear on the cervix, vulva and surrounding skin in women and on the penis in men. In homosexual men rectal lesions are common. Recurrent genital herpes may follow primary infection. Type 2 virus may cause aseptic meningitis. *H. zoster* a local manifestation of reactivation of infection of the varicella zoster virus, the causative agent of chickenpox, characterized by a vesicular rash in the area of distribution of a sensory nerve. Called also shingles.

**herpes virus** one of a group of DNA-containing viruses. They include the causative agents of herpes simplex, herpes zoster, chickenpox, cytomegalic inclusion disease and infective mononucleosis.

**Hess's test** ('hesiz) *A.F. Hess, American physician, 1875–1933.* A test used to diagnose purpura. An inflated blood pressure cuff causes an increase in capillary pressure and rupture of the walls, causing purpuric spots to develop.

**heterochromia** (,hetə.roh'krohmi.ə) a difference in colour in the irises of the two eyes or in different parts of one iris. It may be congenital or secondary due to inflammation.

**heterogeneous** (,hetəroh'jeeni.əs) composed of diverse constituents.

**heterogenous** (,hetə'rojənəs) derived from different sources.

**heterophoria** (,hetə.roh'for.ri.ə) a tendency to squint when fusion is interrupted. It occurs mainly when the person is tired or in poor health.

**heterosexual** (,hetə.roh'seksyooəl) 1. pertaining to, characteristic of or directed towards the opposite sex. 2. a person with erotic interests directed towards the opposite sex.

**heterotropia** (,hetə.roh'trohpi.ə) a marked deviation of the eyes; strabismus or squint.

**heterozygous** (,hetə.roh'ziegəs) possessing dissimilar alternative genes for an inherited characteristic, one gene coming from each parent. One gene is dominant and the other is recessive. *See* HOMOZYGOUS.

**hexachlorophane** (,heksə'klor.rə-fayn) a detergent and germicidal compound commonly incorporated in soaps and dermatological agents. Topical preparations have been associated with severe neurotoxicity and should not be used on children under 2 years old except on medical advice. Avoid on large raw areas.

**hexamine** ('heksə,meen) methenamine; a urinary antiseptic which releases formaldehyde in an acid urine.

**Hg** symbol for *mercury* (L. *hydrargyrum*).

**hiatus** (hie'aytəs) a space or opening. *H. hernia* a protrusion of a part of the stomach through the oesophageal opening in the diaphragm.

**hiccup** ('hikup) hiccough; a spasmodic contraction of the diaphragm causing an abrupt inspiratory sound.

**Hickman line** ('hikmən ,lien) trade name for a central venous line catheter.

**hidrosis** (hi'drohsis) the excretion of sweat.

**high-altitude sickness** (hie'altityood ,siknəs) the condition resulting from difficulty in adjusting to diminished oxygen pressure at high altitudes. It may take the form of mountain sickness, high-altitude pulmonary oedema or cerebral oedema.

**hilum** ('hieləm) hilus; a recess in an organ by which blood vessels, nerves and ducts enter and leave it.

**hindbrain** ('hiend,brayn) that part of the brain consisting of the medulla oblongata, the pons and the cerebellum.

**hip** (hip) 1. the region of the body at the articulation of the femur and the innominate bone at the base of the lower trunk. These bones meet at the hip joint. Called also *coxa*. 2. loosely, the hip joint. *Total h. replacement* replacement of the femoral head and acetabulum with prostheses that are cemented into the bone; called also *total h. arthroplasty*. The procedure is done to replace a severely damaged arthritic hip joint.

**hippus** ('hipəs) alternate contraction and dilatation of the pupils. This occurs in various diseases of the nervous system, e.g. multiple sclerosis.

**Hirschsprung's disease** ('hərshspruhngz) *H. Hirschsprung, Danish physician, 1831–1916. See* MEGACOLON.

**hirsute** ('hərsyoot) hairy.

**hirsutism** ('hərsyoo,tizəm) excessive hairiness.

**hirudin** (hi'roodin) the active principle in the secretion of the leech and certain snake venoms that prevents clotting of blood.

*Hirudo* (hi'roodoh) a genus of leeches. *H. medicinalis* the medical leech.

**histamine** ('histəmeen) an enzyme that causes local vasodilatation and increased permeability of the blood vessel walls. Readily released from body tissues, it is a factor in allergy response, greatly increases gastric secretion of hydrochloric acid and increases the heart rate. *H. test* 1. subcutaneous injection of 0.1% solution of histamine to stimulate gastric secretion in order to measure maximal acid output. 2. after rapid intravenous injection of histamine phosphate, normal persons experience a brief fall in blood pressure, but in those with phaeochromocytoma, after the fall, there is a marked rise in blood pressure.

**histidinaemia** (,histidi'neemi.ə) a hereditary metabolic defect caused by an enzyme defect involving L-histidine ammonia lypase affecting the amino acid histidine. Affected persons show mild mental handicap and disordered speech development.

**histidine** ('histi,deen) one of the ten essential amino acids formed by the

digestion of dietary protein. Histamine is derived from it.

**histiocyte** ('histioh,siet) a stationary macrophage of connective tissue. Derived from the reticuloendothelial cells, it acts as a scavenger, removing bacteria from the blood and tissues.

**histiocytoma** (,histiohsie'tohmə) a tumour containing histiocytes, causing a vascular nodule.

**histiocytosis** (,histiohsie'tohsis) a group of diseases of bone in which granulomata containing histiocytes and eosinophil cells appear. *See* LETTERER–SIWE DISEASE *and* HAND-SCHÜLLER–CHRISTIAN DISEASE.

**histocompatibility** (,histohkəm,patə'bilitee) the ability of cells to be accepted and to function in a new situation. Tissue typing reveals this and ensures a higher success rate in organ transplantation.

**histogram** ('histə,gram) a bar-chart. Statistical values are expressed as blocks on a graph.

**histology** (hi'stoləjee) the science dealing with the minute strcuture, composition and function of tissues.

**histolysis** (hi'stoləjee) the disintegration of tissues.

**histoplasmosis** (,histohplaz'mohsis) infection caused by inhalation of the spores of a yeast-like fungus, *Histoplasma capsulatum*. Usually symptomless, the infection may progress and produce a condition resembling tuberculosis.

**HIV** human immunodeficiency virus.

**hives** (hievz) urticaria.

**Hodge pessary** (,hoj 'pesə.ree) *H.L. Hodge, American gynaecologist, 1796–1873.* A pessary used to maintain the position of the uterus after correction of a retroversion. *See* PESSARY.

**Hodgkin's disease** ('hojkinz) *T. Hodgkin, British physician, 1798–1866.* Lymphadenoma, a malignant condition of the reticuloendothelial cells. There is progressive enlargement of lymph nodes and lymph tissue all over the body. Treated by radiotherapy and cytotoxic drugs. This disease has a good prognosis.

**holism** ('hohlizəm) a philosophy in which the person is considered as a functioning whole rather than as a composite of several systems. May be spelt wholism.

**holistic** (hə'listik) pertaining to holism. *H. health care* a comprehensive approach to health care that implies body–mind–spirit consideration in all actions and interventions for the patient, while recognizing the concept of the uniqueness of the individual and the influence of external and internal environmental factors on health.

**Homans' sign** ('hohmənz) *J. Homans, American surgeon, 1877–1954.* Pain elicited in the calf when the foot is dorsiflexed. Indicative of venous thrombosis.

**homatropine** (hoh'matrə,pin) a short-acting mydriatic used in ophthalmology to dilate the pupil and so allow a better view of the fundus of the eye.

**home help service** (,hohm 'help ,sərvis) a branch of the social services department, which provides domestic and housekeeping assistance to those in need. It is on either a short-term or long-term basis, and payment is according to means.

**homeopathy** (,hohmi'opəthee) a system of medicine promulgated by C.F.S. Hahnemann (*German physician, 1755–1843*) and based upon the principle that 'like cures like'. Remedies are given which can produce in the patient the symptoms of the disease to be cured, but they are administered in minute doses.

**homeostasis** (,hohmioh'staysis, ,hom-) a tendency of biological systems to maintain stability while continually adjusting to conditions that are optimal for survival.

**homicide** ('homi,sied) the killing of a human being. *Culpable h.* covers murder (malice aforethought), manslaughter (without malice aforethought), causing death by reckless driving, and infanticide. *Non-culpable h.* covers justifiable homicide (e.g. lawful execution) and excusable homicide (misadventure or accident). *See* MCNAGHTEN'S RULES ON INSANITY AT LAW.

**homogeneous** (,homə'jeeni.əs) uniform in character. Similar in nature and characteristics.

**homogenize** (ho'mojə,niez) to make homogeneous. To reduce to the same consistency.

**homogenous** (ho'mojənəs) derived from the same source.

**homograft** ('homə,grahft, 'homoh-) a tissue or organ transplanted from one individual to another of the same species. An allograft.

**homolateral** (,homə'latə.rəl, ,hoh-moh-) on the same side; ipsilateral.

**homologous** (hə'moləgəs) 1. in anatomy, having the same embryological origin although performing a different function. 2. in chemistry, possessing a similar structure. *H. chromosomes* those that pair during meiosis and contain an identical arrangement of genes in the DNA pattern.

**homologue** ('homə,log) a part or organ which has the same relative position or structure as another one.

**homoplasty** ('homoh,plastee, 'hohm-) surgical replacement of defective tissues with a homograft.

**homosexual** (,homoh'seksyooəl, ,hohm-) 1. of the same sex. 2. a person who is sexually attracted to a person of the same sex.

**homosexuality** (,homoh,seksyoo'a-litee, ,hohm-) sexual and emotional orientation towards persons of the same sex.

**homozygous** (,homoh'ziegəs) possessing an identical pair of genes

for an inherited characteristic. *See*
HETEROZYGOUS.

**hookworm** ('huhk,wərm) *see* AN-
CYLOSTOMA.

**hordeolum** (hordi'ohləm) a stye;
inflammation of the sebaceous
glands of the eyelashes.

**hormone** ('hawmohn) a chemical
substance that is generated in
one organ and carried by the blood
to another, in which it excites activity. *H. replacement therapy* the
giving of prepared hormones as
a substitute for those hormones
that the body no longer produces
or that have been lost as a result
of surgery. A combination of oes-
trogenic hormones is commonly
given to women for the relief of
menopausal symptoms and the
prevention of osteoporosis. Known
as HRT.

**Horner's syndrome** ('hawnəz) *J.F.
Horner, Swiss ophthalmologist, 1831–
1886.* A condition in which there is a
lesion on the path of sympathetic
nerve fibres in the cervical region.
The symptoms include enophthalmos, ptosis, a contracted pupil and
a decrease in sweating.

**Horton's syndrome** ('hawtənz) *B.T
Horton, American physician, 1895–
1980.* Severe headache caused by
the release of histamine in the body
or by its administration. Histamine
cephalalgia.

**hospice** ('hospis) the concept of a
hospice is that of a caring community of professional and non-
professional people, together with
the family. Emphasis is on dealing
with emotional and spiritual problems as well as the medical problems of the terminally ill. Of
primary concern is control of pain
and other symptoms, keeping the
patient at home for as long as possible or desirable, and making the
remaining days as comfortable and
meaningful as possible. After the
patient dies, family members are

given support throughout their
period of bereavement.

**hospital** ('hospit'l) an institution for
the care, diagnosis and treatment of
the sick and injured. *H.-acquired
infection see* (HOSPITAL-ACQUIRED)
INFECTION.

**host** (hohst) the animal, plant or tissue on which a parasite lives and
multiplies. *Definitive* or *final h.*
one that harbours the parasite
during its adult sexual stage.
*Intermediate h.* one that shelters
the parasite during a non-
reproductive period.

**hourglass contraction** ('owə,glahs)
a contraction near the middle of a
hollow organ, such as the stomach
or uterus, producing an outline
resembling an hourglass shape.

**housemaid's knee** ('howsmaydz)
prepatellar bursitis; inflammation
of the prepatellar bursa, which
becomes distended with serous
fluid.

**HRT** hormone replacement therapy.

**human chorionic gonadotrophin**
('hyoomən) *see* GONADOTROPHIN.

**human immunodeficiency virus**
(,hyoomən) abbreviated HIV. A
lentivirus that belongs to a group of
viruses known as retroviruses and
causes AIDS in humans. There are
two main types of HIV: HIV-1, the
predominant AIDS-causing virus in
the world, and HIV-2, also an AIDS-
causing virus that is found more
commonly in countries on the west
coast of Africa. HIV is transmitted
sexually, parenterally, from mother
to child (during pregnancy, at time
of birth, or in the postnatal period
from breast feeding) and more
rarely, iatrogenically. Most people
become infected sexually through
unprotected penetrative vaginal or
anal sexual intercourse. Unprotected means that the male insertive
partner has not worn a good-
quality, intact rubber latex condom.

Parenteral transmission is usually associated with injecting drug users sharing contaminated injection equipment. Blood tests to identify HIV infection detect antibodies to the virus and may not be positive for 8–12 weeks following primary infection. Because it is not possible to detect all HIV-infected patients, all health-care workers in direct patient contact should practise universal infection control precautions see UNIVERSAL PRECAUTIONS.

**humidity** (hyoo'miditee) the degree of moisture in the air. *H. therapy* the therapeutic use of water to prevent or correct a moisture deficit in the respiratory tract. The principal reasons for employing humidity therapy are: (a) to prevent drying and irritation of the respiratory mucosa; (b) to facilitate ventilation and diffusion of oxygen and other therapeutic gases being administered; and (c) to aid in the removal of thick and viscous secretions that obstruct the air passages. Another important use of water aerosol therapy is to aid in obtaining an induced sputum specimen.

**humour** ('hyooma) any fluid of the body, such as lymph or blood. *Aqueous h.* the fluid filling the anterior chamber of the eye. *Vitreous h.* the jelly-like substance that fills the chamber of the eye between the lens and the retina.

**humour and laughter therapy** ('lahfta) an amusing intervention used by a health-care professional or patient and designed to benefit the patient.

**Huntington's chorea (disease)** ('huntingtanz) *G.S. Huntington, American physician, 1851–1927.* A rare, degenerative inherited disorder of the brain in which there is progressive chorea and mental deterioration (dementia).

**Hurler's syndrome** ('harlaz) *G. Hurler, Austrian paediatrician.* An inherited disorder in which learning difficulties are caused by excess mucopolysaccharides being stored in the brain and reticuloendothelial system. Gargoylism.

**Hutchinson's teeth** ('hutchinsanz) *Sir J. Hutchinson, British surgeon, 1828–1913.* Typical notching of the borders of the permanent incisor teeth occurring in congenital syphilis.

**hyaline** ('hiea lien) resembling glass. *H. degeneration* a form of deterioration that occurs in tumours and is due to deficiency of blood supply. It precedes cystic degeneration. *H. membrane disease* see RESPIRATORY (DISTRESS SYNDROME OF NEWBORN).

**hyaluronidase** ( hiealyuh'roni dayz) an enzyme that facilitates the absorption of fluids in subcutaneous tissues. It is found in the testes of mammals, and a preparation of it is particularly used with subcutaneous infusions to promote absorption.

**hydatid** ('hiedatid) a cystic swelling containing the embryo of *Echinococcus granulosus*. It may be found in any organ of the body, e.g. in the liver. 'Daughter cysts' are produced from the original. Infection is from contaminated foods, e.g. salads. *H. disease* the result of the presence of hydatids in the lungs, liver or brain.

**hydatidiform** ( hieda'tidi fawm) resembling a hydatid cyst. *H. mole see* MOLE.

**hydraemia** (hie'dreemi.a) a modification of the blood in which there is an excess of plasma in relation to the cells. A degree of hydraemia is physiological in pregnancy.

**hydralazine** (hie'drala zeen) a vasodilator and antihypertensive agent used to lower blood pressure.

**hydramnios** (hie'dramnios) an excessive amount of amniotic fluid in the uterus in the later months of pregnancy.

**hydrarthrosis** (,hiedrah'throhsis) a collection of fluid in a joint.

**hydrate** ('hiedrayt) a compound of an element with water.

**hydroa** (hie'droh.ə) a childhood hypersensitivity of the skin to sunlight, resulting in the formation of a vesicular eruption on the exposed parts, with intense irritation.

**hydrocarbon** (,hiedroh'kahbən) a compound of hydrogen and carbon. Fats are of this type.

**hydrocele** ('hiedrə,seel) a swelling caused by accumulation of fluid, especially in the tunica vaginalis surrounding the testicle.

**hydrocephalus** (,hiedroh'kefələs, -'sef-) 'water on the brain'. Enlargement of the skull due to an abnormal collection of cerebrospinal fluid around the brain or in the ventricles. It may be either congenital or acquired from inflammation of the meninges during infancy. The most effective treatment is surgical correction employing a shunting technique. It frequently accompanies spina bifida.

**hydrochloric acid** (,hiedrə'klo.rik, -'klor.rik) HCl, a colourless compound of hydrogen and chlorine. It is present, in 0.2% solution, in gastric juice and aids digestion.

**hydrochlorothiazide** (,hiedrə,-klor.roh'thiəə,zied) a valuable oral diuretic similar to but more potent than chlorothiazide. It is used in the treatment of oedema and hypertension.

**hydrocortisone** (,hiedroh'kawti,zohn) cortisol, the principal GLUCOCORTICOID secreted by the adrenal gland; it is used in the treatment of inflammations, allergies, pruritus, collagen diseases, adrenocortical insufficiency, severe status asthmaticus, shock and certain neoplasms.

**hydroflumethiazide** (,hiedroh,floomi'thiəə,zied) an oral thiazide diuretic used in the treatment of oedema and hypertension.

**hydrogen** ('hiedrəjən) *symbol* H. A combustible gas, present in nearly all organic compounds, which, in combination with oxygen, forms water. *H. ion concentration* the amount of hydrogen in a liquid, which is responsible for its acidity. The degree of acidity is expressed in pH values: the higher the hydrogen ion concentration, the greater the acidity, and the lower the pH value. The concentration in the blood is of importance in acidosis. *H. peroxide* $H_2O_2$, a strong disinfectant cleansing and bleaching liquid used, diluted in water, for cleansing wounds.

**hydrolysis** (hie'drolisis) the process of splitting up into smaller molecules by uniting with water.

**hydrometer** (hie'dromitə) an instrument for estimating the specific gravity of fluids, e.g. a urinometer.

**hydromyelia** (,hiedrohmie'eeli.ə) a dilatation of the central canal of the spinal cord caused by an accumulation of cerebrospinal fluid.

**hydronephrosis** (,hiedrohnə'frohsis) an accumulation of urine in the pelvis of the kidney, resulting in atrophy of the kidney structure, due to an obstruction to the flow of urine from the kidney. The condition may be: (a) congenital, due to malformation of the kidney or ureter; or (b) acquired, due to an obstruction of the ureter by tumour or stone, or to back pressure from stricture of the urethra or an enlarged prostate gland.

**hydropathy** (hie'dropəthee) the treatment of disease by the use of water internally and externally; hydrotherapy.

**hydropericarditis** (,hiedroh,perikah'dietis) inflammation of the pericardium resulting in serous fluid in the pericardial sac.

**hydroperitoneum** (,hiedroh,peritə'neeəm) *see* ASCITES.

**hydrophobia** (,hiedrə'fohbi.ə) 1. rabies. 2. irrational fear of water.

**hydropneumothorax** (ˌhiedroh-ˌnyoomoh'thor.raks) the presence of fluid and air in the pleural cavity.

**hydrops** ('hiedrops) [L.] abnormal accumulation of serous fluid in the tissues or in a body cavity; also called dropsy. *Fetal h., h. fetalis* gross oedema of the entire body of the newborn infant, occurring in haemolytic disease of the newborn.

**hydrotherapy** (ˌhiedroh'therəpee) the treatment of disease by means of water.

**hydrothorax** (ˌhiedroh'thor.raks) fluid in the pleural cavity due to serous effusion, as in cardiac, renal and other diseases.

**hydroureter** (ˌhiedroh.yuh'reetə) an accumulation of water or urine in a ureter.

**hydroxytryptamine** (hieˌdroksi-'triptəˌmeen) serotonin.

**hydroxyurea** (hieˌdroksiyuh'reeə) an orally active cytotoxic agent used mainly in the treatment of melanoma, resistant chronic myelocytic leukaemia and recurrent, metastatic or inoperable ovarian carcinoma.

**hygiene** ('hiejeen) 1. the science of health and its preservation. 2. a condition of practice, such as cleanliness, that is conducive to preservation of health. *Communal h.* the maintenance of the health of the community by the provision of a pure water supply, efficient sanitation, good housekeeping, etc. *Industrial h.* (occupational health) care of the health of workers in an industry. *Mental h.* the science dealing with development of healthy mental and emotional reactions and habits. *Oral h.* the proper care of the mouth and teeth. *Personal h.* individual measures taken to preserve one's own cleanliness and wellbeing.

**hygroma** (hie'grohmə) a swelling caused by fluid. *Cystic h.* a cystic lymphangioma of the neck. *Sub-*

*dural h.* a collection of clear fluid in the subdural space.

**hygrometer** (hie'gromitə) an instrument for measuring the water vapour in the air.

**hygroscopic** (ˌhiegroh'skopik) readily absorbing moisture. An example is glycerin, which is used in suppositories as a means of aiding evacuation by moistening the faeces.

**hymen** ('hiemen) a fold of mucous membrane partially closing the entrance to the vagina. *Imperforate h.* a membrane which completely occludes the vaginal orifice.

**hymenectomy** (ˌhiemə'nektəmee) the surgical removal of the hymen.

**hymenotomy** (ˌhiemə'notəmee) a surgical incision of the hymen.

**hyoid** ('hieoyd) shaped like a U. *H. bone* a U-shaped bone above the thyroid cartilage, to which the tongue is attached.

**hyoscine** ('hieəˌseen) scopolamine; an anticholinergic drug used as an anaesthetic premedicant, antispasmodic, and in the treatment of motion sickness. Should be avoided in the elderly because of its tendency to cause restlessness and confusion (central cholinergic syndrome).

**hypaesthesia** (ˌhiepis'theezi.ə) impairment of the sense of touch.

**hypalgesia** (ˌhiepal'jeezi.ə) a decrease in sensitivity to pain.

**hypamnios** (hiep'amnios) a deficiency of fluid in the amniotic sac.

**hyperacidity** (ˌhiepə.ə'siditee) excessive acidity. *Gastric h.* hyperchlorhydria.

**hyperactive** (ˌhiepə'raktiv) exhibiting hyperactivity; hyperkinetic.

**hyperactivity** (ˌhiepə.rak'tivitee) abnormally increased activity. Developmental hyperactivity of children (hyperkinesia) is characterized by very restless, impulsive behaviour. These children are usually inattentive and have a poor concentration span. Other features that may be associated with hyperactivity include aggression, anxiety, poor eating and sleeping patterns, and social and learning difficulties.

**hyperaemia** (ˌhiepəˈreemi.ə) excess of blood in any part.

**hyperaesthesia** (ˌhiepə.risˈtheezi.ə) excessive sensitiveness to touch or to other sensations, e.g. taste or smell.

**hyperalgesia** (ˌhiepə.ralˈjeezi.ə) excessive sensibility to pain.

**hyperalimentation** (ˌhiepə.ralimen-ˈtayshən) a programme of parenteral administration of all nutrients for patients with gastrointestinal dysfunction; also called total parenteral alimentation (TPA) and total parenteral nutrition (TPN). Although the term hyperalimentation is commonly used to designate total or supplementary nutrition by intravenous feedings, it is not technically correct inasmuch as the procedure does not involve an abnormally increased or excessive amount of feeding. *See* NUTRITION (PARENTERAL).

**hyperasthenia** (ˌhiepə.rasˈtheeni.ə) extreme weakness.

**hyperbaric** (ˌhiepəˈbarik) at a greater pressure than normal; applied to gases under greater than atmospheric pressure. *H. oxygenation* exposure to oxygen under conditions of greatly increased pressure. The patient is placed in a sealed enclosure, called a hyperbaric chamber. Compressed air is introduced; at the same time the patient is given pure oxygen through a face mask. Patients suffering from tetanus and gas gangrene, infections caused by bacteria that are resistant to antibiotics but vulnerable to oxygen, are helped by hyperbaric oxygenation. The technique is also useful in radiotherapy for cancer. When full of oxygen, cancer cells seem more vulnerable to radiation. Carbon

monoxide poisoning can be treated by hyperbaric oxygenation. Carbon monoxide molecules, displacing the oxygen in the erythrocytes, usually cause asphyxiation, but hyperbaric oxygenation can often keep the patient alive until the carbon monoxide has been eliminated from the body's system.

**hyperbilirubinaemia** (ˌhiepə.bili.roobiˈneemi.ə) an excess of bilirubin in the blood.

**hypercalcaemia** (ˌhiepəkalˈseemi.ə) an excess of calcium in the blood. May be caused by overadministration of vitamin D, hyperparathyroidism, thyrotoxicosis, breakdown of bone by malignant disease, or impaired renal function.

**hypercalciuria** (ˌhiepə.kalsiˈyooə.ri.ə) a high level of calcium in the urine leading to renal stone formation.

**hypercapnia** (ˌhiepəˈkapni.ə) an increased amount of carbon dioxide in the blood, causing overstimulation of the respiratory centre. Hypercarbia.

**hypercatabolism** (ˌhiepəkəˈtabə.li.zəm) an excessive rate of catabolism leading to wasting or destruction of a part or tissue.

**hyperchloraemia** (ˌhiepə.kloˈreemi.ə) an excess of chloride in the blood.

**hyperchlorhydria** (ˌhiepəklorˈhie.dri.ə) an excess of hydrochloric acid in the gastric juice.

**hypercholesteraemia, hypercholesterolaemia** (ˌhiepəkə.lestə-ˈreemi.ə, ˌhiepəkə.lestə.roˈleemi.ə) excess of cholesterol in the blood. Predisposes to atheroma and gallstones.

**hypercusis** (ˌhiepəˈkyoosis) excessive sensitivity to sound.

**hyperemesis** (ˌhiepəˈremə.sis) excessive vomiting. *H. gravidarum* an uncommon, serious complication of pregnancy, characterized by severe and persistent vomiting, the aetiology of which is not fully understood.

**hyperextension** (ˌhiepə.rek'stenshən) the forcible extension of a limb beyond the normal. It is used to correct orthopaedic deformities.

**hyperflexion** (ˌhiepə'flekshən) the forcible bending of a joint beyond the normal.

**hypergalactia, hypergalactosis** (ˌhiepəgə'lakti.ə, ˌhiepə.galək'tohsis) excessive secretion of milk.

**hypergammaglobulinaemia** (ˌhiepə.gamə.globyuhli'neemi.ə) increased gamma-globulins in the blood.

**hyperglycaemia** (ˌhiepəglie'seemi.ə) excess of sugar in the blood (normal 2.5–4.7 mmol/litre when fasting); a sign of diabetes mellitus. See HYPOGLYCAEMIA; Table on p. 119.

**hyperhidrosis** (ˌhiepəhi'drohsis) excessive perspiration; hyperidrosis.

**hyperkalaemia** (ˌhiepəkə'leemi.ə) an excess of potassium in the blood. If untreated, this will lead to cardiac arrest.

**hyperkeratosis** (ˌhiepə.kerə'tohsis) hypertrophy of the horny layers of the skin.

**hyperkinesis** (ˌhiepəki'neesis) a condition in which there is excessive motor activity. See HYPERACTIVITY.

**hyperlipaemia** (ˌhiepəli'peemi.ə) an excess of fat or lipids in the blood.

**hypermastia** (ˌhiepə'masti.ə) 1. the presence of one or more supernumerary breasts. 2. overdevelopment of one or both breasts.

**hypermetropia** (ˌhiepəme'trohpi.ə) hyperopia; longsightedness. The light rays entering the eye converge beyond the retina. Clear vision can be obtained by the wearing of spectacles or contact lenses.

**hypermotility** (ˌhiepəmoh'tilitee) excessive movement. *Gastric h.* increased muscle action of the stomach wall, associated with increased secretion of hydrochloric acid.

**hypernatraemia** (ˌhiepənə'treemi.ə) an excess of sodium in the blood, usually diagnosed when the plasma sodium is above 150 mmol/litre. It is the result of loss of water and electrolytes from the body caused by diarrhoea, polyuria, excessive sweating or inadequate fluid intake. May also occur in infants if excessive salt has been added to feeds, resulting in convulsions and brain damage.

**hypernephroma** (ˌhiepəne'frohmə) a malignant tumour of the kidney; renal cell carcinoma.

**hyperostosis** (ˌhiepə.ro'stohsis) a thickening of bone; a bony outgrowth; exostosis.

**hyperparathyroidism** (ˌhiepə.parə-'thieroy.dizəm) excessive activity of the parathyroid glands, causing drainage of calcium from the bones, with consequent fragility and liability to spontaneous fracture.

**hyperphagia** (ˌhiepə'fayji.ə) overeating.

**hyperphasia** (ˌhiepə'fayzi.ə) excessive talkativeness.

**hyperphenylalaninaemia** (ˌhiepə.feenie.laləni'neemi.ə) an excess of phenylalanine in the blood, as in phenylketonuria.

**hyperpituitarism** (ˌhiepəpi'tyuoitə.rizəm) overactivity of the pituitary gland.

**hyperplasia** (ˌhiepə'playzi.ə) excessive formation of normal cells in a tissue or organ, which increases in size.

**hyperpnoea** (ˌhiepə'neeə,-pəp-'neeə) overbreathing; hyperventilation; an abnormal increase in the rate and depth of breathing.

**hyperprolactinaemia** (ˌhiepəproh.lakti'neemi.ə) increased levels of prolactin in the blood; in women, it is associated with infertility and may lead to galactorrhoea, and it has been reported to cause impotence in men.

**hyperpyrexia** (ˌhiepəpie'reksɪə) an excessively high body temperature, i.e. over 41°C.

**hypersensitivity** (ˌhiepəˌsensi'tivitee) abnormal sensitivity, especially to a particular antigen. The reactions include allergies (such as asthma) and anaphylaxis. *Contact h.* produced by contact of the skin with a chemical substance having the properties of an antigen or hapten; it includes contact dermatitis (*see* CONTACT). *Delayed h.* a slowly developing increase in cell-mediated immune response (involving T lymphocytes) to a specific antigen, as occurs in graft rejection, autoimmune disease, etc. *Immediate h.* antibody-mediated hypersensitivity characterized by lesions resulting from release of histamine and other mediators of hypersensitivity from reagin-sensitized mast cells, causing increased vascular permeability, oedema and smooth muscle contraction; it includes anaphylaxis and atopy.

**hypersplenism** (ˌhiepə'splenizəm) overactivity of an enlarged spleen resulting in the destruction of blood cells and platelets.

**hypertelorism** (ˌhiepə'teləˌrizəm) abnormally increased distance between two organs or parts. *Ocular h., orbital h.* increase in the interocular distance, often associated with craniofacial dysostosis and sometimes with mental handicap.

**hypertension** (ˌhiepə'tenshən) persistently high BLOOD PRESSURE. In adults, it is generally agreed that a blood pressure is abnormally high when the resting, supine arterial systolic pressure is equal to or greater than 140 mmHg and the diastolic pressure is equal to or greater than 90 mmHg. A diagnosis of hypertension should be based on a series of readings rather than a single measurement. *Essential h.* high blood pressure without demonstrable change in kidneys, blood vessels or heart. *Malignant h.* a form of hypertension which may develop at a comparatively early age, in which the prognosis is poor. *Portal h.* raised pressure in the portal system. *Pulmonary h.* increased pressure in the arteries of the lung, usually following emphysema or fibrosis.

**hyperthermia** (ˌhiepə'thərmi.ə) an exceedingly high body temperature. *Malignant h.* a serious condition, sometimes arising during general anaesthesia.

**hyperthyroidism** (ˌhiepə'thieroyˌdizəm) excessive activity of the thyroid gland. *See* THYROTOXICOSIS.

**hypertonic** (ˌhiepə'tonik) 1. showing excessive tone or tension, as in a blood vessel or muscle. 2. describing a solution that has greater osmotic pressure than normal physiological tissue fluid. *See* HYPOTONIC.

**hypertrichosis** (ˌhiepətri'kohsis) excessive growth of hair on any part of the body.

**hypertrophy** (hie'pərtrəfee) an increase in the size of a tissue or a structure caused by an increase in the size of the cells that compose it (as opposed to an increase in the number of cells). *See* HYPERPLASIA.

**hyperuricaemia** (ˌhiepəˌyooə–ri.'seemi.ə) an excess of uric acid in the blood. *See* GOUT.

**hyperventilation** (ˌhiepəˌventi'layshən) 1. increase of air in the lungs above the normal amount. 2. abnormally prolonged and deep breathing, usually associated with acute anxiety or emotional tension. Hyperpnoea.

**hypervitaminosis** (ˌhiepəˌvitəmi'nohsis) a condition caused by the intake of an excessive quantity of vitamins, particularly vitamins A and D.

**hypervolaemia** (ˌhiepəvo'leemi.ə) abnormal increase in the volume of circulating fluid (plasma) in the body.

**hyphaema** (hie'feemə) haemorrhage into the anterior chamber of the eye.

**hypnosis** (hip'nohsis) an artificially induced passive state in which there is increased amenability and responsiveness to suggestions and commands. In hypnosis, a drowsy phase is followed by a sleep. It may also be used to produce painless childbirth and tooth extraction.

**hypnotherapy** (ˌhipnoh'therəpee) treatment by hypnosis or by the induction of prolonged sleep.

**hypnotic** (hip'notik) an agent that causes sleep; a soporific.

**hypnotism** ('hipnəˌtizəm) the practice of hypnosis.

**hypocalcaemia** (ˌhiepohkal'seemi.ə) a deficiency of calcium in the blood.

**hypocapnia** (ˌhiepoh'kapni.ə) a deficiency of carbon dioxide in the blood.

**hypochloraemia** (ˌhiepohklo'reemi.ə) a deficiency of chloride in the blood.

**hypochlorhydria** (ˌhiepohklor'hiedri.ə) a lower than normal amount of hydrochloric acid in the gastric juice.

**hypochlorite** (ˌhiepoh'klor.riet) any salt of hypochlorous acid used in solution to yield chlorine, a disinfecting and germicidal agent. Milton, a proprietary preparation, is used in solution for the disinfection of equipment and infant feeding utensils.

**hypochondria** (ˌhiepə'kondri.ə) a morbid preoccupation or anxiety about one's health. The sufferer feels that first one part of the body and then another part is the seat of some serious disease.

**hypochondriac** (ˌhiepə'kondri.ak) one affected by hypochondria. *H. region* the hypochondrium.

**hypochondrium** (ˌhiepoh'kondri.əm) the upper region of the abdomen on each side of the epigastrium.

**hypochromic** (ˌhiepoh'krohmik) deficient in pigmentation or colouring.

**hypodermic** (ˌhiepə'dərmik) beneath the skin; applied to subcutaneous injections and to the syringes used for such injections.

**hypofibrinogenaemia** (ˌhiepohfieˌbrinəjə'neemi.ə) a lack of fibrinogen in the blood. This may occur in severe trauma or haemorrhage or as an inherited condition.

**hypogammaglobulinaemia** (ˌhiepohˌgaməˌglobyuhli'neemi.ə) a deficiency of gamma-globulin in the blood, rendering the person susceptible to infection.

**hypogastrium** (ˌhiepoh'gastri.əm) the lower middle area of the abdomen, immediately below the umbilical region.

**hypoglossal** (ˌhiepoh'glos'l) under the tongue. *H. nerve* the 12th cranial nerve.

**hypoglycaemia** (ˌhiepohglie'seemi.ə) a condition in which the blood sugar level is less than normal. Usually arising in diabetic patients as a result of insulin overdosage, delay in eating or a rapid combustion of carbohydrate. *See* HYPERGLYCAEMIA; Table on p. 119.

**hypokalaemia** (ˌhiepohkə'leemi.ə) a low potassium level in the blood. This is likely to be present in dehydration and with the repeated use of diuretics.

**hypomania** (ˌhiepoh'mayni.ə) a degree of elation, excitement and activity higher than normal but less severe than that present in mania.

**hypometropia** (ˌhiepohme'trohpi.ə) myopia; short-sightedness.

**hypomotility** (ˌhiepohmoh'tilitee) deficient power of movement in any part.

**hyponatraemia** (ˌhiepohnə'treemi ə) a deficiency of sodium in the blood.

**hypoparathyroidism** (ˌhiepohˌparə'thieroyˌdizəm) a lack of parathyroid secretion, leading to a low blood calcium and tetany.

**hypophysis** (hie'pofisis) an outgrowth. *H. cerebri* the pituitary gland.

**hypopituitarism** (ˌhiepohpi'tyooitəˌrizəm) deficiency of secretion from the anterior lobe of the pituitary gland, causing excessive deposition of fat in children. *See* FRÖLICH'S SYNDROME. Dwarfism may result. In adults asthenia, drowsiness and adiposity may occur, together with an impairment of sexual activity and premature senility.

**hypoplasia** (ˌhiepoh'playzi.ə) imperfect development of a part or organ.

**hypopnoea** (ˌhiepoh'neeə, -'popni.ə) shallow breathing.

**hypoproteinaemia** (ˌhiepohˌprohti-'neemi.ə) a deficiency of serum proteins in the blood.

**hypoprothrombinaemia** (ˌhiepohˌprohˌthrombi'neemi.ə) a deficiency of prothrombin in the blood, leading to a tendency to bleed. *See* HAEMOPHILIA.

**hypopyon** (hie'pohpi.ən) an accumulation of pus in the anterior chamber of the eye.

**hyposecretion** (ˌhiepohsi'kreeshən) a deficiency in secretion from any glandular structure or secreting cells.

**hyposensitivity** (ˌhiepohˌsensi'tivitee) a lack of sensitivity, especially to a particular allergen with which the patient may have been overdosed over a period.

**hypospadias** (ˌhiepə'spaydi.əs) a developmental anomaly in the male in which the urethra opens on the underside of the penis or on the perineum.

**hypostasis** (ˌhie'postəsis) 1. a sediment or deposit. 2. congestion of blood in a part, due to slowing of the circulation.

**hypostatic** (ˌhiepoh'statik) relating to hypostasis. *H. pneumonia see* PNEUMONIA.

**hypotension** (ˌhiepoh'tenshən) abnormally low arterial blood pressure; hypopiesis. *Controlled* or *induced h.* an artificially produced lowering of the blood pressure so that an operation field is rendered practically bloodless. *Orthostatic* or *postural h.* temporary hypotension when the patient stands up, producing giddiness and sometimes a faint.

**hypotensive** (ˌhiepoh'tensiv) producing a reduction in tension, especially pertaining to a drug that lowers the blood pressure.

**hypothalamus** (ˌhiepə'thaləməs) the portion of the diencephalon lying beneath the thalamus at the base of the cerebrum, and forming the floor and part of the lateral wall of the third ventricle. It influences peripheral autonomic mechanisms, endocrine activity and many somatic functions, e.g. a general regulation of water balance, body temperature, sleep, thirst and hunger, and the development of secondary sexual characteristics. It plays an important role in the regulation of protein, fat and carbohydrate metabolism, body fluid volume and electrolyte content, and internal secretion of endocrine hormones.

**hypothermia** (ˌhiepoh'thərmi.ə) 1. a severe reduction in the body temperature. The condition usually arises gradually and may prove fatal if untreated. It is most common among babies and elderly people. 2. artificial cooling of the body to reduce the oxygen requirements of the tissues. *Mild h.* a reduction of the body temperature to 34°C, which may be induced by surface cooling with cold air. Generalized lowering of the body temperature is used in three main situations: (a) to control fever, as in malignant hyperthermia; (b) to enable certain cardiac and neurological operations to be carried out; and (c) to protect the brain from raised intracranial pressure in patients with head injuries or following drowning.

**hypothesis** (hie'pothisis) a supposition that appears to explain a group of phenomena and is assumed as a basis of reasoning and experimentation. A starting point for further investigations from known facts.

**hypothrombinaemia** ('hiepoh-'thrombi'neemi.ə) a diminished amount of thrombin in the blood, with a consequent tendency to bleed.

**hypothyroidism** (ˌhiepoh'thieroydi-zəm) an insufficiency of thyroid secretion. In children it may produce cretinism. In adults it leads to myxoedema.

**hypotonia** (ˌhiepoh'tohni.ə) 1. deficient muscle tone. 2. deficient tension in the eyeball.

**hypotonic** (ˌhiepoh'tonik) describing a solution that has a lower osmotic pressure than another one. *See* HYPERTONIC.

**hypoventilation** (ˌhiepoh venti'layshən) hypopnoea; shallow breathing, usually at a very slow rate. It may cause a build-up of carbon dioxide in the blood.

**hypovolaemia** (ˌhiepohvo'leemi.ə) a reduction in the circulating blood volume due to external loss of body fluids or to loss from the blood into the tissues, as in shock.

**hypoxaemia** (ˌhiepok'seemi.ə) an insufficient oxygen content in the blood.

**hypoxia** (hie'poksi.ə) a diminished amount of oxygen in the tissues. *Anaemic h.* low oxygen content due to deficiency of haemoglobin in the blood.

**hysterectomy** (ˌhistə'rektəmee) removal of the uterus. *Abdominal h.* removal via an abdominal incision. *Subtotal h.* removal of the body of the uterus only. *Total h.* removal of the body and cervix. *Vaginal h.* removal through the vagina. *Wertheim's h.* additional excision of the parametrium, upper vagina and lymph glands. Radical abdominal hysterectomy.

**hysteria** (his'tiə.ri.ə) a psychoneurosis in which the individual converts anxiety created by emotional conflict into physical symptoms, e.g. tics, mutism or paralysis of an arm or leg, that have no organic basis; also called conversion reaction or conversion hysteria. The term hysteria is also used to describe a state of tension or excitement in which there is a temporary loss of control over the emotions.

**hysterical** (hi'sterik'l) relating to hysteria.

**hysteromyoma** (ˌhistə.rohmie'ohmə) a fibromyoma of the uterus.

**hysteromyomectomy** (ˌhistə.rohˌmieə'mektəmee) excision of a hysteromyoma.

**hystero-oöphorectomy** (ˌhisteroh-ˌoh.əfə'rektəmee) excision of the uterus and the ovaries.

**hysterosalpingography** (ˌhisterohˌsalping'gogrəfee) radiographic examination of the uterus and uterine tubes after the injection of a radio-opaque dye. Uterosalpingography.

**hysterosalpingostomy** (ˌhisterohˌsalping'gostəmee) the establishment of an opening between the distal portion of the uterine tube and the uterus in an effort to overcome infertility when the medial portion is occluded or excised.

**hysterotomy** (ˌhistə'rotəmee) incision of the uterus, usually in order to remove a fetus in mid-pregnancy when it is too late to perform a therapeutic abortion. *See* CAESAREAN SECTION.

# I

**I** symbol for *iodine*.

**iatrogenesis** (ie͵atroh'jenəsis) additional patient problems, complications or disease brought about by the activities of physicians, surgeons or other health-care professionals, including new infections, unwanted effects of drug therapy and psychological distress.

**ibuprofen** (ie͵byoo'proh͵fen) an antiinflammatory analgesic and antipyretic drug used in the treatment of mild rheumatic and arthritic conditions.

**ice** (ics) water in a solid state, at or below freezing point. *Dry i.* carbon dioxide snow. *I. bag* a rubber or plastic bag half-filled with pieces of ice and applied near or to a part to relieve pain or swelling.

**ichthammol** ('ikthə͵mol) an ammoniated coal tar product, used in ointment form for certain skin diseases.

**ichthyosis** (͵ikthi'ohsis) a congenital abnormality of the skin in which there is dryness and roughness, the horny layer is thickened and large scales appear.

**ICM** International Confederation of Midwives.

**ICN** infection control nurse (*see* INFECTION); International Council of Nurses.

**ICP** intracranial pressure.

**ICSH** interstitial cell stimulating hormone.

**icterus** ('iktə.rəs) jaundice. *I. gravis* a fatal form of jaundice occurring in pregnancy. Acute yellow atrophy. *I. gravis neonatorum* haemolytic disease of the newborn. *See* RHESUS FACTOR.

**ICU** intensive care unit.

**id** (id) that part of the personality, containing the instinctive drives, which leads to gratification of primitive needs and which exists in the unconscious.

**idea** (ie'deeə) a mental impression or conception. *Autochthonous i.* a strange idea that comes into the mind in some unaccountable way, but is not a hallucination. *Compulsive i.* an idea that persists despite reason and will and that drives one to action, usually inappropriate. *Dominant i.* a morbid or other impression that controls or colours every action and thought. *Fixed i.* a persistent morbid impression or belief that cannot be changed by reason. *I. of reference* the incorrect idea that the words and actions of others refer to oneself, or the projection of the causes of one's own imaginary difficulties upon someone else.

**identical** (ie'dentik'l) exactly alike. *I. twins* twins of the same sex developing from a single fertilized ovum.

**identification** (ie͵dentifi'kayshən) a mental mechanism by which an individual adopts the attitudes and ideas of another, often admired, person.

**identity** (ie'dentitee) part of the 'self concept' of being distinguishable and separate from others. *I. crisis* one in which the individual loses the sense of self-distinctiveness and role in society. Occurs most commonly in the transition from one phase of life to the next, e.g. during adolescence.

**ideology** (iedi'oləjee) 1. the science of the development of ideas. 2. the body of ideas characteristic of an individual or of a social unit.

**ideomotion** (ˌiedioh'mohshən) the association of ideas and muscle action, as in involuntary acts.

**idiopathic** (ˌidioh'pathik) self-originated; applied to a condition the cause of which is not known.

**idiosyncrasy** (ˌidioh'singkrəsee) 1. a habit or quality of body or mind peculiar to any individual. 2. an abnormal susceptibility to an agent (e.g. a drug) that is peculiar to the individual.

**idoxuridine** (ˌiedoks'yooə.rideen) abbreviated IDU. An iodine-containing drug used to treat infections caused by herpes virus, particularly keratitis and dendritic corneal ulcer.

**Ig** immunoglobulin of any of the five classes: IgA, IgD, IgE, IgG and IgM.

**ileal** ('ili.əl) referring to the ileum. *I. conduit* a surgical procedure in which the ureters are transplanted into the ileum, an isolated loop of which is then brought to the surface of the abdomen in order to allow the urine to drain into a bag.

**ileitis** (ˌili'ietis) inflammation of the ileum. *Regional i.* Crohn's disease. A chronic condition of the terminal portion of the ileum in which granulation and oedema may give rise to obstruction.

**ileocolitis** (ˌiliohkə'lietis) inflammation of the ileum and colon.

**ileocolostomy** (ˌiliohkə'lostəmee) the making of a permanent opening between the ileum and some part of the colon.

**ileocystoplasty** (ˌilioh'sistoh.plastee) repair of the wall of the urinary bladder with an isolated segment of the ileum.

**ileoproctostomy** (ˌiliohprok'tostə—mee) surgical anastomosis between the ileum and the rectum; ileorectal anastomosis.

**ileorectal** (ˌilioh'rekt'l) referring to the ileum and rectum. *I. anastomosis* ileoproctostomy.

**ileostomy** (ˌili'ostəmee) an artificial opening (stoma) created from the ileum and brought to the surface of the abdomen for the purpose of evacuation. Ileostomy is an inevitable part of proctocolectomy. An ileostomy may be temporary or permanent. *I. bags* disposable bags to collect the liquid faecal matter discharged from an ileostomy. The bags can be adhesive or worn on a belt.

**ileum** ('ili.əm) the last part of the small intestine, terminating at the caecum.

**ileus** ('ili.əs) intestinal obstruction, especially failure of peristalsis. The condition frequently accompanies peritonitis and usually results from disturbances in neural stimulation of the bowel. The principal symptoms of ileus are abdominal pain and distension, vomiting (the vomitus may contain faecal material) and constipation. If the intestinal obstruction is not relieved, the patient becomes extremely ill with SHOCK and DEHYDRATION.

**iliac** ('ili.ak) pertaining to the ilium. *I. artery* the right and left arteries form the terminal branches of the abdominal aorta and supply blood to the pelvic region and the lower limbs. *I. crest* the crest of the hip bone. *I. fossa* the depression on the concave surface of the iliac bone. *I. vein* the right and left veins join to form the inferior vena cava .

**ilium** ('ili.əm) the haunch bone; the upper part of the hip bone.

**illness** ('ilnəs) a condition marked by pronounced deviation from the normal healthy state; sickness. *I. behaviour* the way in which ill individuals regard the structure and function of their own body, interpret symptoms and seek treatment for their condition.

**illusion** (i'loozhən) a mistaken perception due to a misinterpretation of a sensory stimulus; believing something to be what it is not.

**image** ('imij) 1. the mental recall of a former precept. 2. the optical picture transferred to the brain cells by the optic nerve.

**imago** (i'maygoh, i'mahgoh) [L.] 1. in psychoanalysis, a childhood memory or fantasy of a loved person that persists in adult life. 2. the adult or definitive form of an insect.

**imbalance** (im'baləns) lack of balance, e.g. of endocrine secretions, between water and electrolytes, or of muscles.

**imipramine** (i'miprə meen) a drug, chemically related to chlorpromazine, that may be effective in relieving depression. *See* ANTI-DEPRESSANT. Also used to treat nocturnal enuresis in children.

**immature** ( imə'tyooə) unripe; not fully developed, as in a cataract when only a part of the lens is opaque.

**immiscible** (i'misəb'l) incapable of being mixed, e.g. oil and water.

**immobilize** (i'mohbi liez) to render incapable of being moved, as by a plaster of Paris cast.

**immune** (i'myoon) protected against a particular infection or allergy. *I. response* the (in general) helpful events that follow activation of the immune system, including T-lymphocyte activity (cell-mediated responses) and B-lymphocyte activity (humoral responses). Immune responses are involved in protecting persons from disease following infection and are also involved in the rejection of transplanted organs and tissues that the body recognizes as foreign, or non-self.

**immunity** (i'myoonitee) the resistance possessed by the body to infectious diseases, foreign tissues, foreign non-toxic substances and other ANTIGENS. The opposite of susceptibility. Immunological responses in humans can be divided into two broad categories: humoral immunity, which takes place in the body fluids and is concerned with antibody and complement activities; and cell-mediated or cellular immunity, which involves a variety of activities designed to destroy or at least contain cells that are recognized by the body as alien and harmful. Both types of response are instigated by lymphocytes that originate in the bone marrow as stem cells and later are converted into mature cells having specific properties and functions. The two kinds of lymphocyte that are important to the establishment of immunity are T-lymphocytes (T-cells) and B-lymphocytes (B-cells). B-lymphocytes mature into plasma cells that are primarily responsible for forming antibodies, thereby providing humoral immunity. Cellular immunity is dependent upon T-lymphocytes and is primarily concerned with a delayed type of immune response as occurs in the rejection of transplanted organs, defence against some slowly developing bacterial diseases, allergic reactions and certain autoimmune diseases.

**immunization** ( imyuhnie'zay-shən) the act of creating immunity by artificial means. *I. schedule* a standard schedule for immunization against infectious diseases (*see* Appendices).

**immunoassay** (ˌimyuhnoh'asay) a quantitative estimate of the proteins contained in the blood serum.

**immunodeficiency** (ˌimyuhnohdi-'fishənsee) a deficiency of the immune response, either that mediated by humoral antibody or by immune lymphoid cells. *I. disorders* acquired or congenital conditions in which the body's immune system fails to protect against infection, foreign material and some forms of cancer.

**immunoglobulin** (ˌimyuhnoh'globyuhlin) antibody. A variety of chemical compound found mainly in gamma-globulin (*see* GAMMA). Immunoglobulins are major components of the humoral immune response system. They are synthesized by lymphocytes and plasma cells and found in the serum and in other body fluids and tissues. The five classes of immunoglobulin (Ig) are: IgA, IgD, IgE, IgG and IgM. There are two types of IgA and both are known to have antiviral properties. Secretory IgA is present in nonvascular fluids such as colostrum and breast milk. IgD is found in trace quantities in serum. It serves as a B-lymphocyte surface receptor. IgE is called the reaginic antibody and may be increased in persons with allergy. IgG is the most abundant of the five classes of immunoglobulin and is the major antibody in the secondary humoral response of immunity. It is the only immunoglobulin to cross the placenta. IgM is principally concerned with the primary antibody response.

**immunology** (ˌimyuh'nolǝjee) the study of immunity and the body's defence mechanisms.

**immunosuppression** (ˌimyuhnosǝ'preshǝn) inhibition of the formation of antibodies to antigens that may be present; used in transplantation procedures to prevent rejection of the transplanted organ or tissue.

**immunosuppressive** (ˌimyuhnohsǝ-'presiv) 1. pertaining to or inducing immunosuppression. 2. an agent that induces immunosuppression.

**immunotherapy** (ˌimyuhnoh'therǝpee) 1. treatment by immunization. Sometimes used in the treatment of leukaemia. 2. the establishing of passive immunity.

**immunotransfusion** (iˌmyoonoh-trans'fyoozhǝn, -trahns-) transfusion of blood from a donor previously rendered immune to the disease affecting the patient.

**Imodium** (i'mohdiǝm) trade name for preparations of loperamide hydrochloride, an antidiarrhoeal.

**impaction** (im'pakshǝn) a state of being wedged. *Dental i.* the condition in which a tooth, usually a molar, is unable to erupt through the gum because it is lodged in position by bone or the other teeth. *Faecal i.* a collection of putty-like or hardened faeces in the rectum or sigmoid colon.

**impairment** (im'pairmǝnt) any loss or abnormality of psychological, physiological or anatomical structure or function.

**impalpable** (im'palpǝb'l) incapable of being felt by manual examination. May apply to an organ or a tumour.

**imperforate** (im'pǝrfǝ.rǝt) without an opening. *I. anus* a congenital defect in which this opening is closed. *I. hymen* complete closure of the vaginal opening by the hymen.

**impermeable** (im'pǝrmi.ǝb'l) not permitting the passage of fluid or molecules.

**impetigo** (ˌimpǝ'tiegoh) an acute contagious inflammation of the skin marked by pustules and scabs;

of streptococcal or staphylococcal origin. It occurs mainly on the face and limbs, particularly those of children.

**implant** ('implahnt) any substance grafted into the tissues. *Hormone i.* a hormonal pellet which may be implanted subcutaneously. *Intra-ocular lens i.* a plastic lens which may be implanted in the eye after lens extraction. *Plastic i.* a silicone implant which may be used in plastic surgery, e.g. to reshape the breast.

**implantation** (,implahn'tayshən) the act of planting or setting in. 1. the embedding of the fertilized ovum in the wall of the uterus. 2. the placing of a drug within the tissues. 3. the surgical introduction of healthy tissue to replace tissue that has been damaged.

**implementation** (,implimen'tay-shən) the third phase of the nursing process signifying the giving of care in relation to defined nursing interventions and goals. During implementation the nursing care plan is tested for effectiveness and accuracy. Data gathering continues and plans may change on the basis of new information obtained. The implementation phase concludes with the recording of the activities performed and the response of the patient. *See* ASSESSMENT and EVALUATION.

**implosion** (im'plohzhən) in behaviour therapy, a form of desensitization used in the treatment of phobias and related disorders. *See* FLOODING

**impotence** ('impətəns) inability in a man to carry out sexual intercourse from either psychological or physical causes.

**impregnation** (,impreg'nayshən) insemination; rendering pregnant.

**impulse** ('impuls) 1. a sudden pushing force. 2. a sudden uncontrollable act. 3. nerve impulse.

*Cardiac i.* movement of the chest wall caused by the heart beat. *Nerve i.* the electrochemical process propagated along nerve fibres.

**IMV** intermittent mandatory ventilation.

**in situ** (in 'sityoo) [L.] *in the original position.*

**in vitro** (in 'veetroh, 'vit-) [L.] *in a glass.* Refers to observations made outside the body. *See* IN VIVO.

**in vivo** (in 'veevoh) [L.] *within the living body. See* IN VITRO.

**inaccessibility** (,inak,sesə'bilitee) a state of unresponsiveness characteristic of certain psychiatric patients, e.g. schizophrenics.

**inarticulate** (,inah'tikyuhlət) 1. without joints. 2. unable to speak intelligibly.

**incarcerated** (in'kahsə,raytid) held fast. Applied to (a) a hernia that is immovable, and therefore only curable by operation, and (b) a pregnant uterus held under the sacral brim.

**incest** ('insest) sexual intercourse between close blood relatives, e.g. brothers and sisters; marriage between them is legally or culturally prohibited. Some form of incest taboo is found in all known societies, although the relationships prohibited vary.

**incidence** ('insidəns) the number of particular new events which occur in a population in a given period of time. For example, the number of new cases of a disease, such as measles, expressed per 1000 of population per year.

**incipient** (in'sipi.ənt) beginning to exist.

**incision** (in'sizhən) 1. in surgery, a cut into soft tissue. 2. the act of cutting.

**incisor** (in'siezə) one of the four front teeth in the centre of each jaw.

**inclusion** (in'kloozhən) something that is enclosed or the act of enclosing. *I. bodies* particles that are temporarily enclosed in the cytoplasm of a cell. For example, in trachoma virus particles can be seen in the conjunctival epithelial cells.

**incoherent** (inkoh'hiə.rənt) 1. unconnected; inconsistent. 2. uttering speech that is disconnected and rambling.

**incompatibility** (ˌinkəmpatə'bilitee) the state of two or more substances being antagonistic, or destroying the efficiency of each other. Applied to mixtures of drugs, and to blood. *See* BLOOD GROUP.

**incompetence** (in'kompitəns) inefficiency. *Aortic i.* failure of the aortic valves to regulate the flow of blood. *Mitral i.* failure of the mitral valve to close properly.

**incontinence** (in'kontinəns) inability to control natural functions or discharges. *Faecal i.* inability to control the movements of the bowels. *Overflow i.* that from an overfull bladder, most common in elderly men with urinary obstruction. *Paralytic i.* loss of control of anal and urethral sphincters due to injury to nerve centres. *Stress i.* that which is due to a defect in the urethral sphincters and is liable to occur when intra-abdominal pressure is increased, as in coughing or lifting heavy weights; most common in women with weak pelvic muscles. *Urinary i.* inability to control the outflow of urine.

**incoordination** (ˌinkoh.awdi-'nayshən) inability to adjust various muscle movements harmoniously.

**incrustation** (ˌinkru'stayshən) the formation of a crust or scab on a wound.

**incubation** (ˌingkyuh'bayshən) the development and growth of microorganisms and animal embryos. *I. period* the period between the date of infection and the appearance of symptoms of an infectious disease.

**incubator** ('ingkyuh,baytə) 1. a warmed servo-controlled Perspex box for nursing ill and preterm babies. 2. an apparatus used to develop bacteria at a uniform temperature suitable to their growth.

**incus** ('ingkəs) the small anvil-shaped bone of the middle ear. The second auditory ossicle.

**indicator** ('indi,kaytə) 1. the index finger, or the extensor muscle of the index finger. 2. any substance that indicates the appearance or disappearance of a chemical by a colour change or attainment of a certain pH.

**indigenous** (in'dijənəs) occurring naturally in a certain locality.

**indigestion** (ˌindi'jeschən) *see* DYSPEPSIA.

**Indocid** ('indoh,sid) trade name for indomethacin.

**indolent** ('indələnt) slow-growing. Reluctant to heal. Largely painless. *I. ulcer* a chronic ulcer of the skin or mucous membrane.

**indomethacin** (ˌindoh'methəsin) an anti-inflammatory analgesic used in the treatment of arthritis and of acute attacks of gout.

**induction** (in'dukshən) the act of initiating something. *Electromagnetic i.* the production of an electric current in a body because of its nearness to an electrified (or magnetized) body. *I. of abortion* the intentional bringing about of an abortion. *I. of anaesthesia* the start of the administration of a general anaesthetic. *I. of labour* the artificial starting of the process of childbirth.

**induration** (ˌindyuh'rayshən) the abnormal hardening of a tissue or organ.

**industrial** (in'dustri.əl) referring to industry. *I. diseases* those that are caused by the nature of the work. *Prescribed i. diseases* those for which sickness benefit is payable, including those that are notifiable under the Factories Act (1961).

**inebriation** (iˌneebri'ayshən) the condition of being intoxicated by alcohol; drunkenness.

**inert** (i'nərt) having no action. *I. gas* a gas which does not react with other elements, e.g. neon.

**inertia** (i'nərshə) sluggishness; inability to move except when stimulated by an external force. *Uterine i.* lack of muscle contraction during the first and second stages of labour.

**infant** ('infənt) a child under 1 year of age. Educationally, a child under 7 years of age. *Floppy i., floppy i. syndrome* a congenital myopathy of infants, marked clinically by myotonia and muscle weakness. *I. feeding* the supplying of nutrition to an infant. Breast milk is the ideal food for the baby and if breast feeding is established satisfactorily for the first few months it can aid physical and emotional development. Where it is not possible an infant food formula can be given. *I. mortality rate* the number of deaths of children under 1 year of age per 1000 live births in any one year. *Premature i.* one born before the state of maturity. *See* PRETERM INFANT.

**infanticide** (in'fanti,sied) the killing of a child during the first year of its life.

**infantile** ('infən,tiel) concerning an infant; childish. *I. paralysis* poliomyelitis.

**infantilism** (in'fanti,lizəm) persistence of the characteristics of childhood into adult life, marked by underdevelopment of the reproductive organs, and often short stature.

**infarct** ('infahkt) the wedge-shaped area of necrosis in an organ produced by the blocking of a blood vessel, usually due to an embolus. *Red i.* a haemorrhage infarct. Red blood cells infiltrate the area. *White i.* an anaemic infarct. The area is suddenly deprived of blood and is pale.

**infarction** (in'fahkshən) the formation of an infarct. *Myocardial i.* an infarct of the heart muscle following a coronary thrombosis. *Pulmonary i.* an infarct resulting from obstruction of a branch of the pulmonary artery by embolism or thrombosis.

**infection** (in'fekshən) 1. invasion and multiplication of microorganisms in body tissues, especially that causing local cellular injury due to competitive metabolism, toxins, intracellular replication or antigen–antibody response. 2. an infectious disease. *Aerobic i.* infection caused by an aerobe. *Airborne i.* infection by inhalation of organisms suspended in air on water droplets, droplet nuclei or dust particles. *Anaerobic i.* infection caused by an ANAEROBE. *Cross i.* infection transmitted between patients infected with different pathogenic microorganisms. *Droplet i.* infection due to inhalation of respiratory pathogens suspended on liquid particles exhaled by someone already infected. *Hospital-acquired i's* those acquired during hospitalization; also called nosocomial infections. A recent prevalence survey showed that 10% of patients in hospitals in England and Wales acquired an infection while in hospital. The most common causative agents are *Escherichia coli*, *Proteus*, *Pseudomonas* and *Klebsiella*, among the Gram-negative organisms, and *Staphylococcus* and *Enterococcus* among the Gram-positive organisms. *See also* INFECTION (CONTROL). *I. control* the utilization of procedures and techniques in the surveillance, investigation and compilation of statistical data in order to reduce the spread of infection, particularly hospital-acquired infections. Practitioners in infection control are frequently nurses who are employed by NHS trusts. They have titles such as Infection Control Officer and Infection Control Nurse, and

| INFECTIOUS DISEASES | | |
|---|---|---|
| Disease | Incubation period (days) | Period of infectivity |
| Chickenpox (varicella) | 10–20 | 2–3 days before until 10 days after onset of rash |
| Diphtheria | 2–7 | Until culture of three consecutive nose swabs proves negative |
| Enteric fevers Typhoid Paratyphoid | 6–21 | Until at least 1 month after onset of disease and after six consecutive negative stools |
| Measles (morbilli) | 6–12 | 4 days before until 4 days after onset of rash |
| Mumps (parotitis) | 12–28 | 2 days before onset until resolution of symptoms |
| Pertussis (whooping cough) | 7–14 | 7 days before until 3 weeks after onset of cough |
| Rubella (German measles) | 14–21 | During incubation period until 2 days after resolution of symptoms |

they function as liaison between staff, nurses, doctors, department heads, the infection control committee and the health authority. Such practitioners also assume some responsibility for teaching patients and their families, as well as employees. *Mixed i.* infection with more than one kind of organism at the same time. *Opportunistic i.* an infection with a microorganism that does not usually cause disease but may do so when the patient's resistance to infection is lowered, e.g. after surgery. *Secondary i.* infection by a pathogen superimposed upon an infection by a pathogen of another kind. *Sexually transmitted i.* an infection transmitted by sexual intercourse of by intimate contact with the genitals, mouth and rec-

tum. *See* SEXUALLY TRANSMITTED INFECTION. *Subclinical i.* infection associated with no detectable symptoms but caused by microorganisms capable of producing easily recognizable diseases, such as poliomyelitis or mumps; it is detected by the production of antibody, or by delayed hypersensitivity exhibited in a skin test reaction to such antigens as tuberculoprotein.

**infectious** (in'fekshəs) caused by or capable of being communicated by infection (*see* Table). *I. disease* disease resulting from multiplication of microorganisms in the body. Most are communicable, but not all. *See also* COMMUNICABLE DISEASE. *I. mononucleosis* glandular fever. An acute virus infection, characterized by sore throat and glandular enlargement, caused by the Epstein–Barr (EB) virus. A common infection worldwide, particularly prevalent in older children and young adults in Western countries. The source of infection is human and spread is by oropharyngeal secretions: for example, during kissing. The incubation period is 4–6 weeks and infectivity after the disease may be prolonged.

**infective** (in'fektiv) infectious, capable of producing infection; pertaining to or characterized by the presence of pathogens.

**inferior** (in'fiə.ri.ə) lower. *I. vena cava* the lower large vein.

**inferiority** (in fiə.ri'oritee) lesser rank, stature, position or ability. *I. complex see* COMPLEX

**infertility** ( infər'tilətce) inability of a woman to conceive or of a man to bring about conception.

**infestation** ( infe'stayshən) the presence of animal parasites, e.g. mites, ticks or worms, in or on the body, in clothing or in a house.

**infiltration** ( infil'trayshən) the entrance and diffusion of some substance not usually found there, either fluid or solid, into tissues or cells. *I. analgesia* the injection into tissues of a local analgesic solution.

**inflammation** ( inflə'mayshən) a localized protective response elicited by injury or destruction of tissues, which serves to destroy, dilute or wall off both the injurious agent and the injured tissue. The cardinal signs are heat, swelling, pain and redness. *Acute i.* sudden onset of inflammation, with marked and progressive symptoms. *Catarrhal i.* inflammation in which mucous surfaces are attacked, with stimulation of exudation. *Chronic i.* inflammation that develops slowly. Granulation tissue forms and tends to localize the infection. *Diffuse i.* extensive inflammation, as in nephritis and cellulitis. *Suppurative i.* one marked by pus formation. *Traumatic i.* that which follows an injury.

**influenza** ( infloo'enzə) an acute viral infection of the respiratory tract, occurring in isolated cases, epidemics and pandemics. Also called 'flu. Transmission is by droplet inhalation and the period of infectivity lasts from 1 day before the onset of symptoms until up to 7 days later. In the UK, most cases occur between December and May, with the peak incidence being in February. There is fever, headache, pain in the back and limbs, anorexia and sometimes nausea and vomiting. The fever subsides in 2–3 days, leaving a feeling of lassitude There is no specific drug cure for influenza, but an influenza vaccine is available, the formulation of which is changed annually to include recently circulating strains of viruses on recommendation of the WHO. Annual vaccination is advised for persons with chronic heart, lung or renal disease, those with diabetes, and patients on immunosuppressive therapy. It should also be advised for the elderly and residents of residential and nursing homes.

**informed consent** (in'fawmd) *see* CONSENT.

**infrared** ( infrə'red) rays of a lower wavelength than those in the visible spectrum. They can produce radiant heat which is used in the treatment of rheumatic conditions. *See* ULTRAVIOLET RAYS.

**infusion** (in'fyoozhən) 1. the process of extracting the soluble principles of substances (especially drugs) by soaking in water. 2. the solution thus produced. 3. the slow therapeutic introduction by gravity of fluid other than blood into a vein.

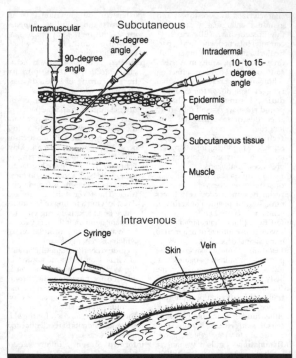

**INTRAMUSCULAR, SUBCUTANEOUS, INTRADERMAL AND INTRAVENOUS INJECTIONS**

**ingestion** (in'jeschən) the taking in of food and drugs by mouth.

**inguinal** ('ing.gwin'l) relating to the groin. *I. canal* the channel through the abdominal wall, above Poupart's ligament, through which the spermatic cord and vessels pass to the testis in the male, and which contains the round ligament of the uterus in the female. *I. ligament* Poupart's ligament; that connecting the anterior superior spine of the ilium to the tubercle of the pubis.

**INH** isoniazid.

**inhalation** (ˌinhə'layshən) 1. the drawing of air or other substances into the lungs. 2. any drug or solution of drugs, administered (as by means of nebulizers or aerosols) by the nasal or oral respiratory route.

**inhaler** (in'haylə) an apparatus used for administering an inhalation.

**inherent** (in'hiə.rənt, -'her-) a characteristic that is innate or natural and essentially a part of a person.

**inheritance** (in'heritəns) the acquisition of qualities and characteristics from parents and ancestors.

**inhibition** (ˌinhi'bishən) arrest or restraint of a process. In psychiatry, the unconscious restraining of an instinctual drive.

**injection** (in'jekshən) 1. the forcing of a liquid into a part, as into the subcutaneous tissues, the vascular tree or an organ (see Figure). 2. a substance so forced or administered; in pharmacy, a solution of a medicament suitable for injection. 3. prominence of small blood vessels on the surface of an organ or tissue, frequently indicating the vascular phase of an inflammatory response. *Depot i.* the giving of a medication by injection, usually intramuscularly, that can be absorbed slowly over a period of time. Many drugs and hormones are given in this way. *Hypodermic i.* that made just below the skin; a subcutaneous injection. *Intramuscular i.* that made into a muscle. *Intrathecal i.* that made into the subarachnoid space of the spinal cord. *Intravenous i.* that made into a vein. *Subcutaneous i.* that made into the subcutaneous tissues; a hypodermic injection.

**inlay** ('in.lay) material inserted to replace a defect in a tissue: for example, a bone graft or a filling cast in metal to fit a hole in a tooth.

**innate** (i'nayt) inborn; present in the individual at birth.

**innervation** (ˌinə'vayshən) nerve supply to a part.

**innocent** ('inəsənt) as applied to a tumour, benign or non-malignant.

**innocuous** (i'nokyooəs) harmless.

**innominate** (i'nominət) unnamed. *I. artery* a branch of the aorta, now termed the brachiocephalic trunk. *I. bone* the hip bone, formed by the union of the ilium, ischium and pubis.

**inoculation** (iˌnokyuh'layshən) 1. introduction of pathogenic microorganisms, injected material, serum or other substances into tissues of living organisms or into culture media. 2. introduction of a disease agent (usually a live infectious agent) into a healthy individual to produce a mild form of the disease, followed by IMMUNITY.

**inorganic** (ˌinaw'ganik) of neither animal nor vegetable origin.

**inositol** (i'nohsi.tol) a form of muscle or plant carbohydrate that has the same formula as simple sugar but not its other properties. *I. nicotinate* a vasodilator used in peripheral vascular disease.

**inotropic** (ˌienə'trohpik, -tropik) affecting the force or energy of muscular contractions, particularly the heart muscle. Beta-blocking drugs are said to be inotropic.

**inquest** ('inkwest) a legal inquiry held by a coroner, with or without a jury, into the cause of sudden or unexpected death.

**insanity** (in'sanətee) a legal term for mental illness, roughly equivalent to PSYCHOSIS and implying inability to be responsible for one's acts.

**insecticide** (in'sekti.sied) one of a large group of chemical compounds that kill insect pests.

**insemination** (inˌsemi'nayshən) 1. fertilization of an ovum by a spermatozoon. 2. introduction of semen into the vagina. *Artificial i.* insemination by means other than sexual intercourse. The semen can be either the husband's (AIH) or some other donor's (AID).

**insensible** (in'sensəb'l) 1. unable to perceive with the senses. 2.

unconscious. 3. imperceptible to the senses.

**insertion** (in'sərshən, -'zər-) 1. the act of implanting. 2. something that is implanted. 3. the attachment of a muscle to the bone that it moves.

**insidious** (in'sidi.əs) approaching by stealth. A term applied to any disease that develops imperceptibly.

**insight** ('in,siet) mental awareness. The capacity of individuals to estimate a situation or their own behaviour or the connection between their present attitudes and past experiences. In psychiatry, a recognition by patients that they are ill. Insight in this connection may be complete, partial or absent, and may alter during the course of the illness.

**insoluble** (in'solyuhb'l) not capable of being dissolved in a liquid.

**insomnia** (in'somni.ə) inability to sleep.

**inspiration** (inspi'rayshən) the act of drawing in the breath.

**inspissated** (in'spisaytid) thickened, through evaporation or absorption of fluid.

**instillation** (,insti'layshən) the act of pouring a liquid into a cavity drop by drop, e.g. into the eye.

**instinct** ('instingkt) a complex of unlearned responses characteristic of a species. *Death i.* in psychoanalysis, the latent instinctive impulse towards death; the drive to reduce tensions by reaching the ultimate tensionless state of death. *Herd i.* the instinct or urge to be one of a group and to conform to its standards of conduct and opinion.

**institutionalization** (,insti,tyoo-shənəlie'zayshən) a condition of apathy and withdrawal occurring in residents of long-stay institutions, prisons, etc., as a result of rigid routines and lack of independence. The person may resist leaving because the routine has become predictable and familiar, making minimal demands.

**insufficiency** (,insə'fishənsee) inadequacy. Used to describe the failure of function of an organ, such as the heart, stomach, liver or muscles.

**insufflation** (,insu'flayshən) the act of blowing air, gas or powder into a cavity of the body.

**insulin** ('insyuhlin) a protein hormone formed in the beta cells of the pancreatic islets of Langerhans. The major fuel-regulating hormone, it is secreted into the blood in response to a rise in concentration of blood glucose or amino acids. A deficiency results in diabetes mellitus. Various types of commercially prepared insulin are available. There are three main groups: rapid-acting, intermediate-acting and long-acting. Diabetic patients react differently in the rate at which they absorb and utilize insulin; therefore the duration of action varies from patient to patient. Insulin is measured in units. The concentration used is 100 units/ml. This strength allows for accurate measurement of dosage and reduces the possibility of error in calculating an individual dose. *I. pump* a device consisting of a syringe filled with a predetermined amount of short-acting insulin, a plastic cannula and a needle, and a pump that periodically delivers the desired amount of insulin.

**insulin sensitivity test** (sensi'tivi-tee) a test used to determine the body's response to hypoglycaemia induced by a small intravenous dose of insulin. It is used to test anterior pituitary function, particularly the ability to secrete growth hormone.

**insulinase** ('insyuhli,nayz) an enzyme that destroys the action of insulin.

**insulinoma** (,insyuhli'nohmə) a benign adenoma of the islet cells of the pancreas, causing hypoglycaemia.

**insult** ('insult) any trauma, irritation, poisoning or injury to the body.

**integument** (in'tegyuhmənt) 1. the skin. 2. a layer of tissue covering a part or organ of the body.

**intellect** ('intə,lekt) the mind, thinking faculty, or understanding.

**intelligence** (in'telijəns) 1. the capacity to understand. 2. general mental ability. *I. quotient* abbreviated IQ. The ratio of the mental age to the chronological age expressed as a percentage. *I. test* a test designed to measure the level of intelligence, usually expressed as an IQ.

**intensive care unit** (in'tensiv) abbreviated ICU. A hospital unit in which are concentrated special equipment and specially trained personnel for the care of seriously ill patients requiring immediate and continuous monitoring and treatment. Also called critical care unit (CCU), intensive therapy unit (ITU). *Neonatal ICU (NICU)* an intensive care unit that is designated solely for small, preterm neonates and those neonates requiring surgery or other specialized care.

**intention** (in'tenshən) a process of healing.

**intercellular** (,intə'selyuhlə) between the cells of a structure. May be applied to the connective tissue or to fluid bathing the cells.

**intercostal** (,intə'kost'l) between the ribs. *I. muscles* muscles situated between the ribs and controlling their movements during inspiration and expiration.

**intercourse** ('intə,kaws) 1. social exchange. 2. coitus.

**intercurrent** (,intə'kurənt) occurring at the same time. Describes a disease occurring during the course of another disease in the same person.

**interdisciplinary** (,intə'disipli,nəree) joint working between professional disciplines: nursing, social work, clergy, medical staff, physiotherapy and other professions allied to medicine (PAMs) or health-care professions (HCPs).

**interferon** (,intə'fiə,ron) a protein, produced by cells infected by a virus, which has an inhibitory effect on the multiplication of the invading viruses.

**interlobular** (,intə'lobyuhlə) between lobules. *I. veins* branches of the portal vein in the liver.

**intermenstrual** (,intə'menstrooəl) occurring between two menstrual periods.

**intermission** (,intə'mishən) a temporary interruption, particularly of a feverish condition.

**intermittent** (,intə'mitənt) occurring at intervals. *I. claudication see* CLAUDICATION. *I. fever* one in which the temperature drops to normal or lower, at times. *I. mandatory ventilation* abbreviated IMV. A type of mechanical ventilation in which the VENTILATOR is set to deliver a prescribed tidal volume at specified intervals, and a high-flow gas system permits the patient to breathe spontaneously between cycles. *I. positive airway ventilation* abbreviated IPAV; also known as intermittent positive pressure ventilation, abbreviated IPPV. A method of assisted ventilation in which oxygen or air is used under pressure to inflate the lungs when the patient is unable to breathe spontaneously.

**internal** (in'tərn'l) situated on the inside. *I. haemorrhage* one occurring in a cavity or into the tissues. *I. secretion* one in which the hormones pass directly into the bloodstream from the secreting gland.

**International Council of Nurses** (intə'nashn'l kownsəl) abbreviated ICN. Founded in 1899 to represent worldwide international nurses' associations as a corporate organization.

**interphase** ('intə͵fayz) the period between two cell divisions during which the chromosomes are not easily visible.

**intersex** ('intə͵seks) 1. a congenital abnormality in which anatomical features of both sexes are evident. 2. a person displaying intersexuality.

**intersexuality** (͵intə͵seksyoo'alitee) an intermingling of the characters of each sex, including physical form, reproductive tissue and sexual behaviour, in one individual, as a result of some flaw in embryonic development.

**interstitial** (͵intə'stishəl) situated within the tissue spaces or between the tissues. *I. cell stimulating hormone* abbreviated ICSH. Luteinizing hormone. *I. fluid* the fluid in which body cells are bathed. It acts as an intermediary between the cells and the blood. Extracellular fluid. *I. keratitis see* KERATITIS. *I. nephritis* chronic nephritis associated with fibrosis and hypertension.

**intertrigo** (͵intə'triegoh) an irritating, eczematous skin eruption caused by the chafing of two moist skin surfaces.

**intervention** (͵intə'venshən) in health care any act carried out to prevent harm to patients or to improve, promote or enhance their physical, mental or spiritual wellbeing.

**intervertebral** (͵intə'vərtibrəl) between the vertebrae. *I. disc* the pad of fibrocartilage between the bodies of the vertebrae. Protrusion of the contents of the disc may give rise to sciatica by exerting pressure on the nerve roots.

**intestinal** (͵inte'stienəl, in'testin'l) referring to the intestine.

**intestine** (in'testin) that part of the alimentary canal that extends from the stomach to the anus. *Small i.* the first 6 m from the pylorus to the caecum, consisting of the duodenum, the jejunum and the ileum. *Large i.* the final 2 m, consisting of the caecum, the ascending, transverse and descending colon, and the rectum.

**intima** ('intimə) the innermost coat of an artery or vein.

**intolerance** (in'tolə͵rəns) lack of power to endure. Applied to the effect of some drugs on individuals, e.g. iodine and quinine. *See* IDIOSYNCRASY.

**intoxication** (in͵toksi'kayshən) 1. poisoning by drugs or harmful substances. 2. the condition produced by excessive use of alcohol.

**intra-abdominal** (͵intrə.əb'domin'l) within the abdomen.

**intra-articular** (͵intrə.ah'tikyuhlə) within a joint capsule. *I-a. injection* injection into a joint capsule, applicable to hydrocortisone, for example.

**intra-atrial** (͵intrə'aytri.əl) within the atrium. *I-a. thrombosis* a blood clot formed in the atrium of the heart.

**intracapsular** (͵intrə'kapsyuhlə) within a capsule, usually of a joint. *I. extraction* the removal of the whole lens with its capsule in the treatment of cataract.

**intracellular** (͵intrə'selyuhlə) within a cell. *I. fluid* the water and its dissolved salts found within the cells.

**intracerebral** (͵intrə'seribrəl) within the brain substance. *I. haemorrhage* an escape of blood in the cerebrum, most often arising from the middle cerebral artery or from an aneurysm.

**intracranial** (͵intrə'krayni.əl) within the skull. *I. abscess* one arising within the brain or meninges. *I. aneurysm* dilatation of one of the cerebral vessels. It may be congenital or acquired. *I. pressure* abbreviated ICP. The pressure exerted by the cerebrospinal fluid within the subarachnoid space and ventricles of the brain.

**intractable** (in'traktəb'l) not able to be relieved, controlled or cured.

**intradermal** (ˌintrə'dərməl) between the layers of the skin.

**intradural** (ˌintrə'dyooə.rəl) within the dura mater. *I. haemorrhage see* HAEMORRHAGE.

**intragastric** (ˌintrə'gastrik) within the stomach.

**intrahepatic** (ˌintrəhi'patik) within the liver. Referring to a condition of the liver cells or connective tissue.

**Intralipid** (ˌintrə'lipid) trade name for an intravenous fat emulsion used to prevent or correct deficiency of essential fatty acids and to provide calories in high density form during total parenteral nutrition.

**intralobular** (ˌintrə'lobyuhlə) within a lobule. *I. veins* veins which collect blood from within the lobules of the liver.

**intramedullary** (ˌintrəmə'dulə.ree) 1. within the medulla oblongata. 2. within the bone marrow. *I. nail* a metal pin used for the internal fixation of fractures.

**intramuscular** (ˌintrə'muskyuhlə) within muscle tissue.

**intranasal** (ˌintrə'nayz'l) within the nose.

**intraocular** (ˌintrə'okyuhlə) within the eyeball.

**intraorbital** (ˌintrə'awbit'l) within the orbit of the eye.

**intraosseous** (ˌintrə'osi.əs) within a bone. *I. infusion* the process of supplying fluid into the narrow cavity of a bone in a life-threatening situation.

**intraperitoneal** (ˌintrəˌperitə'neeəl) within the peritoneal cavity.

**intrathecal** (ˌintrə'theek'l) within the meninges of the spinal cord, usually in the subarachnoid space.

**intratracheal** (ˌintrə'traki.əl, -trə-'keeəl) endotracheal; within the trachea. *I. anaesthesia* inhalation anaesthesia. *See* ANAESTHESIA.

**intrauterine** (ˌintrə'yootə.rien) within the uterus. *I. contraceptive device* abbreviated IUCD. A contraceptive device introduced into the uterine cavity. *I. douche* irrigation of the uterine cavity. A special grooved nozzle is used, so that the fluid can return and is not forced into the uterine tubes. *I. growth retardation* associated with a poor blood supply to the placenta, or maternal disease. Other factors include infection during pregnancy, maternal smoking or drug addiction. The infant at birth is 'small for dates' and falls below the tenth percentile of appropriate gestational age for infants. *I. life* fetal development in the uterus.

**intravenous** (ˌintrə'veenəs) within a vein. *I. flow rate* the rate at which fluids, medications and blood products flow into the bloodstream during intravenous infusion. The flow rate is usually ordered by the doctor as total volume (ml) per total hours or, in the case of drugs, total dose per total hours. *I. infusion* the therapeutic introduction of a fluid, such as saline, into a vein. The infusion works by gravity, in that the container of fluid is higher than the blood vessel into which the fluid is being introduced. *I. urography* radiographic examination of the urinary tract after the injection of a radio-opaque contrast medium into a vein.

**intraventricular** (ˌintrəven'trikyuhlə) within a ventricle; may apply to a cerebral or a cardiac ventricle.

**intrinsic** (in'trinsik, -zik) particular to or contained within an organ. *I. factor* a glycoprotein, contained in the gastric juices, which is necessary for the absorption of extrinsic factor (vitamin $B_{12}$).

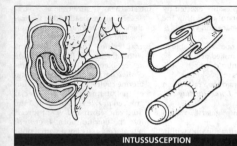

**INTUSSUSCEPTION**

**introitus** (in'troh.itəs) [L.] an opening or entrance into a hollow organ or cavity. *I. vaginae* the vulva.

**introjection** (ˌintrəˈjekshən) a mental process by which individuals take into themselves the personal characteristics of another person, usually those of someone much loved or admired.

**introspection** (ˌintrəˈspekshən) a subjective study of the mind and its processes, in which individuals study their own reactions.

**introversion** (ˌintrəˈvərshən) 1. a turning inwards within itself of a hollow organ. 2. preoccupation with oneself, with reduction of interest in the outside world.

**introvert** ('intrəˌvərt) a person whose interests are turned inwards upon the self. *See* EXTROVERT.

**intubation** (ˌintyuhˈbayshən) the introduction of a tube into a part of the body, particularly into the air passages to allow air to enter the lungs.

**intumescence** (ˌintyuhˈmesəns) a swelling or increase in bulk, as of nasal mucous membrane in catarrh.

**intussusception** (ˌintəsəˈsepshən) prolapse of one part of the intestine into the lumen of an immediately adjacent part (*see* Figure), causing OBSTRUCTION (INTESTINAL).

**inunction** (inˈungkshən) 1. rubbing an oily or fatty preparation containing a medicinal ingredient into the skin, with absorption of the drug. 2. any preparation so applied.

**invagination** (inˌvajiˈnayshən) 1. the folding inwards of a part, thus forming a pouch. 2. intussusception.

**invasion** (inˈvayzhən) 1. the entry of bacteria into the body. 2. the entrance of parasites into the body of a host.

**invasive** (inˈvaysiv, -ziv) 1. having the quality of invasiveness. 2. involving puncture or incision of the skin or insertion of an instrument or foreign material into the body; said of diagnostic techniques.

**invasiveness** (inˈvaysivnəs) 1. the ability of microorganisms to enter the body and spread in the tissues. 2. the ability to infiltrate and actively destroy surrounding tissue, a property of malignant tumours.

**inversion** (inˈvərshən) a turning upside down or inside out. *Sexual i.* homosexuality. *Uterine i.* the condition of the uterus after parturition when a part of its upper segment protrudes through the cervix.

**invertebrate** (inˈvərtiˌbrət, -brayt) 1. without a spinal column. 2. an animal without a spinal column.

**involucrum** (ˌinvəˈlookrəm) new bone which forms a sheath around necrosed bone, as in chronic osteomyelitis.

**involuntary** (inˈvoləntə.ree) independent of the will. *See* VOLUNTARY. *I. muscle* one that acts without conscious control: for instance, the heart and stomach muscles.

**involution** (ˌinvəˈlooshən) 1. turning inwards; describes the contraction of the uterus after labour. The process whereby the uterus returns to its normal size. 2. the progressive degeneration occurring naturally with advancing age, resulting in shrivelling of organs or tissues.

**iodine** (ˈieəˌdeen) *symbol* I. A nonmetallic element with a distinctive odour, obtained from seaweed. Iodine is essential in nutrition, being especially prevalent in the colloid of the THYROID (GLAND). It is used in the treatment of HYPOTHYROIDISM and as a topical antiseptic. It is a frequent cause of poisoning. Iodine is opaque to X-rays and can be combined with other compounds for use as contrast media in diagnostic radiology.

**iodopsin** (ˌieəˈdopsin) a violet pigment found in the retinal cones of the eyes.

**Iodosorb** (ieˈohdohzawb) trade name for a preparation of cadexomer iodide used to cleanse venous leg ulcers and pressure sores.

**iodoxyl** (ˌieəˈdoksil) a radio-opaque contrast medium. *See* INTRAVENOUS (UROGRAPHY).

**ion** (ˈieən) an atom or group of atoms having a positive (cation) or negative (anion) electric charge by virtue of having gained or lost one or more electrons. Substances forming ions are electrolytes (*see* ELECTROLYTE). *See* HYDROGEN.

**ionization** (ˌieənieˈzayshən) the breaking up of molecules into electrically charged particles or ions when an electric current is passed through an electrolytic solution.

**iontophoresis** (ieˌontohfəˈreesis) the introduction through the skin of therapeutic ions by ionization.

**IPAV** intermittent positive airway ventilation.

**ipecacuanha** (ˌipiˌkakyooˈahnə) the dried root of a Brazilian shrub, given in small doses as an expectorant and, in larger doses, as an emetic.

**IPPV** intermittent positive pressure ventilation.

**ipsilateral** (ˌipsiˈlatərəl) occurring on the same side. Applied particularly to paralysis or other symptoms occurring on the same side as the cerebral lesion causing them.

**IQ** intelligence quotient. *See* INTELLIGENCE.

**IRDS** infant respiratory distress syndrome. *See* RESPIRATORY.

**iridectomy** (ˌiriˈdektəmee) excision of a part of the iris, usually for the treatment of glaucoma.

**iridencleisis** (ˌiridenˈkliesis) an operation to make a drain out of a part of the iris, used in the treatment of glaucoma.

**iridium** (iˈridi.əm) *symbol* Ir. A radioactive metal, often used in the form of wires or hairpins to treat superficial malignancies, e.g. those of the tongue, cheek or breast.

**iridocele** (iˈridoh.seel) herniation of a part of the iris through a corneal wound.

**iridocyclitis** (ˌiridohsieˈklietis) inflammation of the iris and ciliary body.

**iridodonesis** (ˌiridohdəˈneesis) trembling of the iris due to lack of support from the lens in dislocation of the lens or after a cataract extraction.

**iridoptosis** (ˌiridopˈtohsis) prolapse of the iris.

**iridotomy** (ˌiriˈdotəmee) the making of a hole in the iris to form an artificial pupil.

**iris** ('ieris) the coloured part of the eye, made of two layers of muscle, the contraction of which alters the size of the pupil and so controls the amount of light entering the eye. *I. bombé* a bulging forwards of the iris due to pressure of the aqueous humour when its passage into the anterior chamber is obstructed.

**iritis** (ie'rietis) inflammation of the iris, causing pain, photophobia, contraction of the pupil and discoloration of the iris. *See* UVEITIS.

**iron** ('ieən) *symbol* Fe. A metallic element, present in the body in small quantities and essential to life. A deficiency may produce anaemia.

**irradiation** (i͟raydi'ayshən) the treatment of disease by electromagnetic radiation.

**irreducible** (͟iri'dyoosəb'l) incapable of being replaced in a normal position. Applied to a fracture or a hernia.

**irrigation** (͟iri'gayshən) the washing out of a cavity or wound with a stream of lotion or water.

**irritable** ('iritəb'l) reacting excessively to a stimulus. *I. bowel syndrome* mucous colitis; spastic colon. The patient complains of disordered bowel function with abdominal pain, but no organic disease can be found.

**irritant** ('iritənt) an agent causing stimulation or excitation.

**irritation** (͟iri'tayshən) 1. a condition of undue nervous excitement resulting from abnormal sensitiveness. 2. itching of the skin. *Cerebral i.* a stage of excitement present in many brain conditions and typical of the recovery stage of concussion.

**ischaemia** (is'keemi.ə) a deficiency in the blood supply to a part of the body. *Myocardial i.* ischaemia of the heart muscles, which causes angina pectoris.

**ischiorectal** (͟iskioh'rekt'l) concerning the ischium and the rectum *I. abscess* a collection of pus in the ischiorectal connective tissue. An anal fistula may result.

**ischium** ('iski.əm) the lower posterior bone of the pelvic girdle.

**Ishihara colour charts** (͟ishi'hahrə) *S. Ishihara, Japanese ophthalmologist, 1879–1963.* Patterns of dots of the primary colours on similar backgrounds which make numbers or patterns. The numbers or patterns can be seen by a normal-sighted person, but one who is colour blind will only be able to identify some of them, depending on the type of colour blindness.

**islet of Langerhans** (͟ielet əv 'langəhanz) *P. Langerhans, German pathologist, 1847–1888.* One of a group of cells in the pancreas that produce insulin and glucagon; islet of the pancreas.

**isocarboxazid** (͟iesohkah'boksə͟zid) a monoamine oxidase inhibitor used in the treatment of depressive illness.

**Isogel** ('iesoh͟jel) proprietary, bulk-forming laxative prepared from the husks of mucilaginous seeds. Used in chronic constipation.

**isograft** ('iesoh͟grahft) a tissue graft from one identical twin to another.

**isoimmunization** (͟iesoh͟imyuhnie-'zayshən) the development of antibodies against an antigen derived from an individual of the same species, e.g. a rhesus-negative woman may immunize herself against her fetus, if it is rhesus-positive, by forming specific ANTIBODY.

**isolation** (͟iesə'layshən) the separation of a person with an infectious disease from those non-infected. *I. period* quarantine; the length of time during which a patient with an infectious fever is considered capable of infecting others by contact.

**isoleucine** (͟iesoh'looseen) one of the ten essential amino acids that are vital for health in the adult.

**isometric** (͟iesoh'metrik) having equal dimensions. *I. exercises* the contraction and relaxation of muscles without producing movement; used to maintain muscle tone after a fracture.

**isoniazid** (ˌiesoh'nieəzid) INH. A drug, given orally in combination with streptomycin or para-amino-salicylic acid (PAS), which is effective in treating tuberculosis. Combined therapy reduces the risk of bacterial resistance.

**isoprenaline** (ˌiesoh'prenəlin) a sympathomimetic drug which has an action like adrenaline and can be used to treat asthma.

**isosorbide dinitrate** (ˌiesoh sorbied die'nietrayt) a short-acting vasodilator similar in action to glyceryl trinitrate and used in the treatment of angina pectoris.

**isotonic** (ˌiesoh'tonik) having uniform tension. *I. solution* a solution of the same osmotic pressure as the fluid with which it is compared. Normal saline (0.9% solution of salt in water) is isotonic with blood plasma.

**isotope** ('iesoh tohp) one of the several forms of an element with the same atomic number but different atomic weights. *Radioactive i.* an unstable isotope which decays and emits alpha, beta or gamma rays. May be used in the diagnosis and treatment of malignant disease.

**isthmus** ('isməs) a narrow connection between two larger bodies or parts, e.g. the band of tissue between the two lobes of the thyroid gland.

**itch** (ich) a skin eruption with irritation. *Baker's i.* eczema of the hands due to the proteins of flour. *Barber's i.* sycosis; tinea barbae. *Dhobi i.* TINEA (CRURIS). The name is derived from the belief in India that the spread of infection was due to washermen (dhobis) wearing their clients' clothes. *I. mite* the cause of scabies, *Sarcoptes scabiei*. *Washerwomen's i.* dermatitis of the hands due to the constant use of detergents.

**ITP** idiopathic thrombocytopenic purpura.

**ITU** intensive therapy unit.

**IUCD** intrauterine contraceptive device.

**IVF** in vitro fertilization. *See* FERTILIZATION.

**IVP** intravenous pyelography (*see* UROGRAPHY).

**IVU** intravenous urography (*see* UROGRAPHY).

# J

**J** symbol for *joule*.

**Jacksonian epilepsy** (jak'sohni.ən) *J. H. Jackson, British neurologist, 1835–1911.* Focal motor EPILEPSY.

**Jacquemier's sign** ('zhahkhmi.ayz) *J.M. Jacquemier, French obstetrician, 1806–1879.* Blueness of the lining of the vagina seen from the early weeks of pregnancy.

**jactitation** (ˌjakti'tayshən) the extreme restlessness of an acutely ill patient.

**jargon** ('jahgən) 1. the terminology used and generally understood only by those who have knowledge of that speciality, e.g. medical jargon, legal jargon. 2. gibberish talked by the insane.

**jaundice** ('jawndis) icterus; a yellow discoloration of the skin and conjunctivae, due to the presence of bile pigment in the blood. It may be one of the following types: (a) *Haemolytic j.* due to excessive destruction of red blood cells, causing increase of bilirubin in the blood. The liver is not involved. *Acholuric j.* is of this type. It is characterized by increased fragility of the red blood cells. (b) *Hepatocellular j.* the liver cells are damaged by either infection or drugs. (c) *Obstructive j.* the bile is prevented from reaching the duodenum owing to obstruction by a gallstone, a growth or a stricture of the common bile duct. (d) *Physiological j.* (icterus neonato-

rum) occurs within the first few days of life, and is caused by the breakdown of the excessive number of red blood cells present in the newborn.

**jaw** (jor) a bone of the face in which the teeth are embedded. *Lower j.* the mandible. *Upper j.* the two maxillae.

**jejunectomy** (ˌjejuh'nektəmee) excision of a part or the whole of the jejunum.

**jejunoileostomy** (ji.joónoh.ili'ostə-mee) the making of an anastomosis between the jejunum and the ileum.

**jejunostomy** (ˌjejuh'nostəmee) the making of an opening into the jejunum through the abdominal wall.

**jejunotomy** (ˌjejuh'notəmee) an incision into the jejunum.

**jejunum** (ji'joonəm) the portion of the small intestine from the duodenum to the ileum; about 2.4 m in length.

**jelly** ('jelee) a soft, coherent, resilient substance; generally, a colloidal semisolid mass. *Contraceptive j.* a non-greasy jelly used in the vagina for prevention of conception (*see also* CONTRACEPTION). *Petroleum j.* a purified mixture of semisolid hydrocarbons obtained from petroleum (also called petrolatum). *Wharton's j.* the soft, jelly-like intracellular substance of the umbilical cord, which insulates the vein and arteries, preventing occlusion and fetal hypoxia.

**jerk** (jərk) a sudden muscular contraction. *Knee j.* a kicking movement produced by tapping the tendon below the patella. Used with other jerks, such as the ankle jerk, to test the nervous reflexes.

**jet lag** ('jet ,lag) the lack of balance that occurs between local time and the person's biological rhythms that results from air travel over a long distance, especially in an easterly direction and to a lesser extent westwards. Sleep, memory and concentration are disturbed and there is a persistent feeling of tiredness usually lasting 2–3 days as the body adjusts to the time change.

**jigger** ('jigə) a sand flea, found in the tropics, which burrows into the soles of the feet and causes severe irritation.

**joint** (joynt) an articulation; the point of junction of two or more bones, particularly one which permits movement of the individual bones relative to each other.

**joule** (jool) *symbol* J. The SI unit of energy.

**judgement** ('jujmənt) the ability of an individual to estimate a situation, to arrive at reasonable conclusions and to decide on a course of action.

**jugular** ('jugyuhlə) relating to the neck. *J. veins* several veins in the neck which drain the blood from the head.

**Jung** (yuhng) *Carl Gustav, Swiss psychologist and psychiatrist, 1875– 1961.*

**junk food** ('junk) convenience or fastfood high in monosodium glutamate.

**jurisprudence** (,jooris'proodəns) the science of law. Medical jurisprudence is another name for forensic medicine.

**juvenile** ('joovə,niel) relating to young people.

**juxta-articular** (,jukstə.ah'tikyuhlə) near a joint.

**juxtaglomerular** (,jukstəglo'meryuhlə) near to a glomerulus of the kidney. *J. cells* specialized cells found in the kidney which appear to play an important part in the control of aldosterone release.

**juxtaposition** (,jukstəpə'zishən) an adjacent, or side by side position.

# K

**K** symbol for *potassium*.

**Kahn test** (kahn) *B.L. Kahn, American bacteriologist, 1887–1979.* An agglutination test for syphilis.

**kala-azar** (ˌkahləˌəˈzah) visceral leishmaniasis. A tropical disease caused by the protozoan parasite *Leishmania donovani* which is carried by the sandfly. Symptoms include enlargement of the liver and spleen, anaemia and wasting. The disease is often fatal.

**kanamycin** (ˌkanaˈmiesin) a broad-spectrum antibiotic for use against severe infections with Gram-negative organisms where penicillin is ineffective.

**kaolin** (ˈkayəlin) powdered clay containing aluminium silicate. It is taken orally in the treatment of diarrhoea and is also used as a dusting powder and for poultices.

**Kaposi's sarcoma** (ˈkapohˌzeez) *M.K. Kaposi, Austrian dermatologist, 1837–1902.* A multifocal, metastasizing, malignant reticulosis with angiosarcoma-like features, involving chiefly the skin. Rarely seen in the developed world until the outbreak of AIDS. Kaposi's sarcoma is a major feature of this disease.

**Kaposi's spots** (spotz) a serious complication of infantile eczema occurring on exposure to herpes simplex virus infection. More commonly known as Kaposi's varicelliform eruption.

**karaya** (kəˈrieˌə) a gum made from certain species of *Sterculia*, a genus of tropical trees and shrubs. Used as an aid to applying ostomy bags to the skin.

**karyotype** (ˈkariohˌtiep) 1. the chromosomal constitution and arrangement of a cell of an individual. 2. the pattern that is seen when human chromosomes are photographed during metaphase. The pictures are then enlarged and paired according to the length of their short arm.

**kcal** kilocalorie.

**Kegel exercises** (ˈkaygəl) specific exercises named after Dr Arnold H. Kegel, a gynaecologist who first developed them to strengthen the pelvic–vaginal muscles as a means of controlling stress incontinence in women.

**Keller's operation** (ˈkeləz) *W.L. Keller, American surgeon, 1874–1959.* An operation for correcting hallux valgus.

**keloid** (ˈkeeloyd) hard, raised scar tissue in the skin, common in people with dark skins. A type occurs in a healed wound due to overgrowth of fibrous tissue, causing the scar to be raised above the skin level.

**Kennedy's syndrome** (ˈkenədiz) *F. Kennedy, American neurologist, 1884–1952.* Ipsilateral optic atrophy caused by a frontal lobe tumour which involves one of the optic nerves.

**keratectasia** (ˌkerətek'tayzi.ə) protrusion of the cornea following inflammation.

**keratectomy** (ˌkerə'tektəmee) excision of a portion of the cornea.

**keratic** (kə'ratik) 1. horny. 2. relating to the cornea. *K. precipitates* inflammatory exudates adhering to the back of the cornea; a sign of iritis and cyclitis.

**keratin** ('kerətin) an albuminoid substance which forms the principal constituent of all horny tissues.

**keratinize** (kə'ratiˌniez) to make or become horny.

**keratitis** (ˌkerə'tietis) inflammation of the cornea. The causes may be physical (trauma, exposure to dust, vapours or ultraviolet light) or due to infectious conditions such as corneal and dendritic ulcers. *Interstitial k.* deep chronic keratitis, usually arising in congenital syphilis. *Striate k.* inflammation that appears in lines due to the folding over of the cornea after injury or operation, particularly one for cataract.

**keratocele** ('kerətohˌseel) descemetocele; protrusion of Descemet's membrane through the base of a corneal ulcer. A horny growth of the skin.

**keratoconjunctivitis** (ˌkerətohkən'jungkti'vietis) inflammation of both the cornea and the conjunctiva of the eye.

**keratoiritis** (ˌkerətoh.ie'rietis) inflammation of both the cornea and iris.

**keratoma** (ˌkerə'tohmə) keratosis.

**keratomalacia** (ˌkerətohmə'layshi.ə) ulceration and softening of the cornea due to a deficiency of vitamin A.

**keratometer** (kerə'tomitə) ophthalmometer. An instrument by which the amount of corneal astigmatism can be measured accurately.

**keratophakia** (ˌkerətoh'fayki.ə) keratoplasty in which a slice of donor's cornea is shaped to a desired curvature and inserted between layers of the recipient's cornea to change its curvature.

**keratoplasty** ('kerətohˌplastee) a plastic operation on the cornea, including corneal grafting.

**keratoscope** ('kerətohˌskohp) an instrument for examining the eye to detect keratoconus. Placido's disc.

**keratosis** (ˌkerə'tohsis) a skin disease marked by excessive growth of the epidermis or horny tissue.

**keratotomy** (ˌkerə'totəmee) incision of the cornea.

**kerion** ('keeri.ən) a complication of ringworm of the scalp, with formation of pustules.

**kernicterus** (kər'niktə.rəs) a condition in the newborn marked by severe neural symptoms, associated with high levels of bilirubin in the blood; it is commonly a sequela of icterus gravis neonatorum.

**Kernig's sign** ('kərnigz) *V.M. Kernig, Russian physician, 1840–1917.* A sign of meningitis. When the thigh is supported at right angles to the trunk, the patient is unable to straighten the leg at the knee joint.

**ketamine** ('ketəˌmeen) a rapidly acting, non-barbiturate general anaesthetic which is given by intramuscular or intravenous injection.

**ketogenic** (ˌkeetoh'jenik) forming or capable of being converted into ketone bodies.

**ketone** ('keetohn) an organic compound containing the carbonyl group (CO) attached to two hydrocarbon groups. Ketones are produced by the metabolization of fats.

**ketonuria** (ˌkeetoh'nyooə.ri.ə) the presence of ketones in urine; acetonuria.

**ketoprofen** (ˌkeetoh'profen) a nonsteroidal anti-inflammatory drug used in the treatment of mild rheumatic and arthritic conditions.

**ketosis** (kee'tohsis) the condition in which ketones are formed in excess in the body and accumulate in the blood. Severe acidosis may occur.

**ketosteroid** (ˌkeetoh'stiə.royd) a steroid hormone which contains a ketone group attached to a carbon atom. *17-k's* are excreted in the urine and formed from the adrenal corticosteroids, testosterone and, to a lesser extent, oestrogens.

**kick chart** ('kik) a method of fetal assessment carried out by the mother. The number of kicks or movements felt during the day is counted and noted. If fewer than 10 kicks are felt in a 12 h daytime period on two consecutive occasions, the mother is advised to contact her midwife or doctor immediately. If no movements are felt in any day, the mother is advised to contact the hospital at once. The value of this test is that it can highlight a potential case of fetal distress and alert medical attention before it is too late.

**kidney** ('kidnee) one of two organs situated in the lumbar region, which purify the blood and secrete urine. The kidney secretes renin and renal erythropoietic factor. *Artificial k.* the apparatus used to remove retained waste products from the blood when kidney function is impaired. *Granular k.* the small fibrosed kidney of chronic nephritis. *Horseshoe k.* a congenital defect producing a fusion of the two kidneys into a horseshoe shape (*see* Figure). *K. failure* the condition in which renal function is severely impaired and the organs are unable to maintain the fluid and electrolyte balance of the body. *K. transplant* the surgical implantation of a kidney taken from a live donor or from one who has recently died. Used in the treatment of renal failure. *Polycystic k.* a congenital bilateral condition of

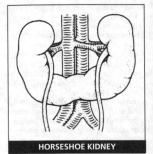

**HORSESHOE KIDNEY**

multiple cysts replacing kidney tissue.

**kilocalorie** ('kiləˌkaləree) *symbol* kcal. One thousand calories, a unit of food energy.

**kilojoule** ('kiləˌjool) *symbol* kJ. One thousand joules, a unit of food energy (1 kcal = 4.184 kJ).

**Kimmelstiel–Wilson syndrome** (ˌkiməlsteel'wilsən) *P. Kimmelstiel, German pathologist, 1900–1970; C. Wilson, British physician, b. 1906.* A degenerative complication of DIABETES (MELLITUS), with albuminuria, oedema, hypertension, renal insufficiency and retinopathy. Called also intercapillary glomerulosclerosis.

**kinaesthesia** (ˌkinis'theezi.ə) the combined sensations by which position, weight and muscular position are perceived.

**kinanaesthesia** (ˌkinanəs'theezi.ə) an inability to perceive the sensation of movements of parts of the body.

**kinase** ('kienayz) an enzyme activator; *see* ENTEROKINASE and THROMBOKINASE.

**kineplasty** ('kiniˌplastee) plastic amputation; amputation in which the stump is so formed as to be utilized for producing motion of the prosthesis.

**kinetic** (ki'netik) producing or pertaining to motion.

**king's evil** (ˌkingz 'eevil) a historic term for tuberculosis of the tonsillar lymph glands in the neck (scrofula) thought to be cured by the touch of the king.

**King's Fund** (fund) King Edward's Hospital Fund for London was founded in 1897 for the support, by the giving of grants, of voluntary hospitals in London. Since the inception of the National Health Service in 1948, it has been concerned with the funding of experimental schemes, particularly relating to the management of services. *K. F. bed* a bed fitted with jointed springs which may be adjusted to various positions, developed as the result of research undertaken on behalf of and funded by the King's Fund.

**kinin** ('kienin) a polypeptide which occurs naturally and is a powerful vasodilator.

**kinship** ('kin.ship) relationship. *K. studies* in anthropology the study of kin (relatives) and their patterns of marriage, descent, inheritance, habitation, social values and economics.

**Kirschner wire** ('kiəshnə ˌwieə) M. *Kirschner, German surgeon, 1879–1942.* A thin wire that may be passed through a bone to apply skeletal traction.

**kiss of life** (ˌkis əv 'lief) the expired air method of artificial respiration, by either mouth-to-nose or mouth-to-mouth breathing. *See* Appendices.

**kJ** kilojoule.

**Klebs–Löffler bacillus** (ˌklebz-'lərflə) *T.A.E. Klebs, German bacteriologist, 1834–1913; F.A.J. Löffler, German bacteriologist, 1852–1915. Corynebacterium diphtheriae*, the causative agent of diphtheria.

**Klebsiella** (ˌklebsi'elə) a genus of Gram-negative bacteria (family Enterobacteriaceae).

**Kleihauer test** ('kliehowə) a microscopic test to detect fetal cells in the maternal circulation, usually done immediately after delivery so that, if the mother is rhesus-negative and the fetus rhesus-positive, anti-D immunoglobulin may be given to prevent isoimmunization.

**kleptomania** (ˌkleptə'mayni.ə) an irresistible urge to steal when there is often no need and no particular desire for the objects. Often associated with depression.

**Klinefelter's syndrome** ('klienfeltəz) *H.F. Klinefelter, American physician, b. 1912.* A congenital chromosome abnormality in which each cell has three sex chromosomes, XXY, rather than the usual XX or XY, making a total of 47 (normal is 46). Affected men have female breast development and small testes and are infertile.

**Klippel–Feil syndrome** (ˌklip'l'fiel) *M. Klippel, French neurologist, 1858–1942; A. Feil, French physician, b. 1884.* A congenital abnormality in which the neck is very short as a result of the absence or fusion of several vertebrae in the cervical region.

**knee** (nee) the joint between the femur and the tibia. *K.cap* the patella. *Housemaid's k.* prepatellar bursitis. *K. jerk* an upward jerk of the leg obtained by striking the patellar tendon when the knee is passively flexed. *Knock-k.* a condition in which the knees turn inwards towards each other; genu valgum.

**kneecap** ('neekap) the patella.

**Koch's bacillus** (ˌkoks) *R. Koch, German bacteriologist, 1843–1910. Mycobacterium tuberculosis*, the causative organism of tuberculosis.

**Köhler's disease** ('kərləz) *A. Köhler, German physician and radiologist, 1874–1947.* Osteochondritis of the navicular bone of the foot, occurring in children.

**koilonychia** (ˌkoylə'niki.ə) the development of brittle, spoon-shaped nails which may occur in iron-deficiency anaemia.

**Koplik's spots** ('kopliks ˌspotz) *H. Koplik, American paediatrician, 1858–1927.* Small white spots that sometimes appear on the mucous membranes inside the mouth in measles on the second day of onset, before the general rash.

**Korotkoff's method** (ko'rotkofs ˌmethəd) *N.S. Korotkoff, Russian physician, 1874–1920.* A method of finding the systolic and diastolic blood pressure by listening to the sounds produced in an artery while the pressure in a previously inflated cuff is gradually reduced.

**Korsakoff's syndrome** or **psychosis** ('kawsəkofs) *S.S. Korsakoff, Russian neurologist, 1854–1900.* A chronic condition in which there is impaired memory, particularly for recent events, and the patient is disorientated for time and place. It may be present in psychosis of infective, toxic or metabolic origin, or in chronic alcoholism.

**kraurosis** (kror'rohsis) dryness and shrinking of a part of the body. *K. vulvae* a degenerative condition of the vulva. May be treated by giving oestrogen preparations.

**Krebs cycle** (krebz) *Sir H.A. Krebs, German–British biochemist, 1900–1981.* A series of reactions during which the aerobic oxidation of pyruvic acid takes place. This is part of carbohydrate metabolism. *K. urea c.* the way in which urea is formed in the liver.

**Küntscher nail** ('koontshə) *G. Küntscher, German orthopaedic surgeon, 1902–1972.* An intramedullary nail used in treating fractures of long bones, especially the shaft of the femur.

**Kupffer's cells** ('kuhpfəz) *K.W. von Kupffer, German anatomist, 1829–1902.* Phagocytic reticulo-endothelial cells of the liver which form bile from haemoglobin released by disintegrated erythrocytes.

**Kveim test** ('kvaym) *M.A. Kveim, Norwegian physician, b. 1892.* A test for sarcoidosis in which antigen from the lymph nodes or spleen of a sarcoidosis patient is injected intradermally.

**kwashiorkor** (ˌkwoshi'awkə) a condition of protein malnutrition occurring in children in underprivileged populations. Fatty infiltration of the liver arises and may cause cirrhosis.

**kymograph** ('kiemə ˌgrahf, - ˌgraf) an instrument for recording variations or undulations, arterial or other.

**kyphoscoliosis** (ˌkiefoh ˌskohli'ohsis) an abnormal curvature of the spine in which there is forward and sideways displacement.

**kyphosis** (kie'fohsis) posterior curvature of the spine; humpback.

# L

**l** symbol for litre.

**labetalol** (lə'beetəlol) an alpha- and beta-adrenergic receptor blocker used in the treatment of hypertension.

**labial** ('laybi.əl) pertaining to the lips or labia.

**labile** ('laybiel) unstable. Applied to those chemicals that are subject to change or readily altered by heat.

**lability** (lə'bilətc) instability. *L. of mood* the tendency to sudden changes of mood of short duration.

**labium** ('laybi.əm) a lip. *L. majus pudendi* the large fold of flesh surrounding the vulva. *L. minus pudendi* the lesser fold within the labium majus.

**labour** ('laybə) parturition or childbirth, which takes place in three stages: (a) dilatation of the cervix uteri; (b) passage of the child through the birth canal; and (c) expulsion of the placenta. *Induced l.* labour brought on by artificial means before term, as in cases of contracted pelvis, or if overdue. *Obstructed l.* labour in which there is a mechanical hindrance. *Precipitate l.* labour in which the baby is delivered extremely rapidly. *Premature l.* labour which occurs before term. *Spurious l.* ineffective labour pains which sometimes precede true labour pains.

**labyrinth** ('labə.rinth) the structures forming the internal ear, i.e. the cochlea and semicircular canals. *Bony l.* the bony canals of the internal ear. *Membranous l.* the soft structure inside the bony canals.

**labyrinthectomy** (,labə.rin'thektəmee) excision of the labyrinth.

**labyrinthitis** (,labə.rin'thietis) inflammation of the labyrinth, causing vertigo.

**laceration** (,lasə'rayshən) a wound with torn and ragged edges.

**lacrimal** ('lakriməl) relating to tears. *L. apparatus* the structures secreting the tears and draining the fluid from the conjunctival sac (see Figure). *L. gland* a gland that secretes tears, which drain through two small openings in the eyelids (*l. puncta*) into a pair of ducts (*l. canaliculi*) into the sac and finally into the nasal cavity through the nasolacrimal duct. Situated in the outer and upper corner of the orbit.

**lacrimation** (,lakri'mayshən) an excessive secretion of tears.

**lacrimator** ('lakri,maytə) a substance that causes excessive secretion of tears, e.g. tear gas.

**lactagogue** ('laktə,gog) any agent that promotes the secretion or flow of milk; galactagogue.

**lactalbumin** (lak'talbyuhmin) an albumin of milk.

**lactase** ('laktayz) an enzyme, produced in the small intestine, which converts lactose into glucose and galactose.

**lactate** ('laktayt, lak'tayt) 1. any substance given to promote lactation.

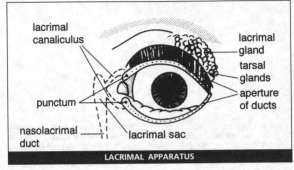

lacrimal
canaliculus

lacrimal
gland

tarsal
glands

aperture
of ducts

punctum

nasolacrimal
duct

lacrimal sac

**LACRIMAL APPARATUS**

2. any salt of lactic acid. 3. to secrete milk. **L. dehydrogenase** abbreviated LD, LDH. An enzyme that catalyses the interconversion of lactate and pyruvate. Widespread in tissues and particularly abundant in kidney, skeletal muscle, liver and myocardium. It has five isoenzymes denoted $LD_1$ to $LD_5$. The 'flipped' pattern, in which the serum $LD_1$ level, is greater than the $LD_2$ level, is indicative of an acute myocardial infarction. This pattern occurs within 12–24 h after the attack.

**lactation** (lak'tayshən) 1. the period during which the infant is nourished from the breast. 2. the process of milk secretion by the mammary glands.

**lacteal** ('lakti.əl) 1. consisting of milk. 2. a lymphatic duct in the small intestine which absorbs chyle.

**lactic** ('laktik) pertaining to milk. **L. acid** an acid formed by the fermentation of lactose or milk sugar. It is produced naturally in the body as a result of glucose metabolism. An excess of the acid accumulating in the muscles may cause cramp.

**lactiferous** (lak'tifə.rəs) conveying or secreting milk.

*Lactobacillus* (ˌlaktohbə'siləs) a genus of Gram-positive, rod-shaped bacteria, many of which produce fermentation.

**lactoferrin** (ˌlaktoh'ferin) an iron-binding protein found in neutrophils and bodily secretions (milk, tears, saliva, bile, etc.), having bactericidal activity and acting as an inhibitor of colony formation by granulocytes and macrophages.

**lactogenic** (ˌlaktə'jenik) stimulating the production of milk. *See* LUTEOTROPHIN.

**lactometer** (lak'tomitə) an instrument for measuring the specific gravity of milk.

**lactose** ('laktohz, -tohs) milk sugar consisting of glucose and galactose. **L. intolerance** the ingestion of milk containing lactose results in the patient experiencing severe abdominal colic and diarrhoea due to a deficiency of the lactose-splitting enzyme (beta-galactosidase) in the lining of the small intestine. Asian and African people who have a change in diet to one with a higher milk content are often affected in this way.

**lactosuria** (ˌlaktə'syooə.ri.ə) lactose in the urine.

**lactovegetarian** (ˌlaktoh vejiˈtair-.ri.ən) 1. a person who subsists on a diet of milk or milk products and vegetables. 2. pertaining to such a diet.

**lactulose** ('laktyuhlohz) a synthetic disaccharide which is used as a laxative.

**lacuna** (ləˈkyoonə) a small cavity or depression in any part of the body.

**Laënnec's disease** (ˌla.eˈnekz) *R.T.H. Laënnec, French physician, 1781–1826*. The most common type of cirrhosis of the liver, frequently attributable to high alcohol consumption.

**Laetrile** ('laytriel) American trade name for a substance derived from apricots, almonds and other fruit; alleged to have antineoplastic activity.

**laevulose** ('levyuhˌlohz) fruit sugar; fructose.

**laking** ('layking) haemolysis of the red blood cells. The cells swell and burst and the haemoglobin is released.

**lallation** (laˈlayshən) a babbling, infantile form of speech.

**Lamaze method** (laˈmayz ˌmethəd) *F. Lamaze, French obstetrician, 1890–1957*. A method of preparing for NATURAL CHILDBIRTH developed by Fernand Lamaze, and based on the technique of training the mind and body for the purpose of modifying perception of pain during labour and delivery.

**lambdoid** ('lamdoyd) shaped like the Greek letter Λ or λ. *L. suture* the junction of the occipital bone with the parietals.

**lambliasis** (lamˈbliəsis) giardiasis.

**lamella** (ləˈmelə) 1. a thin layer, membrane or plate, as of bone. 2. a thin medicated disc of gelatin used in applying drugs to the eye. The gelatin dissolves and the drugs are absorbed.

**lamina** ('laminə) a bony plate or layer.

**laminectomy** (ˌlamiˈnektəmee) excision of the posterior arch of a vertebra, sometimes performed to relieve pressure on the spinal cord or nerves.

**Lancefield's groups** ('lansfeeldz) *R.C. Lancefield, American bacteriologist, 1895–1981*. Divisions of B-haemolytic streptococci, which are classified on the basis of serological action into groups A–R. Most human infections are due to group A.

**Landry's paralysis** (lanˈdreez) *J.B.G. Landry, French physician, 1826–1865*. Guillain–Barré syndrome; acute ascending polyneuritis.

**Landsteiner's classification** ('landstienəz ˌklasifiˈkayshən) *K. Landsteiner, Austrian biologist, 1868–1943*. A system of blood groups; the ABO system, consisting of groups Λ, B, AB and O.

**Lange colloidal gold test** ('langə kəloydˈl) *C.F.A. Lange, German physician, 1883–1953*. A test made on cerebrospinal fluid to detect syphilis, disseminated sclerosis, meningitis and other neurological conditions.

**Langerhans** ('langəˌhanz) *P. Langerhans, German pathologist, 1847–1888*. *Islet of L.* one of the group of cells in the pancreas that produce insulin.

**lanolin** ('lanəlin) a fat obtained from sheep's wool, and used as a basis for ointments, salves, creams and cosmetics.

**lanugo** (ləˈnyoogoh, -noo-) the fine hair that covers the body of the fetus and newly born infants, especially those who are premature. Also called down.

**laparoscopy** (ˌlapəˈroskəpee) viewing of the abdominal cavity by passing an endoscope through the abdominal wall.

**laparotomy** (ˌlapəˈrotəmee) incision of the abdominal wall for exploratory purposes.

**laryngeal** (ləˈrinjiːəl, ˌlarinˈjeeəl) pertaining to the larynx.

**laryngectomy** (ˌlarinˈjektəmee) excision of the larynx.

**laryngismus** (ˌlarinˈjizməs) a spasmodic contraction of the larynx. *L. stridulus* a crowing sound on inspiration, following a period of apnoea, due to spasmodic closure of the glottis. It occurs in children, particularly those suffering from rickets. Croup.

**laryngitis** (ˌlarinˈjietis) inflammation of the larynx causing hoarseness or loss of voice due to acute infection or irritation by gases.

**laryngopharynx** (ləˌringˌgohˈfaringks) the lower portion of the pharynx connecting with the larynx.

**laryngoscope** (ləˈringˌgohˌskohp) an endoscopic instrument for examining the larynx or for aiding the insertion of endotracheal tubes or the bronchoscope.

**laryngospasm** (ləˈringˌgohˌspazəm) a reflex, prolonged contraction of the laryngeal muscles that is liable to occur on insertion or withdrawal of an endotracheal tube.

**laryngostenosis** (ləˌringˌgohstəˈnohsis) contraction or stricture of the larynx.

**laryngostomy** (ˌlaringˈgostəmee) the making of an opening into the larynx to provide an artificial air passage.

**laryngotomy** (ˌlaringˈgotəmee) an incision into the larynx to make a temporary opening in an emergency when the larynx is obstructed. Tracheostomy.

**laryngotracheal** (ləˌringˌgohˈtraki.əl) referring to both the larynx and trachea.

**laryngotracheitis** (ləˌringˌgohˌtrakiˈietis) inflammation of both the larynx and trachea.

**laryngotracheobronchitis** (ləˌringˌgohˌtrakiohbrongˈkietis) an acute viral infection of the respiratory tract which occurs particularly in young children.

**larynx** (ˈlaringks) [Gr.] the muscular and cartilaginous structure, lined with mucous membrane, situated at the top of the trachea and below the root of the tongue and the hyoid bone. The larynx contains the vocal cords and is the source of the sound heard in speech; it is also called the voice box.

**laser** (ˈlayzə) light *a*mplification by *s*timulated *e*mission of *r*adiation. An apparatus producing an extremely concentrated beam of light that can be used to cut metals. Used in the treatment of neoplasms, detached retina, diabetic retinopathy and macular degeneration, and some skin conditions.

**Lassa fever** (ˈlasə) a West African viral haemorrhagic fever with insidious onset and an incubation period of 6–21 days. It is a zoonosis, the reservoir of infection of which is the multimammate rat. Devastating outbreaks of person-to-person transmission have occurred in hospitals in West Africa by accidental inoculation of blood and tissue fluid from infected patients. In the UK prevention is dependent on the early detection of cases and their isolation, and strict precautions to protect health-care staff caring for febrile patients from Africa from inoculation or other accidents.

**Lassar's paste** (ˈlasəz ˌpayst) G. Lassar, German dermatologist, 1849–1907. A soothing paste used in skin diseases, containing salicylic acid, zinc oxide, starch and soft paraffin.

**lassitude** (ˈlasiˌtyood) a feeling of extreme weakness and apathy.

**latent** (ˈlaytənt) temporarily concealed; not manifest. *L. heat* the heat absorbed by a substance during a change in state, e.g. from water into steam. When condensation occurs this heat is released.

**L. period** 1. the incubation period of an infectious disease. 2. the time between the application of a nerve stimulus and the reaction.

**lateral** ('latə.rəl) situated at the side; therefore, away from the centre.

**lateroversion** (,latə.roh'vərshən, -zhən) a turning to one side, such as may occur of the uterus.

**laudanum** ('lawd'nəm) tincture of opium; a preparation formerly used as a narcotic.

**laughing gas** ('lahfing) nitrous oxide.

**lavage** ('lavij, la'vahzh) the washing out of a cavity. *Colonic l.* the washing out of the colon. *Gastric l.* the washing out of the stomach.

**laxative** ('laksətiv) a medicine that loosens the bowel contents and encourages evacuation. A laxative with a mild or gentle effect on the bowels is also known as an aperient; one with a strong effect is referred to as a cathartic or a purgative.

**LE** lupus erythematosus. *LE cell* a mature neutrophilic polymorphonuclear leukocyte that has phagocytized a large, spherical inclusion derived from another neutrophil; a characteristic of lupus erythematosus, but also found in analogous connective tissue disorders.

**lead** (led) *symbol* Pb. A metallic element, many of the compounds of which are highly poisonous. *L. lotion* lead subacetate solution used externally on bruises. *L. poisoning* a condition that usually occurs in children as the result of excessive lead in the atmosphere, or from chewing objects covered with paint containing lead. The symptoms and signs include malaise, diarrhoea and vomiting, and sometimes encephalitis. There is often pallor and a blue line around the gums.

**Leber's disease** ('laybərz) *T.B. Leber, German ophthalmologist, 1840–1917.* Hereditary optic atrophy.

**lecithin** ('lesithin) one of a group of phospholipids that are found in the cell tissues and are concerned in the metabolism of fat.

**leech** (leech) *Hirudo medicinalis,* an aquatic worm which sucks blood and secretes hirudin (an anticoagulant) in its saliva. On rare occasions used to withdraw blood from patients.

**leg** (leg) the lower limb, from knee to ankle. *Barbados l.* elephantiasis. *Bow-l.* genu varum. *Scissor l.* condition in which the patient is cross-legged, such as occurs in cerebral diplegia. *White l.* phlegmasia alba dolens.

*Legionella pneumophila* (,leejə'nelə nyoo'mofilə) a species of Gram-negative, non-acid-fast, rod-shaped bacteria which require both cysteine and iron for growth; it is the causative agent of LEGIONNAIRES' DISEASE and PONTIAC FEVER.

**legionellosis** (,leejənə'lohsis) a disease caused by infection with *Legionella* species, such as *L. pneumophila.* A notifiable disease in Scotland.

**legionnaires' disease** (leejə'nairz) a pulmonary form of legionellosis, resulting from infection with *Legionella pneumophila.* It is contagious and symptoms include fever, pain in the muscles and across the chest, a dry cough and a partial loss of kidney function. The prevalence of legionnaires' disease is not certain but it is estimated that between 5 and 10% of the annual cases of pneumonia in the UK are caused by *L. pneumophila.*

**leiomyoma** (,lieohmie'ohmə) a benign smooth muscle tumour (fibroid) most commonly found in the uterus.

**leiomyosarcoma** (,lieoh,mieohsah-'kohmə) a malignant muscle tumour.

*Leishmania* (leesh'mayni.ə) a genus of parasitic flagellated protozoa which infect the blood of humans and are the cause of leishmaniasis.

**leishmaniasis** (ˌleeshməˈnieəsis) a group of diseases caused by one of the protozoan *Leishmania* parasites. *See* KALA-AZAR.

**Lembert's suture** (lonhˈbairz) *A. Lembert, French surgeon, 1802–1851.* A series of stitches used for wounds of the intestine. So arranged that the edges are turned inwards and the peritoneal surfaces are in contact.

**lens** (lenz) 1. a piece of glass or other material shaped to transmit light rays in a particular direction. 2. the transparent crystalline body situated behind the pupil of the eye. It serves as a refractive medium for rays of light. **Contact l.** a thin sheet of glass or plastic moulded to fit directly over the cornea. Worn instead of spectacles.

**lentigo** (lenˈtiegoh) a brownish or yellowish spot on the skin. A freckle. **L. maligna** Hutchinson's melanotic freckle. *See* FRECKLE.

*Lentivirus* (ˈlentiˌvierəs) from Latin *lentus* (slow) + virus. A group of retroviruses that cause disease in animals and humans, including HIV-1 and HIV-2 (*see* HUMAN IMMUNODEFICIENCY VIRUS). These viruses are associated with slowly progressive diseases.

**leontiasis** (ˌleeənˈtieəsis) an osseous deformity of the face which produces a lion-like appearance. It occurs sometimes in leprosy and rarely in osteitis deformans.

**lepidosis** (ˌlepiˈdohsis) any scaly eruption of the skin.

**leprosy** (ˈleprəsee) Hansen's disease. A chronic infection of the skin, mucous membrane and nerves with *Mycobacterium leprae*. It is predominantly a tropical disease which is transmitted by direct contact. There is an insidious onset of symptoms, mainly involving the skin and nerves, after an incubation

period of between 1 and 30 years. The disease can be classified into three types: (a) Lepromatous, which is a steadily progressive form, often resulting in paralysis, disfigurement and deformity. This form is often complicated by tuberculosis. (b) Tuberculoid, which is often self-limiting and generally runs a more benign course. (c) Indeterminate, in which there are skin symptoms representative of both lepromatous and tuberculoid forms. Leprosy is now treated with a range of drugs including dapsone, rifampicin, clofazimine and thalidomide.

**leptomeningitis** (ˌleptohˌmeninˈjietis) inflammation of the pia mater and arachnoid membranes of the brain and spinal cord.

*Leptospira* (ˌleptohˈspierə) a genus of spirochaetes. *L. icterohaemorrhagiae* the cause of spirochaetal jaundice (Weil's disease).

**leptospirosis** (ˌleptohspieˈrohsis) any of a group of notifiable infectious diseases due to serotypes of *Leptospira*. The best known is Weil's disease, or leptospiral jaundice; others are mud fever, autumn fever and swineherd's disease. The aetiological agent is a spiral organism that is common in water. Initially the symptoms include fever, rigors, vomiting, headache and often jaundice. Diagnosis may be difficult because the symptoms resemble those of several other diseases. Jaundice is a key symptom. Sanitation measures can reduce the spread of the disease in both humans and animals.

**Leriche's syndrome** (ləˈreeshiz) *R. Leriche, French surgeon, 1879–1955.* A condition in which atherosclerosis of peripheral arteries is accompanied by obstruction of the lower end of the aorta.

**lesbianism** (ˈlezbiˌənizəm) sexual and emotional orientation of one woman to another; female homosexuality.

**Lesch–Nyhan syndrome** (ˌlesh 'niehan) *M. Lesch, American physician, b. 1939; W.L. Nyhan Jr, American physician, b. 1926.* A hereditary disorder of purine metabolism transmitted as an X-linked recessive trait with physical and mental handicap, compulsive self-mutilation of fingers and lips by biting, spasticity, cerebral palsy and impaired renal function.

**lesion** ('leezhən) any pathological or traumatic discontinuity of tissue or loss of function of a part. Lesion is a broad term, including wounds, sores, ulcers, tumours, cataracts and any other tissue damage. Lesions range from the skin sores associated with eczema to the changes in lung tissue that occur in tuberculosis.

**lethargy** ('lethəjee) a condition of drowsiness or stupor that cannot be overcome by the will.

**Letterer–Siwe disease** (ˌletə.rə'seevə) *E. Letterer, German physician, 1895–1982; S.A. Siwe, German physician, 1897–1966.* Reticuloendotheliosis of early childhood, marked by a haemorrhagic tendency, eczematoid skin eruption, hepatosplenomegaly with lymph node involvement, and progressive anaemia.

**leucine** ('looseen) a naturally occurring essential amino acid, vital for growth in infants and for nitrogen equilibrium in adults.

**leuco-** ('lookoh) for words beginning thus, see *leuko-*.

**leukaemia** (loo'keemi.ə) a progressive, malignant disease of the blood-forming organs, marked by abnormal proliferation and development of leukocytes and their precursors in the blood and bone marrow. It is accompanied by a reduced number of erythrocytes and blood platelets, resulting in anaemia and increased susceptibil-

ity to infection and haemorrhage. Other typical symptoms include fever, pain in the joints and bones and swelling of the lymph nodes, spleen and liver. Leukaemia is classified clinically on the basis of (a) the duration and character of the disease (acute or chronic), and (b) the cell line involved, i.e. myeloid (myelocytic, myeloblastic, granulocytic) or lymphoid (lymphatic, lymphoblastic, lymphocytic). A widely used classification of acute leukaemia based on cell type is the French American British (FAB) classification. The incidence of the disease is growing and the increase is only partially explained by increased efficiency of detection. Treatment is primarily with chemotherapy but this may also be combined with radiotherapy, removal of the spleen and bone marrow transfusions. Antibiotics are commonly required.

**leukocyte** ('lookəˌsiet) a white blood corpuscle. There are three types: (a) granular (polymorphonuclear cells) formed in bone marrow, consisting of neutrophils, eosinophils and basophils; (b) lymphocytes (formed in the lymph glands); and (c) monocytes (*see* Figure and Table on p. 238).

**leukocytolysis** (ˌlookohsie'tolisis) destruction of white blood cells.

**leukocytopoiesis** (ˌlookohˌsietohpoy'eesis) leukopoiesis.

**leukocytosis** (ˌlookohsie'tohsis) an increase in the number of leukocytes in the blood. Often a response to infection.

**leukoderma** (ˌlookoh'dərmə) an absence of pigment in patches or bands, producing abnormal whiteness of the skin. Vitiligo.

**leukodystrophy** (ˌlookoh'distrəfee) a degenerative disorder of the brain which starts during the first few months of life and leads to mental, visual and motor deterioration.

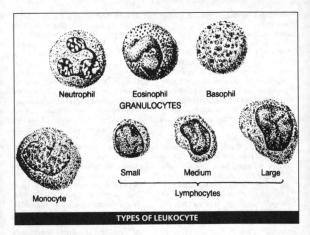

Neutrophil  Eosinophil  Basophil
GRANULOCYTES

Small  Medium  Large
Monocyte  Lymphocytes

**TYPES OF LEUKOCYTE**

| NORMAL LEUKOCYTE COUNT | |
|---|---|
| Cell type | No. cells/litre |
| Neutrophils | $3.5–7.5 \times 10^9$ |
| Eosinophils | $0.04–0.4 \times 10^9$ |
| Basophils | $0.01–0.1 \times 10^9$ |
| Lymphocytes | $1.5–4.0 \times 10^9$ |
| Monocytes | $0.2–0.8 \times 10^9$ |

**leukoma** (loo'kohmə) a white spot on the cornea, usually the result of an injury to the eye.

**leukonychia** (ˌlookoh'niki.ə) white patches on the nails due to air underneath.

**leukopenia** (ˌlookoh'peeni.ə) a decreased number of white cells, usually granulocytes, in the blood.

**leukophoresis** (ˌlookohfə'reesis) withdrawal of blood for the selective removal of leukocytes. The remaining blood is retransfused.

**leukoplakia** (ˌlookoh'playki.ə) a chronic inflammation, characterized by white thickened patches on the mucous membranes, particularly on the tongue, gums and inside of the cheeks. *L. vulvae* thickening of the mucous membrane of the labia with the appearance of scattered white patches.

**leukopoiesis** (ˌlookohpoy'eesis) the formation of white blood cells. Leukocytopoiesis.

**leukorrhoea** (ˌlookə'reeə) a viscid, whitish discharge from the vagina.

**levator** (lə'vaytə) a muscle that raises a structure or organ of the body.

**levels of care** ('lev'lz) the six divisions of the HEALTH CARE SYSTEM; preventive care, primary care, secondary or acute care, tertiary care, restorative care and continuing care.

**levodopa** (ˌleevoh'dohpə) L-dopa; a synthetic drug used in the treatment of Parkinsonism.

**levonorgestrel** (ˌleevohnor'jestrel) a potent progestin used in combination with an oestrogen as an oral contraceptive.

**levorphanol** (le'vorfənol) an analgesic somewhat resembling morphine in its action and addiction potentialities. It is used to relieve severe pain.

**LH** luteinizing hormone.

**Li** symbol for *lithium*.

**liaison** (lee'ayzon) communication and contact between groups, units and/or agencies and organizations. *L. health visitor* appointed to facilitate communications between the hospital and the community services for the benefit of the patient's care at home after discharge from the inpatient unit.

**libido** (li'beedoh) 1. the vital force or impulse which brings about purposeful action. 2. sexual drive in Freudian psychoanalysis, the motive force of all human beings.

**lichen** ('liekən, 'lichən) a group of inflammatory infections of the skin in which the lesions consist of papular eruptions. *L. planus* raised flat patches of dull, reddish-purple colour, with a smooth or scaly surface.

**lichenification** (lie,kenifi'kayshən) the stage of an eruption when it resembles lichen.

**lid** (lid) eyelid. *Granular l.* trachoma. *L. lag* jerky movement of the upper lid when it is being lowered. A sign of exophthalmic goitre (thyrotoxicosis).

**lie** (lie) a position or direction. *L. of fetus* the position of the fetus in the uterus. The normal lie is longitudinal.

**Lieberkühn's glands** ('leebə-,koonz) *J.N. Lieberkühn, German anatomist, 1711–1756.* Tubular glands of the small intestine.

**lien** (lie.en) the spleen.

**lienculus** (lie'engkyuhləs) an accessory spleen.

**lienorenal** (,lieənoh'reen'l) relating to the spleen and kidneys; splenorenal; splenonephric.

**life event** ('lief i,vent) a sociological term used to describe major events in a person's life, e.g. leaving

home for the first time, getting married, moving house, changing a job.

**life expectancy** (eks'pektənsee) the average length of life based upon prevailing mortality trends.

**life support system** (sə'pawt ,sistəm) the equipment and technology used to maintain the life of a patient who is not otherwise able to survive.

**lifestyle** ('lief,stiel) the pattern of daily living that an individual develops. On the initial assessment of a person entering the health-care services this is considered in relation to the delivery of care by health-care workers in order that the aims and objectives for care can be individualized.

**ligament** ('ligəmənt) 1. a band of fibrous tissue connecting bones forming a joint. 2. a layer or layers of peritoneum connecting one abdominal organ to another or to the abdominal wall. *Annular l.* the ringlike band that fixes the head of the radius to the ulna. *Cruciate l.* crossed ligaments within the knee joint. *Inguinal l.* that between the pubic bone and anterior iliac crest. *Round l.* for example, one of the two anterior ligaments of the uterus, passing through the inguinal canal and ending in the labia majora. There are also round ligaments of the femur and of the liver.

**ligation** (lie'gayshən) the application of a ligature.

**ligature** ('ligəchə) a thread of silk, catgut or other material used for tying round a blood vessel to stop it bleeding.

**light** (liet) electromagnetic waves which stimulate the retina of the eye. *L. adaptation* the changes that take place in the eye when the intensity of the light increases or decreases. *L. coagulation* a method of treating retinal detachment by directing a beam of strong light from a carbon arc through the pupil to the affected area.

**lightening** ('lietəning) the relief experienced in pregnancy, 2–3 weeks before labour, when the uterus sinks into the pelvis and ceases to press on the diaphragm.

**lignocaine** ('lignoh,kayn) a local anaesthetic administered by injection and by surface application. Also used intravenously in cases of cardiac arrhythmia, especially myocardial infarction.

**limbus** ('limbəs) an edge or border. *Corneal l.* the border where the cornea joins the sclera.

**liminal** ('limin'l) pertaining to the threshold of perception.

**lincomycin** (,linkoh'miesin) an antibiotic derived from the *Streptomyces* genus. Used in the treatment of streptococcal bone and joint infections, including osteomyelitis.

**linctus** ('lingktəs) a thick syrup given to soothe and allay coughing.

**linea** ('lini.ə) [L.] *a line*. *L. alba* the tendinous area in the centre of the abdominal wall into which the transversalis and part of the oblique muscles are inserted. *L. albicantes* white streaks that appear on the abdomen when it is distended by pregnancy or a tumour. *L. aspera* the rough ridge on the back of the femur into which muscles are inserted. *L. nigra* the pigmented line that often appears in pregnancy on the abdomen between the umbilicus and the pubis.

**linear** ('lini.ə) pertaining to a line. *L. accelerator* a megavoltage machine for accelerating electrons so that powerful X-rays are given off for use in the treatment of deep-seated tumours.

**lingual** ('ling.gwəl) pertaining to the tongue.

**lingula** ('ling.gyuhlə) a tongue-like structure, such as the projection of lung tissue from the left upper lobe.

**liniment** ('linimənt) a liquid to be applied externally by rubbing on to the skin.

**lip** (lip) 1. the upper or lower fleshy margin of the mouth. 2. any lip-like part; labium. *Cleft l.* congenital fissure of the upper lip.

**lip reading** (,reeding) understanding of speech through observation of the speaker's lip movements; called also speech reading.

**lipaemia** (li'peemi.ə) the presence of excess fat in the blood. Sometimes a feature of diabetes. *L. retinalis* condition in which the retinal blood vessels appear to be filled with milk owing to the presence of an excess of fat in the blood.

**lipase** ('lipayz, -pays) fat-splitting enzyme; any enzyme that catalyses the splitting of fats into glycerol and fatty acids. Measurement of the serum lipase level is an important diagnostic test for acute and chronic pancreatitis.

**lipid** ('lipid) one of a group of fatty substances that are insoluble in water but soluble in alcohol or chloroform. They form an important part of the diet and are normally present in the body tissues.

**lipochondrodystrophy** (,lipoh,kondroh'distrəfee) a congenital condition affecting the metabolism of fat and producing bone deformities, short stature, facial abnormalities and learning difficulties. Hurler's syndrome.

**lipodystrophy** (,lipoh'distrəfee) a disorder of fat metabolism. *Progressive l.* a rare condition, occurring mainly in females, in which there is progressive loss of fat over the upper half of the body.

**lipoidosis** (,lipoy'dohsis) any one of a group of diseases in which there is an error in lipoid metabolism producing reticuloendothelial hyperplasia. Xanthomas are common.

**lipolysis** (li'polisis) the breakdown of fats by the action of bile salts and enzymes to a fine emulsion and fatty acids.

**lipoma** (li'pohmə) a benign tumour composed of fatty tissue, arising in any part of the body, and developing in connective tissue. *Diffuse l.* a tumour of fat in an irregular mass, without a capsule, occurring above the pelvis.

**lipoprotein** (,lipoh'prohteen) one of a group of fatty proteins present in blood plasma.

**liposarcoma** (,lipohsah'kohmə) a malignant tumour of the fat cells.

**liquefaction** (,likwi'fakshən) reduction to liquid form.

**liquid** ('likwid) 1. a substance that flows readily in its natural state. 2. flowing readily, neither solid nor gaseous. *L. diet* a diet limited to the intake of liquids or foods that can be changed to a liquid state. A liquid diet may be restricted to clear liquids or it may be a full liquid diet.

**liquor** ('likə, 'liekwor) a watery fluid; a solution. *L. amnii* the fluid in which the fetus floats; amniotic fluid.

***Listeria*** (li'stiə.ri.ə) *Baron J. Lister, British surgeon, 1827–1912.* A genus of Gram-negative bacteria which produce upper respiratory disease, septicaemia and encephalitic disease in humans. They can be transmitted by the consumption of infected, unpasteurized dairy produce, or by direct contact with infected animals or contaminated soil. Newborn infants, pregnant women, the elderly and the immunosuppressed are more susceptible to infection.

**listeriosis** (lis,tiə.ri'ohsis) infection with organisms of the genus *Listeria*.

**lithagogue** ('lithə,gog) a drug that helps to expel calculi.

**lithiasis** (li'thieəsis) the formation of calculi. *Conjunctival l.* the formation of small white chalky areas on the inner surface of the eyelids.

**lithium** ('lithi.əm) *symbol* Li. An alkaline metallic element. *L. carbonate* a drug used in the treatment of manic-depressive illness.

**lithosis** (li'thohsis) pneumoconiosis resulting from inhalation of particles of silica, etc., into the lungs.

**lithotripsy** ('lithoh,tripsee) the crushing of calculi in the bladder; lithotrity.

**lithuresis** (,lithyuh'reesis) passage of small calculi or gravel in the urine.

**litmus** ('litməs) a blue pigment obtained from lichen and used for testing the reaction of fluids. *Blue l.* turned red by an acid. *Red l.* turned blue by an alkali.

**litre** ('leetə) *symbol* l. The SI unit of capacity. One cubic decimetre.

**Little's disease** ('lit'lz) *W.J. Little, British surgeon, 1810–1894.* Spastic diplegia. A congenital muscle rigidity of the lower limbs causing 'scissor leg' deformity.

**liver** ('livə) the large gland situated in the right upper area of the abdominal cavity. Its chief functions are: (a) the secretion of bile; (b) the maintenance of the composition of the blood; and (c) the regulation of metabolic processes. *Cirrhotic l.* fibrotic changes which occur in the liver as the result of degeneration of the liver cells, often as a result of alcoholism. *L. biopsy* the taking of a small core of liver tissue through a liver biopsy needle under a local anaesthetic. Allows for microscopic examination to aid diagnosis of a wide range of disorders of the liver. *L. transplant* the transplantation of a liver from a suitable donor who has recently died.

**livid** ('livid) descriptive of the bluish-grey discoloration of the skin produced by congestion of blood.

**living will** (ˌliving 'wil) a statement signed by a person requesting and indicating what should be done in the event of becoming totally incapacitated or terminally ill. It enables the writer, while still alive, to refuse resuscitation or other measures to maintain life.

**LOA** left occipitoanterior. Refers to a possible position of the fetus in the uterus.

**lobar** ('lohbə) relating to a lobe.

**lobe** (lohb) a section of an organ, separated from neighbouring parts by fissures. The liver, lungs and brain are divided into lobes.

**lobectomy** (loh'bektəmee) removal of a lobe, e.g. of the lung.

**lobular** ('lobyuhlə) relating to a lobule.

**lobule** ('lobyool) a small lobe, particularly one making up a larger lobe.

**local supervising authority** (ˌlohkəl 'soopə.viezing aw'tho.ritee) abbreviated LSA. A local organization, usually the Regional Health Authority, responsible for monitoring midwifery practice within its area. This is done by the appointment of supervisors of midwifery, facilitating their education and training and enabling communication with the supervisors, developing systems to ensure eligibility to practise of each midwife working within the area and, where necessary, suspending from practice any midwife who is felt to have acted in an unsafe or negligent manner. The LSA has a nominated officer, who must be a practising midwife, to carry out its functions.

**localize** ('lohkə.liez) 1. to limit the spread, e.g. of disease or infection, to a certain area. 2. to determine the site of a lesion.

**lochia** ('lohki.ə) the discharge of blood and tissue debris from the uterus after childbirth, lasting for 2–3 weeks. Initially lochia is bright red and gradually becomes paler.

**lochiometra** (ˌlohkioh'meetrə) the retention of lochia in the uterus, causing its distension.

**lockjaw** ('lok.jor) tetanus.

**locomotor** (ˌlohkə'mohtə) pertaining to movement from one place to another. *L. ataxia* tabes dorsalis. *See* ATAXIA.

**loculated** ('lokyuh.laytid) divided into small locules or cavities.

**loculus** ('lokyuhləs) a small cystic cavity, one of a number.

**locum tenens** (ˌlohkəm 'teenenz) a person, usually a doctor, who substitutes for another over a period of time; usually referred to as a locum.

**log roll** ('log .rohl) a nursing technique used to turn a reclining patient from one side to the other. The patient lies on the back with arms folded across the chest, and legs extended. The nurses manipulate the underlying drawsheet so that the patient is rolled on to one side or the other.

**logorrhoea** (ˌlogə'reeə) excessive and often unintelligible volubility.

**loiasis** (loh'ieəsis) infestation of the conjunctiva and eyelids with a parasite worm, *Loa loa*. A tropical condition.

**loin** (loyn) the area of the back between the thorax and the pelvis.

**Lomotil** ('lomətil) trade name for preparations of diphenoxylate, an antidiarrhoeal.

**long sight** (long 'siet) hypermetropia.

**longitudinal study** (ˌlongi'tyoodin'l .studee) an investigation that involves making observations of the same group at sequential time intervals. Longitudinal studies are valuable as a means of studying human development or change and may also be used to observe change over time within an institution or organization.

**loosening** ('loosoning) in psychiatry, a disorder of thinking in which associations of ideas become so shortened, fragmented and disturbed as to lack logical relationship.

**LOP** left occipitoposterior. Refers to a possible position of the fetus in the uterus.

**lorazepam** (lo'razipam, -'rayz-) a minor tranquillizer used to treat anxiety and insomnia.

**lordosis** (lor'dohsis) a form of spinal curvature in which there is an abnormal forward curve of the lumbar spine.

**lotion** ('lohshən) a medicinal solution for external application to the body. Lotions usually have a soothing or antiseptic effect. *Calamine l.* a soothing mixture containing calamine and zinc oxide. *Evaporating l.* a dilute alcoholic solution applied to bruises. *Lead l.* a weak solution of lead acetate used for sprains and bruises where the skin is unbroken.

**loupe** (loop) a magnifying lens, which may be used in eye examination.

**louse** (lows) a general term covering a number of small insects that are parasitic to humans and to other mammals and birds. Three varieties are parasitic to humans: (a) *Pediculus capitis*, the head louse; (b) *Pediculus corporis*, the body louse; and (c) *Phthirus pubis*, which infects the coarse hair on the body and also the eyebrows. Diseases known to be transmitted by lice are typhus fever, relapsing fever and trench fever.

**lozenge** ('lozinj) a medicated tablet with a sugar basis, used to treat mouth and throat conditions.

**LSA** local supervising authority.

**LSD** *see* LYSERGIDE.

**lubb-dupp** (lub'dup) representation of the sounds heard through the stethoscope when listening to the normal heart. *lubb* when the atrioventricular valves shut, and *dupp* when the semilunar valves meet each other.

**lucid** ('loosid) clear, particularly of the mind. *L. interval* period of clear thinking that may occur in cerebral injury between two periods of unconsciousness or as a sane interval in a mental disorder.

**lues** ('looeez) syphilis.

**lumbago** (lum'baygoh) pain in the lower part of the back. It may be caused by muscular strain or by a prolapsed intervertebral disc ('slipped disc').

**lumbar** ('lumbə) pertaining to the loins. *L. puncture* insertion of a trocar and cannula into the spinal canal in the lower back and withdrawal of cerebrospinal fluid for diagnostic purposes.

**lumbosacral** (‚lumboh'saykrəl) relating to both the lumbar vertebrae and the sacrum. *L. support* a corset aimed at both supporting and restricting movement in that region. *L. vertebra* one of the five vertebrae in the lower back lying between the thoracic vertebrae and the sacrum.

**lumen** ('loomin) the space inside a tube.

**lumpectomy** (lum'pektəmee) the surgical excision of only the local lesion (benign or malignant) of the breast.

**lunacy** ('loonəsee) an obsolete term formerly applied to insanity.

**Lund and Browder chart** (‚luhnd ənd 'browdə) a chart that has been adopted by many burn centres in the UK for calculation of the surface area of a burn. At birth the size and area of the head is large compared with the adult, and the legs and thighs constitute a much smaller proportion of the total body surface. On admission to a burns unit or ward the area of the body burned is mapped on to the Lund and Browder chart and the area of the burn affecting each portion of the body surface is calculated.

**lung** (lung) one of a pair of conical organs of the respiratory system, consisting of an arrangement of air tubes terminating in air vesicles (alveoli) and filling almost the whole of the thorax. The right lung has three lobes and the left lung two. They are connected with the air by means of the bronchi and trachea.

**lunula** ('loonyuhlə) the white semi-circle near the root of each nail.

**lupus** ('loopəs) a chronic skin disease having many manifestations. *L. erythematosus* abbreviated LE. An inflammatory disease, affecting both the internal organs and the skin, which finally produces a round plaque-like area of hyperkeratosis. It is thought to be due to an autoimmune reaction to sunlight, infection or other unknown cause. *L. vulgaris* a tuberculous disease of the skin producing brownish nodules, frequently on the nose or cheek, and severe scarring.

**luteinizing hormone** ('lootee.i.niezing) abbreviated LH. One of three hormones produced by the anterior pituitary gland which control the activity of the gonads.

**luteotrophin** (,lootioh'trohfin) an anterior pituitary hormone which stimulates the formation of the corpus luteum and the production of milk. Prolactin.

**luxation** (luk'sayshən) the dislocation of a joint. *L. of the lens* displacement of the lens of the eye into the anterior chamber or posteriorly into the vitreous humour.

**Lyme disease** (liem) a zoonosis transmitted by ticks and characterized by a rash (erythema chronicum migrans), arthritis and aseptic meningitis, caused by the spirochaete *Borrelia burgdorferi*.

**lymph** (limf) the fluid from the blood which has transuded through capillary walls to supply nutriment to tissue cells. It is collected by lymph vessels which ultimately return it to the blood. *L. nodes* or *glands* structures placed along the course of lymph vessels, through which the lymph passes and is filtered of foreign substances, e.g. bacteria. These nodes also make lymphocytes. *Plastic l.* an inflammatory exudate which tends to cause adhesion between structures and so limit the spread of infection. *Vaccine l.* a lymph preparation obtained from calves or other animals and used for vaccination.

**lymphadenectomy** (,limfadə'nektəmee) excision of a lymph gland or nodes.

**lymphadenitis** (,limfadə'nietis) inflammation of a lymph gland.

**lymphadenoma** (,limfadə'nohmə) lymphoma. *Multiple l.* Hodgkin's disease.

**lymphadenopathy** (,limfadə'nopəthee) any disease condition of the lymph nodes.

**lymphangiectasis** (,limfanji'ektasis) dilatation of the lymph vessels due to some obstruction of the lymph flow. It may be congenital.

**lymphangiography** (,limfanji'ogrəfee) radiographic examination of lymph vessels after the insertion of a radio-opaque contrast medium.

**lymphangioma** (,limfanji'ohmə) a swelling composed of dilated lymph vessels.

**lymphangitis** (,limfan'jietis) inflammation of lymph vessels, manifested by red lines on the skin over them. It occurs in cases of severe infection through the skin.

**lymphatic** (lim'fatik) referring to lymph. *L. system* the system of vessels and glands through which the lymph is returned to the circulation. The vessels end in the thoracic duct and the right lymphatic duct.

**lymphoblast** ('limfoh,blast) an early developmental cell that will mature into a lymphocyte.

**lymphocyte** ('limfoh,siet) a white blood cell formed in the lymphoid tissue. Lymphocytes produce immune bodies to overcome and protect against infection.

**lymphocythaemia** (,limfohsie'theemi.ə) an excessive number of lymphocytes in the blood. Lymphocytosis.

**lymphocytopenia** (,limfoh,sietoh'peeni.ə) absence or scarcity of lymphocytes in the blood. Lymphopenia.

**lymphoedema** (,limfi'deemə) a condition in which the intercellular spaces contain an abnormal amount of lymph due to obstruction of the lymph drainage.

**lymphogranuloma** (,limfoh,granyuh'lohmə) Hodgkin's disease. *L. venereum* a sexually transmitted disease, caused by a virus; primarily a tropical condition.

**lymphoma** (lim'fohmə) lymphadenoma. Used to denote any malignant condition of the lymphoid tissue. Generally these diseases are classified as either Hodgkin's or non-Hodgkin's lymphomas. *Burkitt's l.* a type of lymphoma found predominantly in East Africa and affecting the jaws of children.

**lymphopoiesis** (,limfohpoy'eesis) the production of lymphocytes. Occurs chiefly in the bone marrow,

lymph nodes, thymus, spleen and gut wall.

**lymphosarcoma** (,limfohsah'kohmə) a term formerly used to denote a malignant lymphoma (with the exception of Hodgkin's disease).

**lyophilization** (lie,ofilie'zayshən) a method of preserving biological substances in a stable state by freeze-drying. It may be used for plasma, sera, bacteria, viruses and tissues.

**lysergide** (lie'sərjied) lysergic acid diethylamide (LSD). A hallucinogenic drug that can cause visual hallucinations and increased auditory acuity but may prove very disrupting to the personality and affect mental ability.

**lysin** ('liesin) a specific antibody present in the blood that can destroy cells. *See* BACTERIOLYSIN.

**lysine** ('lieseen) an essential amino acid formed by the digestion of dietary protein. It is vital for normal health.

**lysis** ('liesis) 1. the gradual decline of a disease, especially of a fever. The temperature falls gradually, as in typhoid. *See* CRISIS. 2. the destruction of cells.

**lysosome** ('liesə,sohm) a particle, found in the cytoplasm of cells, which causes the breakdown of metabolic substances and foreign particles (e.g. bacteria) within the cell.

**lysozyme** ('liesə,ziem) an enzyme present in tears, nasal mucus and saliva that can kill most bacteria coming into contact with it.

# M

**m** symbol for *metre* and *misce* (mix).

**M** symbol for *molar*.

**McBurney's point** (mək'bɜrniz ˌpoynt) *C. McBurney, American surgeon, 1845–1913.* The spot midway between the anterior iliac spine and the umbilicus where pain is felt on pressure if the appendix is inflamed.

**maceration** (ˌmasə'rayshən) softening of a solid by soaking it in liquid. *Neonatal m.* the natural softening of a dead fetus in the uterus.

**Mackenrodt's ligaments** ('makenˌrohts) *A.K. Mackenrodt, German gynaecologist, 1859–1925.* The transverse or cardinal ligaments that support the uterus in the pelvic cavity.

**Macmillan nurses** (mak'milən) qualified nurses who have also received special training in the management of pain relief, palliative care and the provision of emotional support to cancer patients and their families. This nursing service is provided either in the patient's home through the Macmillan home visiting service, in hospital or in a hospice.

**McNaghten's Rules on Insanity at Law** (mək'nawtənz roolz on in'sanətee at law) the rules that define the factors on which a defence to a charge of murder on grounds of insanity may be established. These were evolved after Sir Robert Peel's Secretary was killed by McNaghten in 1843. He was suffering from delusions and the judge ordered that he be found not guilty. The Homicide Act 1957 provided for a defence based on 'diminished responsibility', i.e. the accused was suffering from such abnormality of mind as to impair mental responsibility and was not responsible for any actions undertaken in that state.

**macrocheilia** (ˌmakroh'kieli.ə) a congenital condition in which there is excessive development of the lips.

**macrocyte** ('makroh ˌsiet) an abnormally large red corpuscle found in the blood in some forms of anaemia.

**macrocythaemia** (ˌmakrohsie'theemi.ə) the presence of abnormally large red cells in the blood. Macrocytosis.

**macromastia** (ˌmakroh'masti.ə) an abnormal increase in the size of the breast.

**macronutrient** (ˌmakroh'nyootri-ˌənt) an essential nutrient that has a large minimal daily requirement (greater than 100 mg); calcium, phosphorus, magnesium, potassium, sodium and chloride are macronutrients.

**macrophage** ('makrohfayj) a large reticuloendothelial cell which has the power to ingest cell debris and bacteria. It is present in connective tissue, especially when there is inflammation.

**macrophthalmia** (ˌmakrofˈthalmi.ə) a congenital condition of abnormally large eyes.

**macroscopic** (ˌmakrohˈskopik) discernible with the naked eye. The opposite of microscopic.

**macrostomia** (ˌmakrohˈstohmi.ə) an abnormal development of the mouth in which the mandibular and maxillary processes do not fuse and the mouth is excessively wide.

**macula** ('makyuhlə) a spot or discoloured area of the skin, not raised above the surface; a macule. *M. corneae* a small area of opacity in the cornea, seen through an ophthalmoscope as a deeper red. *M. lutea* the yellow central area of the retina, where vision is clearest.

**maculopapular** (ˌmakyuhlohˈpapyuhlə) displaying both maculae and papules. *M. eruption* a rash comprised of both maculae and papules, as in measles.

**Madura foot** (məˈdyooə.rə) mycetoma of the foot.

**maduromycosis** (məˌdyooə.rohmie-ˈkohsis) a chronic disease caused by *Madurella mycetoma*. The most common form is Madura foot.

**Magendie's foramen** (ˌmazhon-ˈdeez) *F. Magendie, French physiologist, 1783–1855.* Aperture in the roof of the fourth ventricle of the brain through which cerebrospinal fluid passes into the subarachnoid space.

**maggots** ('magətz) worm-like larvae of flies that feed on organic matter and are occasionally found in wounds. *See* MYIASIS.

**magnesium** (magˈneezi.əm) *symbol* Mg. A bluish-white metallic element. It occurs widely in mineral sources and is present in some of the body tissues. *M. carbonate* and *m. hydroxide* neutralizing antacids used in hyperacidity. *M. sulphate* a saline purgative. Epsom salts. *M. trisilicate* an antacid powder taken after food for dyspepsia and peptic ulceration.

**magnet** ('magnit) in ophthalmology, an instrument used for removing metallic foreign bodies that have penetrated the eye.

**magnetic resonance imaging** (magˈnetik) abbreviated MRI. An imaging technique based on the NUCLEAR MAGNETIC RESONANCE properties of the hydrogen nucleus. Cross-sectional images in any plane of the body for examination may be obtained. MRI is without hazard to the patient.

**Makaton** ('makaˌton) one of the sign languages.

**mal** (mal) [Fr.] *disease.* **Grand m.**, **petit m.** forms of epilepsy. *M. de mer* seasickness.

**malabsorption** (ˌmaləbˈsawpshən, -ˈzaw-) inability of the small intestine to absorb certain substances. It may be the cause of a deficiency disease due to the lack of an essential factor.

**malacia** (məˈlayshi.ə) softening of tissues. *See also* KERATOMALACIA and OSTEOMALACIA.

**maladjustment** (ˌmaləˈjustmənt) in psychiatry, a failure to adjust to the environment.

**malaise** (maˈlayz) a feeling of general discomfort and illness.

**malalignment** (ˌmaləˈlienmənt) displacement, especially of the teeth from their normal relation to the line of the dental arch.

**malaria** (məˈlair.ri.ə) a serious, notifiable infectious illness characterized by periodic chills, fever, sweating and splenomegaly. Serious and often fatal complications may arise in falciparum malaria. It is endemic in parts of Africa, Asia and Central and South America, and is estimated to occur at the rate of 100 million cases each year throughout the world. Some 2000 imported cases per year are reported in the UK. Treatment is with antimalarial drugs. Epidemics usually occur in areas where mosquitoes persist in large numbers. The disease is caused by a parasite of the genus *Plasmodium* introduced into the blood by mosquitoes of the genus *Anopheles*. The attacks are periodic, every 48–72 h according to the type of plasmodium. For *P. vivax* it lasts 48 h, *P. malariae* 72 h, and *P. falciparum* 36–48 h. *Airport m.* a term sometimes used to describe malaria occurring at or near an airport, in a country normally free of the disease, and spread by infected mosquitoes brought in on an aeroplane from an endemic area. Control measures include disinsectization of aircraft where appropriate.

**malformation** (ˌmalfaw'mayshən) deformity; a structural defect.

**malignant** (məˈlignənt) tending to become progressively worse and to result in death; having the properties of anaplasia, invasiveness and metastasis; said of tumours.

**malingering** (məˈlingˈgə.ring) wilful, deliberate and fraudulent feigning or exaggeration of the symptoms of illness or injury to attain a consciously desired end.

**malleolus** (məˈleeələs) one of the two protuberances on either side of the ankle joint. *Lateral m.* that on the outer surface at the lower end of the fibula. *Medial m.* that on the inner surface at the lower end of the tibia.

**malleus** ('mali.əs) the hammer-shaped bone in the middle ear.

**malnutrition** (ˌmalnyoo'trishən) the condition in which nutrition is defective in quantity or quality.

**malocclusion** (ˌmalə'kloozhən) an abnormality of dental development which causes overlapping of the bite.

**Malpighian body** (mal'pigi.ən) *M. Malpighi, Italian anatomist, physician and physiologist, 1628–1694.* The glomerulus and Bowman's capsule of the kidney.

**malposition** (ˌmalpə'zishən) an abnormal position of any part of the body.

**malpractice** (mal'praktis) failure to maintain accepted ethical standards. Professional misconduct.

**malpresentation** (ˌmalprezən'tayshən) any abnormal position of the fetus at birth that renders delivery difficult or impossible.

**Malta fever** ('mawltə) brucellosis; undulant fever.

**maltase** (ˌmawltayz) a sugar-splitting enzyme which converts maltose to glucose. Present in pancreatic and intestinal juice.

**maltose** ('mawltohz, -tohs) the sugar formed by the action of digestive enzymes on starch.

**malunion** (mal'yooni.ən) faulty repair of a fracture.

**mammary** ('mamə.ree) relating to the breasts.

**mammography** (məˈmogrəfee) radiographic or infrared examination of the breast to detect abnormalities.

**mammoplasty** ('mamohˌplastee) a plastic operation to reduce the size of abnormally large, pendulous breasts or augment the size of very small breasts.

**mammothermography** (ˌmamohthər'mogrəfee) an examination of the breast that depends on the more active cells producing heat that can be shown on a thermograph; it may indicate abnormalities of the breast tissue.

**mandible** ('mandib'l) the lower jawbone.

**mania** ('mayni.ə) a disordered mental state of extreme excitement, especially the manic type of manic-depressive psychosis. Also used as a word termination to denote obsessive preoccupation with something, as in kleptomania.

**maniac** ('mayniˌak) colloquial term for one suffering from a violent or extreme form of insanity.

**manic** ('manik) pertaining to mania. *M.-depressive psychosis* a mental illness characterized by mania or endogenous depression. The attacks may alternate between mania and depression or the patient may just have recurrent attacks of mania or depression.

**manipulation** (mə,nipyuh'layshən) use of the hands to produce a desired movement, such as in reducing a fracture or a hernia or changing the position of a fetus. A skilfully applied forced movement upon a joint in order to relocate the joint or increase its range of movements by tearing adhesions round it.

**mannitol** ('mani,tol) a sugar alcohol occurring widely in nature; an osmotic diuretic used for forced diuresis in drug overdose and in cerebral oedema

**manometer** (mə'nomitə) an instrument for measuring the pressure of liquids or gases.

**Mantoux test** (man'too) *C. Mantoux, French physician, 1877–1947.* A tuberculin skin test in which a solution of purified protein derivative (PPD)- tuberculin is injected intradermally into either the anterior or posterior surface of the forearm. The test is read 48–72 h after injection. It is considered positive when the induration at the site of injection is more than 10 mm in diameter.

**manubrium** (mə'nyoobri.əm) the upper part of the sternum to which the clavicle is attached.

**MAOI** *see MONOAMINE OXIDASE.*

**maple syrup urine disease** (,mayp'l 'sirəp) an inborn error of metabolism in which there is an excess in the urine of certain amino acids; the urine smells like maple syrup. There are learning difficulties, spasticity and convulsions.

**marasmus** (mə'razməs) severe and chronic malnutrition producing a gradual wasting of the tissues,

owing to insufficient or unassimilated food, occurring especially in infants. It is not always possible to discover the cause.

**Marburg virus disease** ('mahbərg) a Central African viral haemorrhagic fever with acute onset and characteristic morbilliform rash. The incubation period is 3–7 days. It was first reported in Europe in 1967, associated with the importation of green monkeys from Uganda. Since then several isolated incidents have occurred in Africa. The reservoir of infection is not known. Person-to-person transmission by inoculation of blood and tissue fluid and by sexual intercourse has been reported.

**Marfan's syndrome** (mah'fahnz) *B.J. A. Marfan, French paediatrician, 1858–1942.* A hereditary disorder in which there is excessive height with very long digits, a high arched palate, hypertonus and dislocation of the lens of the eyes; heart disease commonly occurs.

**marihuana** (,mari'hwahnə) *Cannabis indica*; Indian hemp or hashish. *See* CANNABIS.

**marrow** ('maroh) the substance contained in the middle of long bones and in the cancellous tissue of all bones. *M. puncture* investigatory procedure in which marrow cells are aspirated from the sternum or iliac crest. *Red m.* that found in all cancellous tissue at birth. Blood cells are made in it. *Yellow m.* the fatty substance contained in the centre of long bones in later life.

**masculinization** (,maskyuhlinie,zayshən) the development in a woman of male secondary sexual characteristics.

**Maslow's hierarchy of needs** ('mazlohz ,hieə.rahkee əv ,needz) *A.H. Maslow, American psychologist, 1908–1970.* A hierarchical ranking, in ascending order of importance, concerning human needs and the

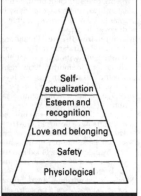

**MASLOW'S HIERARCHY OF NEEDS**

*Self-actualization*

*Esteem and recognition*

*Love and belonging*

*Safety*

*Physiological*

aim of realizing one's full potential. Physiological needs for oxygen, nutrition, shelter, sleep, etc., are the most basic and need to be met first before one is able to deal in successive order with the need for safety, security, love and belonging, self-esteem and ultimately the need for self-actualization (*see* Figure).

**masochism** ('masə‚kizəm) a sexual perversion in which pleasure is derived from suffering mental or physical pain.

**massage** ('masahzh, -sahj) a method of stroking, rubbing, kneading and manipulating the body to stimulate circulation and to promote a sense of wellbeing. *External cardiac m.* the application of rhythmic pressure to the lower sternum to cause expulsion of blood from the ventricles and restart circulation in cases of cardiac arrest.

**masseter** (ma'seetə) the muscle of the cheek chiefly concerned in mastication.

**mast cell** (mahst) a large connective tissue cell found in many body tis-

sues, including the heart, liver and lungs. Mast cells contain granules which release heparin, serotinin and histamine in response to inflammation or allergy.

**mastalgia** (ma'stalji.ə) pain in the breast.

**mastectomy** (ma'stektəmee) amputation of the breast. *Radical m.* removal of the breast, axillary lymph glands and the pectoral muscle.

**mastication** (‚masti'kayshən) the act of chewing food.

**mastitis** (ma'stietis) inflammation of the breast, usually due to bacterial infection.

**mastoid** ('mastoyd) breast- or nipple-shaped. *M. antrum* the cavity in the mastoid process which communicates with the middle ear, and contains air. *M. cells* hollow spaces in the mastoid bone. *M. operation* drainage of mastoid cells when infection spreads from the middle ear. *M. process* the breast-shaped prominence on the temporal bone which projects downwards behind the ear and into which the sternocleidomastoid muscle is inserted.

**mastoidectomy** (‚mastoy'dektəmee) removal of diseased bone and drainage of the mastoid antrum in severe purulent mastoiditis.

**mastoiditis** (‚mastoy'dietis) inflammation of the mastoid antrum and cells.

**masturbation** (‚mastə'bayshən) the production of sexual excitement by friction of the genitals.

**materia medica** (mə‚tiə.ri.ə 'medikə) the science of the source and preparation of drugs used in medicine.

**maternal** (mə'tərn'l) pertaining to the mother. *M. mortality rate* the number of deaths in childbirth per 1000 births.

**matrix** ('maytriks) that tissue in which cells are embedded.

**matter** ('matə) substance. *Grey m.* a collection of nerve cells or non-medullated nerve fibres. *White m.* medullated nerve fibres massed together, as in the brain.

**maturation** (ˌmatyuh'rayshən, ˌma-chuh-) ripening or developing.

**maxilla** (mak'silə) one of the pair of bones forming the upper jaw and carrying the upper teeth.

**maxillary** (mak'silə.ree) pertaining to the upper jawbones.

**maxillofacial** (ˌmaksiloh'fayshəl) pertaining to the maxilla and the face.

**MCHC** mean corpuscular haemoglobin concentration.

**MCV** mean corpuscular volume.

**measles** ('meezəlz) morbilli; rubeola. An acute, infectious, statutorily notifiable disease of childhood caused by a virus spread by droplets. Endemic and worldwide in distribution. Onset is catarrhal before the rash appears on the fourth day. Koplik's spots are diagnostic earlier. Secondary infection may give rise to the serious complication of otitis media or bronchopneumonia. Vaccination provides a high degree of immunity. *German m. see* RUBELLA.

**meatus** (mi'aytəs) an opening or passage. *Auditory m.* the opening leading into the auditory canal. *Urethral m.* the opening of the urethra to the exterior.

**mechanism of labour** ('mekəˌni-zəm) the sequence of movements whereby the fetus adapts itself to pass through the maternal passages during the process of birth.

**Meckel's diverticulum** ('mekəlz) *J. F. Meckel, German anatomist and surgeon, 1781–1833.* The remains of a passage which, in the embryo, connected the yolk sac and intestine, evident as an enclosed sac or tube in the region of the ileum.

**meconium** (mi'kohni.əm) the first intestinal discharges of a newly born child. Dark green and consisting of epithelial cells, mucus and

bile. *M. ileus* intestinal obstruction due to blockage of the bowel by a plug of meconium in a neonate with cystic fibrosis.

**median** ('meedi.ən) 1. placed in the centre. 2. in a series of values, the value middle in position.

**mediastinum** (ˌmeedi.ə'stienəm) the space in the middle of the thorax, between the two pleurae.

**medical** ('medik'l) pertaining to medicine. *M. audit* an evaluative process applied to the quality of clinical practice, often by peer review of routine or specially collected records of individual cases. Judgements are frequently made on the appropriateness of the processes carried out during the management of the case, in light of the outcome. Deaths are frequently the subject of medical audit, two established examples being the Confidential Enquiry into Maternal Deaths (carried out at national level), and local reviews of perinatal deaths. *See* AUDIT. *M. certificate see* MEDICAL STATEMENT below. *M. jurisprudence* medical science as applied to aid the law, e.g. in the case of death by poisoning, violence, etc. *M. laboratory scientific officer* abbreviated MLSO. An allied health professional skilled in the theory and practice of clinical laboratory procedures. *M. model* the traditional approach to the diagnosis and treatment of disease in the Western world. The medical practitioner, using a problem-solving approach, focuses on the disease process and the deficits identified in the body organs and tissues. *M. social worker* a professionally qualified worker who looks after the patients' socioeconomic and welfare needs. *M. statement* replaced the medical certificate in 1976. Advises how long a patient should refrain from work. When the patient is claiming sickness benefit, the statement must be sent to the local social security office. *M. statistics* that branch of statistics concerned with data relating to health and health services. Traditionally these include the use of routine data relating to death, illness and use of hospitals, clinics, etc. The term is also often used to encompass statistics derived from aspects of medical research, such as the conduct of trials of new drugs or procedures.

**medicalization** (ˌmedikˈlieˈzayshən) 1. the extension of medical authority into areas previously regarded as being non-medical, where the lay or a popular approach prevailed, e.g. pregnancy and childbirth. 2. the tendency to view undesirable conduct as illness and therefore requiring medical intervention.

**medicament** (məˈdikəmənt) any medicinal substance used in treatment.

**medicated** (ˈmediˌkaytid) impregnated with a medicinal substance.

**medication** (ˌmediˈkayshən) 1. a substance administered to a patient for therapeutic purposes. 2. the treatment of a patient by means of drugs.

**medicinal** (məˈdisinˈl) 1. having therapeutic qualities. 2. pertaining to a medicine.

**medicine** (ˈmedisin, ˈmedsin) 1. any drug or remedy. 2. the art and science of the diagnosis and treatment of disease and the maintenance of health. 3. the non-surgical treatment of disease. *Community m.* that specialty which deals with all aspects of medical care in the community, including notification and control of infectious diseases, preschool and school health care, and factors affecting the health of the population as a whole. *Emergency m.* that specialty which deals with the acutely ill or injured who

require immediate medical treatment. *Family m.* family practice; the medical specialty concerned with the provision of comprehensive primary health care. *Forensic m.* the application of medical knowledge to questions of law; medical jurisprudence. Also called legal medicine. *Group m.* the practice of medicine by a group of doctors, usually representing various specialties, who are associated together for the cooperative diagnosis, treatment and prevention of disease. *Legal m.* forensic medicine. *Nuclear m.* that branch of medicine concerned with the use of radionuclides in the diagnosis and treatment of disease. *Physical m.* that branch of medicine using physical agents in the diagnosis and treatment of disease. It includes the use of heat, cold, light, water, electricity, manipulation, massage, exercise and mechanical devices. *Preventive m.* the science aimed at preventing disease. *Proprietary m.* any chemical, drug or similar preparation used in the treatment of diseases, if such article is protected against free competition as to name, product, composition or process of manufacture by secrecy, patent, trademark or copyright, or by other means. *Psychosomatic m.* the study of the interrelations between bodily processes and emotional life. *Space m.* that branch of aviation medicine concerned with conditions to be encountered in space. *Sports m.* the field of medicine concerned with injuries sustained in athletic endeavours, including their prevention, diagnosis and treatment.

**medicosocial** (ˌmedikohˈsohshəl) applying to both medicine and the social factors involved.

**medium** (ˈmeediˌəm) in bacteriology, a preparation for the culture of microorganisms. *Contrast m.* a substance used in radiography to make visible structures that could not otherwise be seen.

**medroxyprogesterone** (med,roksi-proh'jestə,rohn) a synthetic female sex hormone used to treat menstrual disorders, endometrial carcinoma and endometriosis, and as a short-term contraceptive.

**medulla** (mə'dulə) 1. bone marrow. 2. the innermost part of an organ, particularly the kidneys, lymph glands and suprarenal glands. *M. oblongata* that portion of the spinal cord that is contained inside the cranium. In it are the nerve centres which govern respiration, the action of the heart, etc.

**medullary** (mə'dulə.ree) pertaining to the marrow or a medulla. *M. cavity* the hollow in the centre of long bones.

**medullated** ('medə,laytid) having a myelin covering. *M. nerve fibre* one enclosed in a myelin sheath.

**medulloblastoma** (mə,dulohbla-'stohmə) a rapidly growing tumour of neuroepithelial origin occurring in childhood and appearing near the fourth ventricle of the brain. The tumour is highly radiosensitive.

**mefenamic acid** (,mefə'namik) an analgesic and antipyretic drug used in the treatment of mild to moderate pain.

**megacolon** (,megə'kohlon) extreme dilatation and hypertrophy of the large intestine. When the condition is congenital it is known as Hirschsprung's disease.

**megakaryocyte** (,megə'karioh,siet) a large cell of the bone marrow, responsible for blood platelet formation.

**megaloblast** ('megəloh,blast) an abnormally large nucleated cell from which mature red blood cells are derived.

**megalocephaly** (,megəloh'kefəlee, -'sef-) 1. abnormal largeness of the head. 2. leontiasis ossea.

**megalomania** (,megəloh'mayni.ə) delusions of grandeur or self-importance characteristic of general paralysis of the insane.

**megaureter** (,megəyuh'reetə) dilatation of the ureter.

**Meibomian cyst** (mie'bohmi.ən) a small swelling of the gland caused by obstruction of its duct. If untreated, it may become infected. A chalazion.

**Meibomian glands** *H. Meibom, German anatomist, 1638–1700.* Small sebaceous glands situated beneath the conjunctiva of the eyelid; tarsal glands.

**meibomianitis** (mie,bohmi.ə'nietis) a bilateral chronic inflammation of the Meibomian glands.

**meiosis** (mie'ohsis) 1. a stage of reduction cell division when the chromosomes of a GAMETE are halved in number ready for union at fertilization. 2. contraction of the pupil of the eye; miosis.

**melaena** (mə'leenə) darkening of the faeces by blood pigments.

**melancholia** (,melən'kohli.ə) a state of extreme DEPRESSION.

**melanin** ('melənin) a dark pigment found in the hair, the choroid of the eye, the skin and in melanotic tumours.

**melanism** ('melə,nizəm) a condition marked by an abnormal deposit of dark pigment in the skin or other tissue. Melanosis.

**melanocyte** ('melənoh,siet) a cell of the skin pigment melanin. *M.-stimulating hormone* abbreviated MSH. Hormone produced in the pituitary gland which stimulates the formation of melanin.

**melanoderma** (,melənoh'dərmə) a patchy pigmentation of the skin.

**melanoma** (,melə'nohmə) a malignant tumour arising in any pigment-containing tissues, especially the skin and the eye. *Amelanotic m.* an unpigmented malignant melanoma. *Juvenile m.* a benign lesion which usually occurs on the face before puberty. May be mistaken for a malignant melanoma.

**melanuria** (ˌmeləˈnyooˌri.ə) the presence of black pigment in the urine. Occurs in melanotic sarcoma and porphyria.

**melasma** (meˈlazmə) dark discoloration of the skin; chloasma.

**melphalan** (ˈmelfələn) a cytotoxic drug that is particularly useful in the treatment of multiple myeloma.

**membrane** (ˈmembrayn) a thin elastic tissue covering the surface of certain organs and lining the cavities of the body. *Basement m.* the interface between epithelial cells and the underlying connective tissue. *Mucous m.* a membrane that secretes mucus and lines all cavities connected directly or indirectly with the skin. *Serous m.* membrane lining the abdominal cavity and thorax and covering most of the organs within.

**memory** (ˈmeməˌree) the mental faculty that enables one to retain and recall previously experienced sensations, impressions, information and ideas. The ability of the brain to retain and to use knowledge gained from past experience is essential to the process of learning. The exact way in which the brain remembers is not completely understood; it is believed that a portion of the temporal lobe of the brain acts as a memory centre, drawing on memories stored in other parts of the brain.

**menarche** (meˈnarkee) the first appearance of menstruation.

**Mendel's theory** (ˈmendˈlz, theeəˈree) *G.J. Mendel, Abbot of Brünn, 1822–1884.* The theory that the characters of sexually reproducing organisms are handed on to the offspring in fixed ratios and without blending.

**Menière's disease** or **syndrome** (ˈmeniˌairz) *P. Menière, French physi-*cian, 1799–1862. A disease of the inner ear causing attacks of vertigo and tinnitus with progressive deafness.

**meninges** (məˈninjeez, ˈmenin-) the membranes covering the brain and spinal cord. There are three: the dura mater (outer), arachnoid mater (middle) and pia mater (inner).

**meningioma** (məˌninjiˈohmə) a slow-growing, usually benign tumour developing from the arachnoid and pia mater.

**meningism** (ˈmeninˌjizəm) a condition in which there are signs of cerebral irritation similar to meningitis but where no causative organism can be isolated.

**meningitis** (ˌmeninˈjietis) inflammation of the meninges due to organisms such as bacteria, viruses and fungi; chemical toxins such as lead and arsenic; contrast media used in myelography; and metastatic malignant cells. Meningitis is a notifiable disease, and its causal organism, if known, should also be stated. *Meningococcal m.* cerebrospinal fever. An epidemic form with a rapid onset caused by *Neisseria meningitidis* infection. *Tuberculous m.* inflammation of tuberculous origin.

**meningocele** (məˈningˌgohˌseel) a protrusion of the meninges through the skull or spinal column, appearing as a cyst filled with cerebrospinal fluid. *See* SPINA (BIFIDA).

**meningococcus** (məˌningˌgohˈkokəs) *Neisseria meningitidis*. A diplococcus, the microorganism of cerebrospinal meningitis.

**meningoencephalitis** (məˌningˌgohˌenˌkefəˈlietis, -ˌsef-) inflammation of the brain and meninges.

**meningomyelocele** (məˌningˌgohˈmieəlohˌseel) a protrusion of the spinal cord and meninges through a defect in the vertebral column. Myelomeningocele. *See* SPINA (BIFIDA).

**meniscectomy** (ˌmenɪˈsektəmeē) surgical removal of a semilunar cartilage from the knee joint.

**meniscus** (məˈnɪskəs) 1. the convex or concave surface of a liquid as observed in its container. 2. a lens having one convex and one concave surface. 3. a semilunar cartilage of the knee joint.

**menopause** (ˈmenəˌpawz) the span of time during which the menstrual cycle wanes and gradually stops; also called change of life and climacteric. It is the period when ovaries stop functioning and therefore menstruation and childbearing cease. Usually occurs between the 45th and 50th years of life. There may be an associated hormonal imbalance which causes symptoms such as night sweats, hot flushes, diminished libido and extreme lethargy. *Artificial m.* an induced cessation of menstruation by surgery or by irradiation.

**menorrhagia** (ˌmenəˈrayjɪ.ə) an excessive flow of the menses; menorrhoea.

**menses** (ˈmenseez) the discharge from the uterus during menstruation.

**menstrual** (ˈmenstrooəl) relating to the menses. *M. cycle* the monthly cycle commencing with the first day of menstruation, when the endometrium is shed, proceeding through a process of repair and hypertrophy till the next period. It is governed by the anterior pituitary gland and the ovarian hormones, oestrogen and progesterone (*see* Figure).

**menstruation** (ˌmenstrooˈayshən) the monthly discharge of blood and endometrium from the uterus, starting at the age of puberty and lasting until the menopause. *Anovular m., anovulatory m.* periodic uterine bleeding without preceding ovulation. *Vicarious m.* discharge of blood at the time of menstruation

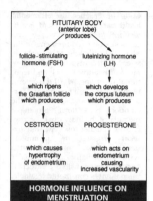

from some organ other than the uterus, e.g. epistaxis, which is not uncommon.

**HORMONE INFLUENCE ON MENSTRUATION**

**mental** (ˈment'l) 1. pertaining to the mind. 2. pertaining to the chin. *M. age* the measurement of the intelligence level of an individual in terms of the average chronological age of children showing the same mental standard, as measured by a scale of mental tests. *M. disorder* a term defined by the Mental Health Acts 1983. The Acts of Parliament govern the care and treatment of the mentally disordered and cover all forms of mental illness and disability including mental impairment and psychopathic disorder. *M. handicap* arrested or incomplete development of mind in which the patient does not require compulsory detention. *M. Health Review Tribunal* a board to whom persons detained under compulsory admission orders or taken into guardianship have the right of appeal at stated intervals for discharge from hospital. Also responsible to the Secretary of State for providing a

Code of Practice for all mental health-care practitioners. *M. health welfare officer* a social worker who carries out the requirements of the Mental Health Acts. *M. hygiene* the science that deals with the development of healthy mental and emotional reactions. *M. illness* a term used to describe a number of disorders of the mind that affect the emotions, perceptions, reasoning or memory of the individual, e.g. psychoses and neuroses. *M. impairment* arrested or incomplete development of mind associated with abnormally aggressive or socially irresponsible conduct. If the patient is considered treatable, hospital admission may be arranged, if necessary compulsorily. *M. mechanism* an unconscious and indirect manner of gratifying a repressed desire. *M. subnormality* this term has been superseded by mental handicap, mental impairment or learning difficulties.

**menthol** ('menthol) a crystalline substance derived from oil of peppermint and used in neuralgia and rhinitis and as a local anodyne and antiseptic.

**mentor** ('mentaw) 1. a wise or trusted adviser or guide. 2. in nursing, a professional colleague who assists with the career development of a colleague, and facilitates and encourages that person's professional growth and awareness.

**mepacrine** ('mepə,krin) a synthetic drug used as an antimalarial agent and in the treatment of giardiasis.

**meprobamate** (mə'prohbə,mayt) a tranquillizer used in the treatment of nervous anxiety.

**mercaptopurine** (mə,kaptoh'pyoo-ə.reen) a drug which prevents nucleic acid synthesis and may be used in the treatment of some types of leukaemia.

**mercury** ('mərkyə.ree) *symbol* Hg. Quicksilver; a heavy liquid metallic element, the salts of which are used occasionally as antiseptics and disinfectants. Also used in the manufacture of various types of thermometer and manometer.

**meridian** (mə'ridiən) a conceptual channel along which qi energy flows in the body. *See* ACUPUNCTURE.

**mescaline** ('meskə,leen) an alkaloid drug which produces intoxication and hallucinations. It is a drug of addiction.

**mesentery** ('mesəntə.ree, 'mez-) a fold of the peritoneum which connects the intestine to the posterior abdominal wall.

**mesmerism** ('mezmə,rizəm) *F.A. Mesmer, Austrian physician, 1734– 1815.* Hypnotism.

**mesoderm** ('mesoh,dərm) the middle of the three primary layers of cells in the embryo from which the connective tissues develop.

**mesometrium** (,mesoh'meetri.əm) the broad ligament connecting the uterus with the abdominal wall.

**mesomorph** ('mesoh,mawf) a stocky individual of medium height with well-developed muscles.

**mesothelioma** (,mesoh,theeli'ohmə) a rapidly growing tumour of the pleura, peritoneum or pericardium which may be seen in patients with asbestosis. However, this tumour may also occur in people who have no history of exposure to asbestos.

**messenger RNA** (,mesinjə) abbreviated mRNA. The ribonucleic acid which acts as a template for the linking of amino acids during the formation of protein in the cells.

**mestranol** ('mestrə,nol) a synthetic oestrogen commonly used in combination with a progesterone in contraceptive pills.

**meta-analysis** (,metə.ə'nalisis) an attempt to improve the findings of research by combining and analysing the results of all discoverable trials on the same subject.

**metabolic** (ˌmetə'bolik) referring to metabolism.

**metabolism** (mə'tabəˌlizəm) the sum of the physical and chemical processes by which living organized substance is built up and maintained (anabolism), and by which large molecules are broken down into smaller molecules to make energy available to the organism (catabolism). Essentially, these processes are concerned with the disposition of the nutrients absorbed into the blood after digestion. *Basal m.* the minimal energy expended for the maintenance of respiration, circulation, peristalsis, muscle tonus, body temperature, glandular activity and the other vegetative functions of the body. *Inborn error of m.* a genetically determined biochemical disorder in which a specific enzyme defect produces a metabolic block that may have pathological consequences at birth, as in phenylketonuria, or in later life.

**metabolite** (mə'tabəˌliet) any product or substance taking part in metabolism. *Essential m.* a substance that is necessary for normal metabolism, e.g. a vitamin.

**metacarpal** (ˌmetə'kahp'l) one of the five bones of the hand which join the fingers to the wrist.

**metacarpophalangeal** (ˌmetəˌkahpohfə'lanji.əl) relating to the metacarpal bones and the phalanges.

**metacarpus** (ˌmetə'kahpəs) the five bones of the hand uniting the carpus with the phalanges of the fingers.

**metamorphosis** (ˌmetə'mawfəsis) a structural change or transformation.

**Metamucil** (ˌmetə'myoosil) tradename for preparations of ispaghula, a bulk laxative.

**metaphase** ('metəˌfayz) the second stage of mitosis or cell division.

**metaphysis** (mə'tafisis) the junction of the epiphysis with the diaphysis in a long bone.

**metaplasia** (ˌmetə'playzi.ə) abnormal change in the structure of a tissue. May be indicative of malignant change.

**metastasis** (mə'tastəsis) the transfer of a disease from one part of the body to another, through the blood vessels, via the lymph channels or across the body cavities. Secondary deposits may occur from a primary malignant growth. Septic infection may arise in other organs from some original focus.

**metatarsal** (ˌmetə'tahs'l) one of the five bones of the foot which join the tarsus to the toes.

**metatarsalgia** (ˌmetətah'salji.ə) pain in the metatarsal bones.

**metatarsus** (ˌmetə'tahsəs) the five bones of the foot uniting the tarsus with the phalanges of the toes.

**Metazoa** (ˌmetə'zoh.ə) the division of the animal kingdom that includes the multicellular animals, i.e. all animals except the PROTO-ZOA.

**metformin** (met'fawmin) a biguanide hypoglycaemic used in the treatment of diabetes mellitus.

**methadone** ('methəˌdohn) a powerful analgesic with no sedative action. Similar in action to morphine, it is used to relieve pain in terminal illness and also in withdrawal programmes for heroin addicts. Methadone is addictive, but less socially disabling than heroin. Amidone.

**methaemalbumin** (ˌmet.heem'albyoomin) a compound of haem with plasma albumin found in the blood in some types of anaemia.

**methaemoglobin** (ˌmet.heemə'glohbin) an altered form of haemoglobin found in the blood and usually produced by the action of a drug on the red blood corpuscles, causing a reduction in their oxygen-carrying ability. May be associated with the use of phenacetin and other aniline derivatives.

**methaemoglobinaemia** (ˌmet-
ˌheeməˌglohbiˈneemi.ə) cyanosis
and inability of the red blood cells
to transport oxygen owing to the
presence of methaemoglobin.

**methane** ('meethayn) marsh gas; an
inflammable explosive gas produced by decomposition of organic
matter.

**methicillin** (ˌmethiˈsilin) a form of
penicillin that is resistant to staphylococcal penicillinase. *M. resistant
Staphylococcus aureus* abbreviated
MRSA. A strain of *S. aureus* that is
distinguished from others by its
resistance to the special beta-lactose
drugs ('methicillin-like' drugs) that
are usually used to treat these
organisms. MRSA can affect people
in different ways. People can carry
the organism in the nose or on
the skin without showing any
symptoms of illness. This is called
MRSA colonization. MRSA also can
cause infections such as boils,
wound infections or infected decubitus ulcers. There is no evidence
that properly treated infections
caused by MRSA are more or less
serious than other *S. aureus* infections. MRSA is spread from person
to person by direct contact. This
means that if persons have MRSA
on their skin (especially on the
hands) and touch another individual, they may spread MRSA. A
person may have MRSA on the
hands as a result of being a carrier
or from touching another person
who is a carrier or infected with
MRSA. General infection control
measures are appropriate for preventing spread. Persons who are
colonized with MRSA do not usually need to be treated but in severe
MRSA infections VANCOMYCIN is
given intravenously. It can have
severe side-effects.

**methionine** (meˈthieohˌneen) 1. a
sulphur-containing essential amino
acid occurring in proteins that is a

vital component of the diet. 2. a
drug used orally in the treatment of
paracetamol poisoning.

**methohexitone** (ˌmethohˈheksi-
tohn) a barbiturate anaesthetic
agent; given intravenously it has a
quick recovery time.

**methotrexate** (ˌmethohˈtreksayt) a
cytotoxic drug that antagonizes
folic acid and prevents cell formation. It is used to treat various types
of malignant disease.

**methotrimeprazine** (ˌmethohtrie-
ˈmeprəzeen) a phenothiazine with
sedative and analgesic properties.
Useful in schizophrenia and terminal illness.

**methoxamine** (meˈthoksəˌmeen) a
sympathomimetic amine used for
its vasopressor effects in restoring
blood pressure during anaesthesia.

**methyl salicylate** (ˌmethil səˈlisi-
ˌlayt, ˌmeethiel) a compound used
externally for rheumatic pains,
lumbago, etc. Oil of wintergreen.

**methylated spirit** (ˌmethiˌlaytid
'spirit) a mixture of 95% ethyl alcohol and 5% methyl alcohol. An
industrial spirit which, taken as a
drink, is poisonous.

**methylcellulose** (ˌmethilˈselyuh-
lohs, -lohz) a bulk-forming drug
used as a laxative and to control
diarrhoea.

**methyldopa** (ˌmethilˈdohpə) a hypotensive drug whose action is increased if used with thiazide
diuretics.

**methylene blue** ('methiˌleen) a synthetic organic compound, in
darkgreen crystals or lustrous crystalline powder, used in treatment of
methaemoglobinaemia, as an antidote in cyanide poisoning, as a
stain in pathology and bacteriology,
and as an antiseptic.

**methylphenobarbitone** (ˌmethilˌfe-
nohˈbahbitohn) a white crystalline
powder used as an anticonvulsant
with a slight hypnotic action. Especially useful for senile tremor.

**methylprednisolone** (ˌmethilpred-ˈnisəˌlohn) a corticosteroid of the glucogenic type, having an anti-inflammatory action similar to that of prednisolone.

**methysergide** (ˌmethiˈsərjied) a potent serotonin antagonist used in the prophylaxis of migraine.

**metoclopramide** (ˌmetohˈklohprə-mied) a drug which speeds up gastric action and is used to treat nausea, heartburn and vomiting.

**metoprolol** (meˈtohprəˌlol) a cardioselective beta blocker having a greater effect on $\beta_1$-adrenergic receptors of the heart than on the $\beta_2$-adrenergic receptors of the bronchi and blood vessels; used for treatment of hypertension. *See* BETA (BLOCKERS).

**metra** (ˈmeetrə) the uterus.

**metre** (ˈmeetə) *symbol* m. The fundamental SI unit of length.

**metritis** (miˈtrietis) inflammation of the uterus.

**metrocolpocele** (ˌmeetrohˈkolpoh-ˌseel) the protrusion of the uterus into the vagina, the wall of the latter also being pushed forwards.

**metronidazole** (ˌmetrohˈnidəˌzohl) a drug that is effective in overcoming *Trichomonas* infection of the genital tract of both sexes. Also used in the treatment of giardiasis, of acute amoebic dysentery and of infection by anaerobic bacteria.

**metrorrhagia** (ˌmeetrəˈrayjiə) irregular uterine bleeding not associated with menstruation.

**mexiletine** (mekˈsiliteen) an antiarrhythmic agent used to treat ventricular arrhythmias.

**mg** milligram(s).

**Mg** Symbol for *magnesium*.

**Michel's suture clips** (miˈshelz) *G. Michel, French surgeon, 1875–1937.* Small metal clips used for suturing wounds.

**miconazole** (mieˈkonəˌzohl) an antifungal agent used topically for dermatophytic infections such as athlete's foot or vulvovaginal candidiasis, orally for candidiasis of the mouth and gastrointestinal tract, and systemically by intravenous infusion for systemic fungal infections.

**microbe** (ˈmiekrohb) a minute living organism, especially one causing disease. A microorganism.

**microbiology** (ˌmiekrohbieˈolǝjee) the study of microorganisms and their effect on living cells.

**microcephalic** (ˌmiekrohkəˈfalik, -sə-) having an abnormally small head.

*Micrococcus* (ˌmiekrohˈkokəs) a genus of bacteria, each of which has a spherical shape. The bacteria occur in pairs or in groups and are Gram-positive. Found in soil and water.

**microcythaemia** (ˌmiekrohsieˈthee-miǝ) the presence of abnormally small red cells in the blood; microcytosis.

**micrognathia** (ˌmiekrohˈnathiə) failure of development of the lower jaw, causing a receding chin.

**microgram** (ˈmiekrohˌgram) *symbol* µg. One millionth of a gram.

**micrometre** (ˈmiekrohmeetə) *symbol* µm. One millionth of a metre. Formerly called micron.

**micron** (ˈmiekron) *see* MICROMETRE.

**micronutrient** (ˌmiekrohˈnyootri-ˌənt) a dietary element essential only in small quantities.

**microorganism** (ˌmiekrohˈawgəˌnizəm) a minute animal or vegetable, particularly a virus, a bacterium, a fungus, a rickettsia or a protozoon.

**microphage** (ˈmiekrohˌfayj) a minute phagocyte.

**microphthalmos** (ˌmiekrofˈthalməs) a condition in which one or both eyes are smaller than normal. Their function may or may not be impaired.

**microscope** (ˈmiekrəˌskohp) an instrument which produces a greatly enlarged image of objects that are normally invisible to the human eye. *Electron m.* a microscope in which a beam of electrons is used instead of a light beam, allowing magnification of as much as 500 000 diameters.

**microscopic** (ˌmiekrəˈskopik) visible only by means of the microscope. The opposite of macroscopic.

*Microsporum* (ˌmiekrohˈspor.rəm) a genus of fungi. The cause of some skin diseases, especially ringworm.

**microsurgery** (ˌmiekrohˈsərjə.ree) the carrying out of surgical procedures using a microscope and miniature instruments.

**micturition** (ˌmiktyuhˈrishən) the act of passing urine.

**midbrain** (ˈmidˌbrayn) that portion of the brain that connects the cerebrum with the pons and cerebellum.

**midlife crisis** (ˈmidˈlief ˈkriesis) experienced by many people during the fifth decade of life, resulting in doubt, anxiety and sometimes depression. During this time men and women may reflect on their lives, review the past and be aware of physiological deterioration associated with ageing. Any children are growing up, moving away from home and establishing their own adult relationships. Empty nest syndrome.

**midwife** (ˈmidˌwief) the title and legal description of a person who is so certified under the MIDWIVES ACTS.

**midwifery** (midˈwifə.ree, ˈmidˌwifə.ree) the art and science of caring for women undergoing normal pregnancy, labour and the period following childbirth (usually 6–8 weeks). *M. process* the application of the nursing process to midwifery. It is the systematic, cyclical method of organizing midwifery care, and is carried out by the assessment of actual and potential problems, and the planning, implementation and evaluation of care.

**Midwife's Code of Practice (1994)** a code issued by the UK Central Council for Nurses, Midwives and Health Visitors (UKCC) as guidance to all midwives practising in the UK. It is not a legal document but failure to comply with its guidance may, in the event of a disciplinary hearing before the UKCC, be used in evidence against the midwife. It covers matters directly relating to the Midwives' Practice Rules, and advice on home births, complementary and alternative therapies, arranging for a substitute, and maternal, intrauterine and neonatal death, as well as notes on other legislation relevant to the practice of a midwife.

**Midwives Acts** (aktz) a number of Acts of Parliament to regulate the practice of midwives, passed in the years 1902, 1918, 1926 and 1936. All this legislation was consolidated by the Midwives Act 1951. The Nurses, Midwives and Health Visitors Acts of 1979 and 1992 replaced the former Midwives Acts, and established a new statutory structure for nursing, midwifery and health visiting in the UK.

**migraine** (ˈmeegrayn, ˈmie-) paroxysmal attacks of severe headache, often with nausea, vomiting and visual disturbance.

**Migravess** (ˈmiegrəves) trade name for combination preparations containing aspirin and metoclopramide, used in migraine.

**Migril** (ˈmiegril) trade name for a combination preparation containing ergotamine, cyclizine and caffeine, used in migraine attacks.

**milestone** (ˈmielˌstohn) one of the 'norms' against which the motor, social and psychological development of a child is measured.

**miliaria** (ˌmiliˈair.ri.ə) prickly heat, an acute itching eruption common among white people in tropical and subtropical areas.

| COMPOSITION OF MILK (%) | | |
|---|---|---|
| | Cows' milk | Human milk |
| Protein | 3.5 | 2.0 |
| Fats | 3.5 | 3.5 |
| Carbohydrates | 4.0 | 6.0 |
| Mineral salts | 0.7 | 0.2 |
| Water | 88.0 | 88.0 |

**miliary** ('milyə.ree) resembling millet seed. *M. tuberculosis see* TUBERCULOSIS.

**milium** ('mili.əm) [L.] a whitish nodule in the skin, especially of the face, usually 1–4 mm in diameter. Milia are spheroidal, epithelial cysts of lamellated keratin lying just under the epidermis, often associated with vellus hair follicles. Popularly called whitehead.

**milk** (milk) 1. a nutrient fluid produced by the mammary gland of many animals for nourishment of young mammals (*see* Table). 2. a liquid (emulsion or suspension) resembling the secretion of the mammary gland. *M. sugar* lactose, a disaccharide present in the milk of all mammals. *M. teeth* the first set of teeth. *Witch's m.* milk secreted from the breast of a newborn child.

**Miller–Abbott tube** (.milə'abət .tyoob) *T.G. Miller, American physician, 1886–1981; W.O. Abbott, American physician, 1902–1943.* A double-channel intestinal tube for treating obstruction, especially that due to paralytic ileus of the small intestine. It has an inflatable balloon at its distal end.

**milligram** ('mili.gram) *symbol* mg. One thousandth of a gram.

**millilitre** ('mili.leetə) *symbol* ml. One thousandth of a litre (one cubic centimetre).

**millimetre** ('mili.meetə) *symbol* mm. One thousandth of a metre.

**millimole** ('mili.mohl) *symbol* mmol. The amount of a sub-

stance that balances or is equivalent in combining power to 1 mg of hydrogen. A method of assessing the body's acid–base balance or needs during electrolyte upset.

**Millipore filter** ('mili.por) trade name for a device used to filter nutrient solutions as they are administered intravenously.

**Milton** ('miltən) trade name for an antiseptic consisting of a standardized 1% solution of electrolytic sodium hypochlorite. It is used especially for the sterilization of babies' feeding bottles and teats in the home.

**Milwaukee brace** (mil'wawkee) a brace consisting of a leather girdle and neck ring connected by metal struts; used to brace the spine in the treatment of SCOLIOSIS.

**mineralocorticoid** (.minə.rəloh'kawti.koyd) a hormone produced by the adrenal cortex. Its function is to maintain the salt and water balance in the body.

**Minims** (minimz) trade name for eye drops packaged in single-use containers.

**minocycline** (.minoh'siekleen) a semisynthetic broad-spectrum antibiotic of the tetracycline group.

**miosis** (mie'ohsis) contraction of the pupil of the eye, as in reaction to a bright light; meiosis.

**miotic** (mie'otik) a drug which causes contraction of the pupil.

**miscarriage** ('miskarij) abortion; the expulsion of the fetus before the

24th week of pregnancy, i.e. before it is legally viable.

**Misuse of Drugs Act (1971)** (mis-yoos əv 'drugz akt) came into effect in 1973 to control the possession, prescription and sale of certain habit-forming drugs, including narcotic drugs such as papaveretum (Omnopon), cocaine, morphine, diamorphine, cannabis indica and amphetamines. These are called controlled drugs and are available for treatment only on medical prescription. Heavy penalties invariably follow the illegal sale or supply of these drugs.

**mite** (miet) a minute animal, frequently parasitic on humans and animals, and causing various forms of dermatitis.

**mithramycin** (ˌmithrə'miesin) an antitumour antibiotic which is particularly helpful in the treatment of hypercalcaemia.

**mitochondrion** (ˌmietoh'kondri.ən) a body which is found in the cytoplasm of cells and is concerned with energy production and the oxidation of food.

**mitomycin C** (ˌmietoh'miesin) a highly toxic antineoplastic; indicated for palliative treatment of certain neoplasms that do not respond to surgery radiation and other drugs.

**mitosis** (mie'tohsis) a method of multiplication of cells by a specific process of division.

**mitral** ('mietrəl) shaped like a mitre. *M. incompetence* the result of a defective mitral valve, when there is a back flow, or regurgitation, after closure of the valve. *M. stenosis* the formation of fibrous tissue, causing a narrowing of the valve; usually due to rheumatic heart disease and endocarditis. *M. valve* the bicuspid valve between the left atrium and left ventricle of the heart. *M. valvotomy* an operation for overcoming stenosis by dividing the fibrous tissue to free the cusps.

**mittelschmerz** ('mit'l shmərts) pain occurring between the menses, accompanying ovulation.

**ml** millilitre(s).

**MLSO** medical laboratory scientific officer.

**mm** millimetre(s).

**mmol** millimole(s).

**Mn** symbol for *manganese*.

**mobilization** (ˌmohbilie'zayshən) the bringing back into mobility of a limb, joint or person following illness or injury.

**molar** ('mohlə) a back tooth used for grinding. There are three on either side of each jaw, making 12 in all (only eight in children). *M. solution* the concentration of a solution expressed in terms of the weight of the dissolved substance in grams per litre divided by its molecular weight.

**mole** (mohl) 1. the molecular weight of a substance expressed in grams. 2. a pigmented naevus or dark-coloured growth on the skin. Moles are of various sizes, and are sometimes covered with hair. 3. a uterine tumour. *Carneous m.* an organized blood clot surrounding a shrivelled fetus in the uterus. *Hydatidiform m.* (*vesicular m.*) a condition in pregnancy in which the chorionic villi of the placenta degenerate into clusters of cysts like hydatids. Malignant growth may follow if any remnants are left in the uterus. *See* CHORIOCARCINOMA.

**molecular** (mə'lekyuhlə) pertaining to or composed of molecules. *M. weight* the weight of a molecule of a substance compared with that of an atom of carbon.

**molecule** ('moli.kyool) the chemical combination of two or more atoms which form a specific chemical substance, e.g. $H_2O$ (water). The smallest amount of a substance that can exist independently.

**molluscum** (mo'luskəm) a skin disease characterized by the development of soft, round tumours. *M. contagiosum* a benign tumour arising in the epidermis caused by a virus, transmitted by direct contact or fomites.

**monarticular** (ˌmonahˈtikyuhlə) referring to one joint only.

**mongolism** ('mongə̩lizəm) outdated term for Down's syndrome.

*Monilia* (moˈniliə) former name for the genus of fungi now known as *Candida*.

**monitor** ('monitə) 1. to check constantly on a given condition, state or phenomenon, e.g. blood pressure, heart, respiration rate or standards of care. 2. an apparatus by which such conditions or phenomena can be constantly observed and recorded. *Patient m.* the use of electrodes or transducers attached to the patient so that information such as temperature, pulse, respiration and blood pressure can be seen on a screen or automatically recorded.

**Monitor** ('monitə) an adaptation for the UK of the USA Rush Medicus system of assessing quality of nursing care. It consists of 'checklists' for quality, leading to a scoring system. The closer the score to 100%, the better the care being given. The master list has over 200 criteria which are divided into four categories based on patient dependency levels. A paediatric version is available: Junior Monitor.

**monoamine oxidase** (ˌmonohˈaymeen 'oksidayz) an enzyme that breaks down noradrenaline and serotonin in the body. *M. o. inhibitor* abbreviated MAOI. A drug that prevents the breakdown of serotonin and leads to an increase in mental and physical activity.

**monochromatism** (ˌmonohˈkrohmə̩tizəm) colour blindness. The patient sees all colours as black, grey or white.

**monoclonal** (ˌmonohˈklohnˈl) derived from a single cell. *M. anti-*

*bodies* antibodies derived from a single clone of cells. All the antibody molecules are identical and will react with the same antigenic site.

**monocular** (moˈnokyuhlə) pertaining to, or affecting, one eye only.

**monocyte** ('monohˌsiet) a white blood cell having one nucleus, derived from the reticular cells, and having a phagocytic action.

**mononucleosis** (ˌmonohˌnyookli'ohsis) an excessive number of monocytes in the blood; monocytosis. *Infectious m.* an infectious disease due to the Epstein–Barr virus; glandular fever.

**monoplegia** (ˌmonohˈpleejiə) paralysis of one limb or of a single muscle or a group of muscles.

**monosaccharide** (ˌmonohˈsakəˌ ried) a simple sugar. The end result of carbohydrate digestion. Examples are glucose, fructose and galactose.

**monosodium glutamate** (ˌmonohˌsohdi.əm 'glootə̩mayt) a chemical food flavour enhancer commonly added to Chinese dishes. May result in nausea, faintness, facial flushing and headache (sometimes called the Chinese restaurant syndrome).

**monosomy** (ˌmonoh'sohmee) a congenital defect in the number of human chromosomes. There is one less than the normal 46.

**mons** (monz) a prominence or mound. *M. pubis* or *m. veneris* the eminence, consisting of a pad of fat, that lies over the pubic symphysis in the female.

**Montgomery's glands** or **tubercles** (məntˈgoməˌriz) *W.F. Montgomery, Irish obstetrician, 1797–1859.* Sebaceous glands around the nipple, which grow larger during pregnancy.

**mood** (mood) emotional reaction. Variations in mood are natural, but in certain psychiatric conditions there is severe depression in some cases and wild excitement in others, or alternations between both.

**moon face** ('moon ˌfays) one of the features occurring in Cushing's syndrome and as a result of prolonged treatment with steroid drugs.

**morbid** ('mawbid) diseased, or relating to an abnormal or disordered condition.

**morbidity** (maw'biditee) the state of being diseased. **M. rate** a figure that shows the susceptibility of a population to a certain disease. Usually shown statistically as the number of cases which occur annually per 1000 or other unit of population.

**morbilli** (mor'bilie) measles.

**morbilliform** (morˈbiliˌfawm) resembling measles.

**moribund** ('moˌriˌbund) in a dying condition.

**morning sickness** ('morning ˌsiknəs) nausea and vomiting which sometimes occurs in early pregnancy.

**Moro reflex** ('moˌroh) *E. Moro, German paediatrician, 1874–1951.* The reaction to loud noise or sudden movement which should be present in the newborn. Startle reflex.

**morphine** ('mawfeen) the principal alkaloid obtained from opium and given mainly to relieve severe pain. It is a drug of addiction. Morphia.

**mortality** (maw'talitee) the state of being liable to die. **M. rate** the number of deaths, per 1000 or other unit of population, occurring annually from a certain disease or condition.

**mortification** (ˌmawtifiˈkayshən) gangrene or death of tissue; necrosis.

**morula** ('moˌryuhlə) an early stage of development of the ovum when it is a solid mass of cells.

**mosaic** (moh'zayik) an individual who has cells of varying genetic composition.

**motile** ('mohtiel) capable of movement.

**motion** ('mohshən) 1. the process of moving. 2. evacuation of the bowels; defecation. **M. sickness** sickness occurring as the result of travel by land, sea or air. Appears to be caused by excessive stimulation of the vestibular apparatus within the inner ear.

**motivation** (ˌmohti'vayshən) the reason or reasons, conscious or unconscious, behind a particular attitude or behaviour.

**motive** ('mohtiv) the incentive that determines a course of action or its direction.

**motor** ('mohtə) something that causes movement. **M. end-plate** the nuclei and cytoplasm of muscle fibres at the termination of motor nerves. **M. nerve** one of the nerves which convey an impulse from a nerve centre to a muscle or gland to promote activity. **M. neurone disease** a disease in which there is progressive degeneration of the anterior cells in the spinal cord, the motor nuclei of cranial nerves and the corticospinal tracts. The cause is unknown.

**mould** (mohld) 1. a species of fungus. 2. the plastic shell used to immobilize a part of the body, usually the head, during radiotherapy.

**moulding** ('mohlding) the alteration in shape of the infant's head as it is forced through the maternal passages during labour.

**mountain sickness** ('mowntin ˌsiknəs) dyspnoea, headache, rapid pulse and vomiting, which occur on sudden change to the rarefied air of high altitudes.

**mouth** (mowth) an opening, particularly the external opening (in the face) of the alimentary canal. **M. ulcers** painful, greyish-white sores occurring inside the mouth. Most are of unknown cause and usually disappear after a few days. Aphthous ulcers. **M.-wash** a solution for rinsing the mouth.

**movement** ('moovmənt) 1. an act of moving; motion. 2. an act of defecation. *Active m.* movement produced by the person's own muscles. *Associated m.* movement of parts that act together, as the eyes. *Passive m.* a movement of the body or of the extremities of a patient performed by another person without voluntary motion on the part of the patient. *Vermicular m's* the worm-like movements of the intestines in peristalsis.

**MRI** magnetic resonance imaging.

**MRSA** methicillin-resistant *Staphylococcus aureus.*

**mucinase** ('myoosi,nayz) an enzyme which acts upon mucin. Contained in some aerosols and useful in the treatment of cystic fibrosis.

**mucocele** ('myookoh,seel) a mucous tumour. *Lacrimal m.* a distension of the lacrimal sac caused by a blockage of the nasolacrimal duct. *M. of the gallbladder* occurs if a stone obstructs the cystic duct.

**mucocutaneous** (,myookohkyoo-'tayni.əs) pertaining to mucous membrane and skin.

**mucoid** ('myookoyd) resembling mucus.

**mucolytic** (,myookoh'litik) a drug that has a mucous-softening effect and so reduces the viscosity of the bronchial secretion in chest disorders.

**mucopurulent** (,myookoh'pyooə.rə-lənt) containing mucus and pus.

**mucosa** (myoo'kohsə) mucous membrane.

**mucous** ('myookəs) pertaining to or secreting mucus. *M. membrane* a membrane that secretes mucus and lines many of the body cavities, particularly those of the respiratory and alimentary tracts.

**mucoviscidosis** (,myookoh,visi-'dohsis) fibrocystic disease of the pancreas. *See* FIBROCYSTIC.

**mucus** ('myookəs) the viscous secretion of mucous membrane.

**multicellular** (,multi'selyuhlə) consisting of many cells.

**multidisciplinary** (,multi'disi-,plinəree) involving two or more professional disciplines.

**multigravida** (,multi'gravidə) a pregnant woman who has had two or more pregnancies.

**multilocular** (,multi'lokyuhlə) having many locules. *M. cyst* a cyst, usually in the ovary, containing many compartments.

**multinuclear** (,multi'nyookli.ə) possessing many nuclei.

**multipara** (mul'tipə.rə) a woman who has had two or more children.

**multiple** ('multip'l) manifold, occurring in many parts of the body at once. *M. myeloma* malignant disease of the plasma cells which invade the bone marrow and suppress its functioning. *M. sclerosis* See SCLEROSIS.

**multivariate analysis** (,multi'vai-reeət ə'nalisis) the analysis of data collected on several different variables but all having a relevance to the study; e.g. in a survey of the provision of community nursing services for a specific population, data may be collected on age, family size and previous use of the services. In analysing the data the effect of each of these variables and their interaction can be examined and considered.

**multivitamin** (,multi'vitamin) a brown, sugar-coated tablet containing vitamin A (2500 units), thiamine hydrochloride (500 μg), ascorbic acid (12.5 mg) and vitamin D (250 units).

**mumps** (mumps) a communicable paramyxovirus disease, which is statutorily notifiable. It attacks one or both of the parotid glands, the largest of the three pairs of salivary glands; also called epidemic parotitis or epidemic parotiditis. Most common amongst children; characterized by inflammation and swelling of the parotid glands. The symptoms are fever, and a painful swelling in front of the ears, making mastication difficult.

**Münchhausen's syndrome** ('muhn-chowzənz) *Baron von Münchhausen, 16th century German traveller noted for his lying tales.* Habitual seeking of hospital treatment for apparent acute illness, the patient giving a plausible and dramatic history, all of which is false. **M. s. by proxy** an uncommon situation in which a parent (usually the mother) or both parents fabricate symptoms or signs in a child, who is then presented for hospital treatment; overlaps with other forms of child abuse, and fatal outcomes have been reported.

**murmur** ('mərmə) a sound, heard on auscultation, usually originating in the cardiovascular system. *Aortic m.* one indicating disease of the aortic valve. *Diastolic m.* one heard after the second heart sound. *Friction m.* one present when two inflamed surfaces of serous membrane rub on each other. *Mitral m.* a sign of incompetence of the mitral valve. *Systolic m.* one heard during systole.

**Murphy's sign** ('mərfeez) *J.B. Murphy, American surgeon, 1857–1916.* A sign denoting inflammation of the gallbladder. Continuous pressure over the organ will cause the patient to 'catch breath' at the zenith of inspiration.

**muscae volitantes** ('muskee ˌvolitanteez) black spots floating before the eyes. They do not obscure the sight.

**muscarine** ('muskə.reen) a poisonous alkaloid found in certain fungi, and causing muscle paralysis.

**muscle** ('mus'l) strong tissue composed of fibres which have the power of contraction, and thus produce movements of the body. *Cardiac m.* muscle composed of

partially striped interlocking cells. Not under the control of the will. *M. relaxant* one of a group of drugs used to reduce muscular spasm and also to relax the muscles during surgery. *Smooth* or *non-striated m.* involuntary muscle of spindle-shaped cells, e.g. that of the intestinal wall. Contracts independently of the will. *Striped* or *striated m.* voluntary muscle. Transverse bands across the fibres give the characteristic appearance. It is under the control of the will.

**muscular** ('muskyuhlə) 1. pertaining to muscle. 2. well provided with strong muscles. *M. dystrophy* one of a number of inherited diseases in which there is progressive muscle wasting. *See* DUCHENNE DYSTROPHY.

**musculocutaneous** (ˌmuskyuhloh-kyoo'tayni.əs) referring to the muscles and the skin. *M. nerve* one of the nerves which supply the muscles and the skin of the arms and legs.

**musculoskeletal** (ˌmuskyuhloh-'skelit'l) referring to both the osseus and muscular systems.

**mustine hydrochloride** (ˌmusteen ˌhiedrə'klor.ried) nitrogen mustard. A cytotoxic drug which may be given intravenously for malignant disease of lymph glands and reticuloendothelial cells, such as Hodgkin's disease.

**mutant** ('myootənt) 1. in genetics, a variation owing to genetic changes. 2. produced by mutation.

**mutation** (myoo'tayshən) a chemical change in the genes of a cell causing it to show a new characteristic. Some produce evolutionary changes, others disease.

**mute** (myoot) without the power of speech. *Deaf m.* one who cannot hear and therefore cannot speak.

**mutilation** (ˌmyooti'layshən) deliberate infliction of bodily injury.

**mutism** ('myootizəm) inability or refusal to speak. In almost all cases, mutes are unable to speak because deafness has prevented them from hearing the spoken word. Speech is learned by imitating the speech of others. May also result from disease, the most common being a stroke. *Elective m.* psychological disorder of childhood.

**myalgia** (mie'alji.ə) pain in the muscles.

**myasthenia** (ˌmieəs'theeni.ə) muscle weakness. *M. gravis* an extreme form of muscle weakness which is progressive. There is a rapid onset of fatigue, thought to be due to the too rapid destruction of acetylcholine at the neuromuscular junction. Commonly affected muscles are those of vision, speaking, chewing and swallowing.

**mycetoma** (ˌmiesi'tohmə) a chronic fungus infection of the tissues, both external and internal but most commonly affecting the hands and feet. There is swelling and the formation of sinuses. Madura foot.

*Mycobacterium* (ˌmiekohbak'tiə.ri.əm) a genus of slender, rod-shaped, acid-fast, Gram-positive bacteria. *M. leprae* the causative organism of leprosy. *M. tuberculosis* the cause of tuberculosis.

**mycology** (mie'koləjee) the study of fungi.

**mycosis** (mie'kohsis) any disease that is caused by a fungus. *M. fungoides* a rare malignant lymphoreticular neoplasm of the skin which later progresses to the lymph nodes and viscera.

**mydriasis** (mi'drieəsis, mie-) abnormal dilatation of the pupil of the eye. Usually caused by injury to the pupil sphincter or by the use of mydriatic drugs.

**mydriatic** (ˌmidri'atik) any drug that causes mydriasis. Used in examination of the eye and in the treatment of inflammatory conditions.

**myelin** ('mieəlin) the fatty covering of medullated nerve fibres.

**myelitis** (ˌmieə'lietis) 1. inflammation of the spinal cord, causing pain in the back and sometimes numbness and paralysis of the legs and the lower part of the trunk. 2. inflammation of the bone marrow; osteomyelitis.

**myeloblast** ('mieəloh,blast) a primitive cell in the bone marrow, from which develop the granular leukocytes.

**myelocyte** ('mieəloh,siet) a cell of the bone marrow, derived from a myeloblast.

**myelography** (ˌmieə'logrəfee) radiographic examination of the spinal cord after the introduction of a radio-opaque substance into the subarachnoid space by means of lumbar puncture.

**myeloid** ('mieə,loyd) 1. pertaining to, derived from or resembling bone marrow. 2. pertaining to the spinal cord. 3. having the appearance of myelocytes, but not necessarily derived from bone marrow. *M. leukaemia* a malignant disease in which there is excessive production of leukocytes in the bone marrow. *M. tissue* red bone marrow.

**myeloma** (ˌmieə'lohmə) a tumour composed of plasma cells. *Multiple m.* a primary malignant tumour of plasma cells, usually arising in bone marrow, and usually associated with anaemia and with a para protein in the blood or Bence Jones protein in the urine.

**myelomatosis** (ˌmieəlohmə'tohsis) a malignant disease of the bone marrow in which multiple myelomas are present.

**myelomeningocele** (ˌmieəlohmə-'ning.goh,seel) meningomyelocele.

**myiasis** (mie'ieəsis) infestation of wounds or body openings by fly larvae (maggots); more commonly seen in the tropics.

**myocardial** (ˌmieoh'kahdi.əl) pertaining to the myocardium. *M.*

*infarction* necrosis of a part of the myocardium, usually following a coronary thrombosis. Ventricular fibrillation may occur, followed by death.

**myocarditis** (͵mieohkah'dietis) inflammation of the myocardium.

**myocardium** (͵mieoh'kahdi.əm) the muscle tissue of the heart.

**myoclonus** (͵mieoh'klohnəs) spasmodic contraction of the muscles.

**myofibrosis** (͵mieohfie'brohsis) a degenerative condition in which there is some replacement of muscle tissue by fibrous tissue.

**myohaemoglobin** (͵mieoh͵heemə-'glohbin) a substance, resembling haemoglobin, which is present in muscle cells. It is a pigment and is responsible for the colour of muscle. It acts as an oxygen store. Myoglobin.

**myokymia** (͵mieoh͵kimi.ə) a benign condition in which there is persistent quivering of the muscles.

**myoma** (mie'ohmə) a benign tumour of muscle tissue. *See* FIBROMYOMA.

**myomectomy** (͵mieə'mektəmee) removal of a myoma; usually referring to a uterine fibroma.

**myometrium** (͵mieoh'meetri.əm) the muscular tissue of the uterus.

**myoneural** (͵mieoh'nyooə.rəl) relating to both muscle and nerve. *M. junction* the point at which nerve endings terminate in a muscle; neuromuscular junction.

**myopathy** (mie'opəthee) any disease of the muscles. Muscular dystrophy is one of a group of inherited myopathies in which there is wasting and weakness of the muscles.

**myopia** (mie'ohpi.ə) shortsightedness. The light rays focus in front of the retina and a biconcave lens is needed to focus them correctly.

**myoplasty** ('mieoh͵plastee) any operation in which muscle is detached and utilized, as may be done to correct deformities.

**myosarcoma** (͵mieohsah'kohmə) a sarcomatous tumour of muscle.

**myosin** ('mieəsin) muscle protein.

**myositis** (͵mieoh'sietis) inflammation of a muscle. *M. ossificans* a condition in which bone cells deposited in muscle continue to grow and cause hard lumps. It may occur after fractures.

**myotomy** (mie'otəmee) the division or dissection of a muscle.

**myotonia** (͵mieə'tohni.ə) lack of muscle tone. *M. congenita* a hereditary disease in which the muscle action has a prolonged contraction phase and slow relaxation.

**myringa** (mi'ring.gə) the eardrum or tympanic membrane.

**myringitis** (͵mirin'jietis) inflammation of the tympanic membrane.

**myringoplasty** (mi'ring.goh͵plastee) a plastic operation to repair the tympanic membrane; tympanoplasty.

**myringotome** (mi'ring.gə͵tohm) an instrument for puncturing the tympanic membrane in myringotomy.

**myringotomy** (͵miring'gotəmee) incision of the tympanic membrane to drain fluid from an infected middle ear.

**myxoedema** (͵miksi'deemə) a condition, caused by hypothyroidism, which is marked by mucoid infiltration of the skin. There is oedematous swelling of the face, limbs and hands, dry and rough skin, loss of hair, slow pulse, subnormal temperature, slowed metabolism and mental dullness. *Congenital m.* cretinism.

**myxoma** (mik'sohmə) a benign mucous tumour of connective tissue.

**myxosarcoma** (͵miksohsah'kohmə) a sarcoma containing mucoid tissue.

**myxovirus** (͵miksoh'vierəs) the group name of a number of related viruses, including the causal viruses of influenza, parainfluenza, mumps and Newcastle disease (of fowl).

# N

**N** symbol for *nitrogen* and *newton*.

**Na** symbol for *sodium*.

**Naboth's follicle** or **cyst** ('nayboths) *M. Naboth, German anatomist, 1675–1721.* Cystic swelling of a cervical gland, the duct of which has become blocked by regenerating squamous epithelium.

**naevus** ('neevəs) a birthmark; a circumscribed area of pigmentation of the skin due to dilated blood vessels. A haemangioma. *N. flammeus* a flat bluish-red area, usually on the neck or face; popularly known as 'port wine stain'. *N. pilosus* a hairy naevus. *Spider n.* a small red area surrounded by dilated capillaries. *Strawberry n.* a raised tumour-like structure of connective tissue containing spaces filled with blood.

**naftidrofuryl** (naf,tidroh'fyooəril) an agent used in the treatment of peripheral and cerebral vascular disorders.

**Nägele's rule** ('naygələz ,rool) rule for calculating the estimated date of labour; subtract 3 months from the first day of the last menstrual period and add 7 days.

**NAI** non-accidental injury.

**nail** (nayl) the keratinized portion of epidermis covering the dorsal extremity of the fingers and toes. *Hang n.* a strip of epidermis hanging at one side or at the root of a nail. *Ingrowing n.* a condition in which the flesh overhangs the edge of the nail, a sharp corner of which may pierce the skin, causing a wound which may become septic. *N. bed* the skin underlying a nail. *Spoon n.* a nail with a depression in the centre and raised edges. Koilonychia.

**nalidixic acid** (,nali'diksik) an antibacterial agent used in the treatment of urinary infections.

**naloxone** (na'loksohn) a narcotic antagonist used as an antidote to narcotic overdosage and as an antagonist for pentazocine overdosage.

**named nurse** (naym'd) a qualified nurse, midwife or health visitor who is known to the patient or client by name and is accountable for care. The aim is to provide maximum continuity and coordination in care for the individual patient or client.

**NANDA** ('nandə) North American Nursing Diagnosis Association.

**nandrolone** ('nandrə,lohn) an anabolic steroid that promotes protein metabolism and skeletal growth.

**nape** (nayp) the back of the neck.

**napkin rash** ('napkin) an erythematous rash which may occur in infants in the napkin area. The many causes include the passage of frequent loose stools, thrush, ammoniacal dermatitis and allergy to washing powders and detergents.

**narcissism** ('nahsi,sizəm) the stage of infant development when children are mainly interested in themselves and their own bodily needs. In adults it may be a symptom of mental disorder. The term is derived from the Greek legend of Narcissus.

**narcoanalysis** (ˌnahkoh.əˈnalisis) a form of psychotherapy in which an injection of a narcotic drug produces a drowsy, relaxed state during which a patient will talk more freely, and in this way much repressed material may be brought to consciousness.

**narcolepsy** (ˈnahkohˌlepsee) a condition in which there is an uncontrollable desire for sleep.

**narcosis** (nahˈkohsis) a state of unconsciousness produced by a narcotic drug. *Basal n.* a state of unconsciousness produced prior to surgical anaesthesia.

**narcosynthesis** (ˌnahkohˈsinthəsis) the inducement of a hypnotic state by means of drugs. An aid to psychotherapy.

**narcotic** (nahˈkotik) a drug that produces narcosis or unnatural sleep.

**nares** (ˈnair.reez) the nostrils. *Posterior n.* the opening of the nares into the nasopharynx.

**nasal** (ˈnayzˈl) pertaining to the nose.

**nascent** (ˈnasˈnt, ˈnay-) 1. at the time of birth. 2. incipient.

**Naseptin** (nayˈseptin) trade name for a combination preparation containing chlorhexidine and neomycin, a nasal cream for the treatment of staphylococcal infections.

**nasogastric** (ˌnayzohˈgastrik) referring to the nose and stomach. *N. tube* one passed into the stomach via the nose.

**nasojejunal feeding** (ˌnayzohjiˈjoonˈl ˌfeeding) a method in which a silicone-coated catheter is passed through the nose into the jejunum to provide sufficient nutrition to a sick baby on a ventilator or receiving continuous inflating pressure

(CIP) by mask or nasal tube. It is used to prevent the dangers of aspiration with a nasogastric tube feed.

**nasolacrimal** (ˌnayzohˈlakrimˈl) concerning both the nose and lacrimal apparatus. *N. duct* the duct draining the tears from the inner aspect of the eye to the inferior meatus of the nose.

**nasopharynx** (ˌnayzohˈfaringks) the upper part of the pharynx; that above the soft palate.

**nasosinusitis** (ˌnayzohˌsienəˈsietis) inflammation of the nose and adjacent sinuses.

**National Board for Nursing, Midwifery and Health Visiting for Northern Ireland** (ˌnawdhən ˈieələnd) *see* NATIONAL BOARDS.

**National Board for Nursing, Midwifery and Health Visiting for Scotland** (ˈskotland) *see* NATIONAL BOARDS.

**National Boards** (ˈnashˌnˈl ˈbawdz) the National Boards for Nursing, Midwifery and Health Visiting were originally set up in England, Wales, Scotland and Northern Ireland by the 1979 Nurses, Midwives and Health Visitors' Act. The key role of the Boards is to approve institutions in relation to the provision of courses. In fulfilling this role, the Boards are required to ensure that the courses so approved meet the standards of the United Kingdom Central Council for Nursing, Midwifery and Health Visiting (UKCC). Each National Board has an important relationship with the UKCC and its respective functions are defined in law.

**National Vocational Qualifications** (vohˈkayshənˈl ˌkwolifikayshənz) abbreviated NVQs. Nationally recognized work-related qualifications that are coordinated by the National Council for Vocational Qualifications. NVQs are based on a system of credits earned after a work-based assessment of skills and the level of competence attained.

**natural childbirth** (nacher'l) a term used to describe an approach to LABOUR and delivery in which the parents are prepared for the event so that the mother is awake and cooperative and the father is able to assume an active and supportive role during the birth of their child. The underlying concept for all methods of natural childbirth is avoidance of medical interference and analgesia in labour, and education of the parents so that they can actively participate in and share the experience of childbirth.

**nature–nurture debate** ('naychə-nərchə də'bayt) the debate surrounding the issue of to what extent human behaviour is the result of hereditary or innate influences (nature) or is determined by the environment and learning (nurture).

**naturopathy** (,naychə'ropəthee) a drugless system of healing by a combination of diet, fasting, exercise, hydrotherapy and positive thinking.

**nausea** ('nawzi.ə) a sensation of sickness with an inclination to vomit.

**navel** ('nayv'l) the umbilicus.

**navicular** (nə'vikyuhlə) boat-shaped. *N. bone* one of the tarsal bones of the foot.

**nebula** ('nebyuhlə) a slight opacity or cloudiness of the cornea, caused by injury or by corneal ulceration.

**nebulizer** ('nebyuh,liezə) an apparatus for reducing a liquid to a fine spray. An atomizer.

**NEC** necrotizing enterocolitis.

**neck** (nek) 1. the narrow part of an organ or bone. 2. the part of the body which connects the head and the trunk. *Derbyshire n.* simple goitre. *Wry n.* torticollis.

**necrobiosis** (,nekrohbie'ohsis) localized death of a part as a result of degeneration.

**necropsy** ('nekropsee) autopsy; a postmortem examination of a body.

**necrosis** (nə'krohsis) death of a portion of tissue.

**necrotizing enterocolitis** ('nekrə-,tiezing) abbreviated NEC. A condition of neonates in which there is severe diarrhoea and blood in the stools. It occurs in preterm or low-birthweight neonates. Exact cause is not known but is often associated with infection.

**necrotizing fasciitis** (,fashi'ietis) a bacterial infection of *Streptococcus* type A underneath the skin in the fascia layer; produces necrosis and toxins, resulting in shock and organ failure. Urgent treatment is required with antibiotics and surgical excision of the infected tissues.

**needlestick injury** ('need'lstik ,injə.ree) an accidental injury with a needle that is contaminated with blood or body fluids. The term is also used sometimes to include other sharps injuries. The injuries have been reported as a means of infecting the nurse or health-care professional with hepatitis or human immunodeficiency virus (HIV).

**needling** ('needling) discission, the operation for cataract of lacerating and splitting up the lens so that it may be absorbed.

**negative** ('negativ) the opposite of positive. The absence of some quality or substance.

**negativism** ('negəti,vizəm) a symptom of mental illness in which the patient does not present what is required and so presents an unco-operative attitude. Common in schizophrenia.

**negligence** ('neglijəns) in law, the failure to do something that a reasonable person of ordinary prudence would do in a certain situation or the doing of something that such a person would not do. Negligence may provide the basis for a lawsuit when there is a legal duty, as in the duty of a doctor or nurse to provide reasonable care to patients, and when the negligence results in damage to the patient.

*Neisseria* (nie'siə.ri.ə) *A.L.S. Neisser, German bacteriologist, 1855–1916.* A genus of paired, spherical, Gram-negative bacteria. *N. gonorrhoeae* the causative organism of gonorrhoea. *N. meningitidis* the cause of meningococcal meningitis.

Nematoda (nemə'tohdə) a phylum of worms, including the *Ascaris* or roundworm and the *Enterobius* or threadworm.

neocortex (neeoh'kawteks) the cerebral cortex, excluding the hippocampal formation and piriform area.

neoglycogenesis (neeoh gliekə-'jenəsis) the formation of liver glycogen from non-carbohydrate sources. Glyconeogenesis.

neologism (nee'olə jizəm) the formation of new words, either completely new ones or ones formed by contraction of two separate words. This is done particularly by schizophrenic patients.

neomycin (neeoh'miesin) an antibiotic drug used against a wide range of bacteria, frequently those affecting the skin or the eyes. Also given orally to sterilize the bowel before surgery.

neonatal (neeə'nayt'l) referring to the first month of life. *N. mortality rate* the number of deaths of infants up to 4 weeks old per 1000 live births in any 1 year. *N. period* the interval from the birth to 28 days of age and the period of greatest risk to the infant.

neonate ('neeə nayt) newborn; specifically pertaining to a baby under 1 month old.

neonatologist (neeənay'toləjist) a medically qualified person specializing in the management, assessment, diseases and intensive care of newborn babies, especially those of low birthweight and those with congenital abnormalities.

neonatology (neeənay'toləjee) the branch of medicine dealing with disorders of the newborn infant.

neoplasm ('neeoh plazəm) a morbid new growth; a tumour. It may be benign or malignant.

neostigmine (neeoh'stigmeen) a synthetic preparation akin to physostigmine used in the treatment of myasthenia gravis and as an antidote to some muscle-relaxant drugs, and as eye drops in the treatment of glaucoma.

Nepenthe (nə'penthee) trade name for a preparation containing opium alkaloids, used as an analgesic.

nephralgic (nə'fraljik) relating to pain arising from the kidney. *N. crises* spasms of pain in the lumbar region in tabes dorsalis.

nephrectomy (nə'frektəmee) excision of a kidney.

nephritis (nə'frietis) inflammation of the kidney; a focal or diffuse proliferative or destructive disease that may involve the glomerulus, tubule or interstitial renal tissue. Also called Bright's disease. The most usual form is glomerulonephritis.

nephroblastoma (nefrohbla-'stohmə) a rapidly developing malignant mixed tumour of the kidneys, made up of embryonic cells, and occurring chiefly in children before the fifth year; Wilms' tumour.

nephrocalcinosis (nefroh kalsi'nohsis) a condition in which there is deposition of calcium in the renal tubules, resulting in calculi formation and renal insufficiency.

nephrocapsulectomy (nefroh kapsyuh'lektəmee) an operation for removal of the capsule of the kidney.

nephrogram ('nefroh gram) a radiograph of the kidney with contrast medium in the renal tubules. Usually the immediate film in an excretion urogram.

**nephrolith** ('nefroh,lith) stone in the kidney; renal calculus.

**nephrolithiasis** (,nefrohli'thieəsis) the presence of a calculus or of gravel in the kidney.

**nephrolithotomy** (,nefrohli'thotəmee) removal of a renal calculus by incising the kidney or by extracorporeal shock wave lithotripsy.

**nephroma** (ne'frohmə) tumour of the kidney.

**nephron** ('nefron) the functional unit of the kidney, comprising Bowman's capsule, the proximal and distal tubules, the loop of Henle and the collecting duct, which conveys urine to the renal pelvis.

**nephropexy** ('nefroh,peksee) the fixation of a floating (mobile) kidney, usually by sutures to neighbouring muscle.

**nephroptosis** (,nefrop'tohsis) downward displacement, or undue mobility, of a kidney.

**nephropyeloplasty** (,nefroh'pieəloh,plastee) a plastic operation on the pelvis of the kidney, performed in cases of hydronephrosis.

**nephropyosis** (,nefrohpie'ohsis) suppuration in the kidney.

**nephrosclerosis** (,nefrohsklə-'rohsis) constriction of the arterioles of the kidney. Seen in benign and malignant hypertension and in arteriosclerosis in old age.

**nephrosis** (ne'frohsis) any disease of the kidney, especially that characterized by oedema, albuminuria and a low plasma albumin. Caused by non-inflammatory degenerative lesions of the tubules.

**nephrostomy** (nə'frostəmee) creation of a permanent opening into the renal pelvis.

**nephrotic** (nə'frotik) referring to or caused by nephrosis. *N. syndrome* a clinical syndrome in which there is albuminuria, low plasma protein and gross oedema. The result of increased capillary permeability in the glomeruli. It may occur as a result of acute glomerulonephritis, in subacute nephritis, diabetes mellitus, amyloid disease, systemic lupus erythematosus and renal vein thrombosis.

**nephrotomogram** (,nefroh'tohmə,gram) a tomogram of the kidney obtained by nephrotomography.

**nephrotomography** (,nefrohtə-'mografee) radiological visualization of the kidney by tomography after introduction of a contrast medium.

**nephrotomy** (nə'frotəmee) incision of the kidney.

**nephrotoxic** (,nefroh'toksik) poisonous or destructive to the cells of the kidney.

**nephroureterectomy** (,nefroh.yuh-,reetə'rektəmee) surgical removal of the kidney and the ureter.

**nerve** (nərv) a bundle of conducting fibres enclosed in a sheath called the epineurium. Its function is to transmit impulses between any part of the body and a nerve centre. *Motor (efferent) n.* one that conveys impulses causing activity from a nerve centre to a muscle or gland. *N. block* a method of producing regional anaesthesia by injecting a local anaesthetic into the nerves supplying the area to be operated on. *N. fibre* the prolongation of the nerve cell, which conveys impulses. Each fibre has a sheath. Medullated nerve fibres have an insulating myelin sheath. *N. gas* a gas that interferes with the functioning of the nerves and muscles. Such gases may cause death from respiratory paralysis; some of them act through the skin and cannot be avoided by the use of gas masks. *Sensory (afferent) n.* one that conveys sensation from an area to a nerve centre.

**nervous** ('nərvəs) 1. pertaining to, or composed of, nerves. 2. apprehensive. *N. breakdown* a popular and misleading term for any type of mental illness that interferes with a person's normal activities. A so-called 'nervous breakdown' can include any of the mental disorders, including NEUROSIS, PSYCHOSIS or DEPRESSION, but is usually used to describe neurosis.

**nervousness** ('nərvəsnəs) excitability of the nervous system, characterized by a state of mental and physical unrest.

**nettle rash** ('net'l ˌrash) an allergic skin condition; urticaria.

**network** ('net ˌwərk) 1. an interconnected group or system of voluntary organizations or of colleagues with similar interests. 2. a system of interconnected computer terminals in which the user has access to others using the system for sharing data, etc.

**networking** ('net ˌwərking) 1. forming and maintaining professional connections and contacts through informal social meetings. 2. the interconnection of two or more computer networks in different places.

**neural** ('nyooə.rəl) pertaining to the nerves. *N. arch* the bony arch on each vertebra which encloses the spinal cord. *N. tube defect* any of a group of congenital malformations involving the neural tube, including anencephaly, hypocephalus and spina bifida.

**neuralgia** (nyuh'raljə, -ji.ə) a sharp stabbing pain, usually along the course of a nerve, owing to neuritis or functional disturbance.

**neurapraxia** (ˌnyooə.rə'praksi.ə) an injury to a nerve resulting in temporary loss of function and paralysis. It is usually caused by compression of the nerve, and there is no lasting damage.

**neurasthenia** (ˌnyooə.rəs'theeni.ə) a neurosis in which there is much mental and physical fatigue, inability to concentrate, loss of appetite, and a failure of memory.

**neurectomy** (nyuh'rektəmee) excision of part of a nerve.

**neurilemma** (ˌnyooə.ri'lemə) the membranous sheath surrounding a nerve fibre.

**neurinoma** (ˌnyooə.ri'nohmə) a benign tumour arising in the neurilemma of a nerve fibre.

**neuritis** (nyuh'rietis) inflammation of a nerve, with pain, tenderness and loss of function. *Multiple n.* that involving several nerves; polyneuritis. *Nutritional (alcoholic) n.* that which may be caused by alcoholism or lack of vitamin B complex. *Optic n.* that affecting the optic disc or nerve. *Peripheral n.* that involving the terminations of nerves. *Sciatic n.* sciatica. *Tabetic n.* a type occurring in tabes dorsalis. *Traumatic n.* that which results from an injury to a nerve.

**neuroblast** ('nyooə.roh ˌblast) an embryonic nerve cell.

**neuroblastoma** (ˌnyooə.rohblə'stohmə) a malignant tumour of immature nerve cells, most often arising in the very young.

**neurodermatitis** (ˌnyooə.roh ˌdərmə'tietis) a localized prurigo of somatic and psychogenic origin. It irritates, and rubbing causes thickening and pigmentation of the skin.

**neuroepithelioma** (ˌnyooə.roh ˌepi ˌtheeli'ohmə) a malignant tumour of the retina of the eye, which may spread into the brain.

**neurofibroma** (ˌnyooə.rohfie' brohmə) a benign tumour of nerve and fibrous tissue.

**neurofibromatosis** (ˌnyooə.roh ˌfiebrohmətoh'sis) von Recklinghausen's disease. A generalized hereditary disease in which there are numerous fibromas of the skin and nervous system.

**neurogenic** (ˌnyooə.rəˈjenik) derived from or caused by nerve stimulation. *N. bladder* a disorder of the urinary bladder caused by a lesion of the nervous system. *N. shock* shock originating in the nervous system.

**neuroglia** (nyuhˈrogli.ə) the special form of connective tissue supporting nerve tissues.

**neurohypophysis** (ˌnyooə.roh.hieˈpofisis) the posterior lobe of the pituitary gland.

**neuroleptic** (ˌnyooə.rohˈleptik) a drug which acts on the nervous system.

**neurological assessment** (ˌnyooə-.rohˈlojikˈl) evaluation of the health status of a patient with a nervous system disorder or dysfunction. Purposes of the assessment include establishing nursing goals to guide the nurse in planning and implementing nursing measures to help the patient cope effectively with daily living activities. Nursing assessment of a patient's neurological status is concerned with identifying functional disabilities that interfere with the person's ability to provide self-care and lead an active life. A functionally oriented nursing assessment includes: (a) consciousness; (b) mental functions; (c) motor function; and (d) sensory function. Evaluation of these functions gives the nurse information about the patient's ability to perform everyday activities such as thinking, remembering, seeing, eating, speaking, moving, smelling, feeling and hearing. A patient with an acute and life-threatening alteration in neurological function is evaluated and monitored in four general areas: (a) level of consciousness; (b) sensory and motor function; (c) pupillary changes; and (d) vital signs and pattern of respiration.

**neurologist** (nyuhˈroləjist) a medical practitioner specializing in neurology.

**neurology** (nyuhˈroləjee) 1. the scientific study of the nervous system. 2. the branch of medicine concerned with diseases of the nervous system.

**neuroma** (nyuhˈrohmə) a tumour consisting of nervous tissue.

**neuromuscular** (ˌnyooə.rohˈmuskyuhlə) appertaining to nerves and muscles. *N. junction* the small gap between the end of the motor nerve and the motor end-plate of the muscle fibre supplied. This gap is bridged by the release of acetylcholine whenever a nerve impulse arrives.

**neuromyelitis** (ˌnyooə.rohˌmieəˈlietis) neuritis associated with myelitis. It is a condition akin to multiple sclerosis. *N. optica* a disease in which there is bilateral optic neuritis and paraplegia.

**neurone (neuron)** (ˈnyooə.rohn, ˈnyooə.ron) a nerve cell. *Lower motor n.* the anterior horn cell and its neurone which convey impulses to the appropriate muscles. *Upper motor n.* that in which the cell is in the cerebral cortex and the fibres conduct impulses to associated cells in the spinal cord.

**neuroparalysis** (ˌnyooə.rohpəˈralisis) paralysis due to disease of a nerve or nerves.

**neuropathy** (nyuhˈropəthee) a disease process of nerve degeneration and loss of function. *Alcoholic n.* neuropathy due to thiamine deficiency in chronic alcoholism. *Diabetic n.* that associated with diabetes. *Entrapment n.* any of a group of neuropathies, e.g. carpal tunnel syndrome, due to mechanical pressure on a peripheral nerve. *Ischaemic n.* that caused by a lack of blood supply.

**neuroplasty** (ˌnyooə.rohˈplastee) the surgical repair of a damaged nerve.

**neuropsychiatry** (ˌnyooə.rohsieˈkieətree) the medical specialism concerned with the effects on mind and behaviour of organic disorders of the nervous system, combining both neurology and psychiatry.

**neurorrhaphy** (nyuh'ro.rəfee) the operation of suturing a divided nerve.

**neurosis** (nyuh'rohsis) a mental disorder, which does not affect the whole personality, characterized by exaggerated anxiety and tension. *Anxiety n.* persistent anxiety and the accompanying symptoms of fear, rapid pulse, sweating, trembling, loss of appetite and insomnia. *Obsessive-compulsive n.* one characterized by compulsions and obsessional rumination.

**neurosurgery** (nyooə.roh'sərjə.ree) that branch of surgery dealing with the brain, spinal cord and nerves.

**neurosyphilis** (nyooə.roh'sifilis) a manifestation of third stage syphilis in which the nervous system is involved. The three most common forms are: (a) meningovascular syphilis, affecting the blood vessels to the meninges; (b) tabes dorsalis (*see* ATAXIA); and (c) general paralysis of the insane.

**neurotic** (nyuh'rotik) a loosely applied adjective denoting association with neurosis.

**neurotoxic** (nyooə.roh'toksik) poisonous or destructive to nervous tissue.

**neurotransmitter** (nyooə.rohtranz-'mitə, -trahnz-) a substance (e.g. noradrenaline, acetylcholine, dopamine) that is released from the axon terminal to produce activity in other nerves.

**neurotripsy** ('nyooəroh,tripsee) the surgical bruising or crushing of a nerve.

**neurotropic** (nyooə.roh'tropik) having an affinity for nerve tissue. *N. viruses* those that particularly attack the nervous system.

**neutropenia** (nyootrə'peeni.ə) a decrease in the number of neutrophils in the blood.

**neutrophil** ('nyootrə,fil) a polymorphonuclear leukocyte which has a neutral reaction to acid and alkaline dyes.

**niacin** ('nieəsin) nicotinic acid.

**niclosamide** (ni'klohsəmied) an anthelmintic used as a single dose in tapeworm infestations.

**nicotine** ('nikə,teen) a poisonous alkaloid in tobacco.

**nicotinic acid** (,nikə'tinik) niacin. A water-soluble vitamin in the B complex. A deficiency of this vitamin causes pellagra.

**nidation** (nie'dayshən) implantation of the fertilized ovum in the uterus.

**nidus** ('niedəs) 1. a nest. 2. a place in which an organism finds conditions suitable for its growth and development. 3. the focus of an infection.

**Niemann–Pick disease** (,neem-ən'pik) *A. Niemann, German paediatrician, 1880–1921; F. Pick, German physician, 1868–1935.* A rare inherited disease occurring primarily in Jewish children and resulting in learning difficulties. There is lipoid storage abnormality and widespread deposition of lecithin in the tissues.

**nifedipine** (nie'fedi,peen) a calcium channel blocker used as a coronary vasodilator in the treatment of angina pectoris, and in the treatment of hypertension.

**night blindness** (niet) nyctalopia; difficulty in seeing in the dark. This may be a congenital defect or be caused by a vitamin A deficiency. Also occurs as a result of retinal degeneration.

**night sweat** profuse perspiration during sleep, associated usually with an acute feverish illness.

**night terror** (,terə) an unpleasant experience in which the subject, usually a young child, screams while asleep and seems terrified. On waking the individual is unable to remember the cause of the fear.

**nihilism** ('niea,lizam) in psychiatry, a term used to describe feelings of not existing and hopelessness, that all is lost or destroyed.

**nikethamide** (ni'ketha,mied) a cardiac and respiratory stimulant given intravenously in cases of respiratory failure.

**nipple** ('nip'l) the small conical projection at the tip of the breast, through which, in the female, milk can be withdrawn. *Accessory n.* a rudimentary nipple anywhere in a line from the breast to the groin. *Depressed n.* one that does not protrude. *N. shield* a shield fitted with a rubber teat which covers the areola of a nursing mother when her nipple is sore or not sufficiently protractile for the baby to suck. *Retracted n.* one that is drawn inwards. It may be a sign of cancer of the breast.

**Nissl granules** ('nis'l) *F. Nissl, German neuropathologist, 1860–1919.* RNA-containing units found in the cytoplasm of cells. Probably associated with protein synthesis.

**nit** (nit) the egg of the head louse, attached to the hair near the scalp.

**nitrazepam** (nie'trazi,pam) a hypnotic and sedative drug used to treat insomnia with early morning wakening.

**nitrofurantoin** (,nietrohfyooa'rantoh.in) a urinary antiseptic which is bactericidal and is effective against a wide range of organisms.

**nitrogen** ('nietrajan) *symbol* N. A gaseous element. Air is largely composed of nitrogen, and it is one of the essential constituents of all protein foods. *N. balance* the state of the body in regard to the rate of protein intake and protein utilization. A negative nitrogen balance occurs when more protein is utilized by the body than is taken in. A positive nitrogen balance implies a net gain of protein in the body. Negative nitrogen balance can be caused by such factors as malnutrition, debilitating disease, blood loss and glucocorticoids. A positive balance can be caused by exercise, growth hormone and testosterone. *N. mustards* a group of toxic, blistering alkylating agents, including nitrogen mustard itself (mechlorethamine hydrochloride) and related compounds; some have been used as antineoplastics in certain forms of cancer.

**nitroglycerin** (,nietroh'glisarin) glyceryl trinitrate. A drug which causes dilatation of the coronary arteries. In angina pectoris a tablet should be dissolved sublingually before exertion.

**nitrous oxide** (,nietras 'oksied) $N_2O$; laughing gas. An inhalation anaesthetic ensuring a brief spell of unconsciousness.

**nociassociation** (,nohsi.a,sohsi'ayshan) the discharge of nervous energy which occurs unconsciously in trauma, as in surgical shock. *See* ANOCI-ASSOCIATION.

**noctambulation** (,noktambyuh'layshan) sleep walking; somnambulism.

**nocturia** (nok'tyooa.ri.a) the production of large quantities of urine at night.

**nocturnal** (nok'tarn'l) referring to the night. *N. enuresis* bed wetting; incontinence of urine during sleep.

**node** (nohd) a swelling or protuberance. *Atrioventricular n.* the specialized tissue between the right atrium and the ventricle, at the point where the coronary vein enters the atrium, from which is initiated the impulse of contraction down the atrioventricular bundle. *N. of Ranvier* a constriction occurring at intervals in a nerve fibre to enable the neurilemma with its blood supply to reach and nourish the axon of the nerve. *Sinoatrial n.* the pacemaker of the heart. The specialized neuromuscular tissue at the junction of the superior vena cava and the right atrium, which, stimulated by the right vagus nerve, controls the rhythm of contraction in the heart.

**nodule** ('nodyool) a small swelling or protuberance.

**noma** ('nohmə) a gangrenous condition of the mouth; cancrum oris.

**nomogram** ('nomə.gram, 'noh-) a graph with several scales arranged so that a ruler laid on the graph intersects the scales at related values of the variables; the values of any two variables can be used to find the values of the others. Increasingly used in the determination of drug therapy dosage, e.g. in paediatrics.

**non compos mentis** (non ˌkompəs 'mentis) [L.] *not of sound mind.* Applied to people whose mental state is such that they are unable to manage their own affairs.

**non-accidental injury** (ˌnonaksi-'dent'l ˌinjə.ree) abbreviated NAI. Injuries inflicted upon children or infants by those looking after them, usually the parents. The injuries are usually physical (beating, burnings, biting) but the term includes the giving of poisons and dangerous drugs, sexual abuse, starvation and any other form of physical assault.

**non-compliance** (ˌnonkəm'pliəans) describes the decision made by a patient not to comply with a drug regimen, even though fully understanding the rationale for such therapy.

**non-maleficence** (ˌnonmə'lefisəns) the concept in the health-care services of the duty to avoid harm to the interests of others.

**non-specific** (ˌnonspə'sifik) 1. not due to any single known cause. 2. not directed against a particular agent, but rather having a general effect. *N. urethritis* abbreviated NSU. A common, sexually transmitted disease which may be due to a variety of agents, e.g. *Chlamydia trachomatis* which causes 40% of cases. Also called non-gonococcal urethritis.

**non-steroidal anti-inflammatory drugs** (non ˌstə'royd'l ˌanti.in'flamətə.ree, - ster-) abbreviated NSAIDs. A group of drugs with analgesic, antipyretic and anti-inflammatory activity due to their ability to inhibit the synthesis of prostaglandins. It includes aspirin, phenylbutazone, indomethacin, tolmetic, ibuprofen and related drugs.

**non-union** in a fracture, failure of the two pieces of bone to unite.

**noradrenaline** (ˌnor.rə'drenəlin) a hormone present in extracts of the suprarenal medulla and at synapses in the peripheral sympathetic nervous system. It causes vasoconstriction and raises both the systolic and the diastolic blood pressure.

**norethisterone** (ˌnor.re'thistə.rohn) an anabolic steroid similar in action to progesterone. Used in the treatment of amenorrhoea. Also used in the combined contraceptive pill.

**normal** ('nawm'l) conforming to a standard; regular or usual. *N. flora* bacteria which normally live on body tissues and have a beneficial effect. *N. saline* isotonic solution of sodium chloride. Physiological solution.

**normoblast** ('nawmoh.blast) a nucleated precursor red blood cell in bone marrow. *See* ERYTHROCYTE.

**normochromic** (ˌnawmoh'krohmik) normal in colour. Applied to the blood when the haemoglobin level is within normal limits.

**normocyte** ('nawmoh.siet) a red blood cell that is normal in size, shape and colour.

**normoglycaemia** (ˌnawmohglie-'seemi.ə) normal blood sugar level.

**normotension** (ˌnawmoh'tenshən) normal tone, tension or pressure.

Usually used in relation to blood pressure.

**North American Nursing Diagnosis Association** (nawth ə'merikən) abbreviated NANDA. Formed as a professional organization of registered nurses in 1982. The purpose of NANDA is 'to develop, refine and promote a taxonomy of nursing diagnostic terminology of general use to the professional'. Meets at regular intervals to review previously approved nursing diagnoses and to further develop the classification systems.

**Norton score** ('nortən ˌskaw) a pressure sore risk assessment scale devised by Norton, McLaren and Exton Smith in 1987. Used primarily in the care of elderly patients and reviewed on a weekly basis. It comprises five health state components, each with a four-point descending scale. Maximum points are 20 and the minimum five; a 'score' of 14 and below indicates that the patient is at risk of developing pressure sores and needs 1–2-hourly changes of posture and the use of pressure-relieving aids.

**nortriptyline** (naw'triptiˌleen) a tricyclic antidepressant drug used for the relief of all types of depression.

**nose** (nohz) the organ of smell and the airway for respiration.

**nosocomial** (ˌnohzə'kohmeeəl) pertaining to, or acquired in hospital. *N. disease* for the patient a new disorder, not related to the original disease, that is caused or precipitated during hospitalization. *N. infection* an infection acquired in hospital at least 72 hours after admission. Also called hospital acquired infection (HAI). *Contact transmitted infection* is the most important and frequent mode of transmission of nosocomial infections and may be either direct or indirect. *Direct contact transmitted infections* involve direct 'body surface-to-body surface' con-

tact, such as occurs in patient care activities, e.g. bathing a patient. Direct contact can also occur between two patients, with one serving as the source of infectious microorganisms, the other being a susceptible host. *Indirect contact transmitted infections* involve contact of a susceptible host with a contaminated intermediate object, usually inanimate (*see* FOMITES), e.g. contaminated instruments, needles, dressings or gloves that are not changed between patients. Unwashed, contaminated hands may also be a source of nosocomial infection.

**nosology** (noh'zolajee) the classification of disease into groups by criteria, based on (expert) agreement of the boundaries of the groups, e.g. by the DELPHI TECHNIQUE.

**nostril** ('nostrəl) one of the anterior orifices of the nose.

**notifiable** ('nohtiˌfieəb'l) applied to such diseases as must by law be reported to the health authorities. These include measles, scarlet fever, typhus and typhoid fever, cholera, diphtheria, tuberculosis, dysentery and food poisoning.

**NSAIDs** non-steroidal anti-inflammatory drugs.

**NSU** non-specific urethritis.

**nuclear** ('nyookli.ə) pertaining to a nucleus. *N. medicine* that branch of medicine concerned with the use of radionuclides in the diagnosis and treatment of disease.

**nuclear magnetic resonance** abbreviated NMR. A phenomenon exhibited by atomic nuclei having a magnetic moment, i.e. those nuclei that behave as if they are tiny bar magnets. In the absence of a magnetic field these magnets are arranged randomly but when a strong magnetic field is applied they align with the field. These signals can be analysed and used for chemical analysis (NMR spectroscopy) or for imaging (magnetic resonance imaging).

**nuclease** ('nyookli,ayz) an enzyme which breaks down nucleic acids.

**nucleic acids** (nyoo'klee.ik, -'klay) deoxyribonucleic acid (abbreviated DNA) and ribonucleic acid (abbreviated RNA), both of which are found in cell nuclei; RNA is also found in the cytoplasm. They are composed of series of nucleotides.

**nucleolus** (,nyookli'ohləs, nyoo-'kleeələs) a small dense body in the cell nucleus which contains ribonucleic acid. It disappears during mitosis.

**nucleoprotein** (,nyooklioh'prohteen) a compound of nucleic acid and protein.

**nucleotide** ('nyooklioh,tied) a compound formed from pentose sugar, phosphoric acid and a nitrogen-containing base (a purine or a pyrimidine).

**nucleus** ('nyookli.əs) 1. the essential part of a cell, governing nutrition and reproduction, its division being essential for the formation of new cells. 2. the positively charged centre portion of an atom. 3. a group of nerve cells in the central nervous system. *Caudate n.* and *lenticular n.* part of the basal ganglia. *N. pulposus* the jelly-like centre of an intervertebral disc.

**nullipara** (nu'lipə.rə) a woman who has never given birth to a child.

**nurse** (nərs) 1. a person who is qualified in the art and science of nursing and meets certain prescribed standards of education and clinical competence. Is registered with the United Kingdom Central Council for Nursing, Midwifery and Health Visiting (UKCC) if practising in the UK. The person so registered is entitled legally to use the title of nurse (*see also* NURSING (PRACTICE)). Prior to 1989 nurse education culminated in qualification as a first-level nurse registered general (RGN), or for mental health, sick children or the mentally handicapped. For second-level nurse, *see* ENROLLED NURSE below. 2. to provide services that are essential to or helpful in the promotion, maintenance and restoration of health and wellbeing. 3. to nourish at the breast (*see also* BREAST (FEEDING)). *Enrolled n.* a nurse who has undertaken a 2-year nurse training course (in Scotland 18 months) meant to provide a practical nurse who works under the supervision of the registered nurse, a second-level nurse. An enrolled nurse may undertake further training to become a first-level registered nurse. *N. practitioner* a qualified nurse who works with general medical practitioners in the clinic, surgery or health centre in the community or in an acute care setting, e.g. accident and emergency services, orthopaedic clinics and minor injuries departments. The patients have a choice of seeing either the doctor or the nurse when they attend. *Practice n.* a qualified nurse who works with a general practitioner (GP), or with a group of GPs, in a health centre or surgery. *Primary n.* a named nurse who is responsible for the overall coordination of the patient's care. *Registered n.* in the UK, one whose name is on the register held by the UKCC. *Wet n.* a woman who breast feeds the infant of another.

**nursing** ('nərsing) the profession of performing the functions of a NURSE. *N. assessment* the systematic collection and analysis of patient data pertaining to the individual's health status, abilities and preferences for care and treatment. The first step of the nursing process leading to a clinical nursing judgement. *See* ASSESSMENT. *N. audit* a systematic procedure for assessing the quality of nursing care rendered to a specific patient population. *N. care plan* devised by a nurse and based upon a nursing assessment and nursing diagnosis for an individual patient. The plan has four essential components: (a) identification of the nursing care problems; (b) an outline of the means/methods of solving these; (c) a statement of the anticipated benefit to the patient; and (d) an account of the specific actions used to achieve the goals specified. *N. diagnosis* a statement of a health problem or of a potential health problem in the patient's/client's health status that a nurse is professionally competent to treat. *N. goal* the objective that the nurse hopes to achieve through nursing interventions and activities related to the patient's health status, needs and abilities, e.g. the development of self-care skills. *N. history* a written record providing data for assessing the nursing care needs of a patient. *N. models* a conceptual framework of nursing practice based on knowledge, ideas and beliefs. A model or theory of nursing clarifies the meaning of nursing, provides criteria for policy and gives direction to team nursing, thereby obviating conflicts in approach and giving the framework for continuity of care. It identifies the nurse's role, highlights areas of practice where research is needed and can be a basis for the nursing curriculum. *N. practice* the performance or compensation of any act in the observation, care and counsel of the ill, injured or infirm, or in the maintenance of health or prevention of illness of others, or in the supervision and teaching of other personnel, or in the administration of medications and treatments as prescribed by a doctor or dentist. This requires substantial specialized judgement and skill and is based on knowledge and application of the principles of biological, physical and social sciences. *N. process* a systematic approach to nursing care derived from many occupational groups. The system itself is not specific to nursing. It has been used as a framework for nursing care by American nurses and subsequently its principles have been adapted to the UK's culture and health-care system by British nurses. It is an organized approach to the identification of a patient's nursing care problems and the utilization of nursing actions that effectively alleviate, minimize or prevent the problems being presented or from developing. *Theories of n.* proposed explanations of the way in which nursing achieves its aims. They require a definition of the nurse's perception of the patient's needs, the nurse's own role and the context in which nursing care is being performed. The understanding of the relationship of these variables enables nursing care to be planned in such a way that the outcome may be predicted and set goals achieved.

**nutation** (nyoo'tayshən) uncontrollable nodding of the head.

**nutrient** ('nyootri.ənt) food; any substance that nourishes. The six classes of nutrient are fats, carbohydrates, proteins, vitamins, minerals and water.

**nutrition** (nyoo'trishən) 1. the sum of the processes involved in taking in nutriments and assimilating and utilizing them. 2. nutriment. *Enteral n.* the provision of nutrients in fluid form to the alimentary tract by mouth, nasogastric tube or via an opening into the tract such as through a gastrostomy. *N. disease* one that is due to the continued absence of a necessary food factor.

*Parenteral n.* a technique for meeting a patient's nutritional needs by means of intravenous feedings; sometimes called hyper-alimentation.

**nutritional status** (nyoo'trishən'l) the condition of the body as a result of its receiving and using nutrients.

**nyctalopia** (ˌniktə'lohpi.ə) night blindness. *See* HEMERALOPIA.

**nymphomania** (ˌnimfə'mayni.ə) excessive sexual desire in a woman.

**nystagmus** (ni'stagməs) an involuntary, rapid movement of the eyeball. It may be hereditary or result from disease of the semicircular canals or of the central nervous system. It can occur from visual defect or be associated with other muscle spasms.

**nystatin** (nie'statin, ni-) an antibiotic drug effective against fungi. Used in the treatment of fungal infections of the ear.

# O

**O** symbol for *oxygen*.

**obese** (oh'bees) very fat; corpulent.

**obesity** (oh'beesətee) corpulence; excessive development of fat throughout the body. A body mass index (BMI) of over $30\,kg/m^2$.

**objective** (ə'bjektiv) 1. in microscopy, the lens nearest the object being looked at. 2. a purpose; a desired end-result. 3. concerning matters outside oneself. *O. signs* signs that the observer notes, as distinct from symptoms of which the patient complains (subjective).

**oblique** (ə'bleek) slanting. *O. muscles* 1. a pair of muscles, the inferior and the superior, which turn the eye upwards and downwards, and inwards and outwards. 2. muscles found in the wall of the abdomen.

**observation register** (ˌobzə'vayshən) a register of children whose development may be adversely affected by problems occurring during the fetal or neonatal period. They should be carefully followed up by the health visitor, general practitioner, social worker and special paediatric department.

**obsession** (əb'seshən) an idea which persistently recurs to an individual, although resisted and regarded as being senseless. A compulsive thought. *See* COMPULSION.

**obstetrician** (ˌobstə'trishən) one who is trained and specializes in obstetrics.

**obstetrics** (ob'stetriks) the branch of medicine and surgery dealing with pregnancy, labour and the puerperium.

**obstipation** (ˌobsti'payshən) intractable constipation.

**obstruction** (əb'strukshən) the act of blocking or clogging; the state of being clogged. *Intestinal o.* any hindrance to the passage of faeces.

**obturator** (ˌobtyuh'raytə) that which closes an opening. *O. foramen* the large hole in the hip bone, closed by fascia and muscle.

**obtusion** (ob'tyoozhən) weakening or blunting of normal sensations, a condition produced by certain diseases.

**occipital** (ok'sipit'l) relating to the occiput. *O. bone* the bone forming the back and part of the base of the skull.

**occipitoanterior** (okˌsipitoh.an'tiə.ri.ə) referring to the position of the fetal occiput when it is to the front of the maternal pelvis as it comes through the birth canal. The opposite of occipitoposterior.

**occipitoposterior** (okˌsipitohpos'tiə.ri.ə) referring to the position of the fetal occiput when it is to the back of the maternal pelvis as it comes through the birth canal. The opposite of occipitoanterior.

**occiput** ('oksiˌput) the back of the head.

**occlusion** (ə'kloozhən) closure, applied particularly to alignment of the teeth in the jaws. *Coronary o.* obstruction of the lumen of a coronary artery. *O. of the eye* covering a good eye to improve the visual acuity of the other, lazy eye. *O. of the pupil* may be congenital or occur in iridocyclitis or after injury.

**occult** ('okult) hidden, concealed. *O. blood* blood excreted in the stools in such a small quantity as to require chemical tests to detect it.

**occupational** (okyuh'payshən'l) relating to work and working conditions. *O. disease* one likely to occur among workers in certain trades. An industrial disease. *O. health nurse* provides immediate care to ill or injured workers and follows up the return to work of the sick and injured. Develops accident prevention programmes and promotes good health amongst the work force. Also has an educational role and a health and safety obligation. *O. health nursing* the branch of nursing that is concerned with the health of people in the workplace. *O. medicine* the branch of medicine concerned with people at work and the effects of work on health. Essentially a branch of preventative or environmental medicine. It is concerned with ensuring that health and safety in the workplace is maintained and legislation complied with. *O. therapy* treatment by provision of interesting and congenial work within the limitations of the patient in cases of mental disability and in order to re-educate and coordinate muscles in physical defect.

**ocular** ('okyuhlə) relating to the eye. *O. myopathy* a gradual bilateral loss of mobility of the eyes. *O. myositis* inflammation of the orbital muscles.

**oculentum** (okyuh'lentəm) an eye ointment.

**oculogyric** (okyuhloh'jierik) causing movements of the eyeballs. *O.*

*crisis* involuntary, violent movements of the eye, usually upwards.

**oculomotor** (okyuhloh'mohtə) relating to movements of the eye. *O. nerves* the third pair of cranial nerves, which control the eye muscles.

**odontoid** (oh'dontoyd) resembling a tooth. *O. process* a tooth-like projection from the axis vertebra upon which the head rotates.

**odontoma** (odon'tohmə) a tumour of tooth structures.

**oedema** (i'deemə) an excessive amount of fluid in the body tissues. If the finger is pressed upon an affected part, the surface pits and slowly regains its original contour. *Angioneurotic o.* temporary oedema suddenly appearing in areas of skin or mucous membrane and occasionally in the viscera. *Brain o.* an excessive accumulation of fluid in the brain substance (wet brain). *Cardiac o.* a manifestation of congestive heart failure, due to increased venous and capillary pressures and often associated with renal sodium retention. *Dependent o.* oedema affecting most severely the lowermost parts of the body. *Famine o.* that due to protein deficiency. *O. neonatorum* a disease of preterm and feeble infants resembling sclerema, marked by spreading oedema with cold, livid skin. *Pitting o.* oedema in which pressure leaves a persistent depression in the tissues. *Pulmonary o.* diffuse extravascular accumulation of fluid in the tissues and air spaces of the lung due to changes in hydrostatic forces in the capillaries or to increased capillary permeability.

**Oedipus complex** ('eedipəs) the suppressed sexual desire of a son for his mother, with hostility towards his father. It is a normal stage in the early development of the child, but may become fixed if the child cannot solve the conflict during his early years or during adolescence. Named after a mythical Greek hero.

**oesophageal** (i.sofə'jeeəl) pertaining to the oesophagus. *O. atresia* a congenital abnormality in which the oesophagus is not continuous between the pharynx and the stomach. May be associated with a fistula into the trachea. *O. varices* varicose veins of the lower oesophagus secondary to portal hypertension.

**oesophagitis** (i.sofə'jietis) inflammation of the oesophagus. *Reflux o.* caused by regurgitation of acid stomach contents through the cardiac sphincter.

**oesophagojejunostomy** (i.sofəgoh.jejuh'nostəmee) an operation to create an anastomosis of the jejunum with the oesophagus after a total gastrectomy.

**oesophagoscope** (i'sofəgoh.skohp) an endoscope for viewing the inside of the oesophagus.

**oesophagus** (i'sofəgəs) the canal that extends from the pharynx to the stomach. It is about 23 cm long. The gullet.

**oestradiol** (.eestrə'dieol) the chief naturally occurring female sex hormone produced by the ovary. Prepared synthetically, it is used to treat menopausal conditions and amenorrhoea.

**oestrogen** ('eestrəjən, -trə.jen) one of several steroid hormones, including oestradiol, all of which have similar functions. Although they are largely produced in the ovary, they can also be extracted from the placenta, the adrenal cortex and the testis. They control female sexual development.

**ointment** ('oyntmənt) an external application with a greasy base in which the remedy is incorporated.

**olecranon** (oh'lekrə.non, .ohli'kraynən) the curved process of the ulna which forms the point of the elbow.

**oleum** ('ohli.əm) an oil.

**olfactory** (ol'faktə.ree) relating to the sense of smell. *O. nerves* the first pair of cranial nerves; those of smell.

**oligaemia** (.oli'geemi.ə) a deficiency in the cellular component of the blood.

**oligocythaemia** (.oligohsie'theemi.ə) a cell deficiency in the blood.

**oligodendroglioma** (.oligoh.dendrohglie'ohmə) a central nervous system tumour of the glial tissue.

**oligohydramnios** (.oligoh.hie'dramnios) a deficiency in the amount of amniotic fluid.

**oligomenorrhoea** (.oligoh.menə-'reeə) 1. a diminished flow at the menstrual period. 2. infrequent occurrence of menstruation.

**oligospermia** (.oligoh'spərmi.ə) a diminished output of spermatozoa.

**oliguria** (.oli'gyooə.ri.ə) a deficient secretion of urine.

**olivary** ('olivə.ree) shaped like an olive. *O. body* a mass of grey matter situated behind the anterior pyramid of the medulla oblongata.

**ombudsman** ('ombudzmən) a person appointed to receive complaints about unfair administration. The officer in the National Health Service, appointed as 'ombudsman' or Health Service Commissioner, investigates complaints about failures in the health services and issues a regular report. Is not able to pass judgement on clinical matters. *See* HEALTH SERVICE COMMISSIONER.

**omentum** (oh'mentəm) a fold of peritoneum joining the stomach to other abdominal organs. *Greater o.* the fold reflected from the greater curvature of the stomach and lying in front of the intestines. *Lesser o.* the fold reflected from the lesser curvature and attaching the stomach to the undersurface of the liver.

**omnivorous** (om'nivərəs) eating food of both plant and animal origin.

**omphalitis** (ˌomfəˈlietis) inflammation of the umbilicus.

**omphalocele** (ˈomfalohˌseel) an umbilical hernia.

*Onchocerca* (ˌongkohˈsərkə) a genus of filarial worms, found in tropical parts of Africa and America, which may give rise to skin and subcutaneous lesions and attack the eye.

**onchocerciasis** (ˌongkohsərˈkieəsis) a tropical skin disease caused by infestation with *Onchocerca*.

**oncogenesis** (ˌongkohˈjenəsis) the causation and formation of tumours.

**oncogenic** (ˌongkohˈjenik) giving rise to tumour formation.

**oncology** (ongˈkoləjee) the scientific study of tumours.

**onychia** (oˈniki.ə) inflammation of the matrix of a nail, with suppuration, which may cause the nail to fall off.

**onychogryphosis** (ˌonikohgriˈfohsis) enlargement of the nails, with excessive ridging and curvature, most commonly affecting the elderly.

**onycholysis** (ˌoniˈkolisis) loosening or separation of a nail from its bed.

**onychomycosis** (ˌonikohmieˈkohsis) infection of the nails by a fungus.

**oöcyte** (ˈoh.əˌsiet) the immature egg cell or ovum in the ovary.

**oögenesis** (ˌoh.əˈjenəsis) the development and production of the ovum.

**oöphorectomy** (ˌoh.əfəˈrektəmee) excision of an ovary; ovariectomy.

**oöphoritis** (ˌoh.əfəˈrietis) inflammation of an ovary.

**oöphorocystectomy** (ohˌofəˌrohsiˈstektəmee) surgical removal of an ovarian cyst.

**oöphorocystosis** (ohˌofəˌrohsiˈstohsis) the development of one or more ovarian cysts.

**oöphoron** (ohˈofəˌron) an ovary.

**oöphoropexy** (ohˈofəˌrohˌpeksee) the surgical fixation of a displaced ovary to the pelvic wall.

**oöphorosalpingectomy** (ohˌofəˌrohˌsalpinˈjektəmee) removal of an ovary and its associated uterine tube.

**opacity** (ohˌpasitee) cloudiness, lack of transparency. Opacities occur in the lens of an eye when a cataract is forming. They also occur in the vitreous humour and appear as floating objects.

**operant conditioning** (ˌopəˌrənt) a form of behaviour therapy in which a reward is given when the subject performs the action required. The reward serves to encourage repetition of the action.

**operation** (ˌopəˈrayshən) a surgical procedure in which instruments or hands are used by the operator.

**ophthalmia** (ofˈthalmi.ə) severe inflammation of the eye or of the conjunctiva or deeper structures of the eye. *O. neonatorum* any hyperacute purulent conjunctivitis which may be caused by the gonococcus, *Escherichia coli*, staphylococci or *Chlamydia trachomatis*, occurring within the first 21 days of life, usually contracted during birth from infected vaginal discharge of the mother. This condition is notifiable except in Scotland. *Sympathetic o.* granulomatous inflammation of the uveal tract of the uninjured eye following a wound involving the uveal tract of the other eye, resulting in bilateral granulomatous inflammation of the entire uveal tract. Also called sympathetic uveitis.

**ophthalmitis** (ˌofthalˈmietis) inflammation of the eyeball.

**ophthalmologist** (ˌofthalˈmoləjist) a specialist in diseases of the eye.

**ophthalmology** (ˌofthalˈmoləjee) the study of the eyes and its diseases.

**ophthalmoplegia** (ofˌthalmohˈpleeji.ə) paralysis of the muscles of the eye.

**ophthalmoscope** (of'thalmə,skohp) an instrument fitted with a light and lenses by which the interior of the eye can be illuminated and examined.

**opiate** ('ohpi.ət, -,ayt) any medicine containing opium.

**opisthotonos** (,ohpis'thotənəs) a muscle spasm causing the back to be arched and the head retracted, with great rigidity of the muscles of the neck and back. This condition may be present in acute cases of meningitis, tetanus and strychnine poisoning.

**opium** ('ohpi.əm) a drug derived from dried poppy juice and used as a narcotic. It produces deep sleep, slows the pulse and respiration, contracts the pupils and checks all secretions of the body except sweat. It is a highly addictive drug. Opium derivatives include apomorphine, codeine, morphine and papaverine.

**opponens** (o'pohnənz) opposing. A term applied to certain muscles controlling the movements of the fingers. *O. pollicis* a muscle that adducts the thumb so that it and the little finger can be brought together.

**opportunistic** (,opətyoo'nistik) 1. denoting a microorganism which does not ordinarily cause disease but becomes pathogenic under certain circumstances. 2. denoting a disease or infection caused by such an organism.

**opsonic index** (op,sonik 'indeks) a measurement of the bactericidal power of the phagocytes in the blood of an individual.

**opsonin** ('opsənin) an antibody, present in the blood, which renders bacteria more easily destroyed by the phagocytes. Each kind of bacterium has its specific opsonin.

**optic** ('optik) relating to vision. *O. atrophy* degeneration of the optic nerve. *O. chiasma* the crossing of the fibres of the optic nerves

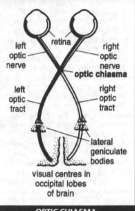

**OPTIC CHIASMA**

at the base of the brain (*see* Figure). *O. disc* the point where the optic nerve enters the eyeball. *O. foramen* the opening in the posterior part of the orbit through which pass the optic nerve and the ophthalmic artery. *O. nerve* a bundle of nerve fibres running from the optic chiasma in the brain to the optic disc on the eyeball.

**optical** ('optik'l) pertaining to sight. *O. density* the refractive power of the transparent tissues through which light rays pass, changing the direction of the ray.

**optician** (op'tishən) a professional trained in the detection of refractive errors and the dispensing of appropriate spectacles or contact lenses.

**optimum** ('optiməm) the best and most favourable.

**optometry** (op'tomətree) the measuring of visual acuity and the fitting of glasses to correct visual defects.

**ora** ('ohrə) [L.] *a margin*. *O. serrata* the jagged edge of the retina.

**oral** ('or.rəl) 1. pertaining to the mouth; taken through or applied in the mouth, as an oral medication or an oral thermometer. 2. denoting that aspect of the teeth which faces the oral cavity or tongue.

**orbit** ('awbit) 1. the bony cavity containing the eyeball. 2. the path of an object moving around another object.

**orchidectomy** (,awki'dektəmee) excision of a testicle. *Bilateral o*. the operation of castration.

**orchidopexy** ('awkidoh,peksee) an operation to free an undescended testicle and place it in the scrotum.

**orchiepididymitis** (,awki,epididi-'mietis) inflammation of a testicle and its epididymis.

**orchitis** (aw'kietis) inflammation of a testicle.

**orf** (awf) a virus infection transmitted from sheep to humans. It may give rise to a boil-like lesion on the hands of meat handlers.

**organ** ('awgən) a part of the body designed to perform a particular function.

**organelle** (,awgə'nel) a structure within a cell which has specialized functions, e.g. nucleus, endoplasmic reticulum, mitochondrion, etc.

**organic** (aw'ganik) 1. pertaining to the organs. 2. pertaining to chemicals containing carbon. *O. disease* disease of an organ, accompanied by structural changes.

**organism** ('awgə,nizəm) an individual living being, animal or vegetable.

**orgasm** ('awgazəm) the climax of sexual excitement.

**orientation** (,or.rien'tayshən) a sense of direction. 1. the ability of a person to estimate position in regard to time, place and persons. 2. the imparting of relevant information at the onset of a course or conference so that its content and objects may be understood. *Reality o.* the way in which older people who may be confused or mentally ill are assisted in keeping in touch with the world around them on a day-to-day basis. This may be achieved in a variety of ways, with large clocks, calendar boards, signs on doors and daily newspapers.

**orifice** ('o.rifis) any opening in the body.

**origin** ('o.rijin) in anatomy: 1. the point of attachment of a muscle. 2. the point at which a nerve or a blood vessel branches from the main stem.

**ornithosis** (,awni'thohsis) a virus disease of birds, usually pigeons, which may be transmitted to humans in a form resembling bronchopneumonia.

**orogenital** (,or.roh'jenit'l) pertaining to the mouth and external genitalia.

**oropharynx** (,or.roh'faringks) the lower portion of the pharynx behind the mouth and above the oesophagus and larynx.

**orphenadrine** (aw'fenə,drin) a drug used to treat Parkinsonism, especially when accompanied by depression.

**orthodontics** (,awthoh'dontiks) dentistry that deals with the prevention and correction of malocclusion and irregularities of the teeth.

**orthopaedics** (,awthə'peediks) the science dealing with deformities, injuries and diseases of the bones and joints.

**orthopnoea** (,awthop'neeə) difficulty in breathing unless in an upright position, e.g. sitting up in bed.

**orthoptics** (aw'thoptiks) the practice of treating by non-surgical methods (usually eye exercises) abnormalities of vision such as strabismus (squint).

**orthostatic** (,awthoh'statik) pertaining to or caused by standing erect. *O. albuminuria see* ALBUMIN-

URIA. *O. hypotension* low blood pressure, occurring when the person stands up.

**orthotic** (aw'thotik) serving to protect or to restore or improve function; pertaining to the use or application of an orthosis (a supportive appliance that can be applied to or around the body in the care/treatment of physical impairment or disability).

**orthotist** ('awtho,tist) a person skilled in orthotics and practising its application in individual cases.

**Ortolani's sign** (,awtoh'lahniz) *M. Ortolani, 20th century Italian orthopaedic surgeon.* A test performed soon after birth to detect possible congenital dislocation of the hip. A 'click' is felt on reversing the movements of abduction and rotation of the hip while the child is lying with knees flexed.

**os** (ohs) [L.] 1. (pl. ora) any body orifice. 2. (pl. ora) the mouth. 3. (pl. ossa) a bone.

**oscillation** (,osi'layshən) 1. a backwards and forwards motion. 2. vibration.

**oscilloscope** (ə'silə,skohp) an apparatus using a cathode-ray tube to depict visibly data fed into it electronically, e.g. the way in which the heart is performing.

**Osler's nodes** ('ohsləz) *Sir W. Osler, Canadian physician, 1849–1919.* Small painful swellings which occur in or beneath the skin, especially of the extremities in subacute bacterial endocarditis, caused by minute emboli. They usually disappear in 1–3 days.

**osmoreceptor** (,ozmohri'septə) one of a group of specialized nerve cells which monitor the osmotic pressure of the blood and the extracellular fluid. Impulses from these receptors are relayed to the hypothalamus.

**osmosis** (oz'mohsis, os-) the passage of fluid from a low concentration solution to one of a higher concentration through a semipermeable membrane.

**osmotic** (oz'motik) pertaining to osmosis. *O. pressure* the pressure exerted by large molecules in the blood, e.g. albumin and globulin proteins, which draws fluid into the bloodstream from the surrounding tissues.

**osseous** ('osi.əs) bony.

**ossicle** ('osik'l) a small bone. *Auditory o.* one of the three bones in the middle ear: the malleus, incus and stapes.

**ossification** (,osifi'kayshən) the process by which bone is developed; osteogenesis.

**osteitis** (,osti'ietis) inflammation of bone. *O. deformans see* PAGET'S DISEASE. *O. fibrosa cystica* or *parathyroid o.* defects of ossification, with fibrous tissue production, leading to weakening and deformity. It affects children chiefly, and is associated with parathyroid tumour, removal of which checks it.

**osteoarthritis** (,ostioh.ah'thrietis) *see* ARTHRITIS.

**osteoarthrotomy** (,ostioh.ah'throtəmee) surgical excision of the jointed end of a bone.

**osteoblast** ('ostioh,blast) a cell which develops into an osteocyte and turns into bone.

**osteochondritis** (,ostiohkon'drietis) inflammation of bone and cartilage, particularly a degenerative disease of an epiphysis, causing pain and deformity. *O. of the hip* Perthes' disease. *O. of the tarsal scaphoid bone* Köhler's disease. *O. of the tibial tuberosity* Osgood–Schlatter disease.

**osteochondroma** (,ostiohkon'drohmə) a tumour consisting of both bone and cartilage.

**osteoclasis** (,osti'okləsis) 1. the surgical fracture of bones to correct a deformity such as bowleg. 2. the restructuring of bone by osteoclasts during growth or the repair of damaged bone.

**osteoclast** ('ostioh₁klast) 1. a large cell that breaks down and absorbs bone and callus. 2. an instrument designed for surgical fracture of bone.

**osteocyte** ('ostioh₁siet) a bone cell.

**osteodystrophy** (₁ostioh'distrəfee) a metabolic disease of bone.

**osteogenesis** (₁ostioh'jenəsis) the formation of bone. *O. imperfecta* a congenital disorder of the bones, which are very brittle and fracture easily. Fragilitas osseum.

**osteoma** (₁osti'ohmə) a benign tumour arising from bone.

**osteomalacia** (₁ostiohmə'layshi.ə) a disease characterized by painful softening of bones. Due to vitamin D deficiency.

**osteomyelitis** (₁ostioh₁mieə'lietis) inflammation of bone, localized or generalized, due to a pyogenic infection. It may result in bone destruction, stiffening of joints, and, in extreme cases occurring before the end of the growth period, in the shortening of a limb if the growth centre is destroyed. Acute osteomyelitis is caused by bacteria that enter the body through a wound, spread from an infection near the bone, or come from a skin or throat infection. The infection usually affects the long bones of the arms and legs and causes acute pain and fever. It most often occurs in children and adolescents.

**osteopath** ('ostioh₁path) one who practises osteopathy.

**osteopathy** (₁osti'opəthee) a system of treatment of disease by bone manipulation. Osteopathic treatment is manipulative and is aimed at freeing and loosening joints and re-establishing proper relationships of the spinal column, its component bones with the pelvis and limb bones.

**osteoperiostitis** (₁ostioh₁perio'stietis) inflammation of bone and periosteum.

**osteopetrosis** (₁ostiohpe'trohsis) a rare congenital disease in which the bones become abnormally dense. Albers–Schönberg disease.

**osteophyte** ('ostioh₁fiet) a small out-growth of bone, usually in a joint damaged by osteoarthritis.

**osteoporosis** (₁ostiohpor'rohsis) abnormal rarefaction of bone which may be idiopathic or secondary to other conditions. The disorder leads to thinning of the skeleton and decreased precipitation of lime salts. There may also be inadequate calcium absorption into the bone and excessive bone resorption. The principal causes are lack of physical activity, lack of oestrogens or androgens, and nutritional deficiency. There is almost always some degree of osteoporosis that occurs with ageing. Symptoms include pathological fractures and collapse of the vertebrae without compression of the spinal cord.

**osteosarcoma** (₁ostiohsah'kohmə) an osteogenic sarcoma; a malignant bone tumour.

**osteosclerosis** (₁ostiohsklə'rohsis) an increase in density and a hardening of bone. *O. congenita* achondroplasia. *O. fragilis* osteopetrosis.

**osteotomy** (₁osti'otəmee) the cutting into or through a bone, sometimes performed to correct deformity. *O. of the hip* a method of treating osteoarthritis by cutting the bone and altering the line of weight-bearing (*see* Figure).

**ostium** ('osti.əm) *Abdominal o.* the opening at the end of the uterine tube into the peritoneal cavity.

**otic** ('ohtik) relating to the ear.

**otitis** (oh'tietis) inflammation of the ear. *Aviation o.* a symptom complex resulting from fluctuations between atmospheric pressure and air pressure in the middle ear; also

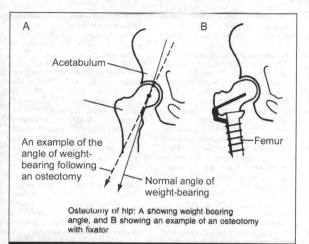

Osteotomy of hip: A showing weight-bearing angle, and B showing an example of an osteotomy with fixator

**OSTEOTOMY OF THE HIP**

called barotitis media. *Furuncular o.* the formation of furuncles in the external ear. *O. externa* inflammation of the external ear. *O. interna, o. labyrinthica* labyrinthitis. *O. mastoidea* inflammation of the mastoid spaces. *O. media* inflammation of the middle ear, occurring most often in infants and young children, and classified as serous, secretory and suppurative.

**otolith** ('otoh‚lith) 1. a calculus in the middle ear. 2. one of a number of small calcareous concretions of the inner ear, at the base of the semicircular canals.

**otomycosis** (‚ohtohmie'kohsis) a fungal infection of the auditory canal.

**otorrhoea** (‚ohtə'reeə) discharge from the ear, especially of pus.

**otosclerosis** (‚ohtohsklə'rohsis) the formation of spongy bone in the labyrinth of the ear, causing

the auditory ossicles to become fixed and less able to pass on vibrations when sound enters the ear. The cause of otosclerosis is still unknown. It may be hereditary, or perhaps related to vitamin deficiency or otitis media. An early symptom is ringing in the ears, but the most noticeable symptom is progressive loss of hearing.

**otoscope** ('ohtoh‚skohp) an auriscope; an instrument for examining the ear.

**Otosporin** (ohtə'spor‚rin) trade name for a combination preparation of ear drops containing hydrocortisone, neomycin and polymyxin.

**ototoxic** (‚ohtoh'toksik) anything which has a deleterious effect on the eighth cranial nerve or on the organs of hearing.

**ouabain** (wah'bah‚in, 'wahbayn) a cardiac glycoside; its effect is similar to that of digitalis, but digitalization is achieved more rapidly.

**outpatient** ('owtpayshənt) a patient who has a medical consultation or receives treatment at a hospital but who does not require to stay overnight in a hospital bed.

**ovarian** (oh'vair.ri.ən) relating to an ovary. *O. cyst* a tumour of the ovary containing fluid.

**ovariectomy** (ˌohvə.ri'ektəmee) oöphorectomy; excision of an ovary.

**ovariotomy** (oh.vair.ri'otəmee) 1. surgical removal of an ovary. 2. excision of an ovarian tumour.

**ovary** ('ohvə.ree) one of a pair of glandular organs in the female pelvis. They produce ova, which pass through the uterine tubes into the uterus, and steroid hormones which control the menstrual cycle.

**over-the-counter drugs** (ˌohvə dhə 'kowntə) abbreviated OTC drugs. Drugs that can be purchased from a pharmacy without a prescription from a doctor. The list of derestricted drugs available to the public is growing and includes corticosteroid ointments, antihistamines, aciclovir, ibuprofen and nicotine patches.

**overbite** ('ohvə.biet) an overlapping of the lower teeth by the upper teeth.

**overcompensation** (ˌohvə.kompən'sayshən) a mental mechanism by which people try to assert themselves by aggressive behaviour or by talking or acting 'big' to compensate for a feeling of inadequacy.

**oviduct** ('ohvi.dukt, 'ovi-) a uterine tube.

**ovulation** (ˌovyuh'layshən, ˌoh-) the process of rupture of the mature Graafian follicle when the ovum is shed from the ovary.

**ovum** ('ohvəm) [L.] *an egg.* The reproductive cell of the female.

**oxidization** (ˌoxsidie'zayshən) oxidation. The process by which combustion occurs and breaking up of

matter takes place, e.g. oxidization of carbohydrates gives carbon dioxide and water: $C_6H_{12}O_6 + 6 O_2 = 6 CO_2 + 6 H_2O$. The opposite of reduction.

**oximeter** (ok'simitə) a photoelectric cell used to determine the oxygen saturation of blood. *Ear o.* one attached to the ear by which the oxygen content of blood flowing through the ear can be measured.

**oxprenolol** (oks'prenoh.lol) a beta-blocking drug used in the treatment of angina, hypertension and cardiac arrhythmias.

**oxygen** ('oksijən) *symbol* O. A colourless, odourless gas constituting one-fifth of the atmosphere. It is stored in cylinders at high pressure or as liquid oxygen. It is used medicinally to enrich the air when either respiration or circulation is impaired. *O. saturation* the amount of oxygen bound to haemoglobin in the blood. *O. tent* a large plastic canopy that encloses the patient in a controlled environment; used for oxygen therapy, humidity therapy or aerosol therapy. *O. therapy* supplementary oxygen administered for the purpose of relieving hypoxaemia and preventing damage to the tissue cells as a result of oxygen lack.

**oxygenation** (ˌoksijə'nayshən) saturation with oxygen; a process which occurs in the lungs to the haemoglobin of blood, which is saturated with oxygen to form oxyhaemoglobin.

**oxygenator** ('oksijə.naytə) a machine through which the blood is passed to oxygenate it during open heart surgery. *Pump o.* a machine which pumps oxygenated blood through the body during heart surgery.

**oxyhaemoglobin** (ˌoksi.heemə'glohbin) haemoglobin that has been oxygenated, as in arterial blood.

**oxyntic** (ok'sintik) acid-forming. *O. cell* a parietal cell of the gastric glands which secretes hydrochloric acid.

**oxypertine** (ˌoksiˈpərteen) an antipsychotic tranquillizing drug used in the treatment of schizophrenia and related psychoses, and of mania and hyperactivity.

**oxytetracycline** (ˌoksiˌtetrəˈsiekleen) a broad-spectrum antibiotic, chiefly used against infections caused by *Chlamydia, Rickettsia* and *Brucella.*

**oxytocic** (ˌoksiˈtohsik) any drug that stimulates uterine contractions and may be used to hasten delivery.

**oxytocin** (ˌoksiˈtohsin) a pituitary hormone which stimulates uterine contractions and the ejection of milk. Synthetically prepared, it is used to induce labour and to control postpartum haemorrhage.

**oxyuriasis** (ˌoksiyuhˈrieəsis) infestation by threadworms of the genus *Enterobius.*

**ozone** ('ohzohn) an intensified form of oxygen containing three O atoms to the molecule (i.e. $O_3$), and often discharged by electrical machines, such as X-ray apparatus. In medicine it is employed as an antiseptic and oxidizing agent.

# P

**P** symbol for *phosphorus*

**Pa** symbol for *pascal*.

**pacemaker** ('pays,mayka) an object or substance that controls the rate at which a certain phenomenon occurs. The natural pacemaker of the heart is the sinoatrial NODE. *Electronic cardiac p.* an electrically operated mechanical device which stimulates the myocardium to contract. It consists of an energy source, usually batteries, and electrical circuitry connected to an electrode which is in direct contact with the myocardium. Pacemakers may be temporary or permanent. Temporary ones usually have an external energy source, whereas permanent ones have a subcutaneously implanted one. The rate at which the pacemaker delivers pulses may be either fixed or on demand. *Fixed* pacing means that pulses are delivered to the heart at a predetermined rate irrespective of any cardiac activity. A *demand* pacemaker is programmed to deliver pulses only in the absence of spontaneous cardiac activity. The need for replacement batteries is usually indicated when the rate of the pulse slows by five beats or more.

**pachydactyly** (,paki'daktilee) abnormal thickening of the fingers or toes.

**pachydermia** (,paki'dərmi.ə) an abnormal thickening of the skin. *P. laryngis* chronic hypertrophy of the vocal cords.

**pachyonychia** (,pakio'niki.ə) abnormal thickening of the nails.

**pachysomia** (,paki'sohmi.ə) abnormal thickening of parts of the body, as in acromegaly.

**Pacini's corpuscles** (pa'cheeniz) *F. Pacini, Italian anatomist, 1812–1883.* Specialized end-organs, situated in the subcutaneous tissue of the extremities and near joints, which react to firm pressure.

**paediatrician** (,peedi.ə'trishən) a medically qualified person specializing in the diseases of children.

**paediatrics** (,peedi'atriks) the branch of medicine dealing with the care and development of children and with the treatment of diseases that affect them.

**paedophilia** (,peedə'fili.ə) a sexual attraction towards young children.

**Paget's disease** ('pajits) *Sir J. Paget, British surgeon, 1814–1899.* 1. a chronic disease of bone in which overactivity of the osteoblasts and osteoclasts leads to dense bone formation with areas of rarefaction. Osteitis deformans. 2. an inflammation of the nipple caused by cancer of the milk ducts of the breast.

**pain** (payn) a feeling of distress, suffering or agony, caused by stimulation of specialized nerve endings. Its purpose is chiefly protective; it acts as a warning that tissues are being damaged and induces the sufferer to remove or withdraw from the source. Pain is a subjective experience and one person's pain cannot be compared to another's experience. *Bearing-down p.* pain accompanying uterine contractions during the second stage of LABOUR. *False p's* ineffective pains during pregnancy which resemble labour pains, but not accompanied by cervical dilatation; also called false labour. *See also* BRAXTON HICKS CONTRACTIONS. *Gas p's* pains caused by distension of the stomach or intestine by accumulations of air or other gases. *Hunger p.* pain coming on at the time of feeling hunger for a meal; a symptom of gastric disorder. *Intermenstrual p.* pain accompanying ovulation, occurring during the period between the menses, usually about midway. Also called mittelschmerz. *Labour p's* the rhythmic pains of increasing severity and frequency due to contraction of the uterus at childbirth. *See also* LABOUR. *Lancinating p.* sharp, darting pain. *Phantom p.* pain felt as if it were arising in an absent (amputated) limb. *See also* AMPUTATION. *Referred p.* pain in a part other than that in which the cause that produced it is situated. Referred pain usually originates in one of the visceral organs but is felt in the skin or sometimes in another area deep inside the body. Referred pain prob-ably occurs because pain signals from the viscera travel along the same neural pathways used by pain signals from the skin. The person perceives the pain but interprets it as having originated in the skin rather than in a deep-seated visceral organ. *Rest p.* a continuous burning pain due to ischaemia of the lower leg, which begins or is aggravated after reclining and is relieved by sitting or standing.

**palate** ('palət) the roof of the mouth. *Artificial p.* a plate made to close a cleft palate. *Cleft p.* a congenital deformity where there is lack of fusion of the two bones forming the palate. *Hard p.* the bony part at the front. *Soft p.* a fold of mucous membrane that continues from the hard palate to the uvula.

**palatine bone** ('palə,tien) one of a pair of bones which form a part of the nasal cavity and the hard palate.

**palliative** ('pali.ətiv) treatment that relieves, but does not cure, disease.

**pallidotomy** (,pali'dotəmee) an operation performed to decrease the activity of the globus pallidus, the medial part of the lentiform nucleus in the base of the cerebrum. It has brought about a marked improvement in severely agitated cases of Parkinsonism.

**pallor** ('palə) abnormal paleness of the skin.

**palmar** ('palmə) relating to the palm of the hand. *Deep p. arches* the deep and superficial palmar arches are the chief arterial blood supply to the hand, formed by the junction of the ulnar and radial arteries. *P. fascia* the arrangement of tendons in the palm of the hand. *Superficial p. arches* see DEEP P. ARCHES above.

**palpation** (pal'payshən) the examination of the organs by touch or pressure of the hand over the part.

**palpebral** ('palpibrəl) referring to the eyelids. *P. ligaments* a band of ligaments which stretches from the junction of the upper and lower lid to the orbital bones, both medially and laterally.

**palpitation** (,palpi'tayshən) rapid and forceful contraction of the heart of which the patient is conscious.

**palsy** ('pawlzee) a historical term for paralysis. *Bell's p.* paralysis of the facial muscles on one side, supplied by the seventh cranial nerve. *Crutch p.* paralysis due to pressure of a crutch on the radial nerve, and a cause of 'dropped wrist'. *Shaking p.* Parkinsonism; paralysis agitans.

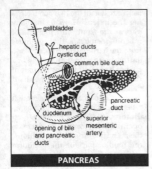

Labels in figure: gallbladder, hepatic ducts, cystic duct, common bile duct, pancreatic duct, duodenum, superior mesenteric artery, opening of bile and pancreatic ducts

**PANCREAS**

**panacea** (ˌpanəˈseeə) a remedy for all diseases.

**panarthritis** (ˌpanahˈthrietis) inflammation of all the joints or of all the structures of a joint.

**Pancoast's tumour** ('pankohsts) *H.K. Pancoast, American radiologist, 1875– 1939.* Pain, wasting and weakness of the arm, which occur as secondary features of carcinoma of the bronchus as a result of neurological involvement. The tumour is at the apex of the lung.

**pancreas** ('pangkri.əs) an elongated, racemose gland about 15 cm long, lying behind the stomach, with its head in the curve of the duodenum and its tail in contact with the spleen (*see* Figure). It secretes a digestive fluid (pancreatic juice) containing ferments which act on all classes of food. The fluid enters the duodenum by the pancreatic duct, which joins the common bile duct. The pancreas also secretes the hormones insulin and glucagon.

**pancreatectomy** (ˌpangkri.əˈtektəmee) surgical excision of the whole or a part of the pancreas.

**pancreatin** ('pangkri.ətin, pangˈkreeə-) an extract from the pancreas containing the digestive enzymes.

Used to treat deficiency, as in cystic fibrosis, and after pancreatectomy.

**pancreatitis** (ˌpangkri.əˈtietis) inflammation of the pancreas. *Acute p.* a severe condition in which the patient experiences sudden pain in the upper abdomen and back. The patient often becomes severely shocked. *Chronic p.* chronic inflammation occurring after acute attacks. Pancreatic failure may lead to diabetes mellitus.

**pancreozymin** (ˌpangkrio'ziemin) a hormone of the duodenal mucosa that stimulates the external secretory activity of the pancreas, especially its production of amylase.

**pancuronium** (ˌpangkyuh'rohni-əm) a neuromuscular blocking agent of the nerve depolarizing type, used as a muscle relaxant during surgery. It has a relatively long duration of action, a single intravenous dose lasting 45–60 min. It is often used in poor-risk patients.

**pancytopenia** (ˌpansietoh'peeni.ə) a reduction in number of all types of blood cell due to failure of bone marrow formation.

**pandemic** (pan'demik) an epidemic spreading over a wide area, sometimes all over the world.

**panic** ('panik) an unreasoning and overwhelming fear or terror. It may occur in anxiety states and acute schizophrenia.

**panniculitis** (pəˌnikyuh'lietis) inflammation of the subcutaneous fat causing tender nodules on the abdomen and thorax and on the thighs.

**pannus** ('panəs) increased vascularity of the cornea leading to granulation tissue formation and impaired vision. It occurs in trachoma after inflammation of the cornea.

**panophthalmia** (ˌpanof'thalmi.ə) panophthalmitis; inflammation of all the tissues of the eyeball.

**pantothenic acid** (ˌpantə'thenik) one of the vitamins in the B complex.

**Papanicolaou test (Pap test)** (ˌpapəˌnikəˈlayoo) *G.N. Papanicolaou, Greek physician, anatomist and cytologist, 1883–1962.* A smear test to detect diseases of the uterine cervix and endometrium.

**papaveretum** (pəˌpahvəˈreetəm) a preparation of the alkaloids of opium with an action similar to morphine. It is used to counteract severe pain.

**papilla** (pəˈpilə) a small nipple-shaped protuberance. *Circumvallate p.* one surrounded by a ridge. A number are found at the back of the tongue arranged in a V-shape, and containing taste buds. *Filiform p.* one of the fine, slender filaments on the main part of the tongue which give it its velvety appearance. *Fungiform p.* a mushroom-shaped papilla of the tongue. *Optic p.* the optic disc, where the optic nerve leaves the eyeball. *Tactile p.* a projection on the true skin which contains nerve endings responsible for relaying sensations of pressure to the brain. A touch corpuscle.

**papillitis** (ˌpapiˈlietis) 1. inflammation of the optic disc. 2. inflammation of a papilla.

**papilloedema** (ˌpapiliˈdeemə) oedema and hyperaemia of the optic disc, usually associated with increased intracranial pressure; also called choked disc.

**papilloma** (ˌpapiˈlohmə) a benign growth of epithelial tissue, e.g. a wart.

**papillomatosis** (ˌpapiˌlohməˈtohsis) the occurrence of multiple papillomas.

**papovavirus** (pəˈpohvəˌvierəs) a family of DNA-producing viruses which cause tumours, usually benign, such as warts.

**papule** (ˈpapyool) a pimple, or small solid elevation of the skin.

**papulopustular** (ˌpapyuhlohˈpustyuhlə) descriptive of skin eruptions of both papules and pustules.

**papulosquamous** (ˌpapyuhlohˈskwayməs) descriptive of skin eruptions that are both papular and scaly. They include such conditions as lichen planus, pityriasis and psoriasis.

**para-aminobenzoic acid** (ˌparəˌaminohˈben'zoh.ik) a member of the B group of vitamins. It is used in creams and lotions to prevent sunburn.

**para-aminosalicylic acid** (ˌparəˌaminoh ˌsaliˈsilik) abbreviated PAS. An acid, the salts of which were used together with other drugs, usually isoniazid (INH) or streptomycin, in the treatment of tuberculosis.

**paracentesis** (ˌparəsenˈteesis) puncture of the wall of a cavity with a hollow needle in order to draw off excess fluid or to obtain diagnostic material.

**paracetamol** (ˌparəˈseetə ˌmol, -ˈsetə-) a mild analgesic drug used to treat headaches, toothache and rheumatic pains, and also to treat pyrexia.

**paracusis** (ˌparəˈkyoosis) a perverted sense of hearing. *P. of Willis* an improvement in hearing when surrounded by noise.

**paradigm** (ˈparəˌdiem) any example or representative instance of a concept or theoretical approach.

**paradoxical sleep** (ˌparəˈdoksikˈl) rapid eye movement (REM) SLEEP.

**paraesthesia** (ˌparisˈtheezi.ə) an abnormal tingling sensation. 'Pins and needles'.

**paraffin** (ˈparəfin) any saturated hydrocarbon obtained from petroleum. *Liquid p.* a mineral oil which is used as a laxative *P. wax* a hard paraffin that can be used for wax treatment for chronic inflammation of joints. *Soft p.* petroleum jelly. Used as a barrier agent to protect the skin.

*Paragonimus* (ˌparəˈgoniməs) a genus of trematode parasites. The flukes infest the lungs and are found mainly in tropical countries.

**paraldehyde** (pə'raldi,hied) a sedative, hypnotic and anticonvulsant that has an unpleasant taste and imparts an unpleasant odour to the breath. It is now little used.

**paralysis** (pə'ralisis) loss or impairment of motor function in a part owing to a lesion of the neural or muscular mechanism; also, by analogy, impairment of sensory function (sensory paralysis). Paralysis is a symptom of a wide variety of physical and emotional disorders rather than a disease in itself. Palsy. *P. agitans* Parkinsonism. *Bulbar p. (labioglossopharyngeal p.)* paralysis due to changes in the motor centre of the medulla oblongata. It affects the muscles of the mouth, tongue and pharynx. *Facial p. (Bell's palsy)* paralysis that affects the muscles of the face and is due to injury or to inflammation of the facial nerve. *Flaccid p.* loss of tone and absence of reflexes in the paralysed muscles. *General p. of the insane* abbreviated GPI. Paralytic dementia occurring in the late stages of syphilis. *Infantile p.* the major form of POLIOMYELITIS. *Spastic p.* paralysis characterized by rigidity of affected muscles.

**paralytic** (,parə'litik) affected by or relating to paralysis. *P. ileus* obstruction of the ileum due to absence of peristalsis in a portion of the intestine.

**paramedian** (,parə'meedi.ən) situated on the side of the median line.

**paramedical** (,parə'medik'l) associated with the medical profession and the delivery of health care. The paramedical services include trained ambulance personnel, occupational and speech therapy, physiotherapy, radiography and social work.

**parametritis** (,parəmi'trietis) inflammation of the parametrium; pelvic cellulitis.

**parametrium** (,parə'meetri.əm) the connective tissue surrounding the uterus.

**paramnesia** (,param'neezi.ə) a defect of memory in which there is a false recollection. The patient may fill in the forgotten period with imaginary events, which are often described in great detail.

**paranoia** (,parə'noyə) a mental disorder characterized by delusions of grandeur or persecution which may be fully systematized in logical form, with the personality remaining fairly well preserved.

**paranoid** ('parə,noyd) resembling paranoia. Refers to a condition that can occur in many forms of mental disease. Delusions of persecution are a marked feature. *P. schizophrenia see* SCHIZOPHRENIA.

**paraparesis** (,parəpə'reesis) an incomplete paralysis affecting the lower limbs.

**paraphasia** (,parə'fayzi.ə) a speech disorder involving the substitution of a similar sound or word for that intended, thereby producing a nonsensical utterance.

**paraphimosis** (,parəfie'mohsis) retraction of the prepuce behind the glans penis, with inability to replace it, resulting in a painful constriction.

**paraphrenia** (,parə'freeniə) schizophrenia occurring for the first time in later life and not accompanied by deterioration of the personality.

**paraplegia** (,parə'pleeji.ə) paralysis of the lower extremities and lower trunk. All parts below the point of lesion in the spinal cord are affected. It may be of sudden onset from injury to the cord or may develop slowly as the result of disease.

**paraprofessional** (,parəprə'feshən'l) 1. a person who is specially trained in a particular field or occupation to assist a professional. 2. an allied health professional. 3. pertaining to a paraprofessional.

**parapsychology** (ˌparəsieˈkolɔjee) the branch of psychology dealing with psychical effects and experiences that appear to fall outside the scope of physical law, e.g. telepathy and clairvoyance.

**paraquat** ('parəˌkwot) a poisonous compound used as a contact herbicide. Contact with concentrated solutions causes irritation of the skin, cracking and shedding of the nails, and delayed healing of cuts and wounds. After ingestion renal and hepatic failure may develop, followed by pulmonary insufficiency and death.

**parasite** ('parəˌsiet) any animal or vegetable organism living upon or within another, from which it derives its nourishment.

**parasiticide** (ˌparəˈsitiˌsied) a drug that kills parasites.

**parasuicide** (ˌparəˈsooˌisied) a suicidal action such as self-mutilation or the taking of a drug overdose which is motivated by a need to attract attention and seek help rather than commit suicide.

**parasympathetic system** (ˌparəˌsimpəˈthetik 'sistəm) the craniosacral part of the autonomic nervous system.

**parasympatholytic** (ˌparəˌsimpəthoˈlitik) anticholinergic; an agent that opposes the effects of the parasympathetic nervous system.

**parathormone** (ˌparəˈthawmohn) the endocrine secretion of the parathyroid glands.

**parathyroid gland** (ˌparəˈthieroyd) one of four small endocrine glands, two of which are associated with each lobe of the thyroid gland, and sometimes embedded in it. The secretion from these has some control over calcium metabolism, and lack of it is a cause of tetany.

**parathyroidectomy** (ˌparəˌthieroy-ˈdektəmee) the surgical removal of the parathyroid glands.

**paratyphoid** (ˌparəˈtiefoyd) a notifiable infection caused by *Salmonella* of all groups except *S. typhi*. The disease is usually milder and has a shorter incubation period, more abrupt onset and lower mortality rate than does typhoid. Clinically and pathologically, the two diseases cannot be distinguished. Also called paratyphoid fever.

**parenchyma** (pəˈrengkimə) the essential active cells of an organ, as distinguished from its vascular and connective tissue.

**parenteral** (pəˈrentəˌrəl) apart from the alimentary canal. Applied to the introduction into the body of drugs or fluids by routes other than the mouth or rectum: for instance, intravenously or subcutaneously.

**paresis** (pəˈreesis, 'parəsis) partial paralysis.

**parietal** (pəˈrieət'l) relating to the walls of any cavity. *P. bones* the two bones forming part of the roof and sides of the skull. *P. cells* the oxyntic cells in the gastric mucosa that secrete hydrochloric acid. *P. pleura* the pleura attached to the chest wall.

**parity** ('parətee) the classification of a woman with regard to the number of children that have been born live to her.

**Parkinson's disease** ('pahkinsənz) *J. Parkinson, British physician, 1755–1824.* Parkinsonism; paralysis agitans. A slowly progressive disease usually occurring in later life, characterized pathologically by degeneration within the nuclear masses of the extrapyramidal system, and clinically by mask-like facies (*see* FACIES (PARKINSON)), a characteristic tremor of resting muscles, a slowing of voluntary movements, a festinating gait, peculiar posture and muscular weakness. When this symptom complex occurs secondarily to another disorder, the condition is called Parkinsonism.

**paronychia** (ˌparo'nikiə) an abscess near the fingernail; a whitlow or felon. *P. tendinosa* a pyogenic infection that involves the tendon sheath.

**parotid** (pə'rotid) situated near the ear. *P. glands* two salivary glands, one in front of each ear.

**parotitis** (ˌparə'tietis) inflammation of a parotid gland. Caused usually by ascending infection via its duct, when hygiene of the mouth is neglected or when the natural secretions are lessened, especially in severe illness or after operation. *Epidemic p.* mumps.

**parous** ('parəs) having borne one or more children.

**paroxysm** ('parokˌsizəm) 1. a sudden attack or recurrence of a symptom of a disease. 2. a convulsion.

**paroxysmal** (ˌparok'sizməl) occurring in paroxysms. *P. cardiac dyspnoea* cardiac asthma. Recurrent attacks of dyspnoea associated with pulmonary oedema and left-sided heart failure. *P. tachycardia* recurrent attacks of rapid heart beats that may occur without heart disease.

**parrot disease** ('parət) *see* PSITTACOSIS.

**parthenogenesis** (ˌpahthənoh'jenəsis) asexual reproduction by means of an egg that has not been fertilized.

**particle** ('pahtik'l) a minute piece of substance.

**parturient** (pah'tyooə.ri.ənt) giving birth; relating to childbirth.

**parturition** (ˌpahtyuh'rishən) the act of giving birth to a child.

**PAS** para-aminosalicylic acid.

**pascal** (pa'skal, 'pask'l) *symbol* Pa. The SI unit of pressure.

**passive** ('pasiv) not active. *P. immunity see* IMMUNITY. *P. movements* in massage, manipulation by a physiotherapist without the help of the patient. *P. smoking* inhaling tobacco smoke exhaled by others;

associated with a significant risk of increase in lung cancer.

**passivity** (pa'sivitee) in psychiatry, a delusional feeling that a person is under some outside control and must therefore be inactive.

**Pasteurella** (ˌpastə'relə) L. *Pasteur, French chemist and bacteriologist, 1833–1895.* A genus of short Gramnegative bacilli. *P. pestis* the causative organism of plague transmitted by rat fleas to humans.

**pasteurization** (ˌpastə.rie'zayshən, ˌpahstyə-) the process of checking fermentation in milk and other fluids by heating them to a temperature of 72°C for 15–20 min or 63°C for 30 min and then rapidly cooling. This kills most pathogenic bacteria.

**patch test** (pach) a test of skin sensitivity in which a number of possible allergens are applied to the skin under a plaster. The causal agent of the allergy will produce an inflammation.

**patella** (pə'telə) the small, circular, sesamoid bone forming the knee-cap.

**patellar** (pə'telə) belonging to the patella. *P. reflex* a knee jerk obtained by tapping the tendon below the patella.

**patellectomy** (ˌpate'lektəmee) excision of the patella.

**patent** ('paytənt) open. *P. ductus arteriosus* failure of the ductus arteriosus to close, causing a shunt of blood from the aorta into the pulmonary artery and producing a continuous heart murmur (*see* Figure).

**pathogen** ('pathə.jen) a microorganism that can cause disease, e.g. *Clostridium tetani* can cause tetanus.

**pathogenicity** (ˌpathəjə'nisitee) the ability of a microorganism to cause disease.

**pathognomonic** (ˌpathəgnə'monik) specifically characteristic of a disease. A sign or symptom by which a

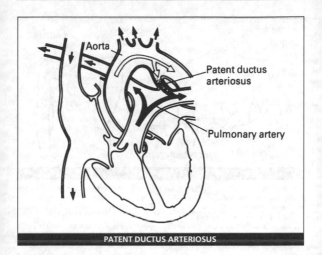

**PATENT DUCTUS ARTERIOSUS**

pathological condition can positively be identified.

**pathological** (‚pathə'lojik'l) 1. pertaining to pathology. 2. causing or arising from disease. *P. fracture* a fracture occurring in diseased bone where there has been little or no external trauma.

**pathology** (pə'tholəjee) the branch of medicine that deals with the essential nature of disease, especially of the structural and functional changes in tissues and organs of the body which cause or are caused by disease.

**pathophobia** (‚pathə'fohbi.ə) an exaggerated dread of disease.

**patient** ('payshənt) a person who is ill or is undergoing treatment for disease.

**patient's rights** ('riets) patients have three basic rights: namely, the right to know, the right to privacy and the right to treatment. The first two are moral rights while the third

is, in the UK, both a moral and legal right.

**Paul–Bunnell test** (‚pawlbə'nel) *J.R. Paul, American physician, 1893–1971; W.W. Bunnell, American physician, 1902–1966.* An agglutination test which, if positive, confirms the diagnosis of glandular fever.

**Pavlov's method** ('pavlovz ‚methəd) *I.P. Pavlov, Russian physiologist, 1849–1936.* A method for the study of the conditioned reflexes. Pavlov noticed that his experimental dogs salivated in anticipation of food when they heard a bell ring.

**Pb** symbol for *lead*.

**peau d'orange** (‚poh do'ronhzh) a dimpled appearance of the overlying skin. Blockage of the skin lymphatics causes dimpling of the hair follicle openings which resembles orange skin. Particularly associated with breast cancer.

**pecten** ('pekten) 1. the middle third of the anal canal. 2. a ridge on the

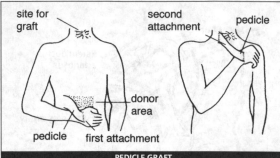

site for graft

second attachment

pedicle

donor area

pedicle

first attachment

**PEDICLE GRAFT**

pubic crest to which the inguinal ligament is attached.

**pectoral** ('pektə.rəl) relating to the chest. *P. muscles* two pairs of muscles, pectoralis major and pectoralis minor, which control the movements of the shoulder and upper arm.

**pectus** ('pektəs) the chest.

**pedicle** ('pedik'l) the stem or neck of a tumour. *P. graft* a tissue graft that is partially detached and inserted in its new position while temporarily still obtaining its blood supply from the original source (*see* Figure).

**pediculosis** (pə.dikyuh'lohsis) the condition of being infested with lice.

*Pediculus* (pə'dikyuhləs) a genus of lice. *P. humanus* a species that feeds on human blood and is an important vector of relapsing fever, typhus and trench fever. Two sub-species are recognized: *P. humanus* var. *capitis* (head louse), found on the scalp hair, and *P. humanus* var. *corporis* (body or clothes louse), found elsewhere on the body.

**peduncle** (pə'dungk'l) a narrow part of a structure acting as a support. *Cerebellar p.* one of the collections of nerve fibres connecting the cerebellum with the medulla oblongata.

**PEEP** positive end-expiratory pressure.

**peer review** (.piə ri'vyoo) a basic component of a quality assurance (see QUALITY) programme in which the results of health and/or nursing care given to a specific patient population are evaluated according to defined criteria established by the peers of the professionals delivering the care. Peer review is focused on the patient and on the results of care given by a group of professionals rather than on individual professional practitioners.

**Pel–Ebstein syndrome** (.pel'eb-stien) *P.K. Pel, Dutch physician, 1852–1919; W. Ebstein, German physician, 1836–1912.* A recurrent pyrexia, having a cycle of 15–21 days, which occurs in cases of lymphadenoma.

**pellagra** (pə'lagrə, -lay-) a syndrome caused by a diet seriously deficient in niacin (or by failure to convert tryptophan to niacin). Most persons with pellagra also suffer from deficiencies of vitamin $B_2$ (riboflavin) and other essential vitamins and minerals. The disease also occurs in persons suffering from alcoholism and drug addiction. Characterized by debility, digestive disorders, peripheral neuritis, ataxia, mental disturbance and erythema with exfoliation of the skin.

**pelvic** ('pelvik) pertaining to the pelvis. *P. exenteration* removal of all the pelvic organs. *P. girdle* the ring of bone to which the lower limbs are jointed. It consists of the two hip bones and the sacrum and coccyx. *P. inflammatory disease* persistent infection of the internal reproductive organs of the female, often resulting in infertility.

**pelvimetry** (pel'vimətree) measurement of the pelvis.

**pelvis** ('pelvis) a basin-shaped cavity. *Bony p.* the pelvic girdle, formed of the hip bones and the sacrum and coccyx. *Contracted p.* narrowing of the diameter of the pelvis. It may be of the true conjugate or the diagonal. Effective antenatal care will recognize this condition, and caesarean section may be necessary. *False p.* the part formed by the concavity of the iliac bones above the ileopectineal line. *Renal p.* the dilatation of the ureter which, by enclosing the hilum, surrounds the pyramids of the kidney substance. *True p.* the basin-like cavity below the false pelvis, its upper limit being the pelvic brim.

**pemphigoid** ('pemfi,goyd) 1. resembling pemphigus. 2. a bullous disease of the elderly with the blisters arising beneath the epidermis. The skin and the mucosa are affected, and sometimes the conjunctiva.

**pemphigus** ('pemfigəs) a distinctive group of rare but serious diseases characterized by successive crops of large bullae ('water blisters'); the name is derived from the Greek word for blister, *pemphix*. Clusters of blisters usually appear first near the nose and mouth (sometimes inside them) and then gradually spread over the skin of the rest of the body. When the blisters burst, they leave round patches of raw and tender skin. Pemphigus is considered to be an autoimmune disorder.

**pendulous** ('pendyuhləs) hanging down. *P. abdomen* the hanging down of the abdomen over the pelvis, due to weakness and laxity of the abdominal muscles.

**penicillamine** (,peni'silə,meen) a chelating agent that is used in heavy metal poisoning to aid excretion of the metal and in the treatment of hepatolenticular degeneration (Wilson's disease). Also used in the treatment of severe rheumatoid arthritis.

**penicillin** (,peni'silin) an antibiotic cultured from certain moulds of the genus *Penicillium*. The drug is used in various forms to treat a wide variety of bacterial infections. Discovered by Fleming in 1929, it was first used therapeutically in 1941. Varieties of the drug include: benethamine penicillin, benzylpenicillin, benzathine penicillin, procaine penicillin, cloxacillin, ampicillin and amoxicillin.

**penicillinase** (,peni'sili,nayz) an enzyme that inactivates penicillin. Many bacteria, particularly staphylococci, produce this enzyme.

*Penicillium* (,peni'sili,əm) a genus of mould-like fungi, from some of which the penicillins are derived. Some species are pathogenic to humans.

**penis** ('peenis) the male organ of copulation and urination.

**pentagastrin** (,pentə'gastrin) a synthetic hormone with a similar structure to gastrin. It has largely replaced histamine in gastric secretion tests as it has no apparent side-effects.

**pentamidine** (pen'tamideen) an anti-protozoal drug used mainly in the treatment of *Pneumocystis carinii* infections.

**pentazocine** (pen'tazoh,seen) an analgesic similar to morphine and used in the treatment of moderate to severe pain.

**pentose** ('pentohz) a monosaccharide containing five carbon atoms in a molecule.

**pentosuria** (,pentoh'syooə.ri.ə) a benign inborn error of metabolism due to a defect in the activity of the enzyme L-xylulose dehydrogenase, resulting in pentose in the urine.

**pepsin** ('pepsin) an enzyme found in gastric juice. It partially digests proteins in an acid solution.

**pepsinogen** (pep'sinəjən) the precursor of pepsin, activated by hydrochloric acid.

**peptic** ('peptik) relating to pepsin or the action of the gastric juices in promoting digestion. *P. ulcer* an ulcer, usually in the stomach or the duodenum, caused by an erosion of the surface to expose the muscle wall by the stomach acid and digestive enzymes. It is often precipitated by HELICOBACTER PYLORI organisms.

**peptide** ('peptied) any of a class of compounds of low molecular weight which yield two or more amino acids on hydrolysis. Peptides form the constituent parts of proteins.

**peptone** ('peptohn) a substance produced by the action of pepsin on protein.

**peptonuria** (,peptə'nyooə.ri.ə) the presence of peptones in the urine.

**per os** (pər 'os) [L.] *by the mouth.*

**percentile** (pə'sentiel) a term used in statistics to show how common some characteristic is. The line represents the percentage of the population who have this characteristic. The 90th percentile (or centile) for height means that 90% of the population will be no taller than the figure. The 50th percentile is the median or average.

**percept, perception** ('pərsept, pə-'sepshən) an awareness and understanding of an impression that has been presented to the senses. The mental process by which we perceive.

**percussion** (pə'kushən) a method of diagnosis by tapping with the fingers or with a light hammer upon any part of the body. Information can thus be gained as to the condition of underlying organs.

**percutaneous** (,pərkyoo'tayni.əs) through the skin, particularly in relation to ointments that are applied to unbroken skin.

**perforation** (,pərfə'rayshən) a hole or break in the containing walls or membranes of an organ or structure of the body. Perforation occurs when erosion, infection or other factors create a weak spot in the organ and internal pressure causes a rupture. It may also result from a deep penetrating wound.

**performance indicators** (pə'form-əns) a 'package' of routine statistics derived nationally by the Department of Health and visually presented in ways that highlight the relative efficiency of health services. Performance indicators are intended to compare services and identify aspects that merit further scrutiny locally with a view to changes in organization or practice.

**perfusion** (pə'fyoozhən) the passage of liquid through a tissue or an organ, particularly the passage of blood through the lung tissue.

**perianal** (,peri'ayn'l) surrounding or located around the anus. *P. abscess* a small subcutaneous pocket of pus near the anal margin.

**periarteritis** (,peri,ahtə'rietis) inflammation of the outer coat and surrounding tissues of an artery.

**periarthritis** (,periah'thrietis) inflammation of the tissues surrounding a joint.

**pericardiectomy** (ˌperiˌkahdiˈekt-əmee) surgical removal of the pericardium; pericardectomy. Used in the treatment of chronic constrictive pericarditis.

**pericarditis** (ˌperikahˈdietis) inflammation of the pericardium. *Adhesive p.* the presence of adhesions between the two layers of pericardium owing to a thick fibrinous exudate. *Bacterial p.* inflammation of the pericardium due to bacterial infection. *Chronic constrictive p.* thickening and sometimes calcification of the pericardium, which inhibits the action of the heart. *Rheumatic p.* pericarditis due to rheumatic fever.

**pericardium** (ˌperiˈkahdi.əm) the smooth membranous sac enveloping the heart, consisting of an outer fibrous and an inner serous coat. The sac contains a small amount of serous fluid.

**perichondrium** (ˌperiˈkondri.əm) the membrane covering cartilaginous surfaces.

**pericranium** (ˌperiˈkrayni.əm) the periosteum of the cranial bones.

**pericyazine** (ˌperiˈsie.əˌzeen) a phenothiazine stronger than chlorpromazine; used in behavioural disturbances, schizophrenia and related psychoses.

**perilymph** (ˈperiˌlimf) the fluid that separates the bony and the membranous labyrinths of the ear.

**perimeter** (pəˈrimitə) 1. the line marking the boundary of any area or geometrical figure; the circumference. 2. an instrument for measuring the field of vision.

**perimetrium** (ˌperiˈmeetri.əm) the peritoneal covering of the uterus.

**perinatal** (ˌperiˈnaytˈl) relating to the period shortly before and 7 days after birth. *P. mortality rate* the number of still births plus deaths of babies under 7 days old per 1000 total births in any one year.

**perinatologist** (ˌperinayˈtoləjist) a medically qualified person specializing in perinatology.

**perinatology** (ˌperinayˈtoləjee) the branch of medicine (obstetrics and paediatrics) dealing with the fetus and infant during the perinatal period.

**perineal** (ˌperiˈnee.əl) relating to the perineum.

**perineorrhaphy** (ˌperiniˈo.rəfee) suture of the perineum to repair a laceration caused during childbirth.

**perineum** (ˌperiˈnee.əm) the tissues between the anus and external genitals. *Lacerated p.* a torn perineum, which may result from childbirth but is often forestalled by performing an episiotomy. Treatment is by perineorrhaphy.

**periodic** (ˌpiə.riˈodik) recurring at regular or irregular intervals. *P. apnoea of the newborn* occurring in the normal full-term infant, periodic episodes of rapid breathing followed by a brief period of apnoea which is associated with rapid eye movements. *P. syndrome* recurrent head, limb or abdominal pains in children for which no organic cause can be found. It often leads to migraine in adult life.

**periodontitis** (ˌperi.ədonˈtietis) inflammation of the periodontium.

**periodontium** (ˌperi.əˈdonshi.əm) the connective tissue between the teeth and their bony sockets.

**perioperative** (ˌperiˈopə.rətiv) pertaining or relating to the period immediately before or after an operation, as in perioperative care.

**periosteal** (ˌperiˈosti.əl) pertaining to or composed of periosteum. *P. elevator* an instrument for separating the periosteum from the bone.

**periosteum** (ˌperiˈosti.əm) the fibrous membrane covering the surface of bone. It consists of two layers: the inner or osteogenetic layer, which is closely adherent and forms new cells (by which the bone grows in girth); and, in close contact with it, the fibrous layer richly supplied with blood vessels.

**periostitis** (,perio'stietis) inflammation of the periosteum, usually as a result of injury.

**peripheral** (pə'rifə.rəl) relating to the periphery. *P. iridectomy* excision of a small piece of iris from its peripheral edge. *P. nervous system* those parts of the nervous system lying outside the central nervous system. *P. neuritis* inflammation of terminal nerves. *P. resistance* the resistance in the walls of the arterioles, which is a major factor in the control of blood pressure.

**periphery** (pə'rifə.ree) the outer surface or circumference.

**peristalsis** (,peri'stalsis) a wavelike contraction, preceded by a wave of dilatation, which travels along the walls of a tubular organ, tending to press its contents onwards. It occurs in the muscle coat of the alimentary canal. *Reversed p.* a wave of contraction in the alimentary canal which passes *towards* the mouth. *Visible p.* a wave of contraction in the alimentary canal that is visible on the surface of the abdomen.

**peritoneal** (,perita'neeəl) referring to the peritoneum. *P. cavity* the cavity between the parietal and the visceral peritoneum. *P. dialysis* a method of removing waste products from the blood by passing a cannula into the peritoneal cavity, running in a dialysing fluid, and after an interval, draining it off.

**peritoneoscopy** (,peritəni'oskəpee) visual examination of the peritoneum by means of a peritoneoscope.

**peritoneum** (,perita'neeəm) the serous membrane lining the abdominal cavity and forming a covering for the abdominal organs. *Parietal p.* that which lines the abdominal cavity. *Visceral p.* the inner layer which closely covers

the abdominal organs and includes the mesenteries.

**peritonitis** (,perita'nietis) inflammation of the peritoneum. *Acute p.* this may be produced by inflammation of abdominal organs, by irritating substances from a perforated gallbladder or gastric ulcer, by rupture of a cyst, or by irritation from blood, as in cases of internal bleeding. *Chronic p.* this is comparatively rare, and is often associated with tuberculosis. Less frequently, it may result from long-standing irritation caused by the presence in the abdomen of a foreign body, such as gunshot, or by chronic peritoneal dialysis.

**peritonsillar** (,peri'tonsilə) around the tonsil. *P. abscess* quinsy.

**perlèche** (pər'lesh) inflammation with fissuring at the angles of the mouth; often due to vitamin B deficiency, poorly fitting dentures or thrush infection.

**permeability** (,pərmi.ə'bilitee) the degree to which a fluid can pass from one structure through a wall or membrane to another.

**pernicious** (pə'nishəs) highly destructive; fatal. *P. anaemia* an anaemia due to lack of absorption of vitamin $B_{12}$ for the formation of red blood cells.

**perniosis** (,pərni'ohsis) a condition, resulting from persistent exposure to cold, which produces vascular spasm in the superficial arterioles of the hands and feet, causing thrombosis and necrosis. Perniosis includes chilblains and Raynaud's disease.

**peroral** (pər'ror.rəl) by the mouth.

**perphenazine** (pər'fenə.zeen) an antiemetic and tranquillizing drug similar to chlorpromazine. Used in the treatment of nausea and vomiting, and of schizophrenia and other psychoses.

**perseveration** (pər,sevə'rayshən) the constant recurrence of an idea or the tendency to keep repeating the same words or actions.

**personality** (ˌpərsəˈnalitee) the sum total of heredity and inborn tendencies, with influences from environment and education, which forms the mental make-up of a person and influences attitude to life. *Antisocial p.* a personality disorder in which repetitive antisocial behaviour is associated with ego eccentricity, lack of guilt or anxiety, and imperviousness to punishment. Also called sociopathic (psychopathic) personality. *Cyclothymic p.* a personality marked by alternate moods of elation and dejection. *Double p., dual p.* multiple personality. *Multiple p.* a dissociative reaction in which an individual adopts two or more personalities alternatively, in none of which is there awareness of the experiences of the other(s). *Psychopathic p.* antisocial personality, sociopathic personality. *Schizoid p.* a personality disorder marked by timidness, self-consciousness, introversion, feelings of isolation and loneliness, and failure to form close interpersonal relationships; the individual is frequently ambitious, meticulous and a perfectionist.

**perspiration** (ˌpərspiˈrayshən) sweat or the act of sweating. *Insensible p.* water evaporation from the moist surfaces of the body, such as the respiratory tract and skin, that is not due to the activity of the sweat glands. It occurs at a constant rate of about 500 ml/day. When treating dehydration this loss must be taken into account. *Sensible p.* sweat that is visible as droplets on the skin. Part of the mechanism for regulation of body temperature.

**Perthes' disease** (ˈpərtayz) *G.C. Perthes, German surgeon, 1869–1927.* Osteochondritis of the head of the femur. Pseudocoxalgia (Legg–Calvé–Perthes disease).

**pertussis** (pəˈtusis) whooping cough.

**perversion** (pəˈvərshən) morbid diversion from a normal course. *Sexual p.* abnormal sexual desires and behaviour. A deviation.

**pes** (payz, peez) the foot, or any foot-like structure. *P. cavus* a foot with an abnormally high arch. Claw foot. *P. malleus valgus* hammer toe. *P. planus* flat foot.

**pessary** (ˈpesə.ree) 1. a plastic or metal ring-shaped device which is inserted in the vagina to support a prolapsed uterus. 2. a medicated suppository inserted into the vagina for antiseptic or contraceptive purposes.

**petechia** (pəˈteeki.ə) a small spot due to an effusion of blood under the skin, as in purpura.

**pethidine** (ˈpethi.deen, .din) a synthetic narcotic analgesic, less potent than morphine with quicker onset but shorter duration of action; used in obstetrics and pre-and postoperative medication. Particularly useful, because it relaxes smooth muscle, in patients with ureteric and biliary colic and as an analgesic in patients with asthma.

**petit mal** (ˌpeti ˈmal) a mild form of epilepsy common in children and characterized by a sudden and brief loss of consciousness.

**pétrissage** (ˌpaytriˈsahzh) a kneading action used in massage.

**petrositis** (ˌpetrohˈsietis) inflammation of the petrous portion of the temporal bone, usually spread from a middle-ear infection.

**petrous** (ˈpetrəs) resembling a stone. *P. bone* that part of the two temporal bones that forms the base of the skull and contains the middle and inner ear.

**Peyer's glands** or **patches** (ˈpieəz) *J. C. Peyer, Swiss anatomist, 1653–1712.* Small lymph nodules situated in the mucous membrane of the lower part of the small intestine.

**Peyronie's disease** ('payrəneez) induration of the corpora cavernosa of the penis, producing a fibrous chordee leading to painful erection.

**pH** a measure of the hydrogen ion concentration, and so the acidity or alkalinity of a solution. Expressed numerically 1 to 14; 7 is neutral, and below this is acid and above alkaline. *See* HYDROGEN (ION CONCENTRATION).

**phaeochromocytoma** (ˌfeeohˌkrohmohsie'tohmə) a tumour of the adrenal medulla which gives rise to paroxysmal hypertension.

**phage** (fayj, fahzh) bacteriophage. A virus that lives on bacteria but is confined to a particular strain. *P.-typing* the identification of certain bacterial strains by determining the presence of strain-specific phages. Used in detecting the causative organisms of epidemics, especially food poisoning.

**phagocyte** ('fagəˌsiet) a blood cell that has the power of ingesting bacteria, protozoa and foreign bodies in the blood.

**phagocytosis** (ˌfagəsie'tohsis) the engulfing and destruction of micro-organisms and foreign bodies by phagocytes in the blood.

**phalanges** (fa'lanjeez) the bones of the fingers or toes.

**phallus** ('faləs) the penis.

**phantasy** ('fantəsee) *see* FANTASY.

**phantom** ('fantəm) 1. an image or impression not evoked by actual stimuli. 2. a model of the body or of a specific part thereof. 3. a device for simulating the in vivo interaction of radiation with tissues. *P. pain* pain felt as if it were arising in an absent (amputated) limb. *P. pregnancy* see PSEUDOCYESIS. *P. tumour* a tumour-like swelling of the abdomen caused by contraction of the muscles or by localized gas.

**pharmacogenetics** (ˌfahməkohjə-'netiks) the study of genetically determined variations in drug metabolism and the response of the individual.

**pharmacology** (ˌfahmə'koləjee) the science of the nature and preparation of drugs and particularly of their effects on the body.

**pharmacopoeia** (ˌfahməkə'pee.ə) an authoritative publication that gives the standard formulae and preparations of drugs used in a given country. *British P.* that authorized for use in the UK.

**pharmacy** ('fahməsee) 1. the art of preparing, compounding and dispensing medicines. 2. the place where drugs are stored and dispensed.

**pharyngeal** (ˌfarin'jeeəl, fə'rinji.əl) relating to the pharynx. *P. pouch* dilatation of the lower part of the pharynx.

**pharyngectomy** (ˌfarin'jektəmee) excision of a section of the pharynx.

**pharyngitis** (ˌfarin'jietis) inflammation of the pharynx.

**pharyngolaryngeal** (fəˌring.goh-ˌlarin'jeeəl) referring to both the pharynx and larynx.

**pharyngotympanic tube** (fəˌring-ˌgohtim'panik) the tube that joins the middle ear to the pharynx; the eustachian tube.

**pharynx** ('faringks) the muscular tube, lined with mucous membrane, situated at the back of the mouth. It leads into the oesophagus, and also communicates with the nose through the posterior nares, with the ears through the pharyngotympanic (eustachian) tubes, and with the larynx. *See* LARYNGOPHARYNX, NASOPHARYNX and OROPHARYNX.

**phenazocine** (fe'nazohˌseen) an analgesic drug used to relieve severe pain. It is a drug of addiction.

**phenelzine** (fe'nelzeen) a monoamine oxidase inhibitor used in the treatment of depressive illness.

**phenindione** (ˌfenin'dieohn) an anticoagulant drug used in the treatment of deep vein thrombosis.

**phenobarbitone** (ˌfeenoh'bahbiˌtohn) a long-lasting barbiturate drug used to treat severe insomnia and also as an anticonvulsant drug in the treatment of epilepsy.

**phenol** ('feenol) carbolic acid. A disinfectant derived from coal tar.

**phenolphthalein** (ˌfeenol'thalee.in, -leen, -'thay-) a cathartic. Its use should be avoided because it may cause rashes, albuminuria and haemoglobinuria. Its laxative effects may continue for several days.

**phenomenon** (fi'nominən) 1. an objective sign or symptom. 2. A noteworthy occurrence.

**phenoperidine** (ˌfeenoh'perideen) a synthetic narcotic analgesic used intraoperatively to supplement general anaesthesia. Also used in the intensive care unit to facilitate patients' acceptance of mechanical ventilation.

**phenothiazine** (ˌfeenoh'thieəzeen) one of a group of drugs used in the treatment of severe psychiatric disorders. The first to be used was chlorpromazine.

**phenotype** ('feenoh.tiep) the characteristics of an individual that are due both to the environment and to genetic make-up.

**phenoxybenzamine** (feˌnoksi'benzəmeen) a vasodilator drug used in the treatment of peripheral conditions such as Raynaud's disease.

**phenoxymethylpenicillin** (feˌnoksiˌmethil.peni'silin) a penicillinase-sensitive antibiotic similar in action to benzylpenicillin. Used mainly against streptococcal infections in children. It is taken orally. Penicillin V.

**phentermine** ('fentə.meen) an appetite-suppressant drug used in the treatment of obesity.

**phentolamine** (fen'tolə.meen) a vasodilator, used to reduce blood pressure in treating phaeochromocytoma.

**phenylalanine** (ˌfeenil'aləneen) an essential amino acid which cannot be properly metabolized in persons suffering from phenylketonuria.

**phenylbutazone** (ˌfeenil'byootəzohn) an analgesic antipyretic drug used in the treatment of gout and rheumatic disorders.

**phenylketonuria** (ˌfeenilˌkeetə'n-yooə.ri.ə) abbreviated PKU. A congenital disease due to a defect in the metabolism of the amino acid phenylalanine. The condition is hereditary. It results from lack of an enzyme, phenylalanine hydroxylase, necessary for the conversion of phenylalanine into tyrosine. Thus there is accumulation of phenylalanine in the blood, with eventual excretion of phenylpyruvic acid in the urine. If untreated, the condition results in learning difficulties and other abnormalities. The condition can be detected soon after birth, and screening of newborns for PKU entails a simple blood test. A sample of blood is taken from infants' heels at approximately 2 weeks and phenylalanine levels are assessed (Guthrie test). Treatment is with a diet low in phenylalanine.

**phenylpyruvic acid** (ˌfeenilpie'roo-vik) an abnormal constituent of the urine present in phenylketonuria.

**phenytoin** (ˌfeni'toh.in) an anticonvulsant drug used in the treatment of major epileptic fits.

**phimosis** (fie'mohsis) constriction of the prepuce so that it cannot be drawn back over the glans penis. The usual treatment is circumcision.

**phlebectomy** (fli'bektəmee) excision of a vein or a portion of a vein.

**phlebitis** (fli'bietis) inflammation of a vein, usually in the leg, which tends to lead to the formation of a thrombus. The symptoms are pain and swelling, and redness along the course of the vein, which is felt later as a hard, tender cord.

**phlebography** (fli'bografee) 1. Radiographic examination of a vein containing a contrast medium. 2. the graphic representation of the venous pulse.

**phlebolith** ('fleboh,lith) a stone formed in a vein by calcification of a blood clot.

**phlebothrombosis** (,flebothrom-'bohsis) obstruction of a vein by a blood clot, without local inflammation. It is usually in the deep veins of the calf of the leg, causing tenderness and swelling. The clot may break away and cause an embolism.

*Phlebotomus* (fla'botomas) a genus of sandflies, the various species of which transmit leishmaniasis in its many forms, and also sandfly fever.

**phlebotomy** (fli'botomee) the puncture of a vein for the withdrawal of blood. Venesection.

**phlegm** (flem) mucus secreted by the lining of the air passages.

**phlegmasia** (fleg'mayzi.ə) an inflammation. *P. alba dolens* acute oedema in a leg due to lymphatic blockage. 'White leg'. Rarely occurs now but was seen most frequently in women after childbirth.

**phlegmatic** (fleg'matik) dull and apathetic.

**phlycten** ('fliktən) 1. a small blister caused by a burn. 2. a small vesicle containing lymph occurring in the conjunctiva or cornea of the eye. Often associated with tuberculosis.

**phobia** ('fohbi.ə) an irrational fear produced by a specific situation which the patient attempts to avoid.

**phocomelia** (,fohkə'meeli.ə) a rare congenital deformity in which the long bones of the limbs are minimal or absent and the individual has hands or feet resembling the flippers of seals, or stump-like limbs of various lengths. The drug thalidomide, taken by the mother early

in pregnancy, has produced this deformity.

**pholcodine** ('folkoh,deen) a linctus for the suppression of a dry or painful cough.

**phonation** (foh'nayshən) the art of uttering meaningful vocal sounds.

**phonocardiogram** (,fohnoh'kahdioh,gram) a record of the heart sounds made by a phonocardiograph.

**phonocardiograph** (,fohnoh'kahdioh,grahf, -graf) an instrument that graphically records heart sounds and murmurs.

**phonology** (fə'noləjee) the study of speech sounds, their production and the relationship between sounds as elements of language.

**phosphatase** ('fosfə,tayz) one of a group of enzymes involved in the metabolism of phosphate. *Alkaline p.* an enzyme formed by osteoblasts in the bones and by liver cells and excreted in the bile.

**phosphate** ('fosfayt) a salt or ester of phosphoric acid.

**phospholipid** (,fosfə'lipid) a lipid of glycerol fats found in cells, especially those of the nervous system.

**phosphorus** ('fosfə.rəs) *symbol* P. Phosphorus is an essential element in the diet. It is a major component of bone, is involved in almost all metabolic processes and also plays an important role in cell metabolism. It is obtained by the body from milk products, cereals, meat and fish. Its use by the body is controlled by vitamin D and calcium. Phosphorus is very inflammable and exceedingly poisonous. Inhalation of its vapour by workers in chemical industries may cause necrosis of the mandible (phosphonecrosis or phossy jaw). Free phosphorus causes fatty degeneration of the liver and other viscera.

**phosphorylase** (fos'fo.ri,layz) an enzyme, found in the liver and kidneys, which catalyses the breakdown of glycogen into glucose 1-phosphate.

**photocoagulation** (ˌfohtohkoh.agˈyuhˈlayshən) the use of a powerful light source to induce inflammation of the retina and choroid to treat retinal detachment.

**photophobia** (ˌfohtohˈfohbi.ə) intolerance of light. It can occur in many eye conditions, including conjunctivitis, corneal ulceration, iritis and keratitis.

**photophthalmia** (ˌfohtofˈthalmi.ə) inflammation of the eye due to overexposure to bright light, especially to ultraviolet light.

**photopic** (fohˈtopik, -ˈtoh-) pertaining to bright light. *P. vision* vision in bright light when the cones of the retina provide the visual appreciation of colour and shape.

**photopsia** (fohˈtopsi.ə) a sensation of flashes of light sometimes occurring in the early stages of retinal detachment.

**photosensitivity** (ˌfohtoh.sensiˈtivitee) an abnormal degree of sensitivity of the skin to sunlight.

**phototherapy** (ˌfohtohˈtherəpee) treatment using fluorescent light, containing a high output of blue light, to reduce the amount of unconjugated bilirubin in the skin of a mildly jaundiced neonate.

**phrenic** (ˈfrenik) 1. relating to the mind. 2. pertaining to the diaphragm. *P. avulsion* the surgical extraction of a part of the phrenic nerve. *P. nerve* one of a pair of nerves controlling the muscles of the diaphragm.

**phthalylsulphathiazole** (ˌthalilˌsulfaˌthiəˌzohl) an insoluble sulphonamide, poorly absorbed in the intestine and so used to kill intestinal bacteria before surgery.

*Phthirus pubis* (ˌthirəs ˈpyoobis) the crab louse.

**phthisis** (ˈthiesis) pulmonary tuberculosis. *P. bulbi* a shrinking of the eyeball following inflammation or injury.

**physical** (ˈfisikˈl) in medicine, relating to the body as opposed to the mental processes. *P. examination* examination of the bodily state of a patient by ordinary physical means, such as inspection, palpation, percussion and auscultation. *P. handicap* a term used when a physical disadvantage is due to impairment of physiological or anatomical structure of function. *P. medicine* the treatment and rehabilitation of patients with physical disabilities. It includes physiotherapy and manipulation. *P. signs* those observed by inspection, percussion, etc.

**physician** (fiˈzishən) a medically qualified person who practises medicine as opposed to surgery. *Community p.* a doctor who practises community medicine (*see* MEDICINE). *Consultant p.* senior doctor in overall charge of patients within a specialist medical field, and responsible for directing junior medical staff working for the same firm. *House p.* a junior doctor, resident in hospital while on duty, acting under the orders of a consultant physician.

**physiological** (ˌfizi.əˈlojikˈl) relating to physiology. Normal, as opposed to pathological. *P. jaundice see* JAUNDICE. *P. solutions* those of the same salt composition and same osmotic pressure as blood plasma.

**physiology** (ˌfiziˈoləjee) the science of the functioning of living organisms.

**physiotherapy** (ˌfiziohˈtherəpee) treatment and rehabilitation by natural forces, e.g. heat, light, electricity, massage, manipulation and remedial exercises.

**physique** (fiˈzeek) the structure of the body.

**physostigmine** (ˌfiesohˈstigmeen) eserine, an alkaloid from the calabar bean. It is an antidote to curare; it constricts the pupils and is used with pilocarpine in the treatment of glaucoma.

**phytomenadione** (ˌfietohˌmenə'die-ohn) an intravenous preparation of vitamin K, effective in treating haemorrhage occurring during anticoagulant therapy.

**pia mater** (ˌpieə 'maytə) [L.] the innermost membrane enveloping the brain and spinal cord, consisting of a network of small blood vessels connected by areolar tissue. This dips down into all the folds of the nerve substance.

**pica** ('piekə) an unnatural craving for strange foods and for things not fit to be eaten. It may occur in pregnancy, and sometimes in children with learning disabilities.

**Pick's disease** (piks) *A. Pick, Czechoslovakian physician, 1851–1924.* A form of presenile brain failure (dementia) with an age of onset between 50 and 60 years. There is shrinkage of the brain and loss of cortical cells.

**Pickwickian syndrome** (pik'wiki.ən) (named after the fat boy 'Joe' in *Pickwick Papers*). A condition in which extreme obesity is associated with severe congestive cardiac failure.

**picornavirus** (pi'kawnəˌvierəs) a family of small RNA-containing viruses including echoviruses and rhinoviruses.

**PID** prolapse of an intervertebral disc.

**pie chart** ('pie) a circular graph divided into sectors proportional to the magnitudes of the quantities represented.

**pigeon breast** ('pijən) a deformity in which the sternum is unduly prominent.

**pigment** ('pigmənt) colouring matter. *Bile p's* bilirubin and biliverdin. *Blood p.* haemoglobin. *Melanotic p.* melanin.

**pigmentation** (ˌpigmen'tayshən) the deposition in the tissues of an abnormal amount of pigment.

**pile** (piel) a haemorrhoid.

**pill** (pil) a rounded mass of one or more drugs, sometimes coated with sugar. Taken orally.

**pilocarpine** (ˌpieloh'kahpeen) an alkaloid prepared from jaborandi leaves. It is used to constrict the pupils in the treatment of glaucoma.

**pilomotor** (ˌpieloh'mohtə) capable of moving the hair. *P. nerves* sympathetic nerves which control muscles in the skin connected with hair follicles. Stimulation causes the hair to be erected, and also the condition of 'gooseflesh' of the skin.

**pilonidal** (ˌpieloh'nied'l) having a growth of hair. *P. cyst* a congenital infolding of hair-bearing skin over the coccyx. It may become infected and lead to sinus formation.

**pilot study** ('pielət ˌstudi) a small-scale version of a planned experiment or observation used to test the design of the larger study. A pilot study is helpful to see if any difficulties or problems arise in order that they can be clarified before embarking on the larger study, thus saving time and resources. A pilot study may also indicate possible extensions to the study or suggest restrictions of those aspects likely to be unhelpful.

**pimple** ('pimp'l) a small papule or pustule.

**pineal** ('pini.əl, 'pie-) shaped like a pine cone. *P. body* a small cone-shaped structure attached by a stalk to the posterior wall of the third ventricle of the brain and composed of glandular substance.

**pinguecula** (ping'gwekyuhlə) [L.] a small, benign, yellowish spot on the bulbar conjunctiva, seen usually in the elderly. Caused by degeneration of the elastic tissue of the conjunctiva.

**pink disease** ('pink) acrodynia.

**pinkeye** ('pingk‚ie) acute contagious conjunctivitis.

**pinna** ('pinə) the projecting part of the external ear; the auricle.

**pinta** ('pintə) a non-venereal skin infection caused by *Treponema carateum* which is similar to the causative agent of syphilis. It is prevalent in the West Indies and Central America.

**pinworm** ('pin‚wərm) a threadworm; *Enterobius vermicularis*.

**piperacillin** (pie‚perə'silin, pi-) a broad-spectrum semisynthetic penicillin active against a wide variety of Gram-negative, Gram-positive and anaerobic bacteria.

**piperazine** (pie'perə‚zeen, pi-) an anthelmintic drug used in the treatment of threadworms and roundworms.

**pirenzepine** (pi'renzə‚peen) a drug which inhibits gastric acid secretion and promotes ulcer healing in the stomach.

**Piriton** ('piriton) trade name for chlorpheniramine maleate; a preparation used for the relief of allergy and the emergency treatment of anaphylactic reactions.

**piroxicam** (pi'roksikam) a nonsteroidal anti-inflammatory drug used in the treatment of rheumatic diseases.

**pituitary** (pi'tyooitə.ree) an endocrine gland suspended from the base of the brain and protected by the sella turcica in the sphenoid bone. It consists of two lobes: (a) the anterior, which secretes a number of different hormones, including adrenocorticotrophic hormone (ACTH), gonadotrophin, thyroid stimulating hormone (TSH) and prolactin; (b) the posterior, which secretes oxytocin and vasopressin. *P. dwarfism* a stunting of growth in the early years of life due to a deficiency of pituitary growth hormone.

**pityriasis** (‚piti'rieəsis) a skin disease characterized by fine scaly desquamation. *P. alba*, a condition, common in children, in which white scaly patches appear on the face. *P. capitis* dandruff. *P. rosea* an inflammatory form, in which the affected areas are macular and ring-shaped.

**PKU** phenylketonuria.

**place of safety order** (plays ov 'sayftee ‚awdə) a court order whereby a child is arbitrarily removed from the care of its parents in the interests of the child's safety.

**placebo** (plə'seeboh) [L.] a substance given to a patient as medicine or a procedure performed on a patient that has no intrinsic therapeutic value and relieves symptoms or helps the patient in some way only because the patient believes or expects that it will. A placebo may be prescribed to satisfy a patient's psychological need for drug therapy and may also be given during controlled experiments. *P. effect* after the administration of a drug or treatment, a change (usually temporary) in a patient's physical or emotional condition following publicity or media interest in the drug or treatment. The placebo response is due more to the patient's expectations or to the expectations of the person giving the drug or treatment than to the result of any direct physiological or pharmacological substance response.

**placenta** (plə'sentə) the afterbirth. A vascular structure inside the pregnant uterus, supplying the fetus with nourishment through the connecting umbilical cord. The placenta develops in about the third month of pregnancy and is expelled after the birth of the child. *Battledore p.* one in which the cord is attached to the margin and not the centre. *P. praevia* one attached to the lower part of the uterine wall. It may cause severe antepartum haemorrhage.

**plagiocephaly** (,playjioh'kefəlee, -'sef-) asymmetry of the head resulting from the irregular closing of the sutures.

**plague** (playg) an acute, febrile, infectious, highly fatal disease caused by the bacillus *Yersinia pestis*. It is a notifiable disease. Transmitted to humans by the bites of fleas that have derived the infection from diseased rats. *Bubonic p.* a type in which the lymph glands are infected and buboes form in the groins and armpits. Known in medieval times as 'The Black Death'. *Pneumonic p.* a type in which the infection attacks chiefly the lung tissues. A fatal form. *Septicaemic p.* a very severe and fatal form when the infection enters the bloodstream.

**plantar** ('plantə) relating to the sole of the foot. *P. arch* the arch made by anastomosis of the plantar arteries. *P. flexion* bending of the toes downwards and so arching the foot. *P. reflex* contraction of the toes on stroking the sole of the foot. *P. wart* a common WART located on the sole of the foot. Plantar warts are epidermal tumours caused by a virus which may be picked up by going barefoot. Also called verruca plantaris.

**plaque** (plak, plahk) 1. a flat patch on the skin. 2. a deposit of food and bacteria on the enamel of teeth which may produce tartar and caries.

**plasma** ('plazmə) the fluid portion of the blood in which corpuscles are suspended. Plasma is to be distinguished from serum, which is plasma from which the fibrinogen has been separated in the process of clotting. *P. proteins* those present in the blood plasma: albumin, globulin and fibrinogen. *P. volume*

*expander* a solution transfused instead of blood to increase the volume of fluid circulating in the blood vessels. Also called artificial plasma extender. *Reconstituted p.* dried plasma when again made liquid by addition of distilled water.

**plasmapheresis** (,plazməfə'reesis) a method of removing a portion of the plasma from circulation. Venesection is performed, the blood is allowed to settle, the plasma is removed, and the red blood cells are returned to the circulation. Used in the treatment of those diseases caused by antibodies circulating in the patient's plasma.

**plasmin** ('plazmin) a fibrinolytic, found in blood plasma, which can dissolve fibrin clots.

**plasminogen** (plaz'minəjən) the inactive precursor of plasmin.

*Plasmodium* (plaz'mohdi.əm) a genus of protozoan parasites in the red blood cells of animals and humans. Four species, *P. falciparrum*, *P. malariae*, *P. ovale* and *P. vivax*, cause the four specific types of human malaria.

**plaster** ('plahstə, 'plastə) 1. a mixture of materials that hardens; used for immobilizing or making impressions of body parts. 2. an adhesive substance spread on fabric or other suitable backing material for application to the skin. *Bohler's p.* plaster for Pott's fracture. A leg splint of plaster of Paris, in which is embedded an iron stirrup extending below the foot, which enables the patient to walk without putting weight on the joint. *Corn p.* an adhesive strip or patch impregnated with salicyclic acid and applied to corns on the feet. *Frog p.* a plaster of Paris splint used to maintain the position after correction of the deformity due to congenital dislocation of the hip. *P. of Paris* calcium sulphate or gypsum which sets hard when water is added to it; it is used to form a plaster cast to immobilize a part, and in dentistry for making dental impressions.

**plastic** ('plastik) 1. constructive; tissue-forming. 2. capable of being moulded; pliable. *P. lymph* the exudate which, in wounds and inflamed serous tissues, is organized into fibrous tissue and promotes healing. *P. surgery* the branch of surgery that deals with the repair and reconstruction of deformed or injured parts of the body, including their replacement, by tissue grafting or other means.

**platelet** ('playtlət) a disc-shaped structure present in the blood and concerned in the process of clotting. A thrombocyte.

**play** (play) an occupation, for either children or adults, which is voluntary and may be a spontaneous or an organized activity providing enjoyment, entertainment, amusement or a diversion. Play is important in childhood as a necessary part of psychological and physical development. *P. group* a session of care and activities for preschool children. It can be organized by any interested person at home or in other premises, but it must be registered by the social services department. *P. specialist* a person who is qualified to use play constructively to help children come to terms with illness and hospitalization. *P. therapist* one trained in the skills of play therapy. *P. therapy* a technique used in child psychotherapy in which play is used to reveal unconscious material. Play is the natural way in which children express and work through unconscious conflicts; thus play therapy is analogous to the technique of free association used in adult psychotherapy.

**pleoptics** (pli'optiks) an orthoptic method of improving the sight in cases of strabismus by stimulating the use of the macular part of the retina.

**plethora** ('pletha.rə) a general term denoting a red, florid complexion or, specifically, an excessive amount of blood.

**plethysmography** (,plethiz'mografee) the measurement of changes in the volume of a limb due to alterations in blood pressure, using an oncometer.

**pleura** ('plooə.rə) the serous membrane lining the thorax and enveloping each lung. *Parietal p.* the layer that lines the chest wall. *Visceral p.* the inner layer which is in close contact with the lung.

**pleurisy, pleuritis** ('plooə.risee, plooə'rietis) inflammation of the pleura; it may be caused by infection, injury or tumour. It may be a complication of lung diseases, particularly of pneumonia, or sometimes of tuberculosis, lung abscess or influenza. The symptoms are cough, fever, chills, sharp, sticking pain that is worse on inspiration, and rapid shallow breathing. *Dry p., fibrinous p.* pleurisy in which the membrane is inflamed and roughened, but no fluid is formed. *P. with effusion* wet pleurisy. A type that is characterized by inflammation and exudation of serous fluid into the pleural cavity. *Purulent p.* empyema. The formation of pus in the pleural cavity. An operation for drainage is usually necessary. *Wet p.* pleurisy with effusion.

**pleurodynia** (,plooə.roh'dini.ə) pain in the intercostal muscles, probably rheumatic in origin.

**plexus** ('pleksəs) a network of veins or nerves. *Auerbach's p.* the nerve ganglion situated between the longitudinal and circular muscle fibres of the intestine. The nerves are motor nerves. *Brachial p.* the network of nerves of the neck and axilla. *Choroid p.* a capillary network situated in the ventricles of the brain which forms the cerebrospinal fluid. *Coeliac p.* solar plexus. *Meissner's p.* the sensory nerve ganglion situated in the submucous layer of the intestinal wall. *Rectal p.* the network of veins which surrounds the rectum and forms a direct communication between the systemic and portal circulations. *Solar p.* coeliac plexus. The network of nerves and ganglia at the back of the stomach, which supply the abdominal viscera.

**plication** (plie'kayshən) the taking of tucks in a structure to shorten it; a folding to decrease the size of a structure or organ during a surgical procedure.

**plumbism** ('plumbizəm) lead poisoning.

**pneumaturia** (ˌnyoomə'tyooə.ri.ə) the passing of flatus with the urine owing to a vesico-intestinal fistula and air from the bowel entering the bladder.

**pneumocephalus** (ˌnyoomoh-'kefələs, -'sef-) the presence of air in the ventricles of the brain caused usually by an anterior fracture of the base of the skull.

**pneumococcus** (ˌnyoomoh'kokəs) the causative agent of lobar and bronchopneumonia and of other bronchial diseases. A Grampositive, ovoid diplococcus, *Streptococcus pneumoniae*.

**pneumoconiosis** (ˌnyoomohˌkohni-'ohsis) an industrial disease of the lung due to inhalation of dust particles over a period of time. *See* ANTHRACOSIS, ASBESTOSIS and SILICOSIS.

*Pneumocystis* (ˌnyoomoh'sistis) a genus of microorganisms of uncertain status, but usually considered to be protozoans. *P. carinii* abbreviated PCP. The causative organism of interstitial plasma cell pneumonia, particularly in immunosuppressed patients, people with human immunodeficiency virus (HIV) infection or small children.

**pneumodynamics** (ˌnyoomohdie-'namiks) the mechanics of respiration.

**pneumoencephalography** (ˌnyoo-moh.enˌkefə'lografee, -ˌsef-) *see* ENCEPHALOGRAPHY.

**pneumogastric** (ˌnyoomoh'gastrik) pertaining to lungs and stomach. *P. nerve* the tenth cranial nerve to the lungs, stomach, etc. The vagus nerve.

**pneumomycosis** (ˌnyoomohmie-'kohsis) infection of the lung by microfungi. *See* BRONCHOMYCOSIS.

**pneumonectomy** (ˌnyoomə'nek-təmee) partial or total removal of a lung.

**pneumonia** (nyoo'mohni.ə) inflammation of the lung with consolidation and exudation. *Aspiration p.* an acute condition caused by the aspiration of infected material into the lungs. *Hypostatic p.* a form which occurs in weak, bedridden patients. *Lobar p.* an acute infectious disease caused by a pneumococcus and affecting whole lobes of either or both lungs. *Virus p.* inflammation of the lung occurring during some virus disease and secondary to it.

**pneumonitis** (ˌnyoomə'nietis) an imprecise term denoting any inflammatory condition of the lung.

**pneumoperitoneum** (ˌnyoomohˌperitə'neeəm) the presence of air or gas in the peritoneal cavity, occurring pathologically or introduced intentionally for diagnostic or therapeutic purposes.

**pneumoradiography** (ˌnyoomohˌraydi'ografee) radiographic examination of a cavity or part after air or a gas has been injected into it.

**pneumotaxic** (ˌnyoomoh'taksik) regulating the rate of respiration. *P. centre* the centre in the pons that influences inspiratory effort during respiration.

**pneumothorax** (,nyoomoh-'thor.raks) accumulation of air or gas in the pleural cavity, resulting in collapse of the lung on the affected side. The condition may occur spontaneously, as in the course of a pulmonary disease, or it may follow trauma to, and perforation of, the chest wall. *Artificial p.* a surgical procedure sometimes used in the treatment of tuberculosis or after pneumonectomy. *Spontaneous p.* sometimes occurs when there is an opening on the surface of the lung allowing leakage of air from the bronchi into the pleural cavity. *Tension p.* a particularly dangerous form of pneumothorax that occurs when air escapes into the pleural cavity from a bronchus but cannot regain entry into the bronchus. As a result, continuously increasing air pressure in the pleural cavity causes progressive collapse of the lung tissue.

**podagra** (pə'dagrə) gout, particularly of the big toe.

**podalic** (pə'dalik) relating to the feet. *P. version* a method of changing the lie of a fetus so that its feet will present.

**podarthritis** (,podah'thrietis) inflammation of any of the joints of the foot.

**podiatry** (po'dieətree) chiropody; a specialty concerned with the care of the feet and the treatment of minor foot complaints.

**pointillage** (,pwanhti'ahzh) [Fr.] a method of massage using the tips of the fingers.

**poison** ('poyzən) any substance which, applied to the body externally or taken internally, can cause injury to any part or cause death.

**poisoning** ('poyzəning) the morbid condition produced by a poison. The poison may be swallowed, inhaled (see CARBON (MONOXIDE)), injected by a stinging insect as in a BEE STING, or spilled or otherwise brought into contact with the skin.

**polioencephalitis** (,pohlioh.en,kefə'lietis, -,sef-) acute inflammation of the cortex of the brain.

**poliomyelitis** (,pohlioh,mieə'lietis) an acute, notifiable, infectious viral disease that attacks the central nervous system, injuring or destroying the nerve cells that control the muscles and sometimes causing paralysis; also called polio or infantile paralysis. Paralysis most often affects the limbs but can involve any muscles, including those that control breathing and swallowing. Since the development and the use of vaccines against poliomyelitis, the disease has been virtually eliminated in developed, wealthy countries, where vaccination rates are high, but is still common in many other parts of the world.

**poliovirus** (,pohlioh'vierəs) a small RNA-containing virus which causes poliomyelitis.

**pollinosis** (,poli'nohsis) hay fever; an allergy caused by various kinds of pollen. Pollenosis.

**pollution** (pə'looshən) the act of destroying the purity of or contaminating something.

**polyarteritis** (,poli,ahtə'rietis) inflammatory changes in the walls of the small arteries.

**polyarthralgia** (,poliah'thralji.ə) pain in several joints.

**polyarthritis** (,poliah'thrietis) inflammation of several joints at the same time, as seen in rheumatoid arthritis.

**polycoria** (,poli'kor.ri.ə) a congenital abnormality in which there are one or more holes in the iris in addition to the pupil.

**polycystic** (,poli'sistik) containing many cysts. *P. ovary disease* Stein–Leventhal syndrome. *P. renal disease* a hereditary disease in which there is massive enlargement of the kidney with the formation of many cysts. Severe bleeding into cysts can occur. End-stage renal disease can affect many members of one family.

**polycythaemia** (ˌpolisie'theemi.ə) an abnormal increase in the number of red cells in the blood. Erythrocythaemia. *P. vera* a rare disease in which there is a greatly increased production of red blood cells and also of leukocytes and platelets. The skin becomes flushed, with cyanosis, thrombosis and splenomegaly.

**polydactylism** (ˌpoli'dakti lizəm) the condition of having more than the normal number of fingers or toes.

**polydipsia** (ˌpoli'dipsi.ə) abnormal thirst. It may be a symptom of diabetes.

**polymorphonuclear** (ˌpoliˌmawfoh-'nyookli.ə) 1. having nuclei of many different shapes. 2. a polymorphonuclear leukocyte.

**polymorphous** (ˌpoli'mawfəs) occurring in several or many different forms.

**polymyalgia rheumatica** (ˌpolimie-ˌalji.ə rooˈmatikə) persistent aching pain in the muscles, often involving the shoulder or the pelvic girdle.

**polymyositis** (ˌpoliˌmieoh'sietis) a generalized inflammation of the muscles with weakness and joint stiffness, particularly around the hips and shoulders.

**polymyxin** (ˌpoli'miksin) an antibiotic drug used in the treatment of Gram-negative bacteria, particularly *Pseudomonas*.

**polyneuritis** (ˌpolinyuh'rietis) inflammation of many nerves at the same time.

**polyneuropathy** (ˌpolinyuh-'ropəthee) a number of disease conditions of the nervous system.

**polyopia** (ˌpoli'ohpi.ə) the perception of two or more images of the same object. Multiple vision.

**polyp** ('polip) a pedunculated tumour of mucous membrane. A polypus.

**polypharmacy** (ˌpoli'fahməsee) 1. the administration of many drugs together. This increases the likelihood of side-effects from drug interactions and of non-compliance by the patient. 2. the administration of excessive medication.

**polyposis** (ˌpoli'pohsis) the presence of many polyps in an organ. *Familial p.* a hereditary condition in which large numbers of polyps develop in the colon, which may become malignant.

**polyuria** (ˌpoli'yooə.ri.ə) an abnormally large output of urine due either to an excessive intake of liquid or to disease, often diabetes.

**pompholyx** ('pomfəliks) an intensely pruritic skin condition in which vesicles appear on the hands and feet, particularly on the palms and soles. Typically occurring in repeated, self-limiting attacks.

**pons** (ponz) a bridge of tissue connecting two parts of an organ. *P. varolii* the part of the brain that connects the cerebrum, cerebellum and medulla oblongata.

**Pontiac fever** ('ponti ak) an influenza-like illness with little or no pulmonary involvement, caused by *Legionella pneumophila*. It is not life-threatening, as is the pulmonary form known as legionnaires' disease. The name Pontiac fever comes from an outbreak of the disease in Pontiac, Michigan.

**popliteal** (ˌpopli'teeəl, pop'liti.əl) relating to the posterior part of the knee joint.

**population** (ˌpopyə'layshən) 1. the total number of persons inhabiting a given geographical area or location. 2. in statistics the aggregate of individuals or items from which a sample for a study is drawn. 3. any group that is distinguished by a particular trait or situation.

**pore** (por) a minute circular opening on a surface. *Sweat p.* an opening of a sweat gland on the skin surface.

**porphyria** (paw'firi.ə) an inborn error in the metabolism of porphyrins, resulting in porphyrinuria. Two general types of porphyria are known: erythropoietic porphyrias, which are concerned with the formation of erythrocytes in the bone marrow; and hepatic porphyrias, which are responsible for liver dysfunction. The manifestations of porphyria include gastrointestinal, neurological and psychological symptoms, cutaneous photosensitivity, pigmentation of the face (and later of the bones) and anaemia, with enlargement of the spleen.

**porphyrin** ('pawfirin) one of a number of pigments used in the production of the haem portion of haemoglobin.

**porphyrinuria** (ˌpawfiri'nyooə.ri.ə) the presence of an excess of porphyrin in the urine.

**porta** ('pawtə) an opening in an organ through which pass the main vessels.

**Portacath** ('pawtəˌkath) a catheter to provide a central venous line; attached to it is an injectable depot which is placed under the skin.

**portacaval** (ˌpawtə'kayv'l) pertaining to the portal vein and the inferior vena cava. *P. anastomosis* the joining of the portal vein to the inferior vena cava so that much of the blood bypasses the liver. It is used in the treatment of portal hypertension.

**portage system** ('pawtij ˌsistəm) a method of behaviour modification taught to family members to enable them to assist a handicapped child in development and acquiring skills for everyday living.

**portfolio** (pawt'fohlioh) a collection of competency evidence assembled by the practitioner/student which demonstrates the owner's professional development. The portfolio may include such material as journals, marked assessments, evidence of reflective practice or other examples that document the acquisition of new skills, knowledge, understanding and achievements relevant to professional practice. *See* PROFILE.

**position** (pə'zishən) attitude or posture. *Dorsal p.* lying flat on the back. *Genupectoral* or *knee-chest p.* resting on the knees and chest with arms crossed above the head. *Lithotomy p.* lying on the back with thighs raised and knees supported and held widely apart. *Prone p.* face down. *Sims' p.* or *semiprone p.* lying on the left side with the right knee well flexed and the left arm drawn back over the edge of the bed. *Trendelenburg p.* lying down on a tilted plane (usually an operating table at an angle of 30°–45° to the floor), with the head lowermost, the shoulders supported and the legs hanging over the raised end of the table.

**positive** ('pozətiv) having a value greater than zero; indicating existence or presence, as chromatin positive or Wassermann positive; characterized by affirmation or co-operation. The opposite of negative.

**positive end-expiratory pressure** abbreviated PEEP. In mechanical ventilation, a positive airway pressure maintained until the end of expiration. A PEEP higher than the critical closing pressure holds alveoli open until the end of expiration and can markedly improve the arterial $Po_2$ in patients with a lowered functional residual capacity (FRC), as in acute respiratory failure.

**posseting** ('positing) regurgitation of a small amount of milk by an infant immediately after a feed.

**Possum** ('posəm) patient-operated selector mechanism; a machine that can be operated with a very slight degree of pressure, or suction, using the mouth, if no other muscle movement is possible. It may transmit messages from a light panel or be adapted for typing, telephoning or working certain machinery.

**post-exposure prophylaxis** (ˌpohsteks'pohzhə) abbreviated PEP. The administration of antibiotics, antiviral agents, or active and/or passive vaccination following exposure to an infectious agent, e.g. antiretroviral drugs after exposure (usually occupationally, but may include sexual exposure) to human immunodeficiency virus (HIV).

**post-traumatic stress disorder** (ˌpohst.traw matik 'stres dis awdə) following the experience of a major incident – personal, such as injury, rape or drowning, or other serious event, such as a natural disaster – the person may experience insomnia, acute anxiety, nightmares and 'flashbacks' resulting in depression, loss of concentration, apathy and guilt. This reaction may be immediate or delayed, and may last for a variable time. Support and counselling are needed.

**postconcussional syndrome** (ˌpohstkən'kushən'l) constant headaches with mental fatigue, difficulty in concentration and insomnia that may persist after head injury.

**posterior** (po'stiə.ri.ə) behind a part. Dorsal. The opposite of anterior. *P. chamber* that part of the aqueous chamber that lies behind the iris, but in front of the lens.

**posteroanterior** (ˌpostə.roh.an'tiə.ri.ə) from the back to the front.

**postganglionic** (ˌpohstgang.gli-'onik) situated posterior or distal to a ganglion. *P. fibre* a nerve fibre posterior to a ganglion of the autonomic nervous system.

**postgastrectomy syndrome** (ˌpohstga'strektəmee) *see* DUMPING.

**posthumous** ('postyuhməs) occurring after death. *P. birth* one occurring after the death of the father, or by caesarean section after the death of the mother.

**postmature** (postmə'tyooə) a state in which the pregnancy is prolonged after the expected date of delivery. Owing to the many variables it is difficult to estimate, but may exist when a pregnancy has lasted 41–42 weeks from the last menstrual period. There is a danger of hypoxia to the fetus.

**postmortem** (pohst'mawtəm) after death. *P. examination* autopsy.

**postnatal** (pohst'nayt'l) after childbirth. *P. care* includes the care of the mother for at least 6 weeks after delivery. *P. clinic* an examination centre where the patient can be examined (postnatally), preferably 6 weeks after childbirth: (a) regarding her general health; (b) specifically, to find out the state of the uterus, pelvic floor and vagina. *P. depression* a low mood experienced by some mothers for a few days after the birth of their baby. Sometimes called 'baby blues'. *P. period* defined in law as a period of not less than 10 days and not more than 28 days after the end of labour, during which the continued attendance of a midwife on the mother and baby is requisite.

**postpartum** (pohst'pahtəm) occurring after labour.

**postprandial** (pohst'prandi.əl) occurring after a meal.

**postural** ('postyuhrəl) relating to a position or posture. *P. drainage* drainage of secretions from specific lobes or segments of the lung, aided by careful positioning of the patient.

**potassium** (pə'tasi.əm) *symbol* K. A metallic alkaline element which is a constituent of all plants and animals. Its salts are widely used in medicine. *P. chloride* a compound used orally or intravenously as an electrolyte replenisher. *P. citrate* a diuretic, expectorant and systemic alkalizer. *P. gluconate* an electrolyte replenisher used in the prophylaxis and treatment of hypokalaemia. *P. iodide* an expectorant and anti-thyroid agent. *P. permanganate* a topical anti-infective, oxidizing agent and antidote for many poisons. *P. sodium tartrate* a compound used as a saline cathartic and also in combination with sodium bicarbonate and tartaric acid.

**Pott's disease** (pots) *P. Pott, British surgeon, 1714–1788.* Tuberculosis of the spine.

**Pott's fracture** a fracture-dislocation of the ankle, involving fracture of the lower end of the tibia, displacement of the talus and sometimes fracture of the medial malleolus.

**pouch** (powch) a pocket-like space or cavity. *Morison's p.* a fold of peritoneum below the liver. *P. of Douglas* the lowest fold of the peritoneum between the uterus and rectum.

**poultice** ('pohltis) a soft, moist mass of about the consistency of cooked cereal, spread between layers of muslin, linen, gauze or towels and applied hot to a given area in order to create moist local heat or to counter irritation.

**Poupart's ligament** ('poopahts) *F. Poupart, French anatomist, 1616–1708.* The inguinal ligament. The tendinous lower border of the external oblique muscle of the abdominal wall, which passes from the anterior spine of the ilium to the os pubis.

**povidone–iodine** (,pohvidohn) a complex of iodine with the polymer povidone; used as a topical anti-infective and in pre-operative skin preparation.

**PPS** pelvic pain syndrome.

**practice** ('praktis) the exercise of a profession. *Family p.* the medical specialty concerned with the planning and provision of comprehensive primary health care, regardless of age or sex, on a continuing basis.

**practitioner** (prak'tishənə) a person who practices a profession. *See* NURSE (PRACTITIONER).

**practolol** ('praktoh,lol) a drug used in the treatment of tachycardia and irregular heart rhythms. It is a beta-blocker and can only be given by injection.

**pre-eclampsia** (,pree.i'klampsi.ə) a condition occurring in late pregnancy. The symptoms include proteinuria, hypertension and oedema.

**precancerous** (pree'kansə.rəs) applied to conditions or histological changes that may precede cancer.

**preceptor** (prə'septə) 1. a teacher, an instructor. 2. a first-level nurse, midwife or health visitor, with at least 12 months (or equivalent) experience in the relevant clinical field, who provides newly registered practitioners with support and guidance in making the transition from student to registered practitioner. Preceptors should be provided with specific preparation for their role.

**preceptorship** (prə'septəship) a period of support, given by a preceptor, of at least the first 4 months of registered practice for the newly registered nurse, midwife or health visitor practitioner or for those returning to nursing after a break of more than 5 years.

**precipitate** (pri'sipi,tayt) a deposit of solid matter which was previously in solution.

**precipitate labour** unusually rapid labour with extremely quick delivery. There is danger to the mother of severe perineal lacerations, and to the child of intracranial trauma as a result of the rapid passage through the birth canal.

**precocious** (pri'kohshəs) developed in advance of the norm, either mentally or physically or both.

**precognition** (ˌpreekog'nishən) a direct perception of a future event which is beyond the reach of inference.

**precordium** (pree'kawdi.əm) the area lying over the heart.

**prediabetes** (ˌpree.die.ə'beetis, -teez) a state which precedes diabetes mellitus, in which the disease is not yet clinically manifest. In pregnancy the diabetes may become evident, or the patient may remain well but give birth to an unsually large child. Screening by urine testing can detect the condition.

**predisposition** (ˌpreedispə'zishən) susceptibility to a specific disease.

**prednisolone** (pred'nisəlohn) a synthetic corticosteroid used in the treatment of inflammatory and rheumatic conditions and of asthma and allergic skin diseases.

**prednisone** ('predniˌsohn) a synthetic drug with an action and usage similar to prednisolone.

**pregnancy** ('pregnənsee) being with child; the condition from conception to the expulsion of the fetus. The normal period is 280 days or 40 weeks. *Ectopic* or *extrauterine p.* pregnancy occurring outside the uterus, in the uterine tube (*tubal p.*) or very rarely in the abdominal cavity. *P. tests* tests used to demonstrate whether conception has occurred. These detect the human chorionic gonadotrophin (HCG) produced by the embryo 8 days after the first missed period. Immunological laboratory tests are more accurate and less likely to give a false positive result than an over-the-counter kit.

**premature** (ˌpremə'tyooə) occurring before the anticipated time.

*P. contraction* a form of cardiac irregularity in which the ventricle contracts before its anticipated time. *See* SYSTOLE. *P. ejaculation* emission of semen before or at the beginning of sexual intercourse. *P. infant* preterm infant. A child born before the 37th completed week of gestation.

**premedication** (ˌpreemedi'kayshən) drugs given preoperatively in order to reduce fear and anxiety and to facilitate the induction and maintenance of, and recovery from, anaesthesia.

**premenstrual** (pree'menstrooəl) preceding menstruation. *P. endometrium* the hypertrophied and vascular mucous lining of the uterus immediately before the menstrual flow starts. *P. tension* feelings of nervousness, depression and irritability experienced by some women in the days before their menstrual periods. Emotional and physical symptoms usually disappear with the onset of menstruation.

**premolar** (pree'mohlə) a bicuspid tooth in front of the molars on each side of the upper and lower jaws.

**prenatal** (pree'nayt'l) preceding birth; antenatal. *P. care* care of the pregnant woman before delivery of the infant.

**prepuce** ('preepyoos) foreskin; the loose fold of skin covering the glans penis.

**presbycusis** (ˌpresbi'kyoosis) progressive bilateral deafness in the higher frequencies in old age.

**presbyopia** (ˌpresbi'ohpi.ə) diminution of accommodation of the lens of the eye, due to a loss of elasticity, occurring normally with ageing and usually resulting in hyperopia, or farsightedness.

**prescription** (pri'skripshən) a formula written by a medically qualified doctor, and in some instances a specially qualified nurse (*see* Nurses' Formulary in Appendices), directing the pharmacist to supply the medication. Also contains instructions to the patient indicating how the medication is to be taken.

**presenile** (pree'seeniel) prematurely aged in mind and body. *See* DEMENTIA.

**presentation** (,prezen'tayshen) in obstetrics, that portion of the fetus that appears in the centre of the neck of the uterus (*see* Figure).

**pressure** ('preshe) stress or strain. The force exerted by one object upon another. *P. areas* areas of the body where the tissues may be compressed between the bed and the underlying bone, especially the sacrum, greater trochanters and heels; the tissues become ischaemic (*see* Figure on p. 324). *P. point* the point at which an artery can be compressed against a bone in order to stop bleeding (*see* Figure on p. 325). *P. sore* a decubitus ulcer; a bedsore. Ulceration of the skin due to pressure, which causes interference with the blood supply to the area.

**presystole** (pree'sistelee) the period in the cardiac cycle just before systole.

**preterm infant** ('preeterm) one with a gestational age of less than 37 weeks.

**priapism** ('priee,pizem) persistent erection of the penis, usually

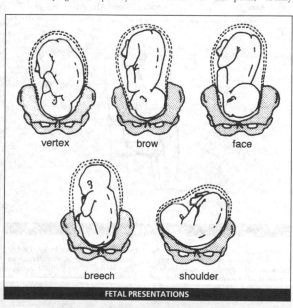

vertex

brow

face

breech

shoulder

**FETAL PRESENTATIONS**

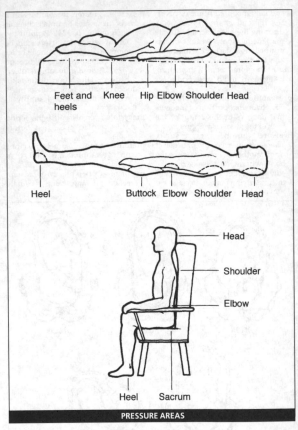

Feet and heels | Knee | Hip | Elbow | Shoulder | Head

Heel | Buttock | Elbow | Shoulder | Head

Head
Shoulder
Elbow

Heel | Sacrum

**PRESSURE AREAS**

without sexual desire. It may be caused by local or spinal cord injury.
**prickly heat** ('priklee) miliaria; heat rash. A skin eruption characterized by minute red spots with central vesicles.

**primaquine** ('primə‚kween) a drug used in the treatment of benign tertian malaria after initial treatment with other antimalarial drugs.
**primary care** ('priem‚ree) the level of care in the HEALTH CARE SYSTEM

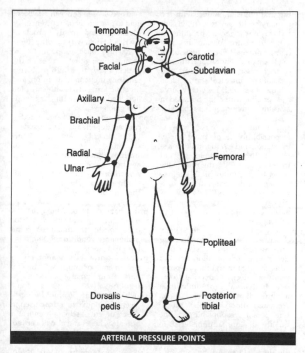

**ARTERIAL PRESSURE POINTS**

that consists of initial care outside institutions. *P. c. groups* abbreviated PCGs. A grouping of general practitioners and their services within a defined area agreed with the health authority and encompassing a natural community of about 100 000 people. PCGs provide a direct means by which general practitioners (and their primary care teams) and community nurses working in cooperation with other health and social care professionals will lead the process of securing appropriate, high-quality care for local people. Responsible also for the commissioning of health services as well as the promotion of good health, to combat inequalities in health in partnership with other agencies, develop primary care services and integrate primary and community services. Known as local health groups in Wales and local health cooperatives in Scotland.

**primary health care** the care given to individuals in the community at the first point of contact with the primary health care team. First contact may be the general practitioner, a health visitor, paramedic or a district nurse. *P. h. c. team* usually made up of a general practitioner, district nurse, health visitors and possibly paramedical staff, such as a physiotherapist. They may serve a geographical area and be based in a health centre or a general practice area.

**primary nurse** a nurse who is responsible for the planning, implementation and evaluation of nursing care for assigned patients and their families for the duration of the patients' stay in hospital. The primary nurse delegates to an associate nurse when off duty but the primary nurse remains responsible and accountable for the patient's nursing care.

**primary nursing** Manthey (1980) described a system for delivering nursing care that consists of four design elements: (a) allocation and acceptance of individual responsibility for decision-making to/by one individual; (b) individual assignment of daily care; (c) direct communication channels; and (d) one person responsible for the quality of care administered to patients on a unit 24 h a day, 7 days a week.

**primidone** ('primi,dohn) an anticonvulsant drug used in the treatment of major epilepsy.

**primigravida** (,priemi'gravidə) a woman who is pregnant for the first time.

**primipara** (prie'mipərə) a woman who has given birth to her first child.

**probability** (,probə'bilitee) a statistical term meaning the likelihood of an association between variables being due to chance.

**probenecid** (proh'benisid) a drug which increases the excretion of uric acid and is used between attacks of gout to prevent their occurrence.

**problem-oriented record** ('probləm-,awrientid ,rekawd) a multiprofessional approach to patient care record-keeping that focuses on the patient's specific health problems requiring immediate attention, and the structuring of a health-care plan designed to cope with the identified problems.

**procainamide** (proh'kaynə,mied) a cardiac depressant drug used in the treatment of abnormal heart rhythms.

**procaine** ('prohkayn) a local anaesthetic used by infiltration. *P. penicillin* a long-acting antibiotic drug, chiefly used in the treatment of venereal diseases.

**procarbazine** (proh'kahbə,zeen) a monoamine oxidase inhibitor used in the treatment of some malignant conditions, such as lymphadenoma.

**process** ('prohses) in anatomy, a prominence or outgrowth of any part. *P. of nursing see* NURSING (PROCESS).

**prochlorperazine** (,prohklor'perə,zeen) a tranquillizing drug used in the treatment of schizophrenia and other psychoses and also of vertigo, nausea and vomiting.

**procidentia** (,prohsi'denshi.ə) complete prolapse of an organ, particularly the uterus so that the cervix extrudes through the vagina.

**proctalgia** (prok'talji.ə) pain in the rectum and anus; proctodynia.

**proctectomy** (prok'tektəmee) surgical removal of the rectum.

**proctitis** (prok'tietis) inflammation of the rectum.

**proctoscope** ('proktə,skohp) an instrument for examination of the rectum. *Tuttle's p.* a speculum illuminated by an electric bulb, combined with an arrangement by which the rectum can be dilated with air.

**proctosigmoiditis** (‚proktoh‚sigmoy'dietis) inflammation of the rectum and sigmoid colon.

**procyclidine** (proh'siekli‚deen) a drug used in the treatment of Parkinsonism because it reduces muscle tremor and rigidity.

**prodrome** ('prohdrohm) a symptom which appears before the true diagnostic signs of a disease.

**prodrug** ('proh‚drug) a compound that, on administration, must undergo chemical conversion by metabolic processes before becoming an active pharmacological agent, thus avoiding gastrointestinal side-effects.

**profession** (prə'fesh'n) 1. an avowed, public declaration or statement of intention or purpose. 2. a calling or vocation requiring specialized knowledge, methods and skills, as well as preparation, in an institution of higher learning, in the scholarly, scientific and historical principles underlying such methods and skills. Members of a profession are committed to continuing study, to enlarging their body of knowledge, to placing service above personal gain and to providing practical services vital to human and social welfare. A profession functions autonomously and is committed to higher standards of achievement and conduct.

**professional** (prə'feshən'l) 1. pertaining to one's profession or occupation. 2. one who is a specialist in a particular field or occupation. *Allied health p.* a person with special training, and licensed where necessary, who works closely with health professionals with responsibilities bearing on patient care.

**profile** ('proh‚fiel) 1. a simple outline, as of the side view of the head or face; by extension, a graph representing quantitatively a set of char-

acteristics determined by tests. 2. a record of achievements developed during a course of study, or subsequently.

**progeny** ('projənee) issue. Descendants.

**progeria** (proh'jeeri.ə) premature senility, the signs of which appear in childhood.

**progesterone** (proh'jestə‚rohn) a hormone of the corpus luteum which plays an important part in the regulation of the menstrual cycle and in pregnancy.

**progestogen** (proh'jestəjən) one of a group of steroid hormones having an action similar to that of progesterone.

**prognathism** ('prognə‚thizəm) enlargement and protrusion of one or both jaws.

**prognosis** (prog'nohsis) a forecast of the probable course and outcome of an attack of disease and the prospects of recovery, as indicated by the nature of the disease and the symptoms of the case. *Nursing p.* the application of information obtained during a nursing assessment in order to determine the prospect for altering, through nursing intervention, a client's/patient's response to illness or injury. The prognosis provides a rationale for setting priorities for meeting a particular client's/patient's nursing care needs and enhances continuity of nursing care by clearly indicating agreed priorities.

**proguanil** (proh'gwahnil) a widely used drug taken daily to prevent malarial infection.

**Project 2000** ('projekt) Diploma in Professional Studies in Nursing (DPNS); a reform of nurse education introduced in the UK in 1988 to meet the changing needs of the population for nursing care. The 3-year educational programme includes a common foundation programme of 18 months, followed by a branch programme in the nursing of either adults, children, people with mental health problems or those with learning disabilities. All student nurses are supernumerary to NHS staffing and receive a student bursary.

**projection** (prəˈjekshən) in psychology, an unconscious process by which painful thoughts or impulses are made acceptable by transferring them on to another person or object in the environment.

**prolactin** (prohˈlaktin) a milk-producing hormone of the anterior lobe of the pituitary body which stimulates the mammary gland.

**prolapse** (ˈprohlaps) the downward displacement of an organ or part of one. *P. of the cord* expulsion of the umbilical cord before the fetus presents. *P. of an intervertebral disc* abbreviated PID. Displacement of part of an intervertebral disc; 'slipped disc'. *P. of the iris* protrusion of a part of the iris through a wound in the cornea. *P. of the rectum* protrusion of the mucous membrane through the anal canal to the exterior. *P. of the uterus* descent of the cervix or of the whole uterus into the vagina owing to a weakening of its supporting ligaments.

**proliferation** (prəˌlifəˈrayshən) rapid multiplication of cells, as may occur in a malignant growth and during wound healing.

**promazine** (ˈprohməˌzeen) a tranquillizing drug used to treat confusion and anxiety in elderly patients.

**promethazine** (ˈprohˈmethəˌzeen) a powerful long-acting antihistamine drug used in conditions of hypersensitivity, e.g. hay fever, contact dermatitis, drug rashes, etc.

**prominence** (ˈprominəns) in anatomy, a projection, usually on a bone.

**pronation** (prohˈnayshən) turning the palm of the hand downwards.

**prone** (prohn) lying face downwards *See* SUPINE.

**propantheline** (prohˈpanthəˌleen) an antispasmodic drug that blocks the impulses from the vagus nerve to the stomach and is used in the treatment of peptic ulcer and spastic colon.

**prophylactic** (ˌprofiˈlaktik) 1. relating to prophylaxis. 2. a drug used to prevent a disease developing.

**prophylaxis** (ˌprofiˈlaksis) measures taken to prevent a disease.

**propranolol** (prohˈpranəˌlol) a beta-blocking drug used in the treatment of cardiac arrhythmias, angina, thyrotoxicosis and also of anxiety states.

**proprietary name** (prəˈprieətə.ree ˌnaym) the name assigned to a drug by the firm that first made it. A drug may have several different proprietary names.

**proprioceptor** (ˌprohprioh'septə) one of the sensory end-organs that provide information about movements and position of the body. They occur chiefly in the muscles, tendons, joint capsules and labyrinth.

**proptosis** (propˈtohsis) forward displacement of the eyeball; exophthalmus.

**propylthiouracil** (ˌprohpil.thieoh-ˈyooə.rəsil) a thyroid inhibitor used in the treatment of thyrotoxicosis.

**prostacyclin** (ˌprostəˈsieklin) an intermediate in the metabolic pathway of arachidonic acid, formed from prostaglandin endoperoxides in the walls of arteries and veins; it is a potent vasodilator and a potent inhibitor of platelet aggregation.

**prostaglandin** (ˌprostəˈglandin) one of several hormone substances produced in many body tissues, including the brain, lungs, uterus and semen. They are active in many ways, having cardiac, gastric and respiratory effects and causing uterine contractions. They are sometimes used for the induction of abortion. Chemically they are fatty acids.

**prostate** ('prostayt) the gland surrounding the male urethra at its junction with the bladder; during ejaculation it produces a fluid which forms part of the semen. It often becomes enlarged after middle age and may require removal if it causes obstruction to the outflow of urine. *P. screening* routine examination and blood testing for prostate-specific antigen (PSA) in older men, as a means to detect cancer of the prostate at an early stage.

**prostatectomy** (,prostə'tektəmee) surgical removal of the whole or a part of the prostate gland. *Retropubic p.* removal of the gland by incising the capsule of the prostate after making a suprapubic abdominal incision. *Transurethral p.* resection of the gland through the urethra using a resectoscope. *Transvesical p.* removal of the gland by incising the bladder after making a low abdominal incision.

**prostatitis** (,prostə'tietis) inflammation of the prostate gland.

**prostatorrhoea** (,prostatə'reeə) a thin urethal discharge from the prostate gland occurring in prostatitis.

**prosthesis** (pros'theesis) [Gr.] 1. the replacement of an absent part by an artificial substitute. 2. an artificial substitute for a missing part.

**prostration** (pro'strayshən) a condition of extreme exhaustion.

**protamine** ('prohtə,meen) one of a number of proteins occurring only in fish sperm. *P. sulphate* a drug used to neutralize circulating heparin, should haemorrhage arise during anticoagulant therapy.

**protease** ('prohti,ayz) a proteolytic enzyme in the digestive juices that causes the breakdown of protein.

**protective isolation** (prə'tektiv) a type of ISOLATION designed to prevent contact between potentially pathogenic microorganisms and uninfected persons who have seriously impaired resistance. Also called reverse isolation.

**protein** ('prohteen) one of a group of complex organic nitrogenous compounds formed from amino acids and occurring in every living cell of animal and vegetable tissue. *Bence Jones p.* an abnormal protein found in the urine of patients suffering from multiple myeloma. *First-class p.* one that provides the essential amino acids. Sources are meat, poultry, fish, cheese, eggs and milk. *P.-bound iodine* the iodine in the plasma which is combined with protein. Measurement of this is made when assessing thyroid function. *P.-losing enteropathy* a condition in which protein is lost from the lumen of the intestine. This causes hypoproteinaemia and oedema. *Second-class p.* one that comes from a vegetable source (e.g. peas, beans and whole cereal) that cannot supply all the body's needs.

**proteinuria** (,prohti'nyooə.ri.ə) an excess of serum proteins in the urine.

**proteolysis** (,prohti'olisis) the processes by which proteins are reduced to an absorbable form by digestive enzymes in the stomach and intestines.

**proteolytic** (,prohtioh'litik) 1. pertaining to, characterized by, or promoting proteolysis. 2. a proteolytic enzyme.

*Proteus* ('prohti.əs) a genus of Gram-negative bacteria common in the intestines of humans and animals and in decaying matter. They are frequently to be found in secondary infections of wounds and in the urinary tract.

**prothrombin** (proh'thrombin) a constituent of blood plasma, the precursor of thrombin, which is formed in the presence of calcium salts and thrombokinase when blood is shed. *P. time* a test to measure the activity of clotting factors. Deficiency of any of these factors leads to a prolongation of clotting time. This test is widely used for the establishment and maintenance of anticoagulant therapy.

**protoplasm** ('prohtə,plazəm) the essential chemical compound of which living cells are made.

**prototype** ('prohtə,tiep) the original form from which all other forms are derived.

**Protozoa** (,prohtə'zoh.ə) a phylum comprising the unicellular eukaryotic organisms; most are free-living but some lead commensalistic, mutualistic or parasitic existences. Pathogenic protozoa include *Entamoeba histolytica* (cause of amoebic dysentery) and *Plasmodium vivax* (cause of malaria). *See* METAZOA.

**protriptyline** (proh'triptə,leen) an antidepressant drug used in the treatment of extreme apathy and withdrawal.

**protuberance** (prə'tyoobə,rəns) in anatomy, a rounded projecting part.

**provider** (prə'viedə) in the health services, a person, group of people or organization supplying a service.

**provitamin** (proh'vitamin) a precursor of a vitamin. *P. 'A'* carotene. *P. 'D'* ergosterol.

**proximal** ('proksiməl) in anatomy, nearest that point which is considered the centre of a system; the opposite to distal.

**prurigo** (prooə'riegoh) a chronic skin disease with an irritating papular eruption.

**pruritus** (prooə'rietis) great irritation of the skin. It may affect the whole surface of the body, as in certain skin diseases and nervous disorders, or it may be limited in area, especially involving the anus and vulva.

**pseudarthrosis** (,syoodah'throhsis) a false joint formed when the two parts of a fractured bone have failed to unite together.

**pseudoangina** (,syoodoh.an'jienə) false angina. Precordial pain occurring in anxious individuals without evidence of organic heart disease.

**pseudocoxalgia** (,syoodohkok-'salji.ə) osteochondritis of the head of the femur. Perthes' disease.

**pseudocrisis** (,syoodoh'kriesis) a false crisis which is sometimes accompanied by the symptoms of true crisis, but in which the temperature rises again almost at once, and there is continuation of the disease.

**pseudocyesis** (,syoodohsie'eesis) false pregnancy; development of all the signs of pregnancy without the presence of an embryo.

**pseudogynaecomastia** (,syoodoh-,gienəkoh'masti.ə) the deposition of adipose tissue in the male breast which may give the appearance of enlarged mammary glands.

**pseudohermaphroditism** (,syoodoh.hər'mafrədi,tizəm) a congenital abnormality in which the external genitalia are characteristic of the opposite sex and confusion may arise as to the true sex of the individual.

**pseudoisochromatic chart** (,syoodoh,iesohkrə'matik) a chart of coloured dots for testing colour blindness. Ishihara colour chart.

*Pseudomonas* (,syoodoh'mohnəs) a genus of Gram-negative motile bacilli commonly found in decaying organic matter. *P. aeruginosa P. pyocyanea*. One found in pus from wounds ('blue pus') and also in urinary tract infections.

**pseudomyopia** (,syoodohmie'ohpi.ə) spasm of the ciliary muscle causing the same focusing defect as in myopia.

**pseudoparalysis** (,syoodohpə'ralisis) apparent loss of muscular power without real paralysis. *Arthritic general p.* a condition resembling dementia paralytica, dependent on intracranial atheroma in arthritic patients. Also called Klippel's disease. *Parrot's p., syphilitic p.* pseudoparalysis of one or more extremities in infants, due to syphilitic osteochrondritis of an epiphysis.

**psittacosis** (ˌsitəˈkohsis) a disease of parrots and budgerigars due to *Chlamydia psittaci*, communicable to humans. The symptoms resemble paratyphoid fever with bronchopneumonia.

**psoas** ('soh.əs) a long muscle originating from the lumbar spine and inserting into the lesser trochanter of the femur. It flexes the hip joint. *P. abscess* one that arises in the lumbar region and is due to spinal caries as a result of tuberculous infection.

**psoriasis** (səˈrieəsis) a chronic, recurrent skin disease characterized by reddish marginated patches with profuse silvery scaling on extensor surfaces, such as the knees and elbow, but which may be more widespread. It is non-infectious and the cause is unknown. It tends to occur in families; about one-third of cases are believed to be related to a hereditary factor.

**psyche** ('siekee) the mind, both conscious and unconscious.

**psychedelic** (ˌsiekəˈdelik) mind-altering; a term applied to hallucinatory or psychotomimetic drugs capable of profound effects upon the nature of the perception and conscious experience. *See also* HALLUCINOGEN.

**psychiatrist** (sieˈkieətrist) a medically qualified doctor who specializes in psychiatry.

**psychiatry** (sieˈkieətree) the branch of medicine that deals with the study, treatment and prevention of mental illness.

**psychoanalysis** (ˌsiekoh.əˈnalisis) 1. a method of investigating mental processes, developed by Sigmund Freud, which uses the techniques of free association, interpretation and dream analysis. 2. a system of theoretical psychology, formulated by Freud, based on the recognition of unconscious mental processes, such as resistance, repression and transference, and of the importance of infantile experience as a determinant of adult behaviour. 3. a method of psychotherapy based on the psychoanalytical method and psychoanalytical psychology.

**psychoanalyst** (ˌsiekohˈanəlist) one who specializes in psychoanalysis.

**psychodrama** (ˌsiekohˈdrahmə) group PSYCHOTHERAPY in which patients dramatize their individual conflicting situations of daily life.

**psychodynamics** (ˌsiekohdie-ˈnamiks) the understanding and interpretation of psychiatric symptoms or abnormal behaviour in terms of unconscious mental mechanisms.

**psychogenic** (ˌsiekohˈjenik) originating in the mind. *P. illness* a disorder that has a psychological as opposed to an organic origin.

**psychogeriatrics** (ˌsiekoh jeriˈatriks) the study and treatment of the psychological and psychiatric problems of the aged.

**psychologist** (sieˈkoləjist) one who studies normal and abnormal mental processes, development and behaviour.

**psychology** (sieˈkoləjee) the study of the mind and mental processes.

**psychometrics** (ˌsiekohˈmetriks) the measurement of mental characteristics by means of a series of tests.

**psychomotor** (ˌsiekohˈmohtə) related to the motor effects of mental activity. The term is applied to those mental disorders that affect muscular activity.

**psychoneurosis** (ˌsiekohnyuh-'rohsis) a mental disorder characterized by an abnormal mental response to a normal stimulus. The psychoneuroses include anxiety states, depression, hysteria and obsessive-compulsive neurosis.

**psychopath** ('siekohˌpath) *see* SOCIO-PATH.

**psychopathic disorder** (ˌsiekoh'pa-thik dis'awdə) a persistent disorder or disability of the mind (whether or not including significant impairment of intelligence) which results in abnormally aggressive or seriously irresponsible conduct on the part of the patient (Mental Health Act 1983).

**psychopathology** (ˌsiekohpə'tho-ləjee) the study of the causes and processes of mental disorders.

**psychopharmacology** (ˌsiekohˌfah-mə'koləjee) the study of drugs that have an action on the mind, and how such action is produced.

**psychoprophylaxis** (ˌsiekohˌprofi-'laksis) 1. a psychological technique used to prevent emotional disturbances. 2. a technique involving breathing control and exercises used to relieve pain during childbirth.

**psychosexual** (ˌsiekoh'seksyooəl) relating to the mental aspects of sex. *P. development* the stages through which an individual passes from birth to full maturity, especially in regard to sexual urges, in the total development of the person.

**psychosis** (sie'kohsis) any major mental disorder of organic or emotional origin, marked by derangement of the personality and loss of contact with reality, often with delusions, hallucinations or illusions. Psychoses are usually classified as functional psychoses, those for which no physical cause has been discovered, and organic psychoses, which are the result of organic damage to the brain.

**psychosomatic** (ˌsiekohsə'matik) relating to the mind and the body. *P. disorders* those illnesses in some individuals in which emotional factors (either causative or aggravating) have a profound influence, including anorexia nervosa and asthma respectively.

**psychotherapy** (ˌsiekoh'therəpee) any of a number of related techniques for treating mental illness by psychological methods. These techniques are similar in that they all mainly rely on establishing communication between the therapist and the patient as a means of understanding and modifying the patient's behaviour. On occasion, drugs may be used, but only in order to make this communication easier.

**psychotrophic** (ˌsiekoh'trohfik) pertaining to drugs that have an effect on the psyche. These include antidepressants, stimulants, sedatives and tranquillizers.

**ptosis** ('tohsis) 1. drooping of the upper eyelid due to paralysis of the third cranial nerve. It may be congenital or acquired. 2. prolapse of an organ, e.g. gastroptosis.

**ptyalin** ('tieəlin) an enzyme (amylase) in saliva which metabolizes starches.

**puberty** ('pyoobətee) the period during which secondary sexual characteristics develop and the reproductive organs become functional. Generally between the 12th and 17th years.

**pubes** ('pyoobeez) pubic hair or the area on which it grows.

**pubic** ('pyoobik) pertaining to the pubis.

**pubiotomy** (ˌpyoobi'otəmee) surgical division of a pubic bone during labour to increase the pelvic diameter.

**pubis** ('pyoobis) the anterior part of a hip bone. The left and right pubic bones meet at the front of the pelvis at the pubic symphysis.

**public health** ('publik) the field of medicine that is concerned with safeguarding and improving the physical, mental and social well-being of the community as a whole. Environmental aspects are the responsibility of the district local authority, whereas communicable disease control is supervised by the Medical Officer for Environmental Health, from the District Health Authority. Central government formulates national policy and is responsible for international aspects. *P.h. laboratory service* a central service within the NHS consisting of over 50 laboratories in the UK that provide the necessary resources for investigation, diagnosis and testing in suspected cases or in outbreaks of infectious disease.

**pudendal block** (pyoo'dend'l) a form of local analgesia induced by injecting a solution of 0.5 or 1% lignocaine around the pudendal nerve. Used mainly for episiotomy and forceps delivery.

**pudendum** (pyoo'dendəm) the external genitalia, especially those of a woman.

**puerperal** (pyoo'ərpə.rəl) pertaining to childbirth. *P. fever* or *sepsis* infection of the genital tract following childbirth.

**puerperium** (,pyooə'piə.ri.əm) a period of about 6 weeks following childbirth when the reproductive organs are returning to their normal state.

*Pulex* ('pyooleks) a genus of fleas. *P. irritans* those parasitic on humans. The type that infests rats may transmit plague to humans.

**pulmonary** ('pulmə.nə.ree, 'puhl-) pertaining to or affecting the lungs. *P. embolism* obstruction of the pulmonary artery or one of its branches by an embolus. *P. hypertension* an increase of blood pressure in the lungs, usually as a result of disease of the lung. *P. oedema* an excess of fluid in the lungs. *P. stenosis* a narrowing of the passage between the right ventricle of the heart and the pulmonary artery. The condition is frequently congenital. *P. tuberculosis see* TUBERCULOSIS. *P. valve* the valve at the point where the pulmonary artery leaves the heart.

**pulp** (pulp) any soft, juicy animal or vegetable tissue. *Digital p.* the soft pads at the ends of the fingers and toes. *P. cavity* the centre of a tooth containing blood tissue and nerves. *Splenic p.* the reddish-brown tissue of the spleen.

**pulsation** (pul'sayshən) a beating or throbbing.

**pulse** (puls) the local rhythmic expansion of an artery, which can be felt with the finger, corresponding to each contraction of the left ventricle of the heart. It may be felt in any artery sufficiently near the surface of the body, which passes over a bone, and the normal adult rate is about 72 beats/min. In childhood it is more rapid, varying from 130 in infants to 80 in older children. *Alternating p.* alternate strong and weak beats; pulsus alternans. *High-tension p.* cordy pulse. The duration of the impulse in the artery is long, and the artery feels firm and like a cord between the beats. *Low-tension p.* one easily obliterated by pressure. *Paradoxical p.* pulsus paradoxus; the pulse rate slows on inspiration and quickens on expiration. It may occur in constrictive pericarditis. *P. deficit* a sign of atrial fibrillation; the pulse rate is slower than the apex beat. *Running p.* there is little distinction between the beats. It occurs in haemorrhage. *Thready p.* thin and almost imperceptible pressure. *Venous p.* that felt in a vein; it is usually taken in the right jugular vein.

**pulseless disease** ('pulsləs) progressive obliteration of the vessels arising from the aortic arch, leading to loss of the pulse in both arms and carotids and to symptoms associated with ischaemia of the brain, eyes, face and arms.

**punctate** ('pungktayt) dotted. *P. erythema* a rash of very fine spots.

**punctum** ('pungktəm) a point or small spot. *P. lacrimalis* one of the two openings of the lacrimal ducts at the inner canthus of the eye.

**puncture** ('pungkchə) 1. the act of piercing with a sharp object. 2. the wound so produced. *Cisternal p.* the withdrawal of fluid from the cisterna magna. *Lumbar p.* the removal of cerebrospinal fluid by puncture between the third and fourth lumbar vertebrae. *Sternal p.* the withdrawal of bone marrow from the manubrium of the sternum. *Ventricular p.* the withdrawal of cerebrospinal fluid from a cerebral ventricle.

**pupil** ('pyoop'l) the circular aperture in the centre of the iris, through which light passes into the eye. *Argyll Robertson p.* absence of response to light but not to accommodation; characteristic of syphilis of the central nervous system. *Artificial p.* one made by cutting a piece out of the iris when the centre part of the cornea or the lens is opaque. *Fixed p.* one that fails to respond to light or convergence. *Multiple p.* two or more openings of the iris. *Tonic p.* one that reacts slowly to light or to convergence or both.

**pupillary** (pyoo'pilə.ree) referring to the pupil.

**purchaser** ('pərchəsə) in the health services, a budget-holder who agrees to buy a service from a PROVIDER.

**purgative** ('pərgətiv) a laxative; an aperient drug. Purgatives may be: (a) irritants, like cascara, senna, rhubarb and castor oil; (b) lubri-

cants, like liquid paraffin; (c) mechanical agents that increase bulk, like bran and agar preparations.

**purine** ('pyooə.reen) a heterocyclic compound that is the nucleus of the purine bases such as adenine and guanine, which occur in DNA and RNA. *See* PYRIMIDINE.

**purpura** ('pərpyuhrə) a condition characterized by extravasation of blood in the skin and mucous membranes, causing purple spots and patches. There are two general types of purpura: primary or idiopathic (usually autoimmune) thrombocytopenic purpura, in which the cause is unknown; and secondary or symptomatic thrombocytopenic purpura, which may be associated with exposure to drugs or other chemical agents, systemic diseases such as systemic lupus erythematosus, diseases affecting the bone marrow, such as leukaemia, and infections such as septicaemia and viral infections. *Allergic p., anaphylactic p.* Schönlein–Henoch purpura; also called Henoch–Schönlein. *Idiopathic thrombocytopenic p.* abbreviated ITP. An acquired thrombocytopenia which may be acute or chronic in its course. Acute ITP is common in young children. The disorder is usually self-limiting and rarely fatal. Chronic ITP is more insidious in onset, and is more common in young adult women. *P. senilis* dark purplish-red ecchymoses occurring on the forearms and backs of the hands in the elderly; the platelet count is normal. *Schönlein–Henoch p.* non-thrombocytopenic purpura of unknown cause, most often seen in children; associated with various clinical symptoms, such as urticaria and erythema, arthropathy and arthritis, gastrointestinal symptoms and renal involvement. *Steroid p.*

purpura secondary to prolonged use of steroids. The platelet count is normal, the basic defect being the loss of supporting connective tissue. *Thrombocytopenic p.* purpura associated with a decrease in the number of platelets in the blood.

**purulent** ('pyooə.rələnt) containing or resembling pus.

**pus** (pus) a thick, yellow semiliquid substance consisting of dead leukocytes and bacteria, debris of cells, and tissue fluids. It results from inflammation caused by invading bacteria, mainly *Staphylococcus aureus* and *Streptococcus haemolyticus*, which have destroyed the phagocytes and set up local suppuration. *Blue p.* that produced by infection with *Pseudomonas pyocyanea.*

**pustule** ('pustyool) a small pimple or elevation of the skin containing pus. *Malignant p. see* ANTHRAX.

**putative** ('pyootətiv) supposed, reputed. *P. father* the man believed to be the father of an illegitimate child.

**putrefaction** (,pyootri'fakshən) decomposition of animal or vegetable matter under the influence of microorganisms, usually accompanied by an offensive odour due to gas formation.

**pyaemia** (pie'eemi.ə) a condition resulting from the circulation of pyogenic microorganisms from some focus of infection. Multiple abscesses occur, the development of which causes rigor and high fever. *Portal p.* pylephlebitis.

**pyarthrosis** (,pieah'throhsis) suppuration in a joint.

**pyelitis** (,pieə'lietis) inflammation of the renal pelvis. Pyelitis is a fairly common disease, particularly among young children, affecting girls more often than boys. The most common presentation includes urgency of micturition,

frequency and dysuria. Pyuria is present.

**pyelography** (,pieə'logrəfee) *see* UROGRAPHY.

**pyelolithotomy** (,pieəlohli'thotəmee) the surgical removal of a stone from the renal pelvis.

**pyelonephritis** (,pieəlohnə'frietis) inflammation of the renal pelvis and renal substance, characterized by fever, acute loin pain and increased frequency of micturition, with the presence of pus and albumin in the urine.

**pyeloplasty** ('pieəloh,plastee) plastic repair of the renal pelvis.

**pylephlebitis** (,pielifli'bietis) inflammation of the portal vein which gives rise to severe symptoms of septicaemia or pyaemia.

**pylethrombosis** (,pielithrom-'bohsis) thrombosis of the portal vein.

**pyloric** (pie'lo.rik) relating to the pylorus. *P. stenosis* stricture of the pyloric orifice. It may be: (a) hypertrophic, when there is thickening of normal tissue; this is congenital and occurs in infants from 4–7 weeks old, usually males and first babies; (b) cicatricial, when there is ulceration or a malignant growth near the pylorus.

**pyloromyotomy** (pie,lo.rohmie-'otəmee) Ramstedt's operation; an incision of the pylorus performed to relieve congenital pyloric stenosis.

**pyloroplasty** (pie'lo.roh,plastee) plastic operation on the pylorus to enlarge the outlet. A longitudinal incision is made and it is resutured transversely (*see* Figure on p. 336).

**pylorospasm** (pie'lo.roh,spazəm) forceful muscle contraction of the pylorus which delays emptying of the stomach and causes vomiting.

**pylorus** (pie'lor.rəs) the opening into the duodenum at the lower end of the stomach. It is surrounded by a circular muscle, the *pyloric*

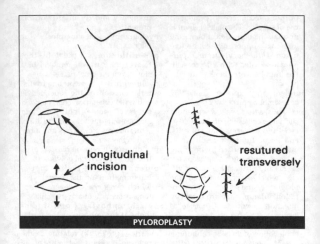

**PYLOROPLASTY**

longitudinal incision

resutured transversely

*sphincter*, which contracts to close the opening.

**pyoderma** (ˌpieoh'dərmə) any purulent skin disease. *P. gangrenosum* a rapidly evolving cutaneous ulcer or ulcers, with undermining of the border. Once regarded as a complication peculiar to ulcerative colitis, it is now known to occur in other wasting diseases.

**pyogenic** (ˌpieoh'jenik) producing pus.

**pyorrhoea** (pieə'reeə) a discharge of pus. *P. alveolaris* pus in the sockets of the teeth; suppurative periodontitis.

**pyramidal** (pi'ramid'l) of pyramid shape. *P. cells* cortical cells shaped like a pyramid from which originate nerve impulses to voluntary muscle. *P. tract* the nerve fibres that transmit impulses from pyramidal cells through the cerebral cortex to the spinal cord.

**pyrazinamide** (ˌpirə'zinəmied) a drug used in the treatment of

tuberculosis, especially tuberculous meningitis.

**pyrexia** (pie'reksi.ə) fever; a rise of body temperature to any point between 37 and 40°C; above this is hyperpyrexia.

**pyridostigmine** (ˌpiridoh'stigmeen) a drug that prevents destruction of acetylcholine at the neuromuscular junctions and is used in treating myasthenia gravis. It is less powerful than neostigmine but has a more prolonged action.

**pyrimethamine** (ˌpieri'methəmeen) a folic acid antagonist used as an antimalarial, especially for suppressive prophylaxis, and also used concomitantly with a sulphonamide in the treatment of toxoplasmosis.

**pyrimidine** (pie'rimi,deen) a nitrogen-containing organic compound. Thymine and cytosine are essential constituents of DNA, and uracil and cytosine of RNA. *See* PURINE.

**pyrixodine** (ˌpiriˈdokseen) vitamin B₆. This vitamin is concerned with protein metabolism and blood formation. It is found in many types of food and deficiency is rare.

**pyrogen** (ˈpierohˌjen) a substance that can produce fever.

**pyromania** (ˌpierohˈmayni.ə) an irresistible desire to set things on fire.

**pyrosis** (pieˈrohsis) heartburn; a symptom of indigestion marked by a burning sensation in the stomach and oesophagus with eructation of acid fluid.

**pyuria** (pieˈyooə.ri.ə) the presence of pus in the urine; more than three leukocytes per high-power field on microscopic examination.

# Q

**Q fever** an acute infectious disease of cattle which is transmitted to humans, usually by infected milk. It is caused by a rickettsia, *Coxiella burnetii*, and has symptoms resembling pneumonia.

**QRS complex** a group of waves depicted on an electrocardiogram; also called the QRS wave. It actually consists of three distinct waves created by the passage of the cardiac electrical impulse through the ventricles and occurs at the beginning of each contraction of the ventricles (*see* Figure). In a normal ELECTROCARDIOGRAM the R wave is the most prominent of the three; the Q and S waves may be extremely weak and are sometimes absent.

**quadratus** (kwod'raytəs) four-sided. The term is used to describe a number of four-sided muscles.

**quadriceps** ('kwodri,seps) four-headed. *Q. femoris muscle* the principal extensor muscle of the thigh.

**quadriplegia** (,kwodri'pleeji.ə) paralysis in which all four limbs are affected; tetraplegia.

**quality** ('kwolətee) 1. a distinguishing characteristic, property or attribute. 2. a degree or standard of excellence. *Q. assurance* in the health-care field, a pledge to the public by those within the various health disciplines that they will work towards the goal of an optimal achievable degree of excellence in the services rendered to every patient. *See* COST EFFECTIVENESS and PERFORMANCE INDICATORS. *Q. indicator* a defined, measurable variable used to monitor the quality or appropriateness of an important aspect of care. Indicators may be activities, events, occurrences or outcomes.

**quarantine** ('kwo.rən,teen) the period of isolation of an infectious or suspected case, to prevent the spread of disease. For contacts, this is the longest incubation period known for the specific disease.

**quartan** ('kwawtan) 1. recurring in 4-day cycles (every third day). 2. a variety of intermittent fever of which the paroxysms recur on every third day (*see* MALARIA).

**Queckenstedt's test** ('kweken,stets) *H.H.G. Queckenstedt, German physician, 1876–1918.* A test, carried out during lumbar puncture, by compression of the jugular veins. When normal there is a sharp rise in pressure, followed by a fall as the compression is released. Blockage of the spinal canal or thrombosis of the jugular vein will result in an absence of rise, or only a sluggish rise and fall.

**quickening** ('kwikəning) the first perceptible fetal movement, felt by the mother usually between the fourth and fifth months of pregnancy.

**quiescent** (kwi'es'nt) inactive or at rest. Descriptive of a time when the

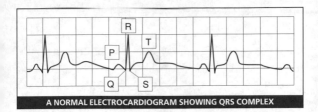

**A NORMAL ELECTROCARDIOGRAM SHOWING QRS COMPLEX**

symptoms of a disease are not evident.

**quinalbarbitone** (ˌkwinalˈbahbiˌtohn) an intermediate-acting barbiturate drug used in the treatment of severe insomnia.

**quinestrol** (kwiˈneestrol) a synthetic oestrogen used for the suppression of lactation after childbirth.

**quinidine** (ˈkwiniˌdeen) an alkaloid obtained from cinchona. It is used in the treatment of cardiac arrhythmias.

**quinine** (ˈkwineen, kwiˈneen) an alkaloid obtained from cinchona. Formerly used in the prevention and treatment of malaria. Still used to treat malignant tertian malaria.

**quinsy** (ˈkwinzee) a peritonsillar abscess; acute inflammation of the tonsil and surrounding cellular tissue with suppuration.

**quotidian** (kwoˈtidiˌən) recurring every day. *Q. fever* a variety of malaria in which the fever recurs daily.

**quotient** (ˈkwohshənt) a number obtained by dividing one number by another. *Intelligence q.* abbreviated IQ. The degree of intelligence estimated by dividing the mental age, reckoned from standard tests, by the age in years. *Respiratory q.* the ratio between the carbon dioxide expired and the oxygen inspired during a specified time.

# R

**R** symbol for the *roentgen* unit.

**Ra** symbol for *radium*.

**rabid** ('rabid) infected with rabies.

**rabies** ('raybeez) hydrophobia; an acute notifiable infectious disease of the central nervous system of animals, especially dogs, foxes, wolves and bats. The virus is found in the saliva of infected animals and is usually transmitted by a bite. Symptoms include fever, muscle spasms and intense excitement, followed by convulsions and paralysis, and death usually occurs. Vaccines are available.

**racemose** ('rasi‚mohz) grape-like *R. gland* a compound gland composed of a number of small sacs, e.g. the salivary gland.

**radiant** ('raydi.ənt) emitting rays.

**radiation** (‚raydi'ayshən) the emanation of energy in the form of electromagnetic waves, including gamma rays, X-rays, infrared and ultraviolet rays, and visible light rays. Radiation may cause damage to living tissues, e.g. in sunburn. *R. pneumonitis* inflammatory changes in the alveoli and interstitial tissue caused by radiation and which may lead to fibrosis later. *R. sickness* a toxic reaction of the body to radiation. Any or all of the following may be present: anorexia, nausea, vomiting and diarrhoea.

**radical** ('radik'l) dealing with the root or cause of a disease. *R. cure* one which cures by complete removal of the cause.

**radioactivity** (‚raydioh.ak'tivitee) disintegration of certain elements to ones of lower atomic weight, with the emission of alpha and beta particles and gamma rays. *Induced r.* that brought about by bombarding the nuclei of certain elements with neutrons.

**radiobiology** (‚raydiohbie'olǝjee) the branch of medical science that studies the effect of radiation on live animal and human tissues.

**radiocolloid** (‚raydioh'koloyd) a radioactive isotope, in the form of a large molecule solution, which can be instilled into the body cavities to treat malignant ascites.

**radiodermatitis** (‚raydioh‚dǝrmǝ-'tietis) a late skin complication of radiotherapy in which there is atrophy, scarring, pigmentation and telangiectases of the skin.

**radiograph** ('raydioh‚grahf, -‚graf) skiagram; the picture obtained, on specially sensitized film, by passing X-rays through the body.

**radiographer** (‚raydi'ogrǝfǝ) a professional health-care worker in a diagnostic X-ray department (diagnostic radiographer) or in a radiotherapy department (therapy radiographer).

**radiography** (‚raydi'ogrǝfee) the making of film records (radiographs) of internal structures of the body by exposure of film specially sensitized to X-rays or gamma rays. *Body-section r.* a special technique to show in detail images and structures lying in a predetermined plane of tissue, while blurring or eliminating detail in images in other planes; various mechanisms and methods for such radiography have been given various names, e.g. laminagraphy, tomography, etc. *Double-contrast r.* a technique for revealing an abnormality of the intestinal mucosa; it involves injection and evacuation of a barium enema, followed by inflation of the intestine with air under light pressure. *Neutron r.* that in which a narrow beam of neutrons from a nuclear reactor is passed through tissues; especially useful in visualizing bony tissue. *Serial r.* the making of several exposures of a particular area at arbitrary intervals.

**radioisotope** (,raydioh'iesə,tohp) an isotope of an element that emits radioactivity. These isotopes may occur naturally or be produced artificially by bombardment with neutrons.

**radiologist** (,raydi'oləjist) a medically qualified doctor who specializes in the science of radiology.

**radiology** (,raydi'oləjee) the science of radiation. In medicine the term refers to its use in the diagnosis and treatment of disease.

**radiomimetic** (,raydiohmi'metik) producing effects similar to those of ionizing radiations.

**radionuclide** (,raydioh'nyooklied) a radioactive substance which is inherently unstable. It is used in both radiodiagnosis and in radiotherapy.

**radioscopy** (,raydi'oskəpee) the examination of X-ray images on a fluorescent screen.

**radiosensitive** (,raydioh'sensitiv) pertaining to those structures that respond readily to radiotherapy.

**radiotherapist** (,raydioh'therəpist) a medically qualified doctor specializing in radiotherapy.

**radiotherapy** (,raydioh'therəpee) treatment of disease by X-rays or radioactive isotopes.

**radium** ('raydi.əm) *symbol* Ra. A radioactive element, obtained from uranium ores, which gives off emanations of great radioactive power. Used in the treatment of some malignant diseases.

**râle** (rahl) an abnormal rattling sound, heard on ausculation of the chest during respiration when there is fluid in the bronchi.

**Ramstedt's operation** ('ramshtets) *W.C. Ramstedt, German surgeon, 1867–1963.* Operation for congenital stricture of the pylorus in which the fibres of the sphincter muscle are divided, leaving the mucous lining intact.

**random sample** ('randəm) a sample from a population, obtained by ensuring that each member of that population has an equal chance of being selected. The sample selected should then demonstrate the same profile as the parent population.

**ranula** ('ranyuhlə) a retention cyst, usually under the tongue when blockage occurs in a submaxillary or sublingual duct, or in a mucous gland.

**rape** (rayp) sexual assault or abuse; criminal forcible sexual intercourse (i.e. penetration) without the consent of the adult or child. Many cases are not reported because of feelings of shame, guilt, embarrassment or fear. Although rape can occur between men, it is usually associated with victims who are women.

**raphe** ('rayfee) a seam or ridge of tissue indicating the junction of two parts.

**rapport** (ra'por) in psychiatry, a satisfactory relationship between two persons, either the doctor and patient or nurse and patient, or the patient with any significant other.

**rarefaction** (ˌrair.riˈfakshən) the process of becoming less dense.

**rash** (rash) a superficial eruption on the skin, frequently characteristic of some specific fever.

**Rashkind catheter** ('rashkint) *W.J. Rashkind, American paediatric cardiologist, b. 1922.* A balloon catheter used to increase the size of the atrial septal defect in children who have transposition of the great vessels.

**rate** (rayt) the speed or frequency with which an event or circumstance occurs per unit of time, population, or other standard of comparison. *Basal metabolic r.* abbreviated BMR. An expression of the rate at which oxygen is utilized in a fasting subject at complete rest as a percentage of a value established as normal for such a subject. *Birth r.* the number of live births in a population in a specified period of time (crude birth rate), for the female population (refined birth rate), or for the female population of childbearing age (true birth rate), usually expressed per year per 1000 of the estimated mid-year population. *Death r.* the number of deaths per stated number of persons (1000, 10 000 or 100 000) in a certain region in a certain time (crude death rate). The death rate calculated with allowances made for age and sex distribution in the population is termed the standardized death rate. Also called *mortality rate. Glomerular filtration r.* an expression of the quantity of glomerular filtrate formed each minute in the nephrons of both kidneys, calculated by measuring the clearance of specific substances, e.g. insulin or creatinine.

**ratio** ('rayshiˌoh) an expression of the quantity of one substance or entity in relation to that of another; the relationship between two quantities expressed as the quotient of one divided by the other. *Lecithin–sphingomyelin r.* the ratio of lecithin to sphingomyelin in amniotic fluid.

**rationalization** (ˌrashənəlieˈzayshən) in psychiatry, the mental process by which individuals explain their behaviour, giving reasons that are advantageous to themselves or are socially acceptable. It may be a conscious or an unconscious act.

**Rauwolfia** (rawˈwuhlfi.ə, row-) a genus of tropical trees and shrubs. The dried root of *R. serpentina* is sometimes used as an antihypertensive and sedative, e.g. reserpine.

**Raynaud's phenomenon** or **disease** ('raynohz) *M. Raynaud, French physician, 1834–1881.* Raynaud's phenomenon is characterized by episodic digital ischaemia provoked by stimuli such as emotion, cold, trauma, hormones and drugs. It includes both Raynaud's disease, where no underlying cause can be found, and Raynaud's syndrome, where there is an associated underlying disorder. These disorders include scleroderma, mixed connective tissue disease, systemic lupus erythematosus (SLE), polymyositis, rheumatoid arthritis, neurovascular entrapment syndromes and occlusive arterial disease.

**re-education** (ˌree.edyuhˈkayshən) the education and training of the physically handicapped or those with learning difficulties to enable them to develop their potential.

**reaction** (riˈakshən) counteraction; a response to the application of a stimulus. *R. time* the interval between the stimulus and the response.

**reactive** (riˈaktiv) in psychiatry, used to describe a mental condition brought about by adverse external circumstances. *R. depression* one that arises in this way and is not endogenous.

**reagent** (riˈayjənt) a substance employed to produce a chemical reaction.

**reality** (ree'alətee) agreed as an absolute by members of the same culture as the total of all things related to perception, meaning and behaviour. Not imaginary, fictitious or pretended. *R. orientation see* ORIENTATION.

**recall** (ri'kawl, 'reekawl) to bring back to consciousness.

**receptor** (ri'septə) 1. a sensory nerve ending that receives stimuli for transmission through the sensory nervous system. 2. a molecule on the surface or within a cell that recognizes and binds with specific molecules, producing some effect in the cell.

**recessive** (ri'sesiv) tending to recede. The opposite to dominant. *R. gene* a gene that will produce its characteristics only when present in a homozygous state; both parents need to possess the particular gene, and there is a 1 in 4 chance of a child inheriting it homozygously.

**recipient** (ri'sipi.ənt) one who receives, as a blood transfusion, or a tissue or organ graft. *Universal r.* a person thought to be able to receive blood of any 'type' without agglutination of the donor cells.

**recrudescence** (,reekroo'des'ns) renewed aggravation of symptoms after an interval of abatement.

**rectal** ('rekt'l) relating to the rectum. *R. examination* inspection by insertion of a glove-covered finger or with the aid of a proctoscope.

**rectopexy** ('rektoh,peksee) the operation for fixation of a prolapsed rectum.

**rectovaginal** (,rektohva'jien'l) concerning the rectum and vagina.

**rectovesical** (,rektoh'vesik'l) concerning the rectum and bladder.

**rectum** ('rektəm) the lower end of the large intestine from the sigmoid flexure to the anus.

**recumbent** (ri'kumbənt) lying down in the dorsal position.

**recuperation** (ri,koopə'rayshən) convalescence; recovery of health and strength.

**recurrent** (ri'kurənt) liable to recur. *R. fever* relapsing fever.

**Redivac drainage tube** ('redi,vak 'draynij) a proprietary closed drainage system used mainly postoperatively for abdominal wounds.

**reduction** (ri'dukshən) 1. the correction of a fracture, dislocation or hernia. 2. the addition of hydrogen to a substance or, more generally, the gain of electrons; the opposite of oxidization. *Closed r.* the manipulative reduction of a fracture without incision. *Open r.* reduction of a fracture after incision into the fracture site.

**referred pain** (ri,fərd) that which occurs at a distance from the place of origin due to the sensory nerves entering the cord at the same level, e.g. the phrenic nerve supplying the diaphragm enters the cord in the cervical region, as do the nerves from the shoulder, and so an abscess on the diaphragm may cause pain in the shoulder. Synalgia.

**reflection** (ri'flekshən) 1. a turning or bending back, as in the folds produced when a membrane passes over the surface of an organ and then passes back to the body wall that it lines. 2. in nursing and health-care practice, conscious and systematic thinking about one's actions; the review, analysis and evaluation of those situations that have occurred, usually after but maybe during an event. An active process by which the practitioner learns from situations with a view to improving future practice.

**reflective practice** (ri'flektiv) an active process by which the health-care professional is able to review, analyse and evaluate events or situations. This conscious monitoring process can be based on any conceptual model, and may utilize

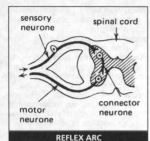

sensory neurone

spinal cord

motor neurone

connector neurone

**REFLEX ARC**

supervision of peers in the process. The aim is to facilitate and enhance professional practice.

**reflex** ('reefleks) reflected or thrown back. *Accommodation r.* the alteration in the shape of the lens according to the distance of the image viewed. *Conditioned r.* that which is not natural, but is developed by association and frequent repetition until it appears natural. *Corneal r.* the automatic reaction of closing the eyelids after exertion of light pressure on the cornea. This is a test for unconsciousness which is absolute when there is no response. *Deep r.* a muscle reflex elicited by tapping the tendon or bone of attachment. *Light r.* alteration of the size of the pupil in response to exposure to light. *R. action* an involuntary action following immediately upon some stimulus, e.g. the knee jerk, or the withdrawal of a limb from a pin-prick. *R. arc* the sensory and motor neurones, together with the connector neurone, which carry out a reflex action (*see* Figure). *R. zone therapy* a system of complementary therapy, similar to reflexology, in which it is believed the body is divided into ten longitudinal and three transverse zones, with corresponding divisions in the feet. Reflex zone therapy can be used to identify areas of disorder or disease in the body and a sophisticated grip technique is used to massage the feet and so treat the problem. The therapy can also be performed on the hands, which correspond closely to the feet, the tongue, the face and the back.

**reflexology** (‚reeflek'soləjee) a technique of deep massage to the soles of the feet, and occasionally the palms of the hands, to relieve somatic symptoms, and promote health and wellbeing.

**reflux** ('reefluks) a backward flow; regurgitation.

**refraction** (ri'frakshən) 1. the bending or deviation of rays of light as they pass obliquely through one transparent medium and penetrate another of different density. 2. in ophthalmology, the testing of the eyes to ascertain the amount and variety of refractive error that may be present in each of them.

**refractory** (ri'fraktəree) not yielding to, or resistant to, treatment. *R. period* the period immediately after some activity during which a nerve or muscle is unable to react to a fresh impulse.

**regeneration** (ri‚jenə'rayshən) renewal, as in new growth of tissue in its specific form after injury.

**register** ('rejistə) an epidemiological term meaning an index or file of all cases with a particular disease or condition in a defined population.

**registrar** (‚reji'strah) 1. an official keeper of records. 2. in British hospitals, a doctor training to be a specialist. *R. of births, marriages and deaths* the official recorder of births, marriages and deaths. In England and Wales, the office comes under the Office for National Statistics. Local registry offices are available in most towns. Births should be registered within 6 weeks in England and Wales (21 days in Scotland). Without a death certificate, which indicates that the death has been registered, it is illegal to dispose of a body.

**registration** (‚reji'strayshən) the act of recording; in dentistry, the making of a record of the jaw relations, present or desired, in order to transfer them to an articulator to facilitate proper construction of a dental prosthesis.

**regression** (ri'greshən) 1. a return to a previous state of health. 2. in psychiatry, a tendency to return to primitive or child-like modes of behaviour. Some degree of regression frequently accompanies physical illness and hospitalization. Patients who are mentally ill may exhibit regression to an extreme degree, reverting all the way back to infantile behaviour (atavistic regression).

**regurgitation** (ri‚gurji'tayshən) backward flow, e.g. of food from the stomach into the mouth. Fluids regurgitate through the nose in paralysis affecting the soft palate. *Aortic r.* backward flow of blood into the left ventricle when the aortic valve is incompetent. *Mitral r.* mitral incompetence. *See* MITRAL.

**REHAB** rehabilitation evaluation of Hall and Baker.

**rehabilitation** (‚reeə‚bili'tayshən) re-education, particularly where an individual has been ill or injured, to enable them to become capable of useful activity. *R. centre* one which provides for organized employment within the capacity of the patient, and with especial regard to the physical influence of the work. *R. evaluation of Hall and Baker* abbreviated REHAB. An assessment system for identifying the patient's level of normal, everyday living and work skills, and of any disturbed behaviour.

**reinforcement** (‚ree.in'fawsmənt) the increasing of force or strength.

In behavioural science, the process of presenting a reinforcing stimulus to strengthen a response. *See* CONDITIONING. A positive reinforcer is a stimulus that is added to the environment immediately after the desired response. It serves to strengthen the response: that is, to increase the likelihood of its occurring again. Examples of a positive reinforcer are food, money, a special privilege, or some other reward that is satisfying to the subject.

**Reiter's syndrome** *H. Reiter, German bacteriologist, 1881–1969.* A non-specific urethritis, affecting males, in which there is also arthritis and conjunctivitis.

**rejection** (ri'jekshən) 1. in immunology, the formation of antibodies by the host against transplanted tissue, with eventual destruction of the transplanted tissue. 2. in psychosocial terms, the denial of acceptance or affection, or the exclusion of another person.

**relapse** (ri'laps, 'ree‚laps) the return of a disease after an interval of convalescence.

**relapsing fever** (ri'lapsing) one of a group of similar notifiable infectious diseases transmitted to humans by the bites of ticks. Marked by alternating periods of normal temperature and periods of fever relapse. The diseases in the group are caused by several different species of spirochaetes belonging to the genus *Borrelia.* Also called recurrent fever.

**relaxant** (ri'laks'nt) a drug or other agent that brings about muscle relaxation or relieves tension.

**relaxation** (‚reelak'sayshən) a lessening of tension, which may be observed when muscles slacken after they have contracted; it is characterized by feelings of peace and calmness. *R. therapy* classes in which patients are taught breathing and other exercises to use for the relief of pain, stress and tension. Used as part of the preparation for childbirth.

**relaxin** (ri'laksin) a hormone that is produced by the corpus luteum of the ovary; it softens the cervix and loosens the pelvic ligaments to aid the birth of the baby.

**releasing factor** (ri'leesing ,faktə) a substance, produced in the hypothalamus, which causes the anterior pituitary gland to release hormones.

**REM** rapid eye movement, a phase of SLEEP associated with dreaming and characterized by rapid movements of the eyes. Paradoxical sleep.

**reminiscence therapy** (remi'nisəns) measures to stimulate long-term elderly patients with memorabilia, films and songs meaningful to their generation. Used in conjunction with or as a prelude to reality orientation therapy. *See* ORIENTATION.

**remission** (ri'mishən) subsidence of the symptoms of a disease for a long time.

**remittent** (ri'mitənt) decreasing at intervals. *R. fever* one in which a partial fall in the temperature occurs daily.

**remotivation** (ree,mohti'vayshən) in psychiatry, a group therapy technique administered by the nursing staff in a psychiatric hospital or department, which is used to stimulate the communication skills and an interest in the environment of long-term, withdrawn patients.

**renal** ('reen'l) relating to the kidney. *R. calculus* stone in the kidney. *R. clearance tests* laboratory tests that determine the ability of the kidney to remove certain substances from the blood. *R. dialysis* the application of the principles of dialysis for treatment of renal failure (*see* below). *See also* HAEMODIALYSIS and PERITONEAL (DIALYSIS). *R. failure* inability of the kidney to maintain normal function. It may be *acute* or *chronic*. Acute renal failure is a sudden, severe interruption of kidney function. It is normally the complication of another disorder and is reversible. Chronic renal failure is a progressive loss of kidney function. In its early stage, renal function can remain adequate but the glomerular filtration rate (GFR) is depressed and plasma chemistry begins to show abnormalities as waste products accumulate. In the later stage, known as end-stage renal disease (ESRD), the GFR deteriorates and when URAEMIA becomes evident and the patient becomes symptomatic, dialysis is started or the patient receives a transplant. *R. threshold* the level of the blood sugar beyond which it is excreted in the urine; normally 10 mmol/l (180 mg/100 ml). *R. tubule* the thin tubular part of a nephron. A uriniferous tubule.

**renin** ('reenin) a proteolytic enzyme released into the bloodstream when the kidneys are ischaemic. It causes vasoconstriction and increases the blood pressure.

**reorganization** (,ri.awgənie'zayshən) healing by formation of new tissue identical to that which was injured or destroyed.

**reovirus** (,reeoh'viərəs) any of a group of RNA viruses isolated from healthy children, children with febrile and afebrile upper respiratory disease, or children with diarrhoea.

**repetitive strain injury** (re,petitiv 'strayn ,injə.ree) a soft-tissue disorder produced by repetitive use of muscle, especially if the muscle activity involves an awkward or uncomfortable position of the body. Particularly affects keyboard operators, musicians, packers and machine operators.

**replication** (,repli'kayshən) 1. the turning back of a tissue on itself. 2.

the process by which DNA duplicates itself when the cell divides.

**replogle tube** (ri'plohg'l) a double-lumen aspiration catheter attached to low pressure suction apparatus.

**repression** (ri'preshən) 1. the act of restraining, inhibiting or suppressing. 2. in psychiatry, a defence mechanism whereby a person unconsciously banishes unacceptable ideas, feelings or impulses from consciousness. A person using repression to obtain relief from mental conflict is unaware that 'forgetting' unpleasant situations is a way of avoiding them (motivated forgetting).

**reproductive system** ( ,reeprə'duktiv ,sistəm) all those parts of the male and female body associated with the production of children.

**resection** (ri'sekshən) surgical removal of a part. *Submucous r.* removal of part of a deflected nasal septum, from beneath a flap of mucous membrane, which is then replaced. *Transurethral r.* a method of removing portions of an enlarged prostate gland via the urethra.

**resectoscope** (ri'sektə,skohp) a telescopic instrument by which pieces of tissue can also be removed. Used for transurethral prostatectomy.

**reserpine** ('rezə,peen) an alkaloid from *Rauwolfia*; a drug used to reduce the blood pressure in hypertension.

**reservoir** ('rezə,vwah) 1. a storage place or cavity. 2. the host or environment in which an organism lives and from which it is able to infect susceptible individuals, e.g. hands, skin, nose and bowel.

**residential care** ( ,rezi'denshəl) the provision of care for frail, elderly people in a variety of settings, e.g. local authority residential homes for the elderly or private residential homes.

**residual** (ri'zidyooəl) remaining. *R. air* residual volume. The amount of

air remaining in the lungs after breathing out fully. *R. urine* urine remaining in the bladder after voiding; seen with bladder outlet obstruction and disorders affecting nerves controlling bladder function. *R. volume* residual air.

**resistance** (ri'zistəns) the degree of opposition to a force. 1. in electricity, the opposition made by a nonconducting substance to the passage of a current. 2. in psychology, the opposition, stemming from the unconscious, to repressed ideas being brought to consciousness. *Drug r.* the ability of a microorganism to withstand the effects of a drug that are lethal to most members of its species. *Peripheral r.* that offered to the passage of blood through small vessels and capillaries. *R. to infection* the natural power of the body to withstand the toxins of disease.

**resolution** ( ,rezə'looshən) 1. in medicine, the process of returning to normal. 2. the disappearance of inflammation without the formation of pus.

**resonance** ('rezənəns) in medicine, the reverberating sound obtained on percussion over a cavity or hollow organ, such as the lung.

**respiration** ( ,respi'rayshən) the gaseous interchange between the tissue cells and the atmosphere. *Artificial r.* the production of respiratory movements by external effort. *External r.* breathing, which comprises inspiration, when the external intercostal muscles and the diaphragm contract and air is drawn into the lungs, and expiration, when the air is breathed out. *Intermittent positive pressure r.* abbreviated IPPR. Respiration produced by a ventilator. *Internal r.* tissue respiration. The interchange of gases that occurs between tissues and blood through the walls of capillaries. *Laboured r.* that which is difficult and distressed. *Stertorous r.* snorting; a noisy breathing. *Tissue r.* internal respiration. *See* CHEYNE– STOKES RESPIRATION.

**respirator** ('respi,raytə) an apparatus to qualify the air breathed through it, or a device for giving artificial respiration or to assist pulmonary ventilation (*see also* VENTILATOR). *R. shock* circulatory SHOCK due to interference with the flow of blood through the great vessels and chambers of the heart, causing pooling of blood in the veins and the abdominal organs and a resultant vascular collapse. The condition sometimes occurs as a result of increased intrathoracic pressure in patients who are being maintained on a mechanical ventilator.

**respiratory** (ri'spirətə.ree, 'respərətree) pertaining to respiration. *Acute r. distress syndrome* abbreviated ARDS. A group of signs and symptoms resulting in acute respiratory failure; characterized clinically by tachypnoea, dyspnoea, tachycardia, cyanosis, and low $PaO_2$ that persists even with oxygen therapy. *R. distress syndrome of newborn* a condition occurring in preterm infants, full-term infants of diabetic mothers, and infants delivered by caesarean section, and associated with pulmonary immaturity and inability to produce sufficient lung surfactant. Also called hyaline membrane disease, idiopathic respiratory distress syndrome, infant respiratory distress syndrome (abbreviated IRDS). *R. failure* a life-threatening condition in which respiratory function is inadequate to maintain the body's need for oxygen supply and carbon dioxide removal while at rest; also called acute ventilatory failure. *R. insufficiency* a condition in which respiratory function is inadequate to meet the body's needs when increased physical activity places extra demands on it. *R. quotient* the ratio of the volume of expired carbon dioxide to the volume of oxygen absorbed by the lungs per unit of time. *R. syncytial virus* a virus isolated from children with bronchopneumonia and bronchitis, characteristically causing severe respiratory infection in very young children but less severe infections as the children grow older. *R. therapy* the technical specialty concerned with the treatment, management and care of patients with respiratory problems, including administration of medical gases.

**resuscitation** (ri,susi'tayshən) restoration to life or consciousness of one apparently dead, or whose respirations have ceased. *See also* ARTIFICIAL (RESPIRATION). *Cardiopulmonary r.* an emergency technique used in cardiac arrest to re-establish heart and lung function until more advanced life support is available.

**retardation** (,reetah'dayshən) delay; hindrance; delayed development. *Mental r.* low general intellectual development, associated with impairment either of learning and social adjustment or of maturation, or of both.

**retching** ('reching) strong, involuntary effort to vomit.

**retention** (ri'tenshən) holding back. *R. cyst see* CYST. *R. defect* a defect of memory. Inability to retain material in the mind so that it can be recalled when required. *R. of urine* inability to pass urine from the bladder, which may be due to obstruction or be of nervous origin.

**reticular** (rə'tikyuhlə) resembling a network. *R. formation* areas in the brain stem from which nerve fibres extend to the cerebral cortex.

**reticulocyte** (rə'tikyuhloh,siet) a red blood cell that is not fully mature; it retains strands of nuclear material.

**reticulocytosis** (rə,tikyuhlohsie'tohsis) the presence of an increased number of immature red cells in the blood, indicating overactivity of the bone marrow.

**reticuloendothelial system** (rə'tikyuhloh,endə'theeli.ə ,sistəm) a collection of endothelial cells in the liver, spleen, bone marrow and lymph glands that produce large mononuclear cells or macrophages. They are phagocytic, destroy red blood cells and have the power of making some antibodies.

**retina** ('retinə) the innermost coat of the eyeball, formed of nerve cells and fibres, from which the optic nerve leaves the eyeball and passes to the visual area of the cerebrum. The impression of the image is focused upon it.

**retinal** ('retinəl) relating to the retina. *R. detachment* partial detachment of the retina from the underlying choroid layer, resulting in loss of vision. It may result from the presence of a tumour, from trauma or from high myopia.

**retinitis** (,reti'nietis) inflammation of the retina. *R. pigmentosa* a group of diseases, frequently hereditary, marked by progressive loss of retinal function, especially associated with contraction of the visual field and impairment of vision. The disorder often follows a slow course over a period of many years, but there is considerable variation in the progression of the disease.

**retinoblastoma** (,retinohbla'stohmə) a malignant tumour arising from retinal cells. Occurs in infancy and may be hereditary. Treatment includes cryosurgery, irradiation and photocoagulation, but enucleation may be required.

**retinopathy** (,reti'nopəthee) any non-inflammatory disease of the retina. *Diabetic r.* a complication of diabetes. Retinal haemorrhages occur, resulting in permanent visu-

al damage, and retinal detachment may follow. *Hypertensive r.* retinal change occurring as a result of high blood pressure.

**retinoscope** ('retinə,skohp) an instrument which illuminates the retina and is used to detect and measure refractive errors.

**retrobulbar** (,retroh'bulbə) pertaining to the back of the eyeball. *R. neuritis* dimness of vision due to inflammation of the optic nerve.

**retroflexion** (,retroh'flekshən) a bending back, particularly of the uterus when it is bent backwards at an acute angle, the cervix being in its normal position. *See* RETROVERSION.

**retrograde** ('retrə,grayd) going backwards. *R. amnesia* forgetfulness of events occurring immediately before an illness or injury. *R. urography* radiographic examination of the kidney after the introduction of a radio-opaque substance into the renal pelvis through the urethra.

**retrolental fibroplasia** (,retroh'lent'l) a fibrous condition of the anterior vitreous body which develops when a premature infant is exposed to high concentrations of oxygen. Both eyes are affected, seriously interfering with vision and leading to retinal detachment. Early treatment with a freezing probe (cryopexy) can prevent retinal detachment.

**retroperitoneal** (,retroh,peritə'nee-əl) behind the peritoneum.

**retropharyngeal** (,retrohfə'rinji.əl, -,farin'jeeəl) behind the pharynx.

**retropubic** (,retroh'pyoobik) behind the pubic bone.

**retrospection** (,retroh'spekshən) a morbid dwelling on memories.

**retrosternal** (,retroh'stərnəl) behind the sternum.

**retroversion** (,retroh'vərshən) a lifting backwards, particularly of the uterus when the whole organ is tilted backwards. *See* RETROFLEXION.

**retrovirus** ('retroh,viərəs) a group of viruses belonging to the family *Retroviridae*, principally infecting and frequently causing diseases in animals, but also including viruses that infect and cause disease in humans, e.g. HUMAN IMMUNODEFICIENCY VIRUS (HIV) and human T-cell leukaemia/lymphoma/lymphotropic virus type I (HTLV-I).

**Reverdin's graft** ('revərdanhz) *J.L. Reverdin, Swiss surgeon, 1842–1929.* A form of skin graft in which pieces of skin are placed as islands over the area. *See* THIERSCH SKIN GRAFT.

**Reye's syndrome** (riez) *R.D.K. Reye, 20th century Australian pathologist.* An acute, potentially fatal illness that may follow a virus infection occurring in children; there is fatty degeneration of the liver and the brain and raised intracranial pressure, accompanied by vomiting, convulsions and coma. The cause of Reye's syndrome is unknown but administration of salicylates in children under the age of 12 years is not recommended. This follows evidence that aspirin may be a contributory factor in the development of Reye's syndrome.

**Rh factor** rhesus factor.

**rhabdomyosarcoma** (,rabdoh,mieohsah'kohmə) a rare malignant growth of striated muscle. It grows rapidly and metastasizes early.

**rhagades** ('ragə,deez) cracks or fissures in the skin, especially those round the mouth.

**rhesus factor** ('reesəs,faktə) abbreviated Rh factor. The red blood cells of most humans carry a group of genetically determined antigens and are said to be rhesus positive (Rh$^+$). Those that do not are said to be rhesus negative (Rh$^-$). This is of importance as a cause of anaemia and jaundice in the newly born when the infant is Rh$^+$ and the mother Rh$^-$. The result of this incompatibility (isoimmunization)

is the formation of an antibody which causes excessive haemolysis in the child's blood. *See* ANTI-RHESUS SERUM.

**rheumatism** ('roomə,tizəm) any of a variety of disorders marked by inflammation, degeneration or metabolic derangement of the connective tissue structures, especially the joints and related structures, and attended by pain, stiffness or limitation of motion. *Acute r.* rheumatic fever. An acute fever associated with previous streptococcal infection and occurring most commonly in children. The onset is usually sudden, with pain, swelling and stiffness in one or more joints. There is fever, sweating and tachycardia, and carditis is present in most cases. Sometimes the symptoms are minor and ignored. This disease is the most common cause of mitral stenosis because scar tissue results from the inflammation.

**rheumatoid** ('roomə,toyd) resembling rheumatism. *R. arthritis see* ARTHRITIS.

**rheumatology** (,roomə'toləjee) the branch of medicine dealing with disorders of the joints, muscles, tendons and ligaments.

**rhinitis** (rie'nietis) inflammation of the mucous membrane of the nose.

**rhinoplasty** ('rienoh,plastee) a plastic operation on the nose; repairing a part of or forming an entirely new nose.

**rhinorrhoea** (,rienə'reeə) an abnormal discharge of mucus from the nose.

**rhinoscopy** (rie'noskəpee) examination of the interior of the nose. *Anterior r.* examination through the nostrils with the aid of a speculum. *Posterior r.* examination through the nasopharynx by means of a rhinoscope.

**rhinovirus** (,rienoh'vierəs) one of a genus of small RNA-containing viruses that cause respiratory diseases, including the common cold.

*Rhipicephalus* (ˌriepiˈkefələs, -ˈsef-) a genus of ticks that can transmit the rickettsiae which cause typhus and relapsing fever.

**rhodopsin** (rohˈdopsin) the visual purple of the retina, the formation of which is dependent upon vitamin A in the diet.

**rhonchus** (ˈrongkəs) a wheezing sound, produced in the bronchial tubes, which is caused by partial obstruction and can be heard on auscultation.

**rhythm** (ˈridhəm) a regular recurring action. *Cardiac r.* the smooth action of the heart when systole is followed by diastole. *R. method* a contraceptive technique in which intercourse is limited to the 'safe period' (avoiding the 2–3 days immediately before and after ovulation).

**rib** (rib) any one of the 12 pairs of long, flat curved bones of the thorax, each united by cartilage to the spinal vertebrae at the back. *Cervical r.* a short extra rib, often bilateral. Pressure on this may cause impairment of nerve or vascular function. *See* SCALENUS (SYNDROME). *False r's* the last five pairs, the upper three of which are attached by cartilage to each other. *Floating r's* the last two pairs, connected only to the vertebrae. *True r's* the seven pairs attached directly to the sternum.

**riboflavin** (ˌriebohˈflavvin) a chemical factor in the vitamin B complex.

**ribonuclease** (ˌriebohˈnyookliˌayz) an enzyme from the pancreas which is responsible for the breakdown of nucleic acid.

**ribonucleic acid** (ˌriebohnyoo-ˈkleeˌik, -ˈklay-) abbreviated RNA. A complex chemical found in the cytoplasm of animal cells and concerned with protein synthesis. Certain viruses contain RNA.

**ribosome** (ˈriebəˌsohm) an RNA- and protein-containing particle which is the site of protein synthesis in the cell.

**rickets** (ˈrikits) a condition of infancy and childhood caused by deficiency of vitamin D, which leads to altered calcium and phosphorus metabolism and consequent disturbance of ossification of bone, resulting in deformity, such as bowing of the legs. Since the action of sunlight on the skin produces vitamin D in the human body, rickets often occurs in parts of the world where the winter is especially long, and where smoke and fog constantly intercept the sun. *Adult r.* OSTEOMALACIA; a rickets-like disease affecting adults. *Fetal r.* achondroplasia. *Late r.* osteomalacia, that occurring in older children. *Vitamin D-resistant r.* a condition almost indistinguishable from ordinary rickets clinically but resistant to unusually large doses of vitamin D; it is often familial.

*Rickettsia* (riˈketsi.ə) a genus of microorganisms which are parasitic in lice and similar insects. The bite of the host is thus the means of transmitting the organisms, some of which are responsible for the typhus group of fevers.

**rifampicin** (riˈfampisin) an antibiotic drug used in leprosy and, with other drugs, in the treatment of tuberculosis.

**rigidity** (riˈjiditee) sustained muscle tension causing the affected part to be stiff and inflexible; may be due to stress, injury or neurological disease.

**rigor** (ˈriegor, ˈrigə) an attack of intense shivering occurring when the heat regulation is disturbed. The temperature rises rapidly and may either stay elevated or fall rapidly as profuse sweating occurs. *R. mortis* stiffening of the body which occurs soon after death.

**Ringer's solution** ('ringəz) *S. Ringer, British physiologist, 1835–1910.* A physiological solution of saline to which small amounts of calcium and potassium salts have been added. Used to replace fluids and electrolytes intravenously.

**ringworm** ('ring.wərm) tinea. A contagious skin disease, characterized by circular patches, pinkish in colour with a desquamating surface, and due to a parasitic fungus.

**risk** (risk) hazard, or chance of developing a disease or of complications during or after treatment. This may arise because of inherent problems with the treatment itself (e.g. drug side-effects) or because of the frailty of the patient. *Relative r.* the likelihood of developing a disease after a given exposure; in epidemiological terms, calculated as incidence rate of disease in an exposed group divided by incidence rate in the non-exposed group. *R. factor* a factor which, when added to others, increases the likelihood of a disease or complication (e.g. smoking and obesity are risk factors for the development of coronary artery disease).

**rite of passage** (.riet əv pasij) the cultural ceremonies and rituals that may accompany the changes in status that occur in the course of a person's life, e.g. 18th birthday parties, bar mitzvah. These ceremonies serve to draw attention to changes in status and social identity and also to the management of the social tensions that such changes may involve.

**RNA** ribonucleic acid. *RNA viruses* viruses which contain ribonucleic acid as their genetic material.

**Rocky Mountain spotted fever** ('rokee .mowntən, -tayn) a tickborne infection caused by a *Rickettsia*, common in the USA, with rash, fever, muscle pain and often an enlarged liver. The disease lasts about 3 weeks.

**rod** (rod) a straight thin structure. *Retinal r.* one of the two types of light-sensitive end-organ of the retina, which contain rhodopsin and are responsible for night vision.

**role** (rohl) a pattern of behaviour developed in response to the demands or expectations of others; the pattern of responses to the persons with whom an individual interacts in a particular situation. *R. play* an educational technique used in teaching interpersonal, communication and practice skills. Students are given roles (or parts) and asked to act these roles out. Some members of the group may be given observational tasks related to the exercise. At the end of the session there is an opportunity for the group to evaluate the exercise. This technique may also be used therapeutically, usually in the psychiatric setting. *Sick r.* the role played by people who have defined themselves as ill. Adoption of the sick role changes the behavioural expectations of others towards the sick person, who is exempted from normal social responsibilities and is not held responsible for the condition. The patient is obliged to 'want to get well' and to seek competent medical help.

**Romberg's sign** ('rombərgz) *M.H. Romberg, German physician, 1795–1853.* Inability to stand erect without swaying if the eyes are closed. A sign of tabes dorsalis.

**Rorschach test** ('rorshahk) *H. Rorschach, Swiss psychiatrist, 1884–1922.* A personality trait test that consists of ten ink-blot designs, some in colours and some in black and white.

**rosacea** (roh'zayshi.ə) *see* ACNE (ROSACEA).

**roseola** (roh'zeeələ) 1. a rose-coloured rash. 2. roseola infantum. *R. infantum* a common acute viral disease that usually occurs in children under 24 months old; it attacks suddenly but disappears in a few days, leaving no permanent marks. *Syphilitic r.* an eruption of rose-coloured spots in early secondary syphilis.

**Roth's spots** ('rohts spotz) *M. Roth, Swiss physician, 1839–1915.* Small white spots seen in the retina early in the course of subacute bacterial endocarditis.

**roughage** ('rufij) coarse vegetable fibres and cellulose that give bulk to the diet and stimulate peristalsis.

**rouleau** ('rooloh) a rounded formation found in blood, caused by red cells piling on each other.

**roundworm** ('rownd,wərm) any of various types of parasitic nematode worm, somewhat resembling the common earthworm, which sometimes invade the human intestinal tract and multiply there. Very common among them is the pinworm, or threadworm.

**Rovsing's sign** ('rohvsingz) *N.T. Rovsing, Danish surgeon, 1868–1927.* A test for acute appendicitis in which pressure in the left iliac fossa causes pain in the right iliac fossa.

**rubefacient** (,roobi'fayshənt) an agent causing redness of the skin.

**rubella** (roo'belə) German measles. An acute, notifiable virus infection of short duration, characterized by pyrexia, enlarged cervical lymph glands and a transient rash. The greatest risk from this disease is to the offspring of mothers who contract it during the early weeks of pregnancy. The child may be born with cataract or deformities, be a deaf mute or have other congenital defects.

**rumination** (,roomi'nayshən) 1. recurring thoughts. 2. voluntary regurgitation of food, which is then chewed and swallowed again. *Obsessional r.* thoughts which persistently recur against the patient's will.

**rupture** ('rupcha) 1. tearing or bursting of a part, as in rupture of an aneurysm; of the membranes during labour; or of a tubal pregnancy. 2. a term commonly applied to hernia.

**Ryle's tube** ('rieəlz) *G.A. Ryle, British physician, 1889–1950.* A thin tube with a weighted end, introduced into the stomach. It may be used for the withdrawal of gastric contents or for the administration of fluids.

# S

**Sabin vaccine** ('saybin) *A.B. Sabin, American biologist, 1906–1993.* A live oral attenuated poliovirus vaccine active against poliomyelitis.

**saccharide** ('sakə,ried) one of a series of carbohydrates, including the sugars.

**saccule** ('sakyool) a small sac, particularly the smaller of the two sacs within the membranous labyrinth of the ear.

**sacral** ('saykrəl) relating to the sacrum.

**sacroiliac** (,saykroh'ili,ak) relating to the sacrum and the ilium.

**sacrum** ('saykrəm) a triangular bone composed of five united vertebrae, situated between the lowest lumbar vertebra and the coccyx. It forms the back of the pelvis.

**sadism** ('saydizem) a form of sexual perversion in which the individual takes pleasure in inflicting mental and physical pain on others.

**SADS** *see* SEASONAL AFFECTIVE DISORDER SYNDROME.

**sagittal** ('sajit'l) arrow-shaped. *S. suture* the junction of the parietal bones.

**salbutamol** (sal'byootəmol) a sympathomimetic drug used in the treatment of bronchospasm.

**salicylate** (sə'lisə,layt) a salt of salicylic acid. *Methyl s.* the active ingredient in ointments and lotions for joint pains and sprains. *Sodium s.* the specific drug used for rheumatic fever. It reduces the pyrexia and relieves the pain but does not prevent cardiac complications.

**salicylic acid** (,sali'silik) a drug with bacteriostatic and fungicidal properties used in the treatment of skin diseases and, in concentrated form, to remove warts and corns.

**saline** ('saylien) a solution of sodium chloride and water. *Hypertonic s.* a greater than normal strength. *Hypotonic s.* a lower than normal strength. *Normal* or *physiological s.* a 0.9% solution which is isotonic with blood.

**saliva** (sə'lievə) the secretion of the salivary glands. When food is taken, saliva moistens and partially digests carbohydrates by the action of its enzyme, ptyalin (amylase).

**salivary** (sə'lievə,ree, 'salivə,ree) relating to saliva. *S. calculus* a duct. *S. fistula* an abnormal opening on the skin of the face, leading into a salivary duct or gland. *S. glands* the parotid, submaxillary and sublingual glands.

**salivation** (,sali'vayshən) 1. the process of salivating. 2. excessive salivation which may lead to soreness of mouth and gums.

**Salk vaccine** (sawlk) *J.E. Salk, American virologist, b. 1914.* The first poliomyelitis vaccine of killed viruses, given by injection. *See* VACCINE.

**Salmonella** (,salmə'nelə) any of the genus of Gram-negative, non-sporing, rod-like bacteria that are parasites of the intestinal tract of humans and animals. *S. typhi* and *S. paratyphi* are exclusively human pathogens which cause typhoid and paratyphoid fevers.

**salmonellosis** (ˌsalməneˈlohsis) infection with the genus *Salmonella*, usually caused by the ingestion of food containing salmonellae or their products. The organisms can be found in raw meats, raw poultry, eggs and dairy products; they multiply rapidly at temperatures between 7 and 46°C. Symptoms of salmonellosis include violent diarrhoea attended by abdominal cramps, nausea and vomiting, and fever. It is rarely fatal and can be prevented by adequate cooking.

**salpingectomy** (ˌsalpinˈjektəmee) excision of one or both of the uterine tubes.

**salpingitis** (ˌsalpinˈjietis) 1. inflammation of the uterine tubes. 2. inflammation of the pharyngotympanic (eustachian) tubes. *Acute s.* most often a bilateral ascending infection due to a streptococcus or a gonococcus. *Chronic s.* a less acute form that may be blood-borne.

**salpingo-oöphorectomy** (salˌpingˌgohˌoh.ofəˈrektəmee) removal of a uterine tube and its ovary.

**salpingography** (ˌsalpingˈgogrəfee) radiographic examination of the uterine tubes after injection of a radio-opaque substance to determine their patency.

**salpingostomy** (ˌsalpingˈgostəmee) the making of a surgical opening in a uterine tube near the uterus to restore patency.

**salpinx** (ˈsalpingks) a tube. Applied to the uterine or pharyngotympanic (eustachian) tubes.

**salt** (sawlt) 1. sodium chloride, common salt, used in solution as a cleansing lotion, a stimulating bath, or for infusion into the blood, etc. 2. any compound of an acid with an alkali or base. 3. a saline purgative such as Epsom salts. *S. depletion* a

loss of salt from the body due to sweating or persistent diarrhoea or vomiting. Common in hot climates when it may be prevented by the taking of salt tablets. *Smelling s's* aromatic ammonium carbonate. A restorative in fainting.

**salve** (salv, sahv) an ointment.

**sample** (sahmpˈl) 1. a selection of individuals made for research purposes from a larger population and intended to reflect that population in all significant aspects. 2. a small part of anything intended as representative of the whole, e.g. blood specimen.

**sandfly** (ˈsandˌflie) a very small fly of the genus *Phlebotomus*, common in tropical climates and the vector of most types of leishmaniasis. *S. fever* a fever transmitted by the bites of sandflies, and common in Mediterranean countries. Similar to dengue and sometimes known as three-day fever.

**sanguineous** (sangˈgwiniəs) pertaining to or containing blood.

**saphena** (səˈfeenə) one of two superficial veins that carry blood from the foot upwards.

**saphenous** (səˈfeenəs) relating to the saphena veins.

**sapphism** (ˈsafizəm) female homosexuality; lesbianism.

**sarcoid** (ˈsahkoyd) 1. tuberculoid; characterized by non-caseating epithelioid cell tubercles. 2. pertaining to or resembling sarcoidosis. 3. sarcoidosis.

**sarcoidosis** (ˌsahkoyˈdohsis) a chronic, progressive, generalized disease resembling tuberculosis which may affect any part of the body but most frequently involves the lymph nodes, liver, spleen, lungs, skin, eyes and small bones of the hands and feet.

**sarcoma** (sahˈkohmə) a malignant tumour developed from connective tissue cells and their stroma. *Kaposi's s.* one principally involving the skin, although visceral lesions may be present; it usually begins on the distal parts of the extremities, most often on the toes or feet, as reddish-blue or brownish soft nodules and tumours. It is viral in origin and is frequently seen in AIDS. *Melanotic s.* a highly malignant type, pigmented with melanin. *Round-celled s.* a highly malignant growth, composed of a primitive type of cell.

**sarcomatosis** (ˌsahkohməˈtohsis) multiple sarcomatous growths in various parts of the body.

*Sarcoptes* (sah'kopteez) a genus of mites. *S. scabiei* the cause of scabies.

**sartorius** (sah'tor.ri.əs) a long muscle of the thigh, which flexes both the thigh and the lower leg.

**satyriasis** (ˌsati'rieəsis) abnormally excessive sexual appetite in men.

**scab** (skab) the crust on a superficial wound consisting of dried blood, pus, etc.

**scabies** ('skaybeez) 'the itch'; a contagious skin disease caused by the itch mite (*Sarcoptes scabiei*), the female of which burrows beneath the skin and deposits eggs at intervals. It is intensely irritating, and the rash is aggravated by scratching. The sites affected are chiefly between the fingers and toes, the axillae and groins. Acquired by close direct contact and may spread in institutions. All members of the family should be treated.

**scald** (skawld) a burn caused by hot liquid or vapour.

**scale** (skayl) 1. a scheme or instrument by which something can be measured. A pair of scales is a balance for measuring weight. 2. compact layers of dead epithelial tissue shed from the skin. 3. to scrape deposits of tartar from the teeth.

**scalenus** (skə'leenəs) one of four muscles which move the neck to either side and raise the first and second ribs during inspiration. *S. syndrome* symptoms of pain and tenderness in the shoulder, with sensory loss and wasting of the medial aspect of the arm. It may be caused by pressure on the brachial plexus, by spasm of the scalenus anterior muscle or by a cervical rib.

**scalp** (skalp) the hairy skin that covers the cranium.

**scalpel** ('skalp'l) a small, pointed surgical knife with a convex edge to the blade.

**scan** (skan) an image produced using a moving detector or a sweeping beam of radiation, as in scintiscanning, B-mode ultrasonography, scanography or computed tomography.

**scanning** ('skaning) 1. visual examination of an area. 2. a speech disorder that may be present in cerebellar disease. The syllables are inappropriately separated from each other and are evenly stressed with rhythmically occurring pauses between them.

**scaphoid** ('skafoyd, 'skay-) boat-shaped. *S. bone* a boat-shaped bone of the wrist which articulates with the radius and with the trapezium and the trapezoid bones.

**scapula** ('skapyuhlə) the large flat triangular bone forming the shoulder-blade.

**scar** (skah) the mark left after a wound has healed with the formation of connective tissue.

**scarlet fever** ('skahlət) scarlatina; an acute, notifiable, rare, infectious disease of childhood. It is caused by a group A beta-haemolytic streptococcus. There is sore throat, high fever and a punctate rash. It is readily treated by antibiotics and the complications of nephritis and middle ear infection are less common.

**Schick test** (shik) *B. Schick, Austrian paediatrician, 1877–1967.* A skin test of susceptibility to diphtheria. A small amount of diphtheria toxin is injected intradermally.

**Schilling test** ('shiling) *R.F. Schilling, American haematologist, b. 1919.* A test used to confirm the diagnosis of pernicious anaemia by estimating the absorption of ingested radioactive vitamin $B_{12}$.

**Schistosoma** (,shistoh'sohmə) a genus of minute blood flukes, some of which are parasitic in humans. *S. haematobium* a species which infests the urinary bladder; widely found in Africa and the Middle East, especially in Egypt. *S. japonicum* and *S. mansoni* species which infest the large intestine. They are found respectively in China, Japan and the Philippines, and in Africa, the West Indies and tropical America.

**schistosomiasis** (,shistəsoh'mieəsis) a parasitic infection of the intestinal or urinary tract by *Schistosoma*. The parasite enters the skin from contaminated water, and causes diarrhoea, haematuria and anaemia. The secondary hosts are freshwater snails. Bilharzias.

**schizoid** ('skitsoyd) resembling schizophrenia *S. personality* one that is marked by introspection, self-consciousness, solitariness and a failure in affection towards others. Some schizophrenics have this personality, but only a few who are schizoid become schizophrenic.

**schizophrenia** (,skitsoh'freeni.ə) a general term encompassing a large group of mental disorders (the schizophrenic disorders) characterized by mental deterioration from a previous level of functioning and characteristic disturbances of multiple psychological processes, including delusions, loosening of associations, poverty of the content of speech, auditory hallucinations, inappropriate affect, disturbed sense of self and withdrawal from the external world. *Paranoid s.* predominance of delusions of a persecutory nature. *Simple s.* a progressive deterioration of the patient's efficiency with increasing social withdrawal. *See* HEBEPHRENIA and CATATONIA.

**Schlemm's canal** (shlemz) *F. Schlemm, German anatomist, 1795–1858.* A venous channel at the junction of the cornea and sclera for the draining of aqueous humour.

**Schönlein–Henoch purpura** or **syndrome** (,shərnlien'henok) *J.L. Schönlein, German physician, 1793–1864; E.H. Henoch, German paediatrician, 1820–1910. See* PURPURA.

**school health service** (,skool 'helth ,sərvis) the provision of medical and dental inspection and treatment, immunization and health programmes in schools.

**school nurse** a registered nurse who has undertaken further training to specialize in the health care of school-age children. Responsibilities include health promotion and education, monitoring growth and development, screening and caring for those with special educational needs.

**sciatica** (sie'atikə) pain down the back of the leg in the area supplied by the sciatic nerve. It is usually caused by pressure on the nerve roots by a protrusion of an intervertebral disc.

**scintigraphy** (sin'tigrəfee) the recording of the distribution of radioactivity in an organ after injection of a small dose of a radioactive substance specifically taken up by that organ.

**sclera** ('skliə.rə) the fibrous coat of the eyeball, the white of the eye, which covers the posterior part and in front becomes the cornea.

**scleroderma** (,skliə.roh'dərmə) a disease marked by progressive hardening of the skin in patches or diffusely, with rigidity of the underlying tissues. It is often a chronic condition. *See* RAYNAUD'S PHENOMENON.

**sclerosis** (sklə'rohsis) the hardening of any part from an overgrowth of fibrous and connective tissue, often due to chronic inflammation. *Amyotrophic lateral s.* rapid degeneration of the pyramidal (motor nerves) tract and anterior horn cells in the spinal cord. Characterized by weakness and spasm of limb muscles, with wasting of the muscle, and difficulty with talking and swallowing. *Disseminated s.* multiple sclerosis. *Mönckeberg's s.* extensive degeneration with atrophy and calcareous deposits in the middle muscle coat of arteries, especially the small ones. *Multiple s.* scattered (disseminated) patches of degeneration in the nerve sheaths in the brain and spinal cord. Characterized by relapses and remissions. Symptoms include disturbances of speech, vision, micturition and muscular weakness of a limb or limbs. *Systemic s. (scleroderma)* a generalized multisystem disease characterized by dense fibrosis of involved organs and a widespread vascular disorder. *See* RAYNAUD'S PHENOMENON.

**sclerotherapy** (ˌskliə.roh'therəpee) treatment of varicose veins and haemorrhoids by the injection of sclerosing solutions to produce fibrosis.

**sclerotic** (sklə'rotik) 1. hard; indurated; affected by sclerosis. 2. pertaining to the sclera of the eye. *S. coat* the tough membrane forming the outer covering of the eyeball, except in front of the iris, where it becomes the clear horny cornea.

**sclerotomy** (sklə'rotəmee) incision of the sclerotic coat, usually for the removal of a foreign body or for the relief of glaucoma.

**scoliosis** (ˌskohli'ohsis) lateral curvature of the spine (*see* Figure). *See* LORDOSIS and KYPHOSIS.

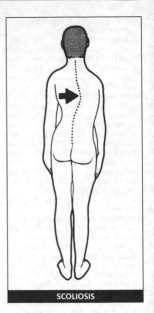

SCOLIOSIS

**scopolamine** (skoh'polə.meen) hyoscine; used in premedication as a sedative and to dry up secretions.

**scorbutic** (skaw'byootik) affected with or related to scurvy.

**scotoma** (skoh'tohmə) a blind area in the field of vision, due to some lesion of the retina. It is also found in glaucoma and in detachment of the retina.

**screening** ('skreening) 1. fluoroscopy. 2. the carrying out of a test on a large number of people to determine the proportion of them that have a particular disease.

**scrotum** ('skrohtəm) the pouch of skin and soft tissues containing the testicles.

**scurf** (skərf) dandruff.

**scurvy** ('skɜːvee) avitaminosis C. A deficiency disease caused by lack of vitamin C, which is found in raw fruits and vegetables. Clinical features include fatigue, oozing of blood from the gums and bruising. The condition rapidly improves with adequate diet.

**seasonal affective disorder syndrome** (ˌseezən'l əˌfektiv dis'awdə) abbreviated SADS. A condition in which the person notices a change in mood or feelings according to the season of the year and hence the amount of exposure to (sun)light.

**sebaceous** (si'bayshəs) fatty, or pertaining to the sebum. *S. cyst* see CYST. *S. glands* found in the skin, communicating with the hair follicles and secreting sebum.

**seborrhoea** (ˌsebə'reeə) a disease of the sebaceous glands, marked by an excessive secretion of sebum which collects on the skin in oily scales.

**sebum** ('seebəm) the fatty secretion of the sebaceous glands.

**secondary** ('sekəndree) second in order of time or importance. *S. deposits* see METASTASIS.

**secretin** (si'kreetin) the hormone originating in the duodenum which, in the presence of bile salts, is absorbed into the bloodstream and stimulates the secretion of pancreatic juice.

**secretion** (si'kreeshən) a substance formed or concentrated in a gland and passed into the alimentary tract, the blood or to the exterior. The secretions of the endocrine glands include various hormones and are important in the overall regulation of body processes.

**sedation** (si'dayshən) the allaying of irritability, the relief of pain or mental distress, and the promotion of sleep, particularly by drugs.

**sedative** ('sedətiv) a drug or agent that lessens excitement and relieves tension. Sedative drugs are used to induce sleep.

**sedentary** ('sed'nt.ə.ree) pertaining to sitting; physically inactive.

**sedimentation** (ˌsedimen'tayshən) the deposit of solid particles at the bottom of a liquid. *Erythrocyte s. rate* abbreviated ESR. *See* ERYTHROCYTE.

**segregation** (ˌsegri'gayshən) the separation during meiosis of allelic genes as the chromosomes migrate towards opposite poles of the cell.

**self** (self) 1. a term used to denote an animal's own antigenic constituents, in contrast to 'not-self', denoting foreign antigenic constituents. 2. the complete being of an individual, comprising both physical and psychological characteristics, and including both conscious and unconscious components.

**self-actualization** (ˌselfˌaktyooəlie-'zayshən) a level of psychological development in which innate potential is realized to the full, allowing transcendence of the environment.

**self-care** (ˌself'kair) the personal care carried out by the patient, e.g. bathing, personal grooming, eating and toilet hygiene. May be with assistance or instruction from a health-care worker. The aim of rehabilitative care is to maximize self-care and personal independence.

**self-examination of breast** (egˌzami'nayshən) *see* BREAST.

**self-examination of testes** *see* TESTICULAR SELF- EXAMINATION.

**self-governing trusts** (ˌselfˌguvəning 'trustz) hospitals, or other establishments or facilities which assume responsibility for their own ownership and management by 'opting out' of direct National Health Service (NHS) control. Trust status is approved by the Secretary of State and each trust has a board of executive and non-executive directors and a chair who is approved by the Secretary of State.

**self-image** (ˌselfˈimij) an individual's concept of their own personality and abilities based on their own ideas and perceptions.

**sella turcica** (ˌselə ˈtɔrsikə) a depression in the sphenoid body which protects the pituitary gland.

**semen** (ˈseemən) the secretion of the testicles containing spermatozoa, which is ejaculated from the penis during sexual intercourse. Seminal fluid.

**semicircular** (ˌsemiˈsərkyuhlə) formed in a half-circle. *S. canals* part of the labyrinth of the internal ear, consisting of three canals in the form of arches which contain fluid and are connected with the cerebellum by their nerve supply. Impressions of change of position of the body are registered in these canals by oscillation of the fluid, and are conveyed by the nerves to the cerebellum.

**semicomatose** (ˌsemiˈkohmətohs, -tohz) in a condition of unconsciousness from which the patient can be roused.

**semilunar** (ˌsemiˈloonə) shaped like a half-moon. *S. cartilages* two crescent-shaped cartilages in the knee joint. *S. valve see* VALVE.

**seminoma** (ˌsemiˈnohmə) a malignant tumour of the testis that is highly radiosensitive.

**semipermeable** (ˌsemiˈpərmi.əbˈl) of a membrane, permitting the passage of some molecules and hindering that of others.

**semiprone** (ˌsemiˈprohn) partly prone. Applied to a position in which the patient is lying face down but the knees are turned to one side.

**senescence** (səˈnesˈns) the process of growing old.

**Sengstaken–Blakemore tube** (ˌsengztaykenˈblaykmor) *R.W. Sengstaken, American neurosurgeon,*

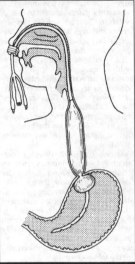

**SENGSTAKEN–BLAKEMORE TUBE**

*b. 1923; A.H. Blakemore, American surgeon, 1879–1970.* A compression tube used in the treatment of bleeding oesophageal varices (*see* Figure).

**senile** (ˈseeniel) related to the involutional changes associated with old age. *S. dementia* deterioration of mental activity in the elderly, associated with an impaired blood supply to the brain.

**senna** (ˈsenə) a laxative derived from the cassia plant. Proprietary standardized preparations are available as tablets or granules.

**sensation** (senˈsayshən) a feeling resulting from impulses sent to the brain by the sensory nerves.

**sense** (sens) the faculty by which conditions and properties of things are perceived, e.g. hunger or pain. *S. organ* one that receives a sensory stimulus: for instance, the eyes and ears. *Special s.* any one of the faculties of sight, hearing, touch, smell, taste and muscle sense, through which the consciousness receives impressions from the environment.

**sensible** ('sensib'l) 1. capable of being perceived. 2. sensitive. *S. perspiration* that obvious on the skin as moisture.

**sensitization** (,sensitie'zayshən) 1. the process of rendering susceptible. 2. an increase in the body's response to a certain stimulus, as in the development of an allergy. *Protein s.* the condition occurring in an individual when a foreign protein is absorbed into the body, e.g. shell-fish causing urticaria when eaten. *See* DESENSITIZATION.

**sensory** ('sensə.ree) relating to sensation. *S. cortex* that part of the cerebral cortex to which information is relayed by the sensory nerves. *S. deprivation* the effecting of a major reduction of sensory information received by the body. This is damaging to the person's ability to function normally, which is dependent upon constant stimulation. *S. nerve* an afferent nerve conveying impressions from the peripheral nerve endings to the brain or spinal cord.

**sentiment** ('sentimənt) an emotion directed towards some object or person. Sentiments are acquired and profoundly influence a person's actions.

**sepsis** ('sepsis) an infection of the body by pus-forming bacteria. *Focal s.* a local focus of infection which produces general symptoms. *Oral s.* infection of the mouth which causes general ill-health by absorption of toxins. *Puerperal s.* infection of the uterus occurring after labour.

**septicaemia** (,septi'seemi.ə) the presence in the blood of large numbers of bacteria and their toxins. The symptoms are: a rapid rise of temperature, which is later intermittent, rigors, sweating, and all the signs of acute fever.

**septum** ('septəm) a division or partition. *Atrial s., atrioventricular s.* along with ventricular septum, the partitions dividing the various cavities of the heart. *Nasal s.* the structure made of bone and cartilage which separates the nasal cavities. *Ventricular s. see* ATRIAL SEPTUM above.

**sequela** (si'kweelə) a morbid condition occurring after a disease and resulting from it.

**sequestrum** (si'kwestrəm) a piece of dead bone. Inflammation in bone leads to thrombosis of blood vessels, resulting in necrosis of the affected part, which separates from the living structure.

**serological** (,siə.rə'lojik'l) relating to serum. *S. tests* those that are dependent on the formation of antibodies in the blood as a response to specific organisms or proteins.

**serology** (si'roləjee) the scientific study of serum.

**serosa** (si'rohsə) a serous membrane. It consists of two layers: the visceral, in close contact with the organ, and the parietal, lining the cavity.

**serotonin** (,siə.roh'tohnin, ,serə-) an amine present in blood platelets, the intestine and the central nervous system, which acts as a vasoconstrictor. It is derived from the amino acid tryptophan and is inactivated by monoamine oxidase.

**serous** ('siə.rəs) related to serum. *S. effusion* an effusion of serous exudate.

**serum** ('siə.rəm) the clear, fluid residue of blood, from which the corpuscles and fibrin have been removed. *S. hepatitis* jaundice caused by hepatitis B virus, usually after a blood transfusion or an inoculation with contaminated material. *S. sickness* an allergic reaction usually 8–10 days after a serum injection. It may be manifest by an irritating urticaria, pyrexia and painful joints. It readily responds to adrenaline and antihistaminic drugs. *See* ANAPHYLAXIS.

**sex** (seks) 1. either of the two divisions of organic organisms described respectively as male and female. 2. to discover the sex of an organism. *S. chromosome* a chromosome that determines sex. Women have two X chromosomes and men have one X chromosome and one Y chromosome. *S. hormone* a steroid hormone produced by the ovaries or the testes and controlling sexual development. *S.-limited* pertaining to a characteristic found in only one sex. *S.-linked* pertaining to a characteristic that is transmitted by genes that are located on the sex chromosomes, e.g. haemophilia.

**sexual** ('seksyooəl) pertaining to sex. *S. development* the biological and psychosocial changes that lead to sexual maturity. *S. deviation* aberrant sexual activity; expression of the sexual instinct in practices which are socially prohibited or unacceptable, or biologically undesirable. *S. intercourse* coitus.

**sexuality** (ˌseksyoo'alitee) 1. the characteristic quality of the male and female reproductive elements. 2. the constitution of an individual in relation to sexual attitudes and behaviour.

**sexually transmitted infection** ('seksyooəlee trans'mitid) abbreviated STI. An infection transmitted either by means of sexual intercourse between heterosexual or homosexual individuals, or by intimate contact with the genitals, mouth and rectum. STIs include

syphilis, gonorrhoea, human immunodeficiency virus (HIV) infection, acquired immunodeficiency syndrome (AIDS), chlamydial infection, genital herpes, non-specific urethritis, trichomoniasis, genital lice, scabies, genital warts, hepatitis B infection and yaws. 'Sexually transmitted infection' is now the preferred term for what was formerly known as sexually transmitted disease (STD).

**SGOT** serum glutamic–oxalacetic transaminase, an enzyme excreted by damaged heart muscle. A raised serum level occurs in myocardial infarction.

**SGPT** serum glutamic–pyruvic transaminase, an enzyme excreted by the parenchymal cells of the liver. There is a raised blood level in infectious hepatitis.

**shaken baby syndrome** ('shaykən) the presence of unexplained fractures in the long bones, together with evidence of a subdural haematoma (bleeding under the membrane surrounding the brain) in a baby. These injuries, a result of child abuse, are caused by the violent shaking of the baby which produces a whiplash effect and a rotational movement of the head resulting in vomiting, convulsions, irritability, coma and death.

**shared care** (shaird) in obstetrics, a term used to describe antenatal care carried out by an obstetrician and a general practitioner. The latter usually carries out the care from the time of the booking until some time in the third trimester.

**sheath** (sheeth) 1. an enveloping tubular structure or part. 2. a condom, worn on the erect penis during sexual intercourse to trap seminal fluid, preventing the transmission of human immunodeficiency virus (HIV) and other viruses and also reducing the risk of pregnancy.

**shiatsu** (shee'atsoo) a form of manipulation in which the practitioner uses the thumbs, fingers and palms of the hands, knees, forearms, elbows and feet to apply pressure to the client's body in order to promote and maintain health.

*Shigella* (shi'gelə) a genus of Gramnegative rod-like bacteria. Some species cause bacillary dysentery. *S. flexneri* and *S. shigae* are common in Asia, *S. dysenteriae* in the USA and *S. sonnei* in Western Europe.

**shin** (shin) the bony front of the leg below the knee. The tibia.

**shingles** (shing.g'lz) herpes zoster.

**Shirodkar's suture** (shi'rodkəz) *Shirodkar, Indian obstetrician.* A 'purse-string' suture that is placed round an incompetent cervix during pregnancy to prevent abortion. It is removed at the 38th week.

**shock** (shok) a condition produced by severe illness or trauma in which there is a sudden fall in blood pressure. This leads to lack of oxygen in the tissues and greater permeability of the capillary walls, so increasing the degree of shock by greater loss of fluid. The patient has a cold, moist skin, a feeble pulse and a low blood pressure, and is distressed, thirsty and restless. *Cardiogenic s.* shock as a result of an acute heart condition such as myocardial infarction. *Hypovolaemic s.* shock resulting from a reduction in the volume of blood in the circulation after haemorrhage or severe burns. *Neurogenic s.* shock due to nervous or emotional factors. *Shell s.* a psychoneurotic condition caused by the stresses of warfare.

**short-sightedness** (shawt'sietidnəs) myopia.

**shoulder** ('shohldə) the junction of the clavicle and the scapula where the arm joins the body.

**show** (shoh) the blood-stained discharge that occurs at the onset of labour.

**shunt** (shunt) a diversion, particularly of blood, due to a congenital defect, disease or surgery.

**sialography** (,sieə'logrəfee) radiographic examination of the salivary ducts after the introduction of a radio-opaque contrast medium.

**sialolith** ('sieəloh,lith) a salivary calculus.

**sibling** ('sibling) one of a family of children having the same parents. Applied in psychology to one of two or more children of the same parent or substitute parent figure. *S. rivalry* jealousy, compounded of love and hate of one child for its sibling.

**sickle-cell anaemia** ('sik'l) an inherited blood disease. *See* ANAEMIA.

**siderosis** (,sidə'rohsis) 1. chronic inflammation of the lung due to inhalation of particles of iron. 2. excess iron in the blood. 3. the deposit of iron in the tissues.

**sigmoid** ('sigmoyd) shaped like the Greek letter sigma, Σ. *S. colon* or *flexure* that part of the colon in the left iliac fossa just above the rectum.

**sigmoidoscope** (sig'moydə,skohp) an instrument by which the interior of the rectum and sigmoid colon can be seen.

**sign** (sien) 1. any objective evidence of disease or dysfunction. 2. an observable physical phenomenon so frequently associated with a given condition as to be considered indicative of its presence. *S. language* hand and body language used by totally deaf people to communicate with others. *Vital s's* the signs of life, namely pulse, respiration and temperature.

**silicosis** (,sili'kohsis) fibrosis of the lung due to the inhalation of silica dust particles. It occurs in miners, stone masons and quarry workers.

**Sims' position** (simz) *J.M. Sims, American gynaecologist, 1813–1883.* A semiprone position. *See* POSITION.

**sinoatrial** (ˌsienoh'aytri.əl) situated between the sinus venosus and the atrium of the heart. **S. node** the pacemaker of the heart. *See* NODE.

**sinus** ('sienəs) 1. a cavity in a bone. 2. a venous channel, especially within the cranium. 3. an unhealed passage leading from an abscess or internal lesion to the surface. *Air s.* a cavity in a bone containing air. *Cavernous s.* a venous sinus of the dura mater which lies along the body of the sphenoid bone. *Coronary s.* the vein that returns the blood from the heart muscle into the right atrium. *Ethmoidal s.* air spaces in the ethmoid bone. *Frontal s.* air spaces in the frontal bone. **S. arrhythmia** *see* ARRHYTHMIA. **S. thrombosis** clotting of blood in a cranial venous channel. In the lateral sinus it is a complication of mastoiditis. *Sphenoidal s.* air spaces in the sphenoid bone.

**sinusitis** (ˌsienə'sietis) inflammation of the lining of a sinus, especially applied to the bony cavities of the face.

**skeleton** ('skelitən) the bony framework of the body, supporting and protecting the organs and soft tissues.

**skill mix** ('skil ˌmiks) the ratio of staff employed in an area of healthcare activity, whether qualified, trained or untrained, representing the availability of skills possessed by these staff.

**skin** (skin) the outer protective covering of the body. It consists of an outer layer, the epidermis or cuticle, and an inner layer, the dermis or corium, which is known as 'true skin'. **S. grafting** transplantation of pieces of healthy skin to an area where loss of surface tissue has occurred. **S. patch** a drug-impregnated adhesive patch which is applied to the skin. The drug is slowly absorbed, allowing its level in the blood to be maintained over a given period of time. **S. test** application of a substance to the skin, or intradermal injection of a substance, to permit observation of the body's reaction to it.

**skull** (skul) the bony framework of the head, consisting of the cranium and facial bones.

**sleep** (sleep) a period of rest for the body and mind, during which volition and consciousness are in partial or complete abeyance and the bodily functions partially suspended. It occurs in a 24-h biological rhythm. Sleep occurs in cycles which have two distinct phases. Each phase lasts approximately 60–90 min: orthodox or non-rapid eye movement sleep (NREM), and paradoxical or rapid eye movement sleep (REM). Sleeping requirements vary, with each individual averaging between 4–10 hours in a 24-hour period. The purpose of sleep is unknown but sleep deprivation is harmful.

**sleeping sickness** ('sleeping ˌsiknəs) trypanosomiasis. A tropical fever occurring in parts of Africa, caused by a protozoal parasite (*Trypanosoma*) which is conveyed by the tsetse fly.

**slipped disc** (slipt) a prolapsed intervertebral disc which causes pressure on the spinal nerves. It may be very painful.

**slit lamp** ('slit ˌlamp) a special light source so arranged with a microscope that examination of the interior of the eye can be carried out at the level of each layer.

**slough** (sluf) dead tissue caused by injury or inflammation. It separates from the healthy tissue and is ultimately washed away by exuded serum, leaving a granulating surface.

**smallpox** ('smawl ˌpoks) variola. Eradicated from the world in 1980.

Smallpox vaccination is no longer required for travellers to any part of the world.

**smear** (smiə) a specimen for microscopic examination that has been prepared by spreading a thin film of the material across a glass slide.

**smegma** ('smegmə) the secretion of sebaceous glands of the clitoris and prepuce.

**smell** (smel) one of the five senses. Air-borne particles are deposited and dissolved in the mucous membrane lining the nose, stimulating the endings of the olfactory nerve. The nose is able to distinguish a wide range of odours.

**Smith-Petersen nail** (,smith'peetəsən) M.N. Smith-Petersen, American surgeon, 1886–1953. A metal nail used to fix the fragments of bone in intracapsular fracture of the head of the femur (see Figure).

**smoking** ('smohking) the act of drawing into the mouth and puffing out the smoke of tobacco contained in a cigarette, cigar or pipe. A close relationship between smoking and lung cancer, heart disease and bronchitis and emphysema has definitely been established. Smoking is also harmful in pregnancy because the inhaled carbon monoxide reduces oxygen transportation in the body and the nicotine causes vasoconstriction of the arterioles. The result is a diminished supply of food and oxygen to the fetus, leading to fetal growth retardation.

**snake** (snayk) a limbless reptile; a serpent. The bites of many snakes are poisonous to humans. *S. venom antitoxin* antivenin. A serum made from animals, usually horses, which have been immunized against the venom of a specific type of snake.

**Snellen's test letters** ('snelən test ,letəz) H. Snellen, Dutch ophthalmologist, 1834–1908. Square-shaped let-

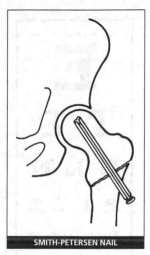

**SMITH-PETERSEN NAIL**

ters on a chart, used for sight testing (see Figure on p. 366).

**snow** (snoh) frozen water vapour. *Carbon dioxide s.* solid $CO_2$, which is used as a refrigerant; 'dry ice'. *S. blindness* photophobia due to the glare of snow.

**snuffles** ('snuflz) a chronic discharge from the nose, occurring in children, as a result of infection of the nasal mucous membrane.

**social class** ('sohshəl ,klahs) a category arising from the division of society into economic or occupational groupings. The most widely used grouping of social class or occupational scale in the UK is the Registrar General's Classification designed originally for use in the 1911 Census but extensively modified for use in later censuses (see Table on p. 367). Occupations are now coded to be comparable with

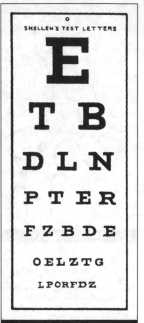

SNELLEN'S TEST LETTERS

the International Standard Classification of Occupations.

**social worker** ('wərkə) a professional trained in the treatment of individual and social problems of patients and their families. *See also* MEDICAL (SOCIAL WORKER).

**socialization** (,sohshəlie'zayshən) the process by which society integrates the individual, and the individual learns to behave in socially acceptable ways.

**sociology** (,sohsi'oləjee) the scientific study of the development of human social relationships and organization, i.e. interpersonal and intergroup behaviour as distinct from the behaviour of an individual.

**sociopath** ('sohsioh,path) a person with an antisocial personality; a psychopath.

**sodium** ('sohdi.əm) *symbol* Na. A metallic alkaline element widely distributed in nature, and forming an important constituent of animal tissue. *S. aminosalicylate* an anti-tuberculous drug used in conjunction with streptomycin and isoniazid. *S. bicarbonate* an antacid widely used to treat digestive disorders, especially flatulence. Repeated use can cause alkalosis. *S. chloride* common salt. Its presence in the diet is necessary to health. *S. citrate* compound used to prevent clotting of blood during blood transfusions. *S. cromoglycate* a drug used as an inhalant in the treatment of asthma. *S. fluoride* a salt used in the fluoridation of water and also in toothpastes to prevent the formation of carries. *S. hydroxide* caustic soda. A powerful corrosive drug used to destroy warts. It can cause severe chemical burns. *S. hypochlorite* a compound with germicidal properties used in solution to disinfect utensils, and diluted as a topical antibacterial agent. *S. phosphate* a purgative. *S. salicylate* an antipyretic drug used in the treatment of rheumatic fever. *S. sulphate* a purgative; also used in 25% solution as a wound dressing. *S. valproate* a drug used in the treatment of epilepsy.

**solar plexus** ('sohlə) coeliac plexus. A network of sympathetic nerve ganglia in the abdomen; the nerve supply to abdominal organs below the diaphragm.

**solution** (sə'looshən) a liquid in which one or more substances have been dissolved.

| REGISTRAR GENERAL'S CLASSIFICATION OF SOCIAL CLASSES | | | | |
|---|---|---|---|---|
| | | | % of economically active and retired | |
| Social class | Description | Examples | Males | Females |
| I | Professional | Accountant Doctor Lawyer | 5 | 1 |
| II | Intermediate | Manager School teacher Nurse | 22 | 21 |
| IIIN | Skilled non-manual | Clerical worker Secretary Shop assistant | 12 | 39 |
| IIIM | Skilled manual | Bus driver Coal-face worker Carpenter | 36 | 9 |
| IV | Semi-skilled manual | Agricultural worker Bus conductor Postman | 18 | 22 |
| V | Unskilled manual | Labourer Cleaner Dock worker | 7 | 7 |

Reproduced with permission from HarperCollins Publishers Ltd from Reid: Tables 2.6 and 3.1., I. (1989) Social class differences in Britain, 3rd edn. London, Fontana

**solvent** ('solvənt) a liquid that dissolves or has power to dissolve. *S. abuse* see ABUSE.

**soma** ('sohmə) 1. the body as distinct from the mind. 2. the body tissue as distinct from the germ cells.

**somatic** (soh'matik) 1. relating to the body as opposed to the mind. 2. relating to the body wall as distinct from the viscera.

**somnambulism** (som'nambyuh‚lizəm) walking and carrying out other complex activities during a state of sleep.

**Somogyi effect** (soh'mohge i‚fekt) *M. Somogyi, American biochemist,* *1883–1971.* A rebound phenomenon occurring in diabetes mellitus; overtreatment with insulin induces hypoglycaemia, resulting in rebound hyperglycaemia and ketosis.

**Sonne dysentery** ('soni) *C.O. Sonne, Danish bacteriologist, 1882–1948.* Bacillary dysentery which is common in the UK. The symptoms are diarrhoea, vomiting and abdominal pain. The causative agent is *Shigella sonnei.*

**sorbitol** ('sawbi‚tol) a sweetening agent which is converted into sugar in the body although it is slowly absorbed from the intestine. It is used in some diabetic foods and in intravenous feeding.

**sordes** ('sawdeez) brown crusts which form on the teeth and lips of unconscious patients, or those suffering from acute or prolonged fevers.

**sore** (sor) a general term for any ulcer or open skin lesion. *Cold s.* herpes simplex. *Hard s.* a syphilitic chancre. *Pressure s.* a sore caused by pressure on the bed (decubitus ulcer) or a splint. *Soft s.* a chancroid ulcer. *S. throat* inflammation of the larynx or pharynx, including tonsillitis.

**souffle** ('soof'l) a blowing sound heard on auscultation. *Uterine s.* a sound due to the blood passing through the uterine arteries of the mother, particularly over the placental site. It is synchronous with the maternal pulse.

**sound** (sownd) an instrument shaped like a probe for exploring cavities, detecting the presence of foreign bodies or dilating a stricture.

**spasm** ('spazəm) a sudden involuntary muscle contraction. *Carpopedal s.* spasm of the hands and feet. A sign of tetany. *Clonic s.* alternate muscle rigidity and relaxation. *Habit s.* a tic. *Nictitating s.* spasmodic twitching of the eyelid. *Tetanic s.* violent muscle spasm, including opisthotonos. *Tonic s.* a sustained muscle rigidity.

**spastic** ('spastik) 1. caused by spasm; convulsive. 2. one affected by spasticity; often applied to persons suffering from congenital paralysis due to some cerebral lesion or impairment. *S. colon* irritable bowel syndrome. *S. paralysis* paralysis associated with lesions of the upper motor neurone, as in cerebral vascular accidents, and characterized by increased muscle tone and rigidity.

**spasticity** (spa'stisitee) marked rigidity of muscles.

**spatial** ('spayshəl) pertaining to space.

**spatula** ('spatyuhlə) 1. a flexible, blunt blade used for spreading ointment. 2. a rigid blade-shaped instrument for depressing the tongue in throat examination, etc.

**specific** (spə'sifik) 1. relating to a species. 2. a remedy that has a distinct curative influence on a particular disease, e.g. quinine in malaria. 3. related to a unit mass of a substance. *S. gravity* the density of fluid compared with that of an equal volume of water.

**specimen** ('spesimən) a sample or part taken to show the nature of the whole, e.g. for chemical testing or microscopic survey.

**spectacles** ('spektək'lz) a frame containing lenses worn in front of the eyes to correct errors of vision or to protect from glare.

**spectrometer** (spek'tromitə) an instrument for measuring the strength and wavelengths of visible or invisible electromagnetic radiations.

**spectroscope** ('spektrə‚skohp) an instrument used for analysing the spectra of light and other radiations.

**speech** (speech) the act of communicating by sounds by means of a linguistic code. *Clipped s.* speech in which the words are cut short. *Deaf s.* the characteristic utterance of people with severe hearing loss. *Explosive s.* loud, sudden utterances; a sign of mental disorder. *Incoherent s.* disconnected utterances made when the sequence of thought is disturbed, as in delirium. *Oesophageal s.* speech produced after laryngectomy by swallowing air and using it to vibrate within the oesophagus against the closed cricopharyngeal sphincter. *Scanning s.* speech in which the syllables are inappropriately separated from each other and are evenly stressed.

Characteristic of cerebellar damage. **S. therapist** a professional trained to identify, assess and rehabilitate persons with speech or language disorders and feeding difficulties. **Staccato s.** speech in which each syllable is separately pronounced. Characteristic of multiple sclerosis.

**sperm** ('spərm) 1. a spermatozoon. 2. the semen. **S. count** a method of determining the concentration of spermatozoa in a semen sample. **S. donation** seminal fluid provided by donors for the fertilization of women whose partners are sterile.

**spermatocele** ('spərmətoh,seel) a cystic swelling in the epididymis, containing semen.

**spermatozoon** (,spərmətoh'zoh.on) a mature male germ cell consisting of a flat-shaped head, a short middle part and a long tail. There are 300–500 billion sperms in a normal ejaculate.

**spermicide** ('spərmi,sied) any agent that will destroy spermatozoa.

**sphenoid** ('sfeenoyd) wedge-shaped. **S. bone** the central part of the base of the skull.

**spherocytosis** (,sfiə,rohsie'tohsis) the presence in the blood of erythrocytes that are more nearly spherical than biconcave. Characteristic of acholuric jaundice. It may also be hereditary.

**sphincter** ('sfingktə) a ring-shaped muscle, contraction of which closes a natural orifice.

**sphincterectomy** (,sfingktə'rektə-mee) 1. the excision of a sphincter. 2. in ophthalmology, an operation to free the sphincter of the iris when it has become attached to the back of the cornea.

**sphygmomanometer** (,sfigmohmə-'nomitə) an instrument for measuring the arterial blood pressure.

**spica** ('spiekə) a bandage applied to a joint in a series of 'figures of eight'.

**spigot** ('spigət) a small peg or bung to close the opening of a tube.

**spina** ('spienə) spine; a slender, thorn-like projection that occurs on many bones. **S. bifida** a congenital defect of non-union of one or more vertebral arches, allowing protrusion of the meninges and possibly their contents. *See* MENINGOCELE and MENINGOMYELOCELE.

**spinal** ('spien'l) relating to the spine. **S. anaesthesia** *see* ANAESTHESIA. **S. canal** the hollow in the spine formed by the neural arches of the vertebrae. It contains the spinal cord, meninges and cerebrospinal fluid. **S. caries** disease of the vertebrae, usually tuberculous. *See* POTT'S DISEASE. **S. column** the backbone; the vertebral column. **S. cord** *see* CORD. **S. curvature** abnormal curving of the spine. If associated with caries, it is known as Pott's disease. *See* KYPHOSIS, LORDOSIS and SCOLIOSIS. **S. jacket** a support for the spine, made of plaster of Paris or other material, used to give rest after injury to or operation on the spine. **S. nerves** the 31 pairs of nerves which leave the spinal cord at regular intervals throughout its length. They pass out in pairs, one on either side between each of the vertebrae, and are distributed to the periphery. **S. puncture** lumbar or cisternal puncture.

**spine** (spien) 1. the backbone or vertebral column, consisting of 33 vertebrae, separated by fibrocartilaginous discs, and enclosing the spinal cord. 2. a sharp process of bone.

**Spinhaler** ('spinhaylə) a nebulizing device which delivers a preset dose of the contained drug.

**spinnbarkeit** ('spinbah,kiet) [Ger.] a thread of mucus secreted by the cervix uteri. Used to determine ovulation as this usually coincides with the time at which the mucus can be drawn out on a glass slide to its maximum length.

**spirochaete** ('spieroh,keet) one of a group of microorganisms in the form of a spiral, some of which are found in impure fresh or salt water. The group includes the species *Treponema, Borrelia* and *Leptospira.*

**spirograph** ('spieroh,grahf, -,graf) an instrument for registering respiratory movements.

**spirometer** (spie'romitə, spi-) an instrument for measuring the air capacity of the lungs.

**spironolactone** (,spierənoh'laktohn) a diuretic drug used when there is excess secretion of aldosterone. It promotes the excretion of sodium and water but the retention of potassium.

**Spitz–Holter valve** (,spits'holtə) *Spitz, American engineer; J.W. Holter, American engineer.* A device used in the treatment of hydrocephalus to drain the cerebrospinal fluid from the ventricles into the superior vena cava or the right atrium.

**splanchnic** ('splangknik) pertaining to the viscera. *S. nerves* sympathetic nerves to the viscera.

**spleen** (spleen) a large, vascular, gland-like but ductless organ, coloured a reddish purple and situated in the left hypochondrium under the border of the stomach. It manufactures lymphocytes and breaks down red blood corpuscles.

**splenectomy** (spli'nektəmee) excision of the spleen.

**splenomegaly** (,spleenoh'megəlee) enlargement of the spleen.

**splenorenal** (,spleenoh'reen'l) relating to the spleen and the kidney. *S. anastomosis* an operation carried out to treat portal hypertension. The spleen is excised and the splenic vein is inserted into the renal vein.

**splint** (splint) an appliance used to support or immobilize a part while healing takes place or to correct or prevent deformity.

**spondylitis** (,spondi'lietis) inflammation of the vertebrae. *Ankylosing s.* a rheumatic disease, chiefly of young males, in which there is abnormal ossification with pain and rigidity of the intervertebral, hip and sacroiliac joints.

**spondylolisthesis** (,spondilohlis-'theesis) a sliding forwards or displacement of one vertebra over another, usually the fifth lumbar over the sacrum, causing symptoms such as low back pain, as a result of pressure on the nerve roots.

**spondylosis** (,spondi'lohsis) ankylosis of the vertebral joints, usually caused by a degenerative disease of the intervertebral discs, such as osteoarthritis.

**spongioblastoma** (,spunjiohbla'stohmə) a rapidly growing brain tumour that is highly malignant. A glioma.

**spontaneous** (spon'tayni.əs) occurring without apparent cause. Applied to certain types of fracture and to recovery from a disease without any specific treatment.

**sporadic** (spə'radik) pertaining to isolated cases of a disease that occurs in various and scattered places (compare ENDEMIC and EPIDEMIC).

**spore** (spor) 1. a reproductive stage of some of the lowest forms of vegetable life, e.g. moulds. 2. a protective state which some bacteria are able to assume in adverse conditions, such as lack of moisture, food or heat. In this form the organism can remain alive, but inert, for years.

**spotted fever** ('spotid) a febrile disease characterized by a skin eruption, such as Rocky Mountain spotted fever, boutonneuse fever, and other infections due to tick-borne rickettsiae.

**sprain** (sprayn) wrenching of a joint, producing laceration of the capsule or stretching of the ligaments, with consequent swelling, which is due to effusion of fluid into the affected part.

**sprue** (sproo) a disease of malabsorption in the intestine, which may be tropical or non-tropical in form. There is steatorrhoea, diarrhoea, glossitis and anaemia.

**sputum** ('spyootəm) material expelled from the air passages through the mouth. It consists chiefly of mucus and saliva; in diseased conditions of the air passages it may be purulent, blood-stained and frothy and may contain many bacteria. It must always be regarded as highly infectious. *Rusty s.* that in which altered blood permeates the mucus. Characteristic of acute lobar pneumonia.

**squamous** ('skwayməs) scaly. *S. bone* the thin part of the temporal bone which articulates with the parietal and frontal bones. *S. cell carcinoma* a malignancy of the squamous cells of the bronchus. *S. epithelium* epithelium composed of flat and scale-like cells.

**squint** (skwint) *see* STRABISMUS.

**staging** ('stayjing) 1. the determination of distinct phases or periods in the course of a disease. 2. the classification of neoplasms according to the extent of the tumour. *TNM s.* staging of tumours according to three basic components: primary tumour (T), regional nodes (N) and metastasis (M). Subscripts are used to denote size and degree of involvement; for example, 0 indicates undetectable, and 1, 2, 3 and 4 a progressive increase in size or involvement.

**stammering** ('stamə.ring) stuttering; a speech disorder in which the utterance is broken by hesitation and repetition or prolongation of words and syllables.

**standard deviation** ('standəd) a measure of the dispersion of a random variable: the square root of the average squared deviation from the mean. For data that have a normal distribution, about 68% of the data points fall within one standard deviation from the mean and about 95% fall within two standard deviations.

**standard precautions** (pri'kawshənz) the current model of best practice in infection control, a synthesis of UNIVERSAL PRECAUTIONS and BODY SUBSTANCE ISOLATION (published 1999). Standard precautions are designed to reduce the risk of transmission of blood-borne and other pathogens in hospital, from both recognized and unrecognized sources of infection, and apply to all patients all the time. Their implementation requires that nurses and other health-care professionals take appropriate measures, e.g. wear gloves, to avoid contact with (a) blood; (b) all body fluids, secretions and excretions except sweat, regardless of whether or not they contain visible blood; (c) non-intact skin; and (4) mucous membranes. Standard precautions are used in association with new concepts of TRANSMISSION-BASED PRECAUTIONS. *See also* INFECTION CONTROL and Appendices.

**standards** statements of the levels of service or care related to specific topics which staff agree to provide. Often accompanied by a description of the structure (staff, equipment, etc.) and process needed to attain specified observable outcomes.

**stapedectomy** (.staypi'dektəmee) removal of the stapes and insertion of a vein graft or other device to re-establish conduction of sound waves in otosclerosis.

**stapediolysis** (stə.peedi'olisis) an operation in which the footpiece of the stapes is mobilized to aid conduction in deafness from oto-sclerosis.

**stapes** ('staypeez) the stirrup-shaped bone of the middle ear.

**Staphylococcus** (,stafiloh'kokəs) a genus of Gram-positive non-mobile bacteria which, under the micro-scope, appear grouped together in small masses like bunches of grapes. They are normally present on the skin and mucous mem-branes. *S. pyogenes* (or *S. aureus*) is a common cause of boils, carbuncles and abscesses.

**staphyloma** (,stafi'lohmə) a protru-sion of the cornea or the sclerotic coat of the eyeball as the result of inflammation or a wound.

**stasis** ('staysis) the stagnation or stoppage of the flow of a fluid. *Intestinal s.* sluggish movement of faeces through the bowel, owing to partial obstruction or to impair-ment of the action of the intestinal muscles. *Venous s.* congestion of blood in the veins.

**statistical process control** (stə'tis-tik'l) abbreviated SPC. The use of statistical concepts which place the emphasis on the continuous moni-toring of a process rather than the reliance on a single outcome as the sole measure for quality assurance in the delivery of a service.

**statistical significance** (sig'nifi-kəns) in research, a conclusion that the results achieved have little probability of occurring by chance alone. If the result is statistically significant, e.g. below 1 in 20 or the 0.05 level, then something other than chance produced the result.

**statistics** (stə'tistiks) 1. numerical facts pertaining to a particular sub-ject or body of objects. 2. the science dealing with the collection, tabu-lation and analysis of numerical facts.

**status** ('staytəs) condition. *S. asth-maticus* a severe and prolonged attack of asthma. *S. epilepticus* a

condition in which there is rapid succession of epileptic fits. *S. lym-phaticus* a condition in which all lymphatic tissues are hypertro-phied, especially the thymus gland.

**statutory bodies** ('statyuhtree, -təri) the statutory control of the practice of nurses, midwives and health visitors is the responsibility of the United Kingdom Central Council for Nursing, Midwifery and Health Visiting (UKCC) and four National Boards for Nursing, Midwifery and Health Visiting: the National Board for Nursing, Midwifery and Health Visiting for Scotland, the National Board for Nursing, Midwifery and Health Visiting for Northern Ireland, the Welsh National Board for Nursing, Midwifery and Health Visiting, and the English National Board for Nursing, Midwifery and Health Visiting. These five bodies are called statutory bodies because they are established in accordance with the Nurses, Midwives and Health Visitors Act 1979.

**STD** sexually transmitted disease.

**steapsin** (sti'apsin) the fat-splitting enzyme (LIPASE) of the pancreatic juice.

**steatoma** (stiə'tohmə) 1. a seba-ceous cyst. 2. a lipoma; a fatty tumour.

**steatorrhoea** (,stiətə'reeə) the pres-ence of an excess of fat in the stools owing to malabsorption of fat by the intestines.

**Stein–Leventhal syndrome** (,stien-'levəntahl) *I.F. Stein, American gynaecologist, 1887–1976; M.L. Leventhal, American gynaecologist, 1901–1971.* Condition affecting females in which obesity, hirsutism and sterility are associated with polycystic ovaries and menstrual irregularities.

**Steinmann pin** ('stienmən ,pin) *F. Steinmann, Swiss surgeon, 1872–1932.* A fine metal rod, passed through a bone, by which extension is applied to overcome muscle contraction in certain fractures. *See* KIRSCHNER WIRE.

**stellate** ('stelayt) star-shaped. *S. fracture* a radiating fracture of the patella. *S. ganglion* the inferior cervical ganglion. A star-shaped collection of nerve cells at the base of the neck.

**stenosis** (stə'nohsis) abnormal narrowing or contraction of a channel or opening. *Aortic s.* narrowing of the opening of the aortic valve due to scar tissue formation as the result of inflammation. *Mitral s.* narrowing of the orifice of the mitral valve, usually following rheumatic fever. *Pulmonary s.* a congenital narrowing of the opening from the right ventricle of the heart into the pulmonary artery. *Pyloric s.* narrowing of the pyloric orifice of the stomach due to scar tissue, new growth or congenital hypertrophy.

**Stensen's duct** ('stensənz) *H. Stensen, Danish physician, 1638–1686.* The duct of the parotid gland, opening into the mouth opposite the second upper molar.

**stent** (stent) a device or splint of rubber, stainless steel or plastic mesh or a coil of wire placed inside a canal, duct or artery to keep the passageway open.

**stercobilin** (ˌstərkoh'bielin) a brown-orange pigment derived from bile and present in faeces.

**stereognosis** (ˌsteriog'nohsis, ˌstiə-) the ability to visualize the shape of an object by touch alone.

**stereotypy** ('steriohˌtiepee, ˌstiə-) repetitive actions carried out or maintained for long periods in a monotonous fashion.

**Sterets** (ste'rets) a proprietary brand of swabs impregnated with 70% isopropyl alcohol. These swabs are rubbed on to a skin site before an injection.

**Steri-Strips** ('steriˌstrips) a proprietary brand of skin closure strips which are placed across a wound with a space between the edges to allow for drainage. A final strip is placed on either side parallel to the wound.

**sterile** ('steriel) 1. aseptic; free from microorganisms. 2. barren; incapable of producing young.

**sterility** (stə'rilətee) 1. the state of being free from microorganisms. 2. the inability of a woman to become pregnant, or of a man to produce potent spermatozoa.

**sterilization** (ˌsterilie'zayshən) 1. rendering dressings, instruments, etc. aseptic by destroying or removing all microbial life. 2. rendering incapable of reproduction by any means.

**sterilizer** ('steriˌliezə) an apparatus in which objects can be sterilized. *See* AUTOCLAVE.

**sternotomy** (stər'notəmee) the operation in which the sternum is cut through to enable the heart to be reached.

**sternum** ('stərnəm) the breastbone; the flat narrow bone in the centre of the anterior wall of the thorax.

**steroid** ('steroyd, 'stiə-) one of a group of hormones chemically related to cholesterol. They include oestrogen and androgen, progesterone and the corticosteroids. They may be naturally occurring or they may be synthesized.

**sterol** ('sterol, 'stiə.rol) one of a group of steroid alcohols which includes cholesterol and ergosterol.

**stertorous** ('stərtə.rəs) snore-like; applied to a snoring sound produced in breathing during sleep or in a coma.

**stethoscope** ('stethəˌskohp) the instrument used for listening to internal body sounds, especially from the heart and lung. It consists of a hollow tube, one end of which is placed over the part to be examined and the other at the ear of the examiner.

**Stevens–Johnson syndrome** (ˌsteevənzˈjonsən) *A.M. Stevens, American paediatrician, 1884–1945; F.C. Johnson, American paediatrician, 1894–1934.* A severe form of erythema multiforme in which the lesions may involve the oral and anogenital mucosa, eyes and viscera, associated with such constitutional symptoms as malaise, headache, fever, arthralgia and conjunctivitis.

**STI** sexually transmitted infection.

**stigma** (ˈstigmə) 1. a small spot or mark on the skin. 2. any mark characteristic of a condition or defect, or of a disease. It refers to visible signs rather than symptoms.

**stilboestrol** (stilˈbeestrol) a synthetic oestrogen preparation used in the treatment of cancer of the prostate and less commonly for postmenopausal breast cancer.

**stillbirth** (ˈstilˌbərth) a baby which has issued forth from its mother after the 24th week of pregnancy and has not, at any time after being completely expelled from its mother, breathed or shown any sign of life. *S. certificate* a certificate issued to the parents by a registered medical practitioner who was present at the birth or examined the body.

**Still's disease** (stilz) *Sir G.F. Still, British paediatrician, 1868–1941.* A form of rheumatoid arthritis in children, sometimes associated with enlargement of the lymph glands.

**stimulant** (ˈstimyuhlənt) an agent that causes increased energy or functional activity of any organ.

**stimulus** (ˈstimyuhləs) *pl. stimuli* (L.) any agent, act or influence that produces functional or trophic reaction in a receptor in an irritable tissue. *Conditioned s.* a neutral object or event that is psychologically related to a naturally stimulating object or event and which causes a CONDITIONED RESPONSE (*see also* CONDITIONING). *Discriminative s.* a stimulus, associated with reinforcement, which exerts control over a particular form of behaviour; the subject discriminates between closely related stimuli and responds positively only in the presence of that stimulus. *Eliciting s.* any stimulus, conditioned or unconditioned, that elicits a response. *Structured s.* a well-organized and unambiguous stimulus, the perception of which is influenced to a greater extent by the characteristics of the stimulus than by those of the perceiver. *Threshold s.* a stimulus that is just strong enough to elicit a response. *Unconditioned s.* any stimulus that is capable of eliciting an unconditioned response (*see also* CONDITIONING). *Unstructured s.* an unclear or ambiguous stimulus, the perception of which is influenced to a greater extent by the characteristics of the perceiver than by those of the stimulus.

**stitch** (stich) 1. a popular term used to describe a sudden sharp pain usually due to spasm of the diaphragm. 2. a suture. *S. abscess* pus from a formation where a stitch has been inserted.

**Stokes–Adams syndrome** (ˌstohksˈadəmz) *Sir W. Stokes, Irish surgeon, 1804–1878; R. Adams, Irish physician, 1791–1875.* Attacks of syncope or fainting due to cerebral anaemia in some cases of complete heart block. The heart stops temporarily but breathing continues. The syndrome is treated by using an artificial pacemaker.

**stoma** (ˈstohmə) 1. a mouth or mouth-like opening. 2. an artificial opening in the skin surface leading into one of the tubes forming the alimentary canal. *See* COLOSTOMY and ILEOSTOMY.

**stomach** ('stumək) the dilated portion of the alimentary canal between the oesophagus and the duodenum, just below the diaphragm. *Bilocular* or *hourglass s.* one divided into two parts by a constriction. *S. pH electrode* apparatus used to measure gastric contents in situ. *S. pump* a pump that removes the contents of the stomach by suction. *S. tube* a flexible tube used for washing out the stomach or for the administration of liquid food.

**stomatitis** (,stohmə'tietis) inflammation of the mouth, either simple or with ulceration, caused by a vitamin deficiency or by a bacterial or fungal infection. *Angular s.* cracking at the corners of the mouth, usually due to riboflavin deficiency. *Aphthous s.* that characterized by small, white, painful ulcers on the mucous membrane. *Ulcerative s.* painful shallow ulcers on the tongue, cheeks and lips. A severe type that may produce serious constitutional effects.

**stone** (stohn) a calculus.

**stool** (stool) a motion or discharge from the bowels. *Fatty s.* that which contains undigested fat. *Hunger s.* stool passed by underfed infants: frequent, small and green. *Ricewater s.* the water stool, containing small white flakes, seen in cholera. *Tarry s.* a black tarry stool due to the presence of blood from a peptic ulcer.

**strabismus** (strə'bizməs) squint; heterotropia. A deviation of the eye from its normal direction. It is called convergent when the eye turns in towards the nose, and divergent when it turns outwards. *Concomitant s.* a squint in which the angle of deviation stays constant.

**strabotomy** (strə'botəmee) the division of ocular muscles in the treatment of strabismus.

**strain** (strayn) 1. overuse or stretching of a part, e.g. a muscle or tendon. 2. a group of microorganisms within a species. 3. to pass a liquid through a filter.

**strangulated** (,strang.gyuh'laytid) compressed or constricted so that the circulation of the blood is arrested. *S. hernia see* HERNIA.

**strangulation** (,strang.gyuh'layshən) 1. choking caused by compression of the air passages. 2. arrested circulation to a part, which will result in gangrene.

**strangury** ('strang.gyuhree) a painful, frequent desire to micturate, but in which only a few drops of urine are passed with difficulty.

**stratified** ('strati,fied) arranged in layers. *S. tissue* a covering tissue in which the cells are arranged in layers. The germinating cells are the lowest, and as surface cells are shed there is continual replacement.

**stratum** ('strahtəm, 'stray-) a layer; applied to structures such as the skin and mucous membranes. *S. corneum* the outer, horny layer of the epidermis.

**Streptococcus** (,streptoh'kokəs) a genus of Gram-positive spherical bacteria occurring in chains or pairs. Divided into various groups. The first group includes the beta-haemolytic human and animal pathogens; the second and third include alpha-haemolytic parasitic forms occurring as normal flora in the body; and the fourth is made up of saprophytic forms. *S. mutans* implicated in dental caries. *S. pneumoniae* pneumococcus, the most common cause of lobar pneumonia; also causes serious forms of meningitis, septicaemia, empyema and peritonitis. *S. pyogenes* beta-haemolytic, toxigenic, pyogenic streptococci causing septic sore throat, scarlet fever, rheumatic fever, puerperal fever and acute glomerulonephritis.

**streptokinase** (ˌstreptoh'kienayz) an enzyme derived from a streptococcal culture and used to liquefy clotted blood and pus.

**Streptomyces** (ˌstreptoh'mieseez) a genus of soil bacteria from which a large number of antibiotics are derived.

**streptomycin** (ˌstreptoh'miesin) an antibiotic drug derived from *Streptomyces griseus*; used particularly in the treatment of tuberculosis, when treatment is combined with other drugs to reduce drug resistance.

**stress** (stres) any factor, mental or physical, the pressure of which can adversely affect the functioning of the body. **S. disorders** those resulting from an individual's inability to withstand stress. **S. incontinence** incontinence, usually of urine, when the intra-abdominal pressure is raised, such as in coughing, sneezing or laughing.

**stria** ('striea) *pl.* striae. A line or stripe. **Striae gravidarum** the lines that appear on the abdomen of pregnant women. They are red in first pregnancy, but white subsequently, and are due to stretching and rupture of the elastic fibres.

**striated** (strie'aytid) striped. **S. muscle** voluntary muscle. *See* MUSCLE.

**stricture** ('strikchə) a narrowing or local contraction of a canal. It may be caused by muscle spasm, new growth, or scar tissue formation after inflammation.

**stridor** ('striedor) a harsh, vibrating, shrill sound, produced during respiration when there is partial obstruction of the larynx or trachea.

**stroke** (strohk) a popular term to describe the sudden onset of symptoms, especially those of cerebral origin affecting movement, sensation, speech and vision. There may be paralysis and loss of sensation down one side of the body or one side of the face. **Apoplectic s.** cerebral haemorrhage. **Heat s.** a hyperpyrexia accompanied by cerebral symptoms. It may occur in someone newly arrived in a very hot climate.

**stroma** ('strohmə) the connective tissue forming the ground substance, framework or matrix of an organ, as opposed to the functioning part or parenchyma.

**Strongyloides** (stronji'loydeez) a genus of nematode worms, one of which, *S. stercoralis*, is common in tropical countries and causes diarrhoea and intestinal ulcers.

**strontium** ('stronti.əm) *symbol* Sr. A metallic element. Isotopes of strontium are used in bone scanning to detect abnormalities. **S.-90** a radioactive isotope used in radiotherapy in the treatment of skin and eye malignancies.

**strychnine** ('strikneen) a highly poisonous alkaloid made from the seeds of *Strychnos nux-vomica*. Formerly used in small amounts in 'tonics'.

**Stryker frame** ('striekə) an apparatus specially designed for care of patients with injuries of the spinal cord or paralysis. It is constructed of pipe and canvas and is designed so that one nurse can turn the patient without difficulty.

**stupor** ('styoopə) a state of semiunconsciousness, occurring in the course of many varieties of mental illness, in which the patient does not move or speak, and makes no response to stimuli.

**Sturge–Weber syndrome** (stərj 'webə) *W.A. Sturge, British physician, 1850–1919; Sir H.D. Weber, British physician, 1824–1918.* A congenital abnormality in which there is a port wine stain on the face with an angioma of the meninges on the same side. Common symptoms are epilepsy, hemiplegia and associated learning difficulties.

**stuttering** ('stutə.ring) *see* STAMMER-ING.

**stye** (stie) *see* HORDEOLUM.

**stylet** ('stielit) a wire or rod for keeping clear the lumen of catheters, cannulae and hollow needles.

**styloid** ('stieloyd) like a pen. *S. process* a long pointed spine, particularly one projecting from the temporal bone. Also processes on the ulna and radius.

**styptic** ('stiptik) an astringent which, applied locally, arrests haemorrhage, e.g. alum and tannic acid.

**subacute** (ˌsubə'kyoot) moderately acute. Applied to a disease that progresses moderately rapidly, but does not become acute.

**subarachnoid** (ˌsubə'raknoyd) below the arachnoid. *S. space* between the arachnoid and pia mater of the brain and spinal cord, and containing cerebrospinal fluid.

**subclavian** (sub'klayvi.ən) beneath the clavicle. *S. artery* the main vessel of supply to the neck and arms.

**subclinical** (sub'klinik'l) without clinical manifestations; said of the early stages or a very mild form of a disease.

**subconscious** (sub'konshəs) 1. not conscious yet able to be recalled to consciousness. 2. in psychoanalysis, the part of the mind that retains memories which cannot without much effort be recalled to mind.

**subcutaneous** (ˌsubkyoo'tayni.əs) beneath the skin. *S. injection* one given hypodermically.

**subdural** (sub'dyooə.rəl) below the dura mater. *S. haematoma* a blood clot between the arachnoid and dura mater. It may be acute or arise slowly from a minor injury.

**subinvolution** (ˌsubinvə'looshən) incomplete or delayed return of the uterus to its pregravid size during the puerperium, usually as the result of retained products of conception and infection.

**subjective** (sub'jektiv) related to the individual. *S. symptoms* those of which the patient is aware by sensory stimulation, but which cannot easily be seen by others. *See also* OBJECTIVE.

**sublimate** ('subli.mayt) a substance obtained by sublimation.

**sublimation** (ˌsubli'mayshən) 1. the vaporization of a solid and its condensation into a solid deposit. 2. in psychoanalysis, a redirecting of energy at an unconscious level. The transference into socially acceptable channels of tendencies that cannot be expressed. An important aspect of maturity.

**subliminal** (sub'limin'l) below the threshold of perception.

**sublingual** (sub'ling.gwəl) beneath the tongue. *S. glands* two small salivary glands in the floor of the mouth.

**subluxation** (ˌsubluk'sayshən) partial dislocation of a joint.

**submaxillary** (ˌsubmak'silə.ree) beneath the lower jaw. *S. glands* two salivary glands situated under the lower jaw.

**submucous** (sub'myookəs) beneath mucous membrane. *S. resection* an operation to correct a deflected nasal septum.

**subnormal** (sub'norm'l) below normal.

**subphrenic** (sub'frenik) beneath the diaphragm. *S. abscess* one that develops below the diaphragm, usually after peritonitis or from postoperative infection.

**substitution** (ˌsubsti'tyooshən) the act of putting one thing in place of another. In psychology, this may be the nurse or foster mother in the place of the child's own mother. In psychotherapy, the nurse or therapist may be substituted for someone in the patient's background.

**substrate** ('substrayt) a substance on which an enzyme acts.

**succus** ('sukəs) a juice. *S. entericus* a digestive fluid secreted by intestinal glands. *S. gastricus* gastric juice.

**succussion** (su'kushən) a method of determining when free fluid is present in a cavity in the body. A sound of splashing is heard when the patient moves or is deliberately moved.

**sucrose** ('sookrohz, -ohs) a disaccharide obtained from cane or beet sugar.

**suction** ('sukshən) 1. the process of sucking. 2. the removal of gas or fluid from a cavity or other container by means of reduced pressure. *Post-tussive s.* a sucking noise heard in the lungs just after a cough.

**sudamen** (soo'daymən) a small white vesicle formed in the sweat glands after prolonged sweating.

**sudden infant death syndrome** (sud'n) abbreviated SIDS. The sudden and unexpected death of an apparently healthy infant, typically occurring between the ages of 3 weeks and 5 months, and not explained by careful postmortem studies. Called crib or cot death because the infant often is found dead in the cot. The prone position, tobacco smoke and overheating have been found to increase the risk of cot death, so these should be avoided.

**sudor** ('syoodor) sweat; perspiration.

**sudorific** (,syoodə'rifik) diaphoretic; an agent causing sweating.

**suffocation** (,sufə'kayshən) asphyxiation; a cessation of breathing caused by occlusion of the air passages, leading to unconsciousness and ultimately to death.

**suffusion** (sə'fyoozhən) a process of diffusion or overspreading, as in flushing of the skin; blushing.

**sugar** ('shugə) a group of sweet carbohydrates classified chemically as monosaccharides or disaccharides. The following are included: *beet s.* obtained from sugar beet; *cane s.* obtained from sugar cane; *fructose* fruit sugar; *grape s.* dextrose, glucose; *milk s.* lactose. *Muscle s.* inositol; a sugar-like compound found in animal tissue, particularly in muscle, and also in many plant tissues.

**suggestibility** (sə,jestə'bilətee) inclination to act on suggestions of others.

**suggestion** (sə'jeschən) a tool of psychotherapy in which an idea is presented to and accepted by a patient. *Posthypnotic s.* one implanted in a patient under hypnosis, which lasts after return to a normal condition.

**suicide** ('sooi,sied) the intentional taking of one's own life. Legally, a death suspected of being due to violence that is self-inflicted is not termed a suicide unless the victim leaves positive evidence of the intention to commit suicide, or the method of death is such that a verdict of suicide is inevitable. Some religious faiths consider it to be a sin and may refuse a consecrated burial.

**sulcus** ('sulkəs) a furrow or fissure; applied especially to those of the brain.

**sulphacetamide** (,sulfə'setə,mied) a soluble sulphonamide used as eye drops to treat corneal and conjunctival infections.

**sulphadiazine** (,sulfə'dieə,zeen) a slow-acting sulphonamide drug which is relatively non-toxic. Used in the treatment of meningococcal meningitis.

**sulphadimidine** (,sulfə'diemi,deen) a sulphonamide of which a high blood level can be obtained with reduced incidence of side-effects.

Used in the treatment of urinary tract infections.

**sulphamethizole** (,sulfə'methi,zohl) a sulphonamide used in urinary infection as it is rapidly excreted in an active form.

**sulphasalazine** (,sulfə'salə,zeen) a sulphonamide used in the treatment of ulcerative colitis.

**sulphonamide** (sul'fonə,mied) the generic term for all aminobenzenesulphonamide preparations, including the bactericidal sulpha drugs.

**sulphone** ('sulfohn) one of a group of drugs which with prolonged use have been successful in treating leprosy. Dapsone is the most widely used.

**sulphonylurea** (,sulfoni'lyooə.ri.ə) one of a group of oral hypoglycaemic agents used in the treatment of diabetes mellitus.

**sulthiame** (sul'thie,aym) an anticonvulsant drug used in the treatment of epilepsy.

**sunburn** ('sun,bərn) a dermatitis due to exposure to the sun's rays, causing burning and redness.

**sunstroke** ('sun,strohk) a profound disturbance of the body's heat-regulating mechanism caused by prolonged exposure to excessive heat from the sun. Persons over 40 and those in poor health are most susceptible to it.

**superego** (,soopə'reegoh, -'regoh) that part of the personality that is concerned with moral standards and ideals that are derived unconsciously from parents, teachers and environment, and influence the person's whole mental make-up, acting as a control on impulses of the ego.

**superfecundation** (,soopə,fekən-'dayshən, - ,fee-) the fertilization of two or more ova, produced during the same menstrual cycle, by spermatozoa from separate coital acts.

**superfetation** (,soopəfee'tayshən) the fertilization of a second ovum when pregnancy has already started, producing two fetuses of different maturity.

**superior** (soo'piə.ri.ə) above; the upper of two parts.

**supine** ('soopien) 1. lying on the back, with the face upwards. 2. with the palm of the hand upwards. *See* PRONE.

**suppository** (sə'pozitə.ree) a medicated solid substance, prepared for insertion into the rectum or vagina, which will dissolve at body temperature.

**suppression** (sə'preshən) 1. complete cessation of a secretion. 2. in psychology, conscious inhibition as distinct from repression, which is unconscious. *S. of urine* no secretion of urine by the kidneys.

**suppuration** (,supyuh'rayshən) the formation of pus.

**supracondylar** (,sooprə'kondilə) above the condyles. *S. fracture* one above the lower end of the humerus or femur.

**supraorbital** (,soopra'awbit'l) above the orbit of the eye.

**suprapubic** (,soopra'pyoobik) above the pubic bones. *S. cystotomy* surgical incision of the urinary bladder just above the pubic bones.

**suprarenal** (,soopra'reen'l) above the kidney. *S. gland* adrenal gland. One of a pair of triangular endocrine glands situated on the upper surface of the kidneys. *See* ADRENAL.

**surfactant** (sər'faktənt) a surface-active agent. A mixture of phospholipids that is secreted into the pulmonary alveoli and reduces the surface tension of pulmonary fluids, thus contributing to the elastic properties of pulmonary tissue. Surfactant can be given via a tracheal catheter as treatment for respiratory distress syndrome. *See also*

RESPIRATORY (DISTRESS SYNDROME OF NEWBORN).

**surgeon** ('sərjən) a medical practitioner who specializes in surgery. By custom the surgeon's title is Mr, Mrs, Miss or Ms, as opposed to physicians who are called Doctor.

**surgery** ('sərjə.ree) the branch of medicine that treats disease by operative measures.

**surrogate** ('surəgət) a real or imaginary substitute for a person or object in someone's life. *S. mother* a woman who carries a child for another (the commissioning parent) with the intention that the child be handed over after birth.

**survey** ('sərvay) the systematic collection of information, not forming part of a scientific epidemiological study.

**susceptibility** (sə,septə'bilitee) lack of resistance to infection. The opposite to immunity.

**suspensory** (sə'spensə.ree) supporting a part. *S. bandage* one applied to support a part of the body, particularly the scrotum or the lower jaw. *S. ligament* a ligament that supports or suspends an organ, e.g. that of the lens of the eye.

**suture** ('soochə) 1. a stitch or series of stitiches used to close a wound (*see* Figure). 2. the jagged line of junction of the bones of the cranium. *Atraumatic s.* a suture fused to the needle to obtain a single thickness through each puncture of the needle. *Continuous s.* a form of oversewing with one length of suture. *Coronal s.* the junction between the frontal and parietal bones. *Everting s.* a type of mattress stitch that turns the edges outwards to give a closer approximation. *Fascial s.* a strip of fascia taken from the patient and used to form a suture. *Interrupted s.* a series of

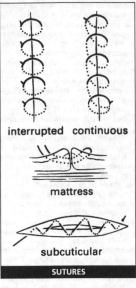

interrupted  continuous

mattress

subcuticular

**SUTURES**

separate sutures. *Lambdoid s.* the junction between the parietal and occipital bones. *Mattress s.* one in which each suture is taken twice through the wound, giving a loop one side and a knot the other. *Purse-string s.* a circular continuous suture round a small wound or appendix stump. *Sagittal s.* the junction between the two occipital bones. *Subcuticular s.* a continuous suture placed just below the skin. *Tension s.* or *relaxation s.* one taking a large bite and relieving the tension on the true stitch line.

**suxamethonium** (,suksəmee'thohni.əm) a short-acting muscle-relaxant drug primarily used in intubation of a patient.

**swab** (swob) 1. a small piece of cotton wool or gauze. 2. in pathology, a dressed sterile stick used in taking bacteriological specimens.

**swallowing** ('swoloh.ing) the taking in of a substance through the mouth and pharynx and into the oesophagus. It is a combination of a voluntary act and a series of reflex actions. Once begun, the process operates automatically. Also called deglutition.

**sweat** (swet) perspiration; a clear watery fluid secreted by the sweat glands. *S. glands* coiled tubular glands situated in the dermis with long ducts to the skin surface.

**sycosis** (sie'kohsis) a pustular inflammation of the hair follicles, usually of the beard and moustache.

**Sydenham's chorea** ('sid'n'mz) *T. Sydenham, British physician, 1624–1689.* A disorder of the central nervous system closely linked with rheumatic fever; called also Saint Vitus' dance. The condition, usually self-limited, is characterized by purposeless, irregular movements of the voluntary muscles that cannot be controlled by the patient.

**symbiosis** (simbie'ohsis) in parasitology, an intimate association between two different organisms for the mutual benefit of both.

**symblepharon** (sim'blefə.ron) adhesion of an eyelid to the eyeball.

**symbolism** ('simbə,lizəm) in psychology, an abnormal mental condition in which events or objects are interpreted as symbols of the patient's own thoughts. In psychiatry, the re-entry into consciousness of repressed material in an acceptable form.

**sympathectomy** (simpə'thektə-mee) division of autonomic nerve fibres which control specific involuntary muscles. An operation performed for many conditions, among them Raynaud's disease.

**sympathetic** (simpə'thetik) 1. exhibiting sympathy. 2. relating to the autonomic nervous system. *S. nervous system* one of the two divisions of the autonomic nervous system. It supplies involuntary muscle and glands; it stimulates the ductless glands and the circulatory and respiratory systems, but inhibits the digestive system. *S. ophthalmia* inflammation leading to loss of sight in the opposite eye after a perforating injury in the ciliary region.

**sympathomimetic** (simpəthohmi'metik) pertaining to drugs that produce effects similar to those caused by a stimulation of the sympathetic nervous system.

**symphysis** ('simfisis) a cartilaginous joint along the line of union of two bones. *S. pubis* the cartilaginous junction of the two pubic bones.

**symptom** ('simptəm) any indication of disease perceived by the patient. *Cardinal s's* 1. symptoms of greatest significance to the doctor, establishing the identity of the illness. 2. the symptoms shown in the temperature, pulse and respiration. *Dissociation s.* anaesthesia to pain and to heat and cold, without impairment of tactile sensibility. *Objective s.* one perceptible to others than the patient, such as pallor, rapid pulse or respiration, restlessness, etc. *Presenting s.* the symptom or group of symptoms about which the patient complains or from which relief is sought. *Signal s.* a sensation, aura or other subjective experience indicative of an impending epileptic or other seizure. *Subjective s.* one perceptible only to the patient, as pain, pruritus, vertigo, etc. *Withdrawal s's* symptoms that follow sudden abstinence from a drug on which a person is dependent.

**symptomatology** (simptəmə'tolojee) 1. the study of the symptoms of a disease. 2. the symptoms of a particular disease, taken together.

**synalgia** (si'nalji.ə) pain felt in one part of the body but caused by inflammation of or injury to another part. Referred pain.

**synapse** ('sienaps) the junction between the termination of an axon and the dendrites of another nerve cell. Chemical transmitters pass the impulse across the space.

**syncope** ('singkəpee) a simple faint or temporary loss of consciousness due to cerebral ischaemia, often caused by dilatation of the peripheral blood vessels and a sudden fall in blood pressure.

**syndactylism** (sin'dakti.lizəm) possessing webbed fingers or toes. A condition in which two or more fingers or toes are joined together.

**syndrome** ('sindrohm) a group of signs or symptoms typical of a distinctive disease, which frequently occur together and form a distinctive clinical picture.

**synergist** ('sinə.jist, si'nər-) 1. a muscle that works in conjunction with another muscle. 2. a drug that works in combination with another drug, the two drugs having a greater effect when taken together than when taken separately.

**synovectomy** (.sienoh'vektəmee, .si-) excision of a diseased synovial membrane to restore joint movement.

**synovial fluid** (sie'nohvi.əl, si-) the fluid that surrounds a joint and is secreted by the synovial membrane. It is a thick, colourless, lubricating substance.

**synovial membrane** a serous membrane lining the articular capsule of a movable joint and terminating at the edge of the articular cartilage.

**synovitis** (.sienoh'vietis) inflammation of a synovial membrane, usually with an effusion of fluid within the joint.

**synthesis** ('sinthəsis) the building up of a more complex structure from simple components. This may apply to drugs or to plant or animal tissues.

**syphilis** ('sifilis) an infectious venereal disease leading to many structural and cutaneous lesions; called also lues. Syphilis is caused by a spiral-shaped bacterium (spirochaete), *Treponema pallidum*. It is a SEXUALLY TRANSMITTED INFECTION, with the exception of congenital syphilis acquired by an infant from the mother in utero. There is an early infectious stage, followed by a latent period of many years before the non-infectious late stage, when serious disorders of the nervous and vascular systems arise. *Congenital s.* that transmitted by the mother to the fetus; it is preventable if the mother receives a full course of penicillin during her pregnancy. *Non-venereal s.* a chronic treponemal infection mainly seen in children, occurring in many areas of the world; it is caused by an organism indistinguishable from *Treponema pallidum* and transmitted by direct non-sexual contact. Lesions are usually oral mucous patches; subsequent lesions occur in the axillae, inguinal region and rectum. Then, after a latent period, destructive lesions of the skin and bones develop.

**syringe** (si'rinj) an instrument for injecting fluids or for aspirating or irrigating body cavities. It consists of a hollow tube with a tight-fitting piston. A hollow needle or a thin tube can be fitted to the end.

**syringomyelia** (si.ring.gohmie'ee-li.ə) the formation of cavities filled with fluid inside the spinal cord. Impairment of muscle function and sensation result at the level of and below the lesion. Painless injury may be the first symptom. It is a progressive disease.

**syringomyelitis** (si͵ring.goh͵mie-ə'lietis) inflammation of the spinal cord, as the result of which cavities are formed in it.

**syringomyelocele** (si͵ring.goh'mie-əloh͵seel) a type of spina bifida in which the protruded sac of fluid communicates with the central canal of the spinal cord.

**systemic** (si'stemik) pertaining to or affecting the body as a whole. *S. circulation* circulation of the blood throughout the whole body, other than the pulmonary circulation. *See* SCLEROSIS.

**systole** ('sistəlee) the period of contraction of the heart. *See* DIASTOLE.

*Atrial s.* the contraction of the heart by which the blood is pumped from the atria into the ventricles. *Extra-s.* a premature contraction of the atrium or ventricle, without alteration of the fundamental rhythm of the pacemaker. *Ventricular s.* the contraction of the heart by which the blood is pumped into the aorta and pulmonary artery.

**systolic** (si'stolik) relating to a systole. *S. murmur* an abnormal sound produced during systole in heart infections. *S. pressure* the highest pressure of the blood reached during systole.

# T

**T** symbol for *thymine*.

**T cell** a lymphocyte which is derived from the thymus and is responsible for cell-mediated immunity.

**TAB** typhoid–paratyphoid A and B vaccine; paratyphoid C may now be included. A sterile suspension of the killed salmonellae causing these diseases. Used as a preventative, it provides an active immunity.

**tabes** ('taybeez) a wasting away. *T. dorsalis* locomotor ataxia. A slowly progressive disease of the nervous system affecting the posterior nerve roots and spinal cord. It is a late manifestation of syphilis.

**taboo** (tə'boo) any ritual prohibition of certain activities, e.g. incest in many societies, or the open discussion of death and dying.

**taboparesis** (,taybohpə'reesis) the presence of the symptoms of both tabes dorsalis and general paralysis of the insane in a patient suffering from late syphilis.

**tachycardia** (,taki'kahdi.ə) abnormally rapid action of the heart and consequent increase in pulse rate. *See* BRADYCARDIA. *Paroxysmal t.* spasmodic increase in cardiac contractions of sudden onset lasting a variable time, from a few seconds to hours.

**tachyphasia, tachyphrasia** (,taki'fay zi.ə, ,taki'frayzi.e) extreme volubility of speech. It may be a sign of mental disorder.

**tachyphrenia** (,taki'freeni.ə) hyperactivity of the mental processes.

**tachypnoea** (,takip'neeə) rapid, shallow respirations; a reflex response to the vagus nerve endings in the pulmonary vessels.

**tactile** ('taktiel) relating to the sense of touch.

*Taenia* ('teeni.ə) a genus of tapeworms. *T. saginata* the beef tapeworm. The most common type of tapeworm found in the human intestine. *T. solium* the pork tapeworm. Can also be parasitic in humans, causing cysticercosis. *See* TAPEWORM.

**taeniasis** (tee'nieəsis) an infestation with tapeworms.

**TAF** toxoid–antitoxin floccules. A vaccine used for diphtheria immunization. *See* TOXOID.

**t'ai chi** (,tie 'chee) a system of movement, Chinese in origin, promoting general health and wellbeing.

**talipes** ('talipeez) clubfoot. A deformity caused by a congenital or acquired contraction of the muscles or tendons of the foot (*see* Figure). *T. calcaneus* the heel alone touches the ground on standing. *T. equinus* the toes touch the ground but not the heel. *T. valgus* the inner edge of the foot only is in contact with the ground. *T. varus* the person walks on the outer edge of the foot.

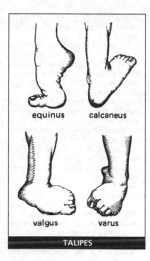

equinus    calcaneus

valgus    varus

**TALIPES**

**talus** ('taylǝs) the astragalus or ankle bone.

**tampon** ('tampon) a plug of absorbent material inserted in the vagina, the nose or other orifice to restrain haemorrhage or absorb secretion.

**tamponade** ('tampǝ,nayd) the surgical use of tampons. *Cardiac t.* impairment of heart action by haemorrhage or effusion into the pericardium; may be due to a stab wound or follow surgery.

**tantalum** ('tantǝlǝm) *symbol* Ta. A metallic element used for prostheses and wire sutures.

**tantrum** ('tantrǝm) an outburst of ill temper. *Temper t.* a behaviour disorder of childhood. A display of bad temper in which the child performs uncontrolled actions in a state of emotional stress.

**tapeworm** ('taypwǝrm) any of a group of cestode flatworms, including the *Taenia* genus, which are parasitic in the intestines of humans and many animals. The adult consists of a round head with suckers or hooklets for attachment (scolex). From this, numerous segments (proglottids) arise, each of which produces ova capable of independent existence for a considerable length of time. Treatment is by anthelmintic drugs.

**tapotement** (,tapoht'monh) [Fr.] a tapping movement used in massage.

**tapping** ('taping) *see* PARACENTESIS.

**tarsal** ('tahs'l) relating to a tarsus. *T. bones* the seven small bones of the ankle and instep. *T. cyst* Meibomian cyst; chalazion. *T. glands* Meibomian glands of the eyelids. *T. plates* small cartilages in the upper and lower eyelids.

**tarsalgia** (tah'salji.ǝ) pain in the foot, usually associated with flattening of the arch.

**tarsorrhaphy** (tah'so.rǝfee) stitching of the eyelids together to protect the cornea or to allow healing of an abrasion.

**tartar** ('tahtǝ) a hard incrustation deposited on the teeth and on dentures. *T. emetic* antimony potassium tartrate. A salt used in the treatment of schistosomiasis and leishmaniasis.

**task allocation** (tahsk ,alǝ'kayshǝn) a method of organizing care whereby each specific type of care is carried out by a separate nominated nurse, e.g. for the same patient one nurse will record the blood pressure and another nurse will give the prescribed medications.

**taste** (tayst) the sense by which it is possible to identify what is eaten and drunk. Taste receptors (buds) lie on the tongue and give the sensations of sweet, sour, salt and bitter.

**tattoo** (tǝ'too) a permanent discoloration of the skin due to a foreign pigment.

**tattooing** (tə'tooing) the deliberate (usually for decorative purposes) or accidental insertion of coloured material into the deeper layers of the skin, perhaps as a result of an explosion.

**taxis** ('taksis) manipulation by hand to restore any part to its normal position. It can be used to reduce a hernia or a dislocation.

**taxonomy** (tak'sonəmee) the theory and practice of the classification of animals and plants.

**Tay–Sachs disease** ( ˌtay'saks) *W. Tay, British physician, 1843–1927; B. Sachs, American neurologist, 1858–1944. See* AMAUROTIC (FAMILIAL IDIOCY).

**team nursing** (teem) a method of organizing care based on the allocation of each nurse to a team that cares for a group of patients, usually for a number of shifts.

**tears** (tiəz) the watery, slightly alkaline and saline secretion of the lacrimal glands that moistens the conjunctiva.

**teat** (teet) 1. a nipple of the breast. 2. a manufactured nipple used on infants' feeding bottles.

**technetium** (tek'neeshi.əm) *symbol* Tc. A metallic element. *Radioactive t.* an isotope ($^{99m}$Tc) used in a number of diagnostic tracer tests. As it has a short half-life (6 h), a high dose may be given for scanning organs, but the patient receives only a low radiation dose.

**teeth** (teeth) *see* DENTITION.

**tegument** ('tegyuhmənt) the skin.

**telangiectasis** (tə ˌlanji'ektəsis) a group of dilated capillary blood vessels, web-like or radiating in form.

**telangioma** (tə ˌlanji'ohmə) a tumour of the blood capillaries.

**telepathy** (tə'lepəthee) the transmission of thought without any normal means of communication between two persons.

**telereceptor** ( ˌteliri'septə) a sensory nerve ending which can respond to distant stimuli. Those of the eyes, ears and nose are examples. Teleceptor.

**telophase** ('teloh ˌfayz) the last stage in the division of cells when the chromosomes have been reconstituted in the nuclei at either end of the cell and the cell cytoplasm divides to form two new cells.

**temperature** ('temprəchə) the degree of heat of a substance or body as measured by a thermometer. *Normal t.* the normal temperature of the human body is 37°C, with a slight decrease in the early morning and a slight increase at night. It indicates the balance between heat production and heat loss.

**template** ('templayt) a mould or pattern. In radiotherapy, a map of the area of the patient requiring treatment and of those areas to be protected from radiation.

**temple** ('temp'l) the region on either side of the head above the zygomatic arch.

**temporal** ('tempə.rəl) pertaining to the side of the head. *T. arteritis* giant cell arteritis. A chronic inflammatory condition of the carotid arterial system, occurring usually in elderly people. There is persistent headache and partial or total blindness may result. *T. bone* one of a pair of bones on either side of the skull containing the organ of hearing. *T. lobe* the part of the cerebrum below the lateral sulcus.

**temporomandibular** ( ˌtempə.rohman'dibyuhlə) relating to the temporal bone and the mandible. *T. joint* the hinge of the lower jaw. *T. joint syndrome* painful dysfunction of the temporomandibular joint, marked by a clicking or grinding sensation in the joint; commonly caused by malocclusion of the teeth.

**tenacious** (tə'nayshəs) thick and viscid, as applied to sputum or other body fluids.

**tendinitis** (ˌtendi'nietis) inflammation of a tendon and its attachments.

**tendon** ('tendən) a band of fibrous tissue forming the termination of a muscle and attaching it to a bone. *Achilles t.* that inserted into the calcaneum. *T. grafting* an operation which repairs a defect in one tendon by a graft from another. *T. insertion* the point of attachment of a muscle to a bone which it moves. *T. reflex* the muscular contraction produced on percussing a tendon.

**tenesmus** (tə'nezməs) a painful, ineffectual straining to empty the bowel or bladder.

**tennis elbow** ('tenis) a painful disorder which affects the extensor muscles of the forearm at their attachment to the external epicondyle.

**Tenon's capsule** (tə'nonhz) *J.R. Tenon, French surgeon, 1724–1816.* The fibrous tissue in which the eyeball is situated.

**tenonitis** (ˌtenə'nietis) inflammation of Tenon's capsule. Proptosis of the eyeball occurs, often accompanied by pain and pyrexia.

**tenorrhaphy** (te'no.rəfee) the suturing together of the ends of a divided tendon.

**tenosynovitis** (ˌtenoh sienoh'vietis) inflammation of a tendon sheath.

**TENS** (tenz) abbreviation for transcutaneous electrical nerve stimulation. A method of treating persistent pain by passing small electrical currents into the spinal cord or sensory nerves by means of electrodes applied to the skin. TENS is non-invasive and non-addictive, with no known side-effects. The UKCC has approved the use of TENS by midwives and first-level nurses on their own responsibility, provided they have been instructed in its use.

**tension** ('tenshən) the act of stretching or the state of being stretched.

*Arterial t.* the pressure of blood on the vessel wall during cardiac contraction. *Intraocular t.* the pressure of the contents of the eye on its walls, measured by a tonometer. *Intravenous t.* the pressure of blood within the veins. *Premenstrual t.* symptoms of abdominal distension, headache, emotional lability and depression, occurring a few days before the onset of menstruation. *See* PREMENSTRUAL. *Surface t.* tension or resistance which acts to preserve the integrity of a surface, particularly the surface of a liquid.

**teratogen** ('terətoh jen) an agent or influence that causes physical defects in the developing embryo.

**teratoma** (ˌterə'tohmə) a solid tumour containing tissues similar to those of a dermoid cyst. Found most often in the ovaries and testes, many of these tumours are malignant.

**tertian** ('tərshən) recurring every 48 h. *See* MALARIA.

**tertiary** ('tərshə.ree) third. *T. prevention* prevention of ill health, mitigating the effects of illness and disease that have already occurred. *T. syphilis* the non-infectious stage of neurosyphilis.

**test** (test) 1. an examination or trial. 2. analysis of the composition of a substance by the use of chemical reagents. *Agglutination t.* one whose results depend on agglutination of bacteria or other cells. Used in diagnosing certain infectious diseases and rheumatoid arthritis, the cross-matching of blood and in pregnancy tests; in the latter no agglutination indicates a positive pregnancy test, whereas when agglutination occurs the result is negative. *Complement-fixation t's* tests that utilize antigen–antibody reaction, and result in haemolysis, to determine the presence of various organisms in the blood. *Concentration t.* a test of renal function based on the patient's ability to concentrate urine. *Creatinine clearance t.* a test for renal function based on the rate at which ingested creatinine is filtered through the renal glomeruli. *Early pregnancy t.* a do-it-yourself immunological test for pregnancy, performed as early as 9 days after menstruation was expected. *Glucose tolerance t.* a metabolic test of carbohydrate tolerance used to diagnose diabetes mellitus. *Glycosylated haemoglobin t.* measurement of the percentage of haemoglobin $A_1$ ($HbA_1$) molecules, which helps to assess diabetic control. $HbA_1$ is a type of adult haemoglobin where one part of the beta chain has been combined with glucose; it increases in diabetes, especially when the blood glucose control is poor. *Histamine t.* after a rapid intravenous injection of histamine phosphate, the blood pressure normally falls, but in patients with phaeochromocytoma, after the fall, there is a marked rise in blood pressure. *Pregnancy t's* laboratory procedures for early determination of pregnancy. *Sickling t.* a method to demonstrate haemoglobin S and the sickling phenomenon in erythrocytes, performed by reducing the oxygen concentration to which the red cells are exposed. *T. weighing* a method of determining the amount of breast milk taken by weighing the baby before and after the feed without changing any of its clothes, so that the difference equals the feed. Sometimes called test feeding. With successful demand feeding there should be no need for this scheme. *Treponema pallidum haemagglutination (TPHA) t., Treponema pallidum immobilization (TPI) t.* serological tests related directly to the causative organism, used in the diagnosis of syphilis. *VDRL t.* a slide flocculation test for syphilis

designed by the Venereal Disease Research Laboratory, USA.

**testicle** ('testik'l) a testis; one of the two glands in the scrotum which produce spermatozoa. *Undescended t.* a condition in which the organ remains in the pelvis or inguinal canal.

**testicular self-examination** (tes'ti-kyoolə) should be performed regularly once a month for the detection of early tumours of the testis, which are highly curable if detected at an early stage. Self-examination should take place after a warm bath or shower, which relaxes the scrotal skin. It is performed as follows: (a) Standing in front of a mirror, look for any swelling. One testicle may appear larger than the other or hang lower; this is usually perfectly normal. (b) Examine each testicle with both hands and gently roll each testicle between the fingers and thumb. A small lump is felt for and, if found, almost always occurs in only one testis and is usually painless. (c) A cord-like structure found on the top and back of each testicle should be found and examined for any swelling.

**testis** ('testis) a testicle.

**testosterone** (tes'tostə,rohn) the hormone produced by the testes which stimulates the development of sex characteristics. It can now be made synthetically, and is used medicinally in cases of failure of sex function and as a palliative treatment in some cases of advanced metastatic breast cancer in females.

**tetanus** ('tetənəs) an acute disease of the nervous system caused by the contamination of wounds by the spores of a soil bacterium, *Clostridium tetani.* Muscle stiffness around the site of the wound occurs, followed by rigidity of face and neck muscles; hence 'lockjaw'. All muscles are then affected and opisthotonos may occur. *T. antito-*

*xin* a serum that gives a short term passive immunity and may be used with penicillin for immediate treatment of a case of tetanus. *T. vaccine* or *toxoid* will give an active immunity.

**tetany** ('tetənee) an increased excitability of the nerves due to a lack of available calcium, accompanied by painful muscle spasm of the hands and feet (carpopedal spasm). The cause may be hypoparathyroidism or alkalosis owing to excessive vomiting or hyperventilation.

**tetracycline** (,tetrə'siekleen) an antibiotic drug belonging to the group known as the tetracyclines which are effective against many different microorganisms, including rickettsiae, Gram-negative and Gram-positive organisms and certain viruses.

**tetralogy** (te'traləjee) a series of four. *T. of Fallot see* FALLOT'S TETRALOGY.

**tetraplegia** (,tetrə'pleeji.ə) quadriplegia. Paralysis of all four limbs.

**thalamus** ('thaləməs) a mass of nerve cells at the base of the cerebrum. Most sensory impulses from the body pass to this area and are transmitted to the cortex.

**thalassaemia** (,thalə'seemi.ə) a group of haemolytic anaemias mostly found in the Mediterranean region and the Far East, caused by the inheritance of abnormal haemoglobin. *T. major* Cooley's anaemia; the severest form of thalassaemia with death usually occurring before adolescence. *T. minor* a mild form of the disease with few symptoms. Those suffering from it can pass the disease on to their children.

**thalassotherapy** (thə,lasoh-'therəpee) treatment involving sea bathing or a sea voyage.

**thanatology** (,thanə'toləjee) 1. the study of death and dying. 2. the forensic study of the causes of death.

**theca** ('theekə) a sheath, such as the covering of a tendon. *T. folliculi* the covering of a Graafian follicle. *T. vertebralis* the membranes enclosing the spinal cord; the dura mater.

**thenar** ('theenah) 1. the palm of the hand. 2. the fleshy part at the base of the thumb.

**theophylline** (thi'ofi,leen) an alkaloid derived from tea-leaves, which increases the heart rate and the excretion of urine, thus reducing oedema. Used mainly in the treatment of bronchospasm and asthma.

**therapeutic** (,therə'pyootik) pertaining to therapeutics or treatment of disease; curative. *T. abortion see* ABORTION. *T. community* any treatment setting (usually psychiatric) which provides a living–learning situation through group processes emphasizing social, environmental and personal interactions and which encourages the individual to learn socially from these processes. *T. use of self* the ability of the psychiatric nurse to use therapy and experimental knowledge along with self-awareness and the ability to explore, and use, one's personal impact on others.

**therapeutics** (,therə'pyootiks) the science and art of healing and the treatment of disease.

**therapy** ('therəpee) the treatment of disease.

**thermal** ('thərməl) relating to heat.

**thermocautery** (,thərmoh-'kawtə.ree) the deliberate destruction of tissue by means of heat. *See* CAUTERY.

**thermography** (thər'mogrəfee) a method of measuring the amount of heat produced by different areas of the body, using infrared photography. Used as a diagnostic aid in the detection of breast tumours and the assessment of rheumatic joints; also used in the study of pain.

**thermolysis** (thər'molisis) the loss of body heat by radiation, by excretion and by the evaporation of sweat.

**thermometer** (thə'mɒmitə) an instrument for measuring temperature. *Clinical t.* one used to measure the body temperature. *Electronic t.* a clinical thermometer which works electrically. It contains electronic devices whose characteristics change with temperature. The reading is recorded within seconds and displayed visually.

**thermoreceptor** (ˌthərmohri'septə) a nerve ending that responds to heat and cold.

**thermostat** ('thərməˌstat) an apparatus which automatically regulates the temperature and maintains it at a specified level.

**thermotaxis** (ˌthərmoh'taksis) the normal regulation of body temperature by the maintenance of the balance between heat production and heat loss.

**thermotherapy** (ˌthərmoh'therəpee) the treatment of disease by application of heat.

**thiamine** ('thieəˌmeen) vitamin B₁, or aneurine. An essential vitamin involved in carbohydrate metabolism. A deficiency causes beriberi. The source is liver and unrefined cereals.

**thiazides** ('thieəˌziedz) any of a group of diuretics that act by inhibiting the reabsorption of sodium in the proximal renal tubule and stimulating chloride excretion, with resultant increase in excretion of water.

**Thiersch skin graft** ('teeəsh) I. *Thiersch, German surgeon, 1822–1895.* The transplantation of areas of partial thickness skin. *See* GRAFT.

**thioguanine** (ˌthieoh'gwahneen) an antimetabolite used in the treatment of acute leukaemia.

**thiopentone** (ˌthieoh'pentohn) a basal narcotic of the barbiturate group given intravenously as a short-acting anaesthetic and in preoperative preparation.

**thiouracil** (ˌthieoh'yooəˌrəsil) a drug used in the treatment of thyrotoxicosis. A derivative, propylthiouracil, which is more active and less toxic, is now more often used.

**thirst** (thərst) an uncomfortable sensation of dryness of the mouth and throat with a desire for oral fluids. *Abnormal t.* polydipsia.

**Thomas splint** ('tɒməs) *H.O. Thomas, British orthopaedic surgeon, 1834–1891.* A splint consisting of an oval iron ring that fits over the lower limb. Attached to the ring are two round iron rods which are bent into a **W** shape at the lower end. It is used to support the limb and move the weight from the knee joint to the pelvis.

**thoracic** (thor'rasik) relating to the thorax. *T. duct* the large lymphatic vessel situated in the thorax along the spine. It opens into the left subclavian vein.

**thoracocentesis** (ˌthor.rəkohsen'teesis) puncture of the wall of the thorax to allow aspiration of pleural fluid.

**thoracoscopy** (ˌthor.rə'koskəpee) examination of the pleural cavity by means of an endoscopic instrument.

**thoracotomy** (ˌthor.rə'kotəmee) a surgical incision into the thorax.

**thorax** ('thor.raks) the chest; a cavity containing the heart, lungs, bronchi and oesophagus. It is bounded by the diaphragm, the sternum, the thoracic vertebrae and the ribs. *Barrel-shaped t.* a development in emphysema, when the chest is malformed like a barrel.

**threadworm** ('thredˌwərm) a species of roundworm, *Enterobius vermicularis*, parasitic in the large intestine, particularly of children.

**threonine** ('threeəˌneen) one of the essential amino acids.

**thrill** (thril) a tremor discerned by palpation.

**throat** (throht) 1. the anterior surface of the neck. 2. the pharynx. *Clergyman's sore t.* laryngitis. *Sore t.* pharyngitis.

**thrombin** ('thrombin) an enzyme that converts fibrinogen to fibrin during the later stages of blood clotting.

**thromboangiitis** (,thromboh,anji'ietis) inflammation of blood vessels with clot formation. *T. obliterans* inflammation of the arteries, usually of the legs of young males, causing intermittent claudication and gangrene. Buerger's disease.

**thrombocyte** ('thromboh,siet) a disc-shaped blood platelet; essential for the clotting of shed blood.

**thrombocytopenia** (,thromboh,sietoh'peeni.ə) a reduction in the number of platelets in the blood; bleeding may occur. Destruction of platelets can be caused by infections, certain drugs, transfusion related purpuras, idiopathic thrombocytopenic purpura and disseminated intravascular coagulation.

**thrombocytosis** (,thromboh sie'tohsis) an increase in the number of platelets in the blood.

**thrombokinase** (,thromboh'kienayz) thromboplastin. A lipid-containing protein, activated by blood platelets and injured tissues, which is capable of activating prothrombin to form thrombin, which, combined with fibrinogen, forms a clot.

**thrombolysis** (throm'bolisis) the disintegration or dissolving of a clot by the infusion of an enzyme such as streptokinase into the blood.

**thrombophlebitis** (,thrombohfli'bietis) the formation of a clot, associated with inflammation of the lining of a vein.

**thromboplastin** (,thromboh'plastin) *see* THROMBOKINASE.

**thrombosis** (throm'bohsis) the formation of a thrombus. *Cavernous sinus t.* thrombosis of the cavernous sinus, usually the result of infection of the face, when the veins in the sinus are affected via ophthalmic vessels. *Cerebral t.* the occlusion of a cerebral artery, the most common cause of cerebral infarction (a 'stroke'). *Coronary t.* the occlusion of a coronary vessel, by which the heart muscle is deprived of blood, causing myocardial ischaemia and often leading to myocardial infarction (a 'heart attack'). *Lateral sinus t.* a complication of mastoiditis when infection of the lateral sinus of the dura mater occurs and there is clot formation.

**thrombus** ('thrombəs) a stationary blood clot caused by coagulation of the blood in the heart or in an artery or a vein.

**thrush** (thrush) an infection of the mucous membranes, most commonly of the mouth and vagina, by a fungus, *Candida albicans*. *See* CANDIDIASIS.

**thymectomy** (thie'mektəmee) surgical removal of the thymus.

**thymine** ('thiemeen) symbol T. One of the pyrimidine bases found in DNA.

**thymol** ('thiemol) an aromatic antiseptic used in solution as a mouthwash.

**thymoma** (thie'mohmə) a tumour that originates in thymus tissue.

**thymus** ('thieməs) a gland-like structure situated in the upper thorax and neck. Present in early life, it reaches its maximum development during puberty and continues to play an immunological role throughout life, even though its function declines with age.

**thyroglossal** (,thieroh'glos'l) relating to the thyroid and the tongue. *T. cyst see* CYST.

**thyroid** ('thieroyd) 1. shaped like a shield. 2. pertaining to the thyroid gland. *Intrathoracic* or *retrosternal t.* position of the gland low in the neck and wholly or in part behind the sternum. *T. cartilage* the largest cartilage of the larynx. It forms the 'Adam's apple' in the front of the throat. *T. gland* a ductless gland, consisting of two lobes, situated in front and on either side of the trachea. It secretes the hormones thyroxine and triiodothyronine which are concerned in regulating the metabolic rate. *T.-stimulating hormone* abbreviated TSH. Thyrotrophin; a hormone, produced by the anterior pituitary gland, which controls the activity of the thyroid gland.

**thyroidectomy** (ˌthieroy'dektəmee) partial or complete removal of the thyroid gland.

**thyroiditis** (ˌthieroy'dietis) inflammation of the thyroid. Acute thyroiditis, usually due to a virus infection, is characterized by sore throat, fever and painful enlargement of the gland. *Hashimoto's t.* a progressive autoimmune disease of the thyroid gland with degeneration of its epithelial elements and replacement by lymphoid and fibrous tissue.

**thyroparathyroidectomy** (ˌthierohˌparəˌthieroy'dektəmee) surgical removal of the thyroid and parathyroid glands.

**thyrotoxicosis** (ˌthierohˌtoksi'kohsis) hyperthyroidism. The symptoms arise when there is overactivity of the thyroid gland. The metabolism is speeded up and there is enlargement of the gland and exophthalmos.

**thyrotrophin** (ˌthieroh'trohfin) *see* THYROID-(STIMULATING HORMONE).

**thyroxine** (thie'rokseen) one of the two hormones secreted by the thyroid gland. It is used in the treatment of hypothyroidism.

**TIA** transient ischaemic attack.

**tibia** ('tibi.ə) the shin bone; the larger of the two bones of the leg, extending from knee to ankle.

**tic** (tik) a spasmodic twitching of certain muscles, usually of the face, neck or shoulder. *T. douloureux* paroxysmal trigeminal neuralgia.

**tick** (tik) a blood-sucking parasite which may transmit the organisms of disease.

**tidal volume** ('tied'l) the amount of gas passing into and out of the lungs in each respiratory cycle.

**tine test** (tien) a tuberculin skin test employing a multiple-puncture, disposable device. It is especially useful in mass screening of children, but is less accurate than the Mantoux test.

**tinea** ('tini.ə) a group of skin infections caused by a variety of fungi and named after the area of the body affected, thus: *T. barbae*, the beard; *T. capitis*, the head; *T. circinata* or *T. corporis*, the body; *T. cruris*, the groin; and *T. pedis*, the feet. *See* RINGWORM.

**tinnitus** (ti'nietəs) a ringing, buzzing or roaring sound in the ears.

**tissue** ('tisyoo, 'tishoo) a group or layer of similarly specialized cells that together perform certain special functions.

**titration** (tie'trayshən) determination of a given component in solution by addition of a liquid reagent of known strength until a given endpoint, e.g. change in colour, is reached, indicating that the component has been consumed by reaction with the reagent.

**tobacco** (tə'bakoh) the dried leaves of the plant *Nicotiana tabacum*, containing the drug nicotine, which may be smoked, chewed or inhaled. All these activities are potentially dangerous to health. Cigarette smoking in particular is responsible for an increase in cancer of the lungs and mouth and bronchitis. Smoking increases the likelihood of emphysema and coronary artery disease. It is also harmful during pregnancy, leading to smaller and less healthy babies. *T. withdrawal syndrome* a change in mood or behaviour associated with the stopping of or reduction in cigarette smoking.

**tobramycin** (ˌtobrəˈmiesin) an antibiotic drug used chiefly in the treatment of *Pseudomonas* infection.

**tocography** (toˈkogrəfee) the measurement of alterations in the intrauterine pressure during labour.

**tocopherol** (toˈkofəˌrol) vitamin E, present in wheatgerm, green leaves and milk.

**token economy programme** (ˌtohkən iˈkonəmee ˌprohgram) a behavioural approach to modifying troublesome behaviours and restoring lost self-help behaviours by the systematic rewarding of desired behaviour by giving tokens which may be exchanged for goods or privileges.

**tolazamide** (toˈlazəˌmied) an oral hypoglycaemic drug used in the treatment of diabetes mellitus.

**tolazoline** (toˈlazohˌleen) a vasodilator drug of the peripheral blood vessels, used in the treatment of peripheral vascular disease.

**tolbutamide** (tolˈbyootəˌmied) an oral drug that stimulates the release of insulin from the pancreas. Used in the treatment of diabetes mellitus.

**tolerance** (ˈtoləˌrəns) the ability to endure without effect or injury. *Drug t.* decrease of susceptibility to the effects of a drug due to its continued administration. *Immunological t.* specific nonreactivity of lymphoid tissues to a particular antigen capable, under other conditions, of inducing immunity.

**tomography** (təˈmogrəfee) body section radiography in which X-rays or ultrasound waves are used to produce an image of a layer of tissue at any depth.

**tone** (tohn) 1. the normal degree of tension, e.g. in a muscle. 2. a particular quality of sound.

**tongue** (tung) a muscular organ attached to the floor of the mouth and concerned in taste, mastication, swallowing and speech. It is covered by a mucous membrane from which project numerous papillae.

**tonic** (ˈtonik) 1. a term popularly applied to any drug supposed to brace or tone up the body or any particular part or organ. 2. possessing tone in a state of contraction, e.g. muscles. *T. spasm* a prolonged contraction of one or several muscles, as seen in epilepsy, for example. *See* CLONIC.

**tonography** (tohˈnogrəfee) the measurement made by an electric tonometer recording the intraocular pressure and so, indirectly, the drainage of aqueous humour from the eye.

**tonsil** (ˈtonsil) a mass of lymphoid tissue, particularly one of two small, almond-shaped bodies, situated one on each side between the pillars of the fauces. It is covered by mucous membrane, and its surface is pitted with follicles. *Pharyngeal t.* the lymphadenoid tissue of the pharynx between the pharyngotympanic tubes. Adenoids. *T. test* a small sample of tonsil obtained in suspected cases of CREUTZFELDT–JAKOB DISEASE (CJD) for the identification of the prion found in new variant CJD, a spongiform encephalopathy.

**tonsillectomy** (ˌtonsiˈlektəmee) excision of one or both tonsils.

**tonus** (ˈtohnəs) the normal state of partial contraction of the muscles.

**tooth** (tooth) a structure in the mouth designed for the mastication of food. Each is composed of a crown, neck and root with one or more fangs. The main bulk is of dentine enclosing a central pulp; the crown is covered with a hard white substance called enamel. *See* DENTITION.

**tophus** ('tohfəs) a small, hard, chalky deposit of sodium urate in the skin and cartilage, occurring in gout and sometimes appearing on the auricle of the ear.

**topical** ('topik'l) relating to a particular spot; local. *T. lotion* one for local or external application.

**topography** (tə'pogrəfee, toh-) the study of the surface of the body in relation to the underlying structures.

**TORCH** (tawch) acronym for *t*oxo plasmosis, *o*ther, *r*ubella, *c*ytomegalovirus and *h*erpes simplex infections.

**torpor** ('tawpə) a sluggish condition in which response to stimuli is absent or very slow.

**torsion** ('tawshən) twisting: (a) of an artery to arrest haemorrhage; (b) of the pedicle of a cyst, which produces venous congestion in the cyst and consequent gangrene (a possible complication of ovarian cyst).

**torso** ('tawsoh) the body, excluding the head and the limbs; the trunk.

**torticollis** (ˌtawti'kolis) wryneck, a contracted state of the cervical muscles, producing torsion of the neck. The deformity may be congenital or secondary to pressure on the accessory nerve, to inflammation of glands in the neck, or to muscle spasm.

**tourniquet** ('tooəniˌkay, 'tawni-) a constrictive band applied to a limb to arrest arterial haemorrhage. No longer used in first aid because its use may cause permanent damage to muscles or nerve supply.

**toxaemia** (tok'seemi.ə) poisoning of the blood by the absorption of bacterial toxins. *T. of pregnancy* a condition affecting pregnant women and characterized by albuminuria, hypertension and oedema, with the possibility of pre-eclampsia and eclampsia developing.

**toxic** ('toksik) 1. poisonous, relating to a poison. 2. caused by a toxin. *T. shock syndrome* a severe illness characterized by high fever of sudden onset, vomiting, diarrhoea and, in severe cases, death. A sunburn-like rash with peeling of the skin occurs.

**toxicity** (tok'sisitee) the degree of virulence of a poison.

**toxicology** (ˌtoksi'koləjee) the science dealing with poisons.

**toxin** ('toksin) any poisonous compound, usually referring to that produced by bacteria.

*Toxocara* (ˌtoksoh'kahrə) a genus of nematode worms, parasitic in the intestines of dogs and cats, which may also infest humans, especially children. The spleen, liver and lungs are most often affected but the parasite may also infest the retina, causing inflammation and granulation.

**toxoid** ('toksoyd) a toxin which has been deprived of some of its harmful properties but is still capable of producing immunity and may be used in a vaccine.

*Toxoplasma* (ˌtoksoh'plazmə) a genus of protozoa which infests birds and animals and may be transmitted from them to humans.

**toxoplasmosis** (ˌtoksohplaz'mohsis) a disease due to *Toxoplasma gondii*. The congenital form is marked by central nervous system lesions, which may lead to blindness, brain defects and death. The acquired infection is often asymptomatic but may result in pneumonia, skin rashes and nephritis.

**TPA** total parenteral alimentation.

**TPN** total parenteral nutrition.

**trabecula** (trə'bekyuhlə) a dividing band or septum, extending from the capsule of an organ into its interior and holding the functioning cells in position.

**trabeculectomy** (trəˌbekyuh'lektə-mee) an operation to lower the intraocular pressure in glaucoma that cannot be controlled by medication.

**tracer** ('traysə) a means by which something may be followed, as (a) a mechanical device by which the outline or movements of an object can be graphically recorded, or (b) a material by which the progress of a compound through the body may be observed, e.g. a radioactive isotope tracer.

**trachea** (trə'keeə, 'traki.ə) the windpipe; a cartilaginous tube lined with ciliated mucous membrane, extending from the lower part of the larynx to the commencement of the bronchi.

**tracheitis** (,traki'ietis) inflammation of the trachea causing pain in the chest, with coughing.

**tracheobronchitis** (,trakiohbrong-'kietis) acute infection of the trachea and bronchi due to viruses or bacteria.

**tracheostomy** (,traki'ostəmee) a surgical opening into the third and fourth cartilage rings of the trachea. *T. tubes* those used to maintain an airway after tracheotomy, either permanently or until the normal use of the air passages is regained.

**tracheotomy** (,traki'otəmee) surgical incision of the trachea. *High t.* superior tracheotomy. *Inferior* or *low t.* that in which the opening is made below the thyroid isthmus. *Superior t.* high tracheotomy. That in which the opening is made above the thyroid isthmus.

**trachoma** (trə'kohmə) a chronic infectious disease of the conjunctiva and cornea, producing photophobia, pain and lacrimation, caused by an organism once thought to be a virus but now classified as a strain of the bacterium *Chlamydia trachomatis*. Trachoma is more prevalent in Africa and Asia than in other parts of the world.

**traction** ('trakshən) 1. the exertion of a pulling force, such as that applied to a fractured bone or dislocated joint or to relieve muscle spasm, to maintain proper position and facilitate healing. 2. In obstetrics, that along the axis of the pelvis to assist in delivery of a fetal part, or the placenta and membranes. *Hamilton–Russell t.* a form of traction of the leg. *Head t.* traction exerted on the head in the treatment of cervical injury. *Skeletal t.* a method of keeping the fractured ends of bone in position by traction on the bone. A metal pin or wire is passed through the distal fragment or adjacent bone to overcome muscle contraction.

**trait** (trayt) an inherited or developed physical or mental characteristic.

**trance** (trans) a condition of semiconsciousness of hysterical, cataleptic or hypnotic origin. It is not due to organic disease.

**tranquillizer** ('trangkwi,liezə) a drug which allays anxiety, relieves tension and has a calming effect on the patient.

**transactional analysis** (tran'zakshən'l) a theory of personality structure and a psychotherapeutic method. The human personality is viewed as consisting of three ego states: the parent, the adult and the child. The aim is to allow the adult ego to take control over the child and parent egos.

**transaminase** (tran'zami,nayz) one of a group of enzymes which catalyse the transfer of an amine group from one amino acid into another. Transaminases include *glutamic-oxalacetic t.* (GOT) and *glutamic-pyruvic t.* (GPT).

**transcendental meditation** (,transen'dent'l ,medi'tayshən) a technique for attaining a state of physical relaxation and psychological calm by the regular practice of a relaxation procedure which entails the repetition of a mantra. Has been successfully used by some patients to reduce hypertension.

**transcutaneous blood gas monitors** (ˌtranzkyoo'tayneeəs) the application to a baby's skin of a probe which is heated to a temperature of 44°C and enables measurements of $Po_2$ and $Pco_2$ to be made. Accuracy depends on the quality of the peripheral circulation, thus transcutaneous blood gas monitoring is usually used in conjunction with intermittent arterial sampling.

**transcutaneous electrical nerve stimulation** (i'lektrik'l nərv ˌstimyuh-'layshən) see TENS.

**transference** ('transfə.rəns, trans'fər.rəns) in psychiatry, the unconscious transfer by the patient on to the psychiatrist of feelings that are appropriate to other people significant to the patient.

**transfusion** (trans'fyoozhən) the introduction of whole blood or a blood component into a vein, performed in cases of severe loss of blood, shock, septicaemia, etc. It is used to supply actual volume of blood, or to introduce constituents, such as clotting factors or antibodies, that are deficient in the patient. *Direct t.* the transfer of blood directly from a donor to a recipient. *Exchange t.* replacement transfusion. The removal of most or all of the recipient's blood and its replacement with fresh blood. Used with infants suffering from erythroblastosis. *See* RHESUS FACTOR. *Intra-arterial t.* the passing of blood into an artery under positive pressure in cases where large quantities are required rapidly, as in cardiovascular surgery. *Replacement t.* exchange transfusion.

**transient ischaemic attack** ('tranziənt) abbreviated TIA. A sudden episode of temporary or passing symptoms, caused by diminished blood flow through the carotid or vertebrobasilar blood vessels.

**transillumination** (ˌtranziˌloomi-'nayshən) the illumination of a translucent body structure by a strong light as an aid to diagnosis, particularly of tumours of the retina and of abnormalities in the ethmoidal and frontal sinuses.

**translocation** (ˌtranzloh'kayshən) in morphology, the transfer of a segment of a chromosome to a different site on the same chromosome or to a different chromosome. It can be a cause of congenital abnormality.

**translucent** (tranz'loosn't) allowing light rays to pass through indistinctly.

**transmigration** (ˌtranzmie-'grayshən) a movement from one place to another, as in the passage of blood cells through the walls of the capillaries. Diapedesis. *External t.* the passage of an ovum from its ovary to the uterine tube on the opposite side. *Internal t.* the movement of an ovum from one uterine tube to the other through the uterus.

**transmission-based precautions** (trans'mishən bayst pri'kawshənz) precautions, designed to be applied to patients known or suspected to be infected with PATHOGENS that are highly transmissible or epidemiologically important, and for which additional measures beyond STANDARD PRECAUTIONS are needed to interrupt transmission in hospital. There are three types of transmission-based precaution: airborne, droplet and contact precautions. They may be combined for diseases that have multiple routes of transmission. When employed either singly or in combination, they are used in addition to 'standard precautions'.

**transplacental** (ˌtransplə'sentʹl) across the placenta. Movement may be from mother to fetus or vice versa. *T. infection* may affect the unborn child.

**transplant** ('transplahnt) 1. an organ or tissue taken from the body and grafted into another area of the same individual or another individual. 2. to transfer tissue from one part to another or from one individual to another.

**transplantation** (ˌtransplahn'tayshən) the transfer of living organs from one part of the body to another (autotransplant) or from one individual to another (allograft). Transplantation is often called grafting, though the latter is more commonly used to refer to the transfer of skin.

**transposition** (ˌtranzpə'zishən) 1. displacement of any of the viscera to the opposite side of the body. 2. the operation which partially removes a piece of tissue from one part of the body to another, complete severance being delayed until it has become established in its new position. *T. of the great vessels* a congenital abnormality of the heart in which the positions of the pulmonary artery and aorta are reversed.

**transsexualism** (tranz'seksyoooˌlizəm) a disturbance of gender identity; there is a persistent conviction that the person's true gender is opposite to the actual anatomical sex.

**transudate** ('transyuh'dayt) any fluid that passes through a membrane.

**transverse** (trans'vərz) cross-wise. *T. presentation* position of the fetus whereby it lies across the pelvis; this position must be corrected before normal birth can take place.

**transvestite** (tranz'vestiet) a person who experiences a habitual and strongly persistent desire to dress as a member of the opposite sex ('cross-dressing'), often for reasons of sexual gratification. The majority are male and have no desire to physically change sex (by surgery).

**tranylcypromine** (ˌtranil'sieprohmeen) a monoamine oxidase inhibitor used in psychiatry for the treatment of depression.

**trauma** ('trawmə) injury. *Birth t.* an injury to the infant sustained during the process of being born. In some psychiatric theories, the psychological shock produced in an infant by the experience of being born. *Psychological t.* an emotional shock that makes a lasting impression.

**treatment** ('treetmənt) the mode of dealing with a patient or disease. *Active t.* that in which specific medical or surgical treatment is undertaken. *Conservative t.* that which aims at preserving and restoring injured parts by natural means, e.g. rest, fluid replacement, etc., as opposed to radical or surgical methods. *Empirical t.* treatment based on observation of symptoms and not on science. *Palliative t.* that which relieves distressing symptoms but does not cure the disease. *Prophylactic t.* that which aims at the prevention of disease.

**Trematoda** (ˌtremə'tohdə, ˌtree-) a class of fluke worms, some of which are parasitic in humans. Many of them have freshwater snails as secondary hosts.

**tremor** ('tremə) an involuntary, muscular quivering which may be due to fatigue, emotion or disease. Tremor, first of one hand, and later affecting the other limbs, is the first symptom of Parkinsonism. *Intention t.* one that occurs on attempting a movement, as in disseminated sclerosis.

**Trendelenburg's position** (tren'delən bərgz) *F. Trendelenburg,*

*German surgeon, 1844–1924. See* POSITION.

**Trendelenburg's sign** a test of the stability of the hip. The patient stands on the affected leg and flexes the other knee and hip. If there is dislocation the pelvis is lower on the side of the flexed leg, which is the reverse of normal.

**trephine** (tri'fien, -'feen) an instrument for cutting out a circular piece of bone, usually from the skull. *Corneal t.* one used to cut out a piece of cornea in keratoplasty.

*Treponema* (ˌtrepə'neemə) a genus of spirochaetes. Anaerobic bacteria, they are motile, spiral and parasitic in humans and animals. *T. carateum* the causative agent of pinta. *T. pallidum* the causative agent of syphilis. *T. immobilization test* a serological test for syphilis. *T. pertenue* the causative agent of yaws (framboesia).

**tri-iodothyronine** (trieˌieədoh'thierəˌneen) a hormone produced by the thyroid gland together with thyroxine.

**triage** (tree'ahzh) [Fr.] 1. choosing, classifying or sorting. 2. a process by which a patient is assessed upon arrival to determine the urgency of the problem, and to designate appropriate health-care resources to care for the identified problem. *T. nurse* a registered nurse with specialist skills and knowledge who carries out the assessment and classification of casualties according to the type and severity of their injuries in order to assign them for treatment in the accident and emergency department.

**triamcinolone** (ˌtrieam'sinəˌlohn) a glucocorticoid steroid which does not cause salt and water retention; used to treat inflammatory disorders.

**triamterene** (trie'amtəˌreen) a diuretic that acts by antagonizing aldosterone and does not cause

potassium loss. Used in the treatment of oedema.

**triceps** ('trieseps) having three heads. *T. muscle* that situated on the back of the upper arm, which extends the forearm.

**trichiasis** (tri'kieəsis) 1. a condition of ingrowing hairs about an orifice, or ingrowing eyelashes. 2. the appearance of hair-like filaments in the urine.

**trichinosis** (ˌtriki'nohsis) a disease caused by eating underdone pork containing a parasite, *Trichinella spiralis*. This becomes deposited in muscle and causes stiffness and painful swelling. There may also be nausea, diarrhoea and fever. Trichiniasis.

**trichloroethylene** (trieˌklor.roh'ethiˌleen) a weak inhalation anaesthetic. Used in midwifery and for painful dressings and also in general anaesthesia in combination with other anaesthetics.

**trichology** (tri'koləjee) the study of hair.

*Trichomonas* (ˌtrikoh'mohnas) a genus of flagellate protozoa that are parasitic to humans. *T. hominis* infests the bowel and may cause dysentery. *T. tenax* infests the mouth and may be present in cases of pyorrhoea. *T. vaginalis* is commonly present in the vagina and may cause leukorrhoea and vaginitis.

**trichomoniasis** (ˌtrikohmə'nieəsis) infestation with a parasite of the genus *Trichomonas*.

*Trichophyton* (ˌtrikoh'fieton) a genus of fungi that affect the skin, nails and hair.

**trichophytosis** (ˌtrikohfie'tohsis) infection of the skin, nails or hair with one of the genus *Trichophyton*. *See* TINEA.

**trichosis** (tri'kohsis) any abnormal growth of hair.

**trichuriasis** (ˌtrikyuh'rieəsis) infestation by the whipworm.

*Trichuris* (tri'kyoo.ris) a genus of nematode worms which may infest the colon and cause diarrhoea. A whipworm.

**tricuspid** (trie'kuspid) having three flaps or cusps. *T. valve* that at the opening between the right atrium and the right ventricle of the heart.

**trifluoperazine** (‚triefloo.oh'pera‚zeen) a potent tranquillizing drug that is used in the treatment of schizophrenia and of psychoneuroses.

**trifocal** (trie'fohk'l) pertaining to a spectacle lens that has three foci, one for distant, one for intermediate and one for near vision.

**trigeminal** (trie'jemin'l) divided into three. *T. nerves* the fifth pair of cranial nerves, each of which is divided into three main branches and supplies one side of the face. *T. neuralgia* pain in the face which is confined to branches of the trigeminal nerve. Tic douloureux.

**trigger finger** ('trigə) a stenosing of the tendon sheath at the metacarpophalangeal joint, allowing flexion of the finger but not extension without assistance, when it 'clicks' into position.

**triglyceride** (trie'glisə‚ried) 'human fat', an ester of glycerol and three fatty acids.

**trigone** ('triegohn) a triangular area. *T. of the bladder* the triangular space on the floor of the bladder, between the ureteric openings and the urethral orifice.

**trimeprazine** (trie'meprə‚zeen) a sedative drug used for pre-operative medication, in the treatment of pruritus and to sedate children.

**trimester** (trie'mestə) a period of 3 months. *First t. of pregnancy* the first 3 months, during which rapid development is taking place.

**trimipramine** (trie'miprə‚meen) an antidepressant drug used particularly when anxiety and insomnia accompany depression.

**triplopia** (tri'plohpi.ə) a condition in which three images of an object are seen at the same time.

**trismus** ('trizməs) lockjaw; a tonic spasm of the muscles of the jaw.

**trisomy** ('triesəmee) the presence of an extra chromosome in each cell in addition to the normal paired set of 46. The cause of several chromosome disorders including Down's syndrome and Klinefelter's syndrome.

**trocar** ('trohkah) a pointed instrument used with a cannula for performing paracentesis.

**trochanter** (troh'kantə) either of two bony prominences below the neck of the femur. *Greater t.* that on the outer side forming the bony prominence of the hip. *Lesser t.* that on the inner side at the neck of the femur.

**trochlea** ('trokli.ə) any pulley-shaped structure, but particularly the fibrocartilage near the inner angular process of the frontal bone through which passes the tendon of the superior oblique muscle of the eye.

**trochlear** ('trokli.ə) relating to nutrition. *T. nerves* those that control the nutrition of a part. *T. ulcer* one arising from a failure in the nutrition of a part.

**trophoblast** ('trofoh‚blast) the layer of cells surrounding the blastocyst at the time of and responsible for implantation.

**tropia** ('trohpi.ə) a manifest squint, one that is present when both eyes are open.

**tropical** ('tropik'l) relating to the areas north and south of the equator, termed the tropics. *T. medicine* that concerned with diseases that are more prevalent in hot climates.

**Trousseau's sign** ('troosohz) *A. Trousseau, French physician, 1801–1867*. 1. spontaneous peripheral

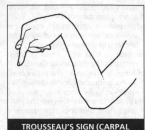

**TROUSSEAU'S SIGN (CARPAL SPASM) WITH HYPOCALCAEMIA**

venous thrombosis. 2. a sign for tetany in which carpal spasm can be elicited by compressing the upper arm and causing ischaemia to the nerves distally (*see* Figure).

**truancy** ('trooənsee) absence of a child from school without leave. A disorder of conduct which may result from emotional insecurity or a feeling of unfairness.

**truncus** ('trungkəs) a trunk; the main part of the body, or a part of it, from which other parts spring. *T. arteriosus* the arterial trunk connected to the fetal heart which develops into the aortic and pulmonary arteries.

**truss** (trus) an apparatus in the form of a belt with a pressure pad for retaining a hernia in place after reduction.

*Trypanosoma* (ˌtripənoh'sohmə) a genus of protozoan parasites which pass some of their life cycle in the blood of vertebrates, including humans. *T. gambiense* and *T. rhodesiense* are transmitted by the bite of the tsetse fly, and are the cause of sleeping sickness.

**trypanosomiasis** (ˌtripənohsə'mieə-sis) a disease caused by infestation with *Trypanosoma*. Sleeping sickness.

**trypsin** ('tripsin) a digestive enzyme that converts protein into amino acids.

**trypsinogen** (trip'sinəjən) the precursor of trypsin. It is secreted in the pancreatic juice and activated by the enterokinase of the intestinal juices into trypsin.

**tryptophan** ('triptəˌfan) one of the essential amino acids.

**tsetse fly** ('tetsee ˌflie, 'tse-) a fly of the genus *Glossina* which transmits the parasite *Trypanosoma* to humans, causing trypanosomiasis.

**TSH** thyroid-stimulating hormone.

**tsutsugamushi disease** (ˌtsoo-tsoogə'mooshee) scrub typhus, which occurs in Japan and is transmitted by the bite of a mite.

**tubal** ('tyoob'l) relating to a tube. *T. ligation* tying of the fallopian tubes as a method of female sterilization. *T. pregnancy* extrauterine pregnancy where the embryo develops in the uterine tube. Ectopic pregnancy.

**tube feeding** ('tyoob ˌfeeding) administration of liquid and semisolid foods through a nasogastric, gastrostomy or enterostomy tube. Tube feeds are administered to patients who are unable to take foods by mouth.

**Tubegauz** ('tyoob ˌgawz) a proprietary brand of woven circular bandage applied with a special applicator.

**tubercle** ('tyoobək'l) 1. a small nodule or a rounded prominence on a bone. 2. the specific lesion (a small nodule) produced by the tubercle bacillus.

**tubercular** (tyuh'bərkyuhlə) pertaining to tubercles.

**tuberculin** (tyuh'bərkyuhlin) the filtrate from a fluid medium in which *Mycobacterium tuberculosis* has been grown and which contains its toxins. *Old t.* prepared from the human bacillus and used in skin tests in diagnosing tuberculosis. *See* MANTOUX TEST and HEAF TEST.

**tuberculosis** (tyuhˌbərkyuh'lohsis) an infectious, inflammatory, notifiable disease, produced by the tubercle bacillus *Mycobacterium tuberculosis*, that is chronic in nature. *Bovine t.* a form found in cattle and spread by infected milk. *Miliary t.* a severe form with small tuberculous lesions spread throughout the body and severe toxaemia. *Open t.* any type of tuberculosis in which the organisms are being excreted from the body. *Pulmonary t.* that affecting the lungs; also termed phthisis. *T. of the spine* Pott's disease.

**tuberosity** (ˌtyoobəˈrositee) an elevation or protuberance on a bone to which tendons are attached.

**tuberous** (ˈtyoobə.rəs) covered with tubers. *T. sclerosis* a familial disease with tumours on the surfaces of the lateral ventricles of the brain and sclerotic patches on its surface; marked by mental deterioration and epileptic attacks.

**tubocurarine** (ˌtyoobohkyooˈrahreen) a preparation of curare used to secure skeletal muscle relaxation.

**tubule** (ˈtyoobyool) a small tube. *Renal* or *uriniferous t.* the essential secreting tube of the kidney.

**tularaemia** (ˌtooləˈreemi.ə) a plague-like disease of rodents, caused by *Francisella* (*Pasteurella*) *tularensis*, which is transmissible to humans. The illness can be contracted by handling diseased animals or their hides, eating infected wild game or being bitten by insects that have fed on infected animals. It causes fever and headache; the lymph glands enlarge and may suppurate.

**tumefaction** (ˌtyoomiˈfakshən) a swelling or the process of becoming swollen. Tumescence.

**tumescence** (ˌtyooˈmesəns) 1. a swelling or enlarging of a part. 2. a swollen condition. 3. a penile erection.

**tumour** (ˈtyoomə) an abnormal swelling. The term is usually applied to a morbid growth of tissue which may be benign or malignant. A neoplasm. *Benign* or *innocent t.* one that does not infiltrate or cause metastases, and is unlikely to recur if removed. *Malignant t.* one that invades and destroys tissue and can spread to neighbouring tissues, and to more distant sites via the blood and the lymphatic systems.

**tunica** (ˈtyoonikə) a coat, a covering, or the lining of a vessel. *T. adventitia, t. media, t. intima* the outer, middle and inner coats of an artery, respectively. *T. vaginalis* the membrane covering the front and sides of the testis.

**tuning fork** (ˈtyooning ˌfawk) a metal instrument used for testing hearing by means of the sounds produced by its vibration.

**tunnel** (ˈtun'l) in anatomy, a canal through a structure. *Carpal t.* the osteofibrous channel in the wrist between the carpal bones and tissue covering the flexor tendons. *C. tunnel syndrome* pain and tingling in the hand and fingers caused by compression of the median nerve in the carpal tunnel. *T. vision* vision that is restricted to the central field. Occurs in chronic glaucoma and in retinitis pigmentosa.

**turbinate** (ˈtərbinət, -ˌnayt) scroll-shaped. *T. bone* one of the three long thin plates that form the walls of the nasal cavity.

**turgid** (ˈtərjid) swollen or distended.

**Turner's syndrome** (ˈtərnəz) *H.H. Turner, American physician, 1892–1970.* A chromosomal defect in females, causing short stature. Classically, an absence of one X chromosome. Affects 1 in 3000 live female births. The majority have streak ovaries leading to an absence of puberty and infertility. Other features may include webbing of the neck, cubitus valgus, nail abnormalities and coarctation of the aorta. Intelligence is usually normal.

**twin** (twin) one of a pair of individuals who have developed in the uterus together. *Binovular (dizygotic) t.* each twin has developed from a separate ovum; fraternal twins. *Uniovular (monozygotic) t.* both twins have developed from the same cell; identical twins.

**tympanectomy** (ˌtimpəˈnektəmee) excision of the tympanic membrane.

**tympanites** (ˌtimpəˈnieteez) distension of the abdomen by accumulation of gas in the intestine or the peritoneal cavity.

**tympanitis** (ˌtimpəˈnietis) inflammation of the middle ear; otitis media.

**tympanoplasty** ('timpənohˌplastee) an operation to reconstruct the eardrum and restore conductivity to the middle ear. Myringoplasty.

**tympanosclerosis** (ˌtimpənohsklə-ˈrohsis) fibrosis and the formation of calcified deposits in the middle ear which lead to deafness.

**tympanum** ('timpənəm) 1. the middle ear. 2. the eardrum or tympanic membrane.

**type** (tiep) the general or prevailing character of any particular case of disease, person, substance, etc. *Asthenic t.* a type of physical constitution, with long limbs, small trunk, flat chest and weak muscles. *Athletic t.* a type of physical constitution with broad shoulders, deep chest, flat abdomen, thick neck and good muscular development. *Blood t's see* BLOOD GROUP. *Phage t.* a subgroup of a bacterial species susceptible to a particular bacteriophage and demonstrated by phagetyping (*see* PHAGE). Also called lysotype and phagotype. *Pyknic t.* a type of physical constitution marked by rounded body, large chest, thick shoulders, broad head and short neck.

**type A behaviour** a behaviour pattern associated with the development of coronary heart disease, characterized by excessive competitiveness and aggression and a fast-paced lifestyle. Research has shown that this type of behaviour is associated with coronary artery disease and myocardial infarction. The opposite type of behaviour, exhibited by individuals who are relaxed, unhurried and less aggressive, is called type B and is associated with a lower risk of heart disease.

**typhoid fever** ('tiefoyd) enteric fever. A notifiable infectious disease caused by *Salmonella typhi*, which is transmitted by water, milk or other foods, especially shellfish, that have been contaminated. There is high fever, a red rash, delirium and sometimes intestinal haemorrhage. Recovery usually begins during the fourth week of the disease. A person who has had typhoid fever gains immunity from it but may become a carrier. Although perfectly well, the person harbours the bacteria and passes them out in the faeces. The typhoid bacillus often lodges in the gallbladder of carriers.

**typhus** ('tiefəs) an acute, notifiable, infectious disease caused by species of the parasitic microorganism *Rickettsia*. There is high fever, a widespread red rash and severe headache. Typhus is likely to occur where there is overcrowding, lack of personal cleanliness and bad hygienic conditions, because the infection is spread by bites of infected lice or by rat fleas. *Scrub t.* a form spread by mites and widespread in the Far East. Tsutsugamushi disease.

**tyramine** ('tierəˌmeen, 'ti-) an enzyme present in cheese, game, broad-bean pods, yeast extracts, wine and strong beer, which has a similar effect in the body to that of adrenaline. Foodstuffs containing tyramine should be avoided by patients taking monoamine oxidase inhibitors.

**tyrosine** ('tieroh,seen, 'ti-) an essential amino acid which is the product of phenylalanine metabolism. In some diseases, especially of the liver, it is present as a deposit in the urine. It is a precursor of catecholamines, melanin and thyroid hormones.

**tyrosinosis** (,tierohsi'nohsis, ,ti-) a congenital condition in which there is an error of metabolism and phenylalanine cannot be reduced to tyrosine. Hepatic failure may occur.

# u

**UKCC** United Kingdom Central Council for Nursing, Midwifery and Health Visiting.

**ulcer** ('ulsə) an erosion or loss of continuity of the skin or of a mucous membrane, often accompanied by suppuration. *Decubitus u.* a pressure sore caused by lying immobile for long periods of time. *Duodenal u.* a peptic ulcer in the duodenum. *Gastric u.* one in the lining of the stomach. *Gravitational u.* a varicose ulcer of the leg which heals with difficulty because of its dependent position and the poor venous return. *Gummatous u.* one arising in late non-infective syphilis; it is slow to heal. *Indolent u.* one that is painless and heals slowly. *Peptic u.* one that occurs on the mucous membrane of either the stomach or duodenum. *Perforating u.* one that erodes through the thickness of the wall of an organ. *Rodent u.* a slow-growing epithelioma of the face which may cause much local destruction and ulceration, but does not give rise to metastases. Basal cell carcinoma. *Trophic u.* one due to a failure of nutrition of a part. *Varicose u.* gravitational ulcer.

**ulcerative** ('ulsə,raytiv) characterized by ulceration (the formation of ulcers). *U. colitis* inflammation and ulceration of the colon and rectum of unknown cause.

**ultrasonic** (,ultrə'sonik) relating to sound waves having a frequency range beyond the upper limit perceived by the human ear. These waves are widely used instead of X-rays, particularly in the examination of structures not opaque to X-rays.

**ultrasonogram** an echo picture obtained from using ultrasound.

**ultrasonography** (,ultrəsə'nogrəfee) a radiological technique in which deep structures of the body are visualized by recording the reflections (echoes) of ultrasonic waves directed into the tissues.

**ultrasound** ('ultrə,sownd) ultrasonic waves used to examine the interior organs of the body. These waves can also be used in the treatment of soft-tissue pain, and to break up renal calculi or the crystalline lens when cataract is present. *U. screening* a method of body imaging based on the reflectivity of sound. Ultrasound scanning is noninvasive and is widely used in obstetrics to detect the site of the placenta, the presence of fetal abnormalities and the sex of the fetus; it will reveal a multiple pregnancy at an early stage. Also used by other medical disciplines.

**ultraviolet light** (,ultrə'violət) used to promote vitamin D formation and for treatment of certain skin conditions.

**ultraviolet rays** short wavelength electromagnetic rays. They are present in sunlight and cause tanning and sunburn.

**umbilical cord** (um'bilik'l) arises from the placenta and enters the fetus at the site of the future navel, providing the nutritional, hormonal and immunological link between mother and fetus during pregnancy.

**umbilicus** (um'bilikəs, ‚umbi'liekəs) the navel; the circular depressed scar in the centre of the abdomen where the umbilical cord of the fetus was attached.

**unconditioned response** (unkən‚dishənd ris'pons) an unlearned response, i.e. one that occurs naturally.

**unconscious** (un'konshəs) 1. insensible; incapable of responding to sensory stimuli and of having subjective experiences. 2. that part of mental activity which includes primitive or repressed wishes, concealed from consciousness by the psychological censor. *Collective u.* in Jungian psychology, the portion of the unconscious which is theoretically common to human beings.

**unconsciousness** (un'konshəsnəs) the state of being unconscious. This may vary in depth from deep unconsciousness, when no response can be obtained, through to lesser degrees of unconsciousness when the patient can be roused by painful stimuli, to a level when the patient can be roused by speech or non-painful stimuli. Deep prolonged unconsciousness is known as COMA.

**undecylenic acid** (‚undeesie'leenik) an antifungal agent used in the treatment of such infections as athlete's foot. May be used in powder, ointment, lotion or spray form.

**undine** (undeen) a glass flask with a spout used for irrigation of the eye.

**undulant** ('undyuhlənt) rising and falling like a wave. *U. fever see* BRUCELLOSIS.

**unguentum** (ung'gwentəm) an ointment.

**unilateral** (‚yooni'latə.rəl) on one side only.

**union** ('yooni.ən) 1. a joining together. 2. the repair of tissue after separation by incision or fracture. *See* CALLUS and HEALING.

**uniovular** (‚yooni'ohvyuhlə, -'ov-) from one ovum. *U. twins* identical twins, developed from one ovum.

**unipara** (‚yooni'parə) a woman who has had only one child.

**unit** ('yoonit) 1. a single thing. 2. a standard of measurement. *Intensive care u.* a hospital department reserved for those with severe medical or surgical disorders. *International insulin u.* a measurement of the pure crystalline insulin arrived at by biological assay. *SI u.* one of the various units of measurement making up the Système International d'Unités (International System of Units).

**United Kingdom Central Council for Nursing, Midwifery and Health Visiting** (yoo‚nietid 'kingdəm ‚sentrəl ‚kownsil) abbreviated UKCC. A statutory body set up as a result of the 1979 Nurses, Midwives and Health Visitors Act. Provides, with the four National Boards of England, Northern Ireland, Wales and Scotland, the statutory organization responsible for the education and training regulations, together with the maintenance of professional standards, of nurses, midwives and health visitors. *See* Appendices.

**universal precautions** (yooni‚vərsəl pri'kawshənz) abbreviated UP. A concept developed by nurses during the mid-1980s (largely as a response to human immunodeficiency virus, or HIV, epidemics) that assumes all patients are potentially infected with BLOOD-BORNE VIRUSES; consequently, universal blood and body fluid infection control precautions are used for all patients, all the time. This concept has been further developed and is known as STANDARD PRECAUTIONS. *See also* BODY SUBSTANCE ISOLATION, INFECTION (CONTROL) and Appendices.

**urachal** (‚yoo'rayk'l) referring to the urachus. *U. cyst* a congenital abnormality in which a small cyst persists along the course of the urachus. *U. fistula* one that forms when the urachus fails to close. Urine may leak from the umbilicus.

**urachus** ('yooə.rəkəs) a tubular canal existing in the fetus, connecting the bladder with the umbilicus. In the adult it persists in the form of a solid fibrous cord.

**uraemia** (yuh'reemi.ə) 1. an excess in the blood of urea, creatinine and other nitrogenous end-products of protein and amino acid metabolism; sometimes referred to as azotaemia. 2. in current usage, the entire complex of signs and symptoms of chronic renal failure. Depending upon the cause it may or may not be reversible. Uraemia leads to vomiting and nausea, headache, weakness, metabolic disturbances, convulsions and coma (*see* RENAL (FAILURE)).

**urate** ('yooə.rayt) a salt of uric acid. *Sodium u.* a compound generally found in concentration around joints in cases of gout.

**urea** (yuh'reeə, 'yooə.ri.ə) carbamide. A white crystalline substance which is an end-product of protein metabolism and the chief nitrogenous constituent of urine. It is a diuretic. The normal daily output is about 33 g. *Blood u.* that which is present in the blood. Normal value is 20–40 mg/100 ml.

**ureter** (yuh'reetə, 'yooə.ritə) one of the two long narrow tubes that convey the urine from the kidney to the bladder.

**ureterectomy** (yuh‚reetə'rektəmee) the surgical removal of a ureter.

**ureteric** (‚yuhree'terik) relating to the ureter. *U. catheter see* CATHETER *U. transplantation* an operation in which the ureters are divided from the bladder and implanted in the colon or loop of ileum. Congenital defects or malignant growth may make this necessary.

**ureterocele** (yuh'reetə.roh‚seel) a cystic enlargement of the wall of the ureter at its entry into the bladder.

**ureterolith** (yuh'reetə.roh‚lith) a calculus in a ureter.

**ureterolithotomy** (yuh‚reetə.rohli-'thotəmee) removal of a calculus from the ureter.

**ureteronephrectomy** (yuh‚reetə.roh-nə'frektəmee) surgical removal of a kidney and its ureter.

**ureterostomy** (yuh‚reetə'rostəmee) the surgical creation of a permanent opening through which the ureter discharges urine.

**ureterovaginal** (yuh‚reetə.rohvə-'jien'l, -'vajin'l) relating to the ureter and vagina. *U. fistula* an opening into the ureter by which urine escapes via the vagina.

**urethra** (yuh'reethrə) the canal through which the urine is discharged from the bladder. The male urethra is about 18 cm long and the female about 3.5 cm.

**urethritis** (‚yooə.ri'thrietis) inflammation of the urethra. The condition is frequently a symptom of gonorrhoea but may be caused by other infectious organisms. *Nonspecific u.* abbreviated NSU. A sexually transmitted inflammation of the urethra caused by a variety of organisms other than gonococci. *See* NON-SPECIFIC (URETHRITIS).

**urethrocele** (yuh'reethroh‚seel) a prolapse of the female urethral wall which may result from damage to the pelvic floor during childbirth.

**urethrography** (ˌyooə.rɪ'throgrəfee) radiographic examination of the urethra. A radio-opaque contrast medium is inserted by catheter.

**urethroscope** (yuh'reethrə ˌskohp) an instrument for examining the interior of the urethra.

**uric acid** ('yooə.rik) lithic acid, the end-product of nucleic acid metabolism, a normal constituent of urine. Its accumulation in the blood produces uricacidaemia. Renal calculi are frequently formed of it.

**uricosuric** (ˌyooə.rikoh'syooə.rik) any drug that promotes the excretion of uric acid in the urine.

**urinalysis** (ˌyooə.ri'nalisis) the bacteriological or chemical examination of the urine.

**urinary** ('yooə.rinə ˌree) relating to urine. **U. tract** the system that conducts urine from the kidneys to the exterior, including the ureters, the bladder and the urethra.

**urination** (ˌyooə.ri'nayshən) micturition. The act of passing urine.

**urine** ('yooə.rin) the clear fluid of a varying straw colour secreted by the kidneys and excreted through the bladder and urethra. It is composed of 96% water and 4% solid constituents, the most important being urea and uric acid. Specific gravity is 1.017–1.020; slightly acidic. **Residual u.** that which remains in the bladder after micturition. **U. retention** the inability to urinate voluntarily or to empty a full bladder.

**urinometer** (ˌyooə.ri'nomitə) an instrument used for measuring the specific gravity of urine.

**urobilin** (ˌyooə.roh'bielin) the main pigment of urine, derived from urobilinogen.

**urobilinogen** (ˌyooə.rohbie'linəjən) a pigment derived from bilirubin which, on oxidation, forms urobilin.

**urochrome** ('yooə.roh ˌkrohm) the yellow pigment which colours urine.

**urodynamics** (ˌyooə.rohdie'namiks) the dynamics of the propulsion and flow of urine in the urinary tract.

**urogenital** (ˌyooə.roh'jenit'l) relating to the urinary and genital organs. Urinogenital.

**urogram** ('yooə.roh ˌgram) a radiographic image obtained by urography.

**urography** (yuh'rogrəfee) radiographic examination of the urinary tract after the injection of a radio-opaque, water-soluble, iodine-containing medium.

**urokinase** (ˌyooə.roh'kienayz) an enzyme in urine which is secreted by the kidneys and causes fibrinolysis. In certain diseases it may cause bleeding from the kidneys.

**urolith** ('yooə.roh ˌlith) a calculus in the urinary tract.

**urology** (yuh'roləjee) the study of diseases of the urinary tract.

**urostomy** (yuh'rostəmee) an artificial urinary conduit for deflecting urine from the ureters to the abdominal wall.

**urticaria** (ˌərti'kair.i.ə) nettle rash or hives. An acute or chronic skin condition characterized by the recurrent appearance of an eruption of weals, causing great irritation. The cause may be certain foods, infection, drugs or emotional stress. *See* ALLERGY.

**uterine** ('yootə ˌrien) relating to the uterus.

**uterosalpingography** (ˌyootə.rohˌsalping'gogrəfee) radiographic examination of the uterus and the uterine tubes.

**uterovesical** (ˌyootə.roh'vesik'l) referring to the uterus and bladder. **U. pouch** the fold of peritoneum between the two organs.

**uterus** ('yootə.rəs) the womb; a triangular, hollow, muscle organ situ-

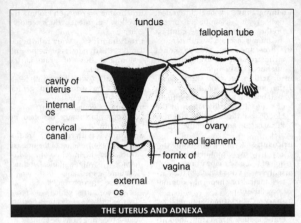

**THE UTERUS AND ADNEXA**

ated in the pelvic cavity between the bladder and the rectum (*see* Figure). Its function is the nourishment and protection of the fetus during pregnancy and its expulsion at term. *Bicornuate u.* one having two horns. A congenital malformation; see BICORNUATE. *Gravid u.* the pregnant uterus. *U. didelphys* a double uterus caused by the failure of union of the two Müllerian ducts from which it is formed.

**utricle** ('yootrik'l) the delicate membranous sac in the bony vestibule of the ear.

**uvea** ('yoovi.ə) uveal tract. The pigmented layer of the eye, consisting of the iris, ciliary body and choroid.

**uveitis** (,yoovi'ietis) inflammation of the uveal tract.

**uvula** ('yoovyuhlə) the small fleshy appendage which is the free edge of the soft palate, hanging from the roof of the mouth.

# V

**vaccination** (ˌvaksiˈnayshən) the introduction of vaccine into the body to produce immunity to a specific disease.

**vaccine** ('vakseen) a suspension of killed or attenuated organisms (viruses, bacteria or rickettsiae), administered for prevention, amelioration or treatment of infectious diseases. *Attenuated v.* one prepared from living organisms which, through long cultivation, have lost their virulence. *Bacille Calmette–Guérin v.* an attenuated bovine bacillus vaccine giving immunity from tuberculosis. *Sabin v.* an attenuated poliovirus vaccine that can be administered by mouth, in a syrup or on sugar. *Salk v.* one prepared from an inactivated strain of poliomyelitis virus. *TAB v.* a sterile solution of the organisms that cause typhoid and paratyphoid A and B. Paratyphoid C may now be included. *Triple v.* one that protects against diphtheria, tetanus and whooping cough.

**vaccinia** (vakˈsinɪ.ə) cowpox; a virus infection of cows, which may be transmitted to humans by contact with the lesions. A local pustular eruption is produced. Also known as cowpox.

**vacuum** ('vakyoom) a space from which air or gas has been extracted. *V. extractor* an instrument known as a Ventouse is used to assist delivery of the fetus. A suction cup is attached to the head and a vacuum created slowly. Gentle traction is applied, which is synchronized with the uterine contractions.

**vagal** ('vaygˈl) relating to the vagus nerve.

**vagina** (vəˈjienə) the canal, lined with mucous membrane, that leads from the cervix of the uterus to the vulva.

**vaginismus** (ˌvajiˈnizməs) a painful spasm of the muscles of the vagina, occurring usually when the vulva or vagina is touched, resulting in painful sexual intercourse or dyspareunia.

**vaginitis** (ˌvajiˈnietis) inflammation of the vagina. *Atrophic* or *postmenopausal v.* inflammation caused by degenerative changes in the mucous lining of the vagina and insufficient oestrogen secretion. Adhesions may occur, partially closing the vagina. *Trichomonas v.* infection caused by T. vaginalis, a protozoon that causes a thin, yellowish discharge, giving rise to local tenderness and pruritus.

**vagotomy** (vayˈgotəmee) surgical incision of the vagus nerve or any of its branches. A treatment for gastric or duodenal ulcer. *Highly selective v.* division of only those vagal fibres supplying the acid-secreting glands of the stomach. *Medical v.* interruption of impulses carried by the vagus nerve by administration of suitable drugs.

**vagus** ('vaygəs) the tenth cranial nerve, arising in the medulla and providing the parasympathetic nerve supply to the organs in the thorax and abdomen. *V. resection* vagotomy.

**valgus** ('valgəs) a displacement outwards, particularly of the feet. *See* GENU, HALLUX, TALIPES.

**validity** (val'lidətee) the extent to which a measure, indicator or method of data collection possesses the quality of being sound or true, as far as can be judged.

**valine** ('valəen) an essential amino acid formed by the digestion of dietary protein.

**Valium** ('vali.əm) trade name for a preparation of diazepam, an anxiolytic and skeletal muscle relaxant.

**Valsalva's manoeuvre** (val'salvəz mə,noovə) *A.M. Valsalva, Italian anatomist, 1666–1723.* Technique for increasing the intrathoracic pressure by closing the mouth and nostrils and blowing out the cheeks, thereby forcing air back into the nasopharynx. When the breath is released, the intrathoracic pressure drops and the blood is quickly propelled through the heart, producing an increase in the heart rate (tachycardia) and the blood pressure. Immediately after this event a reflex bradycardia ensues. Valsalva's manoeuvre occurs when a person strains to defecate or urinate, uses the arm and upper trunk muscles to move up in bed, or strains during coughing, gagging or vomiting. The increased pressure, immediate tachycardia and reflex bradycardia can bring about cardiac arrest in vulnerable heart patients.

**valve** (valv) 1. a means of regulating the flow of liquid or gas through a pipe. 2. a fold of membrane in a passage or tube, so placed as to permit passage of fluid in one direction only. Valves are important structures in the heart, in veins and in lymph vessels. *Semilunar v.* either of two valves at the junction of the pulmonary artery and aorta, respectively, with the heart.

**valvotomy** (val'votəmee) valvulotomy. A surgical operation to open up a fibrosed valve, e.g. mitral valvotomy to relieve mitral stenosis.

**valvulitis** (,valvyuh'lietis) inflammation of a valve, particularly of the heart.

**vancomycin** (,vankoh'miesin) an antibiotic highly effective against Gram-positive bacteria, especially staphylococci. The toxic effects are quite severe and may include damage to the eighth cranial (vestibulocochlear) nerve, and renal disorders.

**vaporizer** ('vaypə,riezə) an apparatus for producing a very fine spray of a liquid.

**variable** ('vairee.əb'l) in social research, a characteristic which can be measured and which may vary along a continuum (e.g. recording of foot size in a population being studied), be more discrete (e.g. in family size) or be bipolar (e.g. sex).

**varicella** (,vari'selə) chickenpox. An infectious disease of childhood with an incubation period of 12–20 days. There is slight fever and an eruption of transparent vesicles on the chest, on the first day of disease; these appear in successive crops all over the body. The vesicles soon dry up, sometimes leaving shallow pits in the skin. The disease is usually mild, but may be severe in neonates, adults and those who are immunocompromised. Chickenpox is a notifiable disease in Scotland.

**varicose** ('vari,kohs) swollen or dilated. *V. ulcer* gravitational ulcer. *See* ULCER. *V. veins* a dilated and twisted condition of the veins (usually those of the leg) caused by structural changes in the walls or valves of the vessels.

**variola** (və'rieələ) smallpox.

**varix** ('vair.riks) an enlarged or varicose vein.

**varus** ('vair.rəs) a displacement inwards. *See* GENU, HALLUX, TALIPES.

**vas** (vas) *pl.* vasa. A vessel or duct. *V. deferens* one of a pair of excretory ducts conveying the semen from the epididymis to the urethra. *V. efferens* one of the many small tubes that convey semen from the testis to the epididymis. *Vasa vasorum* the minute nutrient vessels that supply the walls of the arteries and veins.

**vascular** ('vaskyuhlə) relating to, or consisting largely of, blood vessels. *V. system* the cardiovascular system.

**vascularization** (,vaskyuhlə.rie-'zayshən) the development of new blood vessels within a tissue.

**vasculitis** (,vaskyuh'lietis) angiitis; inflammation of a blood vessel. *Allergic v.* a severe allergic response to drugs or to cold. Arising in small arteries or veins, with fibrosis and thrombi formation.

**vasectomy** (və'sektəmee) excision of a part of the vas deferens. If performed bilaterally, sterility results. Employed as a method of contraception.

**vasoconstrictor** (,vayzohkən'striktə) any agent that causes contraction of a blood vessel wall, and therefore a decrease in the blood flow and a rise in the blood pressure.

**vasodilator** (,vayzohdie'laytə) any agent that causes an increase in the lumen of blood vessels, and therefore an increase in the blood flow and a fall in the blood pressure.

**vasomotor** (,vayzoh'mohtə) controlling the muscles of blood vessels, both dilator and constrictor. *V. centre* nerve cells in the medulla oblongata controlling the vasomotor nerves. *V. nerves* sympathetic nerves regulating the tension of the blood vessels.

**vasopressin** (,vayzoh'presin) antidiuretic hormone (ADH). A hormone from the posterior lobe of the pituitary gland which causes constriction of plain muscle fibres and reabsorption of water in the renal tubules. Used in the treatment of diabetes insipidus and bleeding from oesophageal varices.

**vasovagal** (,vayzoh'vayg'l) vascular and vagal. *V. attack* fainting or syncope, often evoked by emotional stress associated with fear and pain. There is postural hypotension.

**vector** ('vektə) 1. an animal that carries organisms or parasites from one host to another, either to a member of the same species or to one of another species. 2. a quantity with magnitude and direction. *Electrocardiographic v.* the area of the heart that is monitored during electrocardiographic investigation.

**vecturonium** (,vektyuh'rohniəm) a muscle relaxant used in general anaesthesia

**vegan** ('veegən) a vegetarian who excludes all animal protein from the diet.

**vegetarian** (,veji'tair.reeən) a person who eats only food of vegetable origin. *V. diet* one in which no meat is eaten. A *lacto-vegetarian* diet prohibits the intake of meat, poultry, fish and eggs. An *ovo-lacto-vegetarian* diet allows all foods from plants plus eggs, milk and other dairy products. An *ovo-vegetarian* diet allows eggs and foods of plant origin, but prohibits all animal and dairy products.

**vegetation** (,veji'tayshən) in pathology, a plant-like outgrowth. *Adenoid v.* overgrowth of lymphoid tissue in the nasopharynx.

**vehicle** ('veeək'l) in pharmacy, a substance or medium in which a drug is administered.

**vein** (vayn) a vessel carrying blood from the capillaries back to the heart. It has thin walls and a lining endothelium from which the venous valves are formed.

**venepuncture** ('veni,pungkchə) the insertion of a needle into a vein for the introduction of a drug or fluid or for the withdrawal of blood.

**venereal** (və'niə.ri.əl) pertaining to or caused by sexual intercourse. *V. disease* a disease transmitted by sexual intercourse or other genital contact. In the UK, GONORRHOEA, SYPHILIS and CHANCROID are defined in law as venereal diseases. The term venereal disease (VD) is being replaced by the term SEXUALLY TRANSMITTED INFECTION.

**venereology** (və,niə.ri'oləjee) the study and treatment of venereal diseases.

**venesection** ('veni,sekshən) phlebotomy. Surgical blood-letting by opening a vein or introducing a wide-bore needle. Performed on blood donors and occasionally to relieve venous congestion.

**venogram** ('veenə,gram) 1. a graphic recording of the pulse in a vein. 2. a radiograph taken during venography.

**venography** (vee'nogrəfee) radiographic examination of a vein after the instillation of a contrast medium to trace its pathway.

**venom** ('venəm) a poison secreted by an insect, snake or other animal. *Russell's viper v.* the venom of the Russell viper (*Vipera russelli*), which acts in vitro as an intrinsic thromboplastin and is useful in defining deficiencies of clotting factor X.

**venous** ('veenəs) pertaining to the veins. *V. sinus* one of 14 channels, similar to veins, by which blood leaves the cerebral circulation.

**ventilation** (,venti'layshən) 1. the process or act of supplying a house or room continuously with fresh air. 2. in respiratory phy-

siology, the process of exchange of air between the lungs and the ambient air. *Pulmonary v.* (usually measured in litres per minute) refers to the total exchange, whereas *alveolar v.* refers to the effective ventilation of the alveoli, where gas exchange with the blood takes place. 3. in psychiatry, the free discussion of one's problems or grievances.

**ventilator** ('venti,laytə) an apparatus designed to qualify the air that is breathed through it either intermittently or continuously. Ventilators provide an intermittent flow of air and/or oxygen under pressure and are connected to the patient by a tube inserted through the mouth, the nose or an opening in the trachea.

**Ventimask** ('venti,mahsk) an oxygen mask that provides oxygen enrichment of the inspired air while eliminating the need to rebreathe the expired carbon dioxide.

**Ventolin** ('ventohlin) trade name for a salbutamol metered-dose inhaler; a bronchodilator.

**Ventouse** (,ven'tooz) *see* VACUUM EXTRACTOR.

**ventricle** ('ventrik'l) a small pouch or cavity; applied especially to the lower chambers of the heart and to the four cavities of the brain.

**ventricular** (ven'trikyuhlə) pertaining to a ventricle. *V. folds* the outer folds of mucous membrane forming the false vocal cords. *V. septal defect* abbreviated VSD. Congenital abnormality in which there is communication between the two ventricles of the heart as a result of maldevelopment of the intraventricular septum.

**ventriculography** (ven,trikyuh'logrəfee) 1. radiographic examination of the ventricles of the heart using a radio-opaque contrast medium. 2. radiographic examination of the ventricles of the brain after the injection of air or a contrast medium through a burr hole.

**Venturi mask** (ven'tyooə.ree ‚mahsk) *G.B. Venturi, Italian physicist, 1746–1822.* A type of disposable mask used to deliver a controlled oxygen concentration to a patient. The flow of 100% oxygen through the mask draws in a controlled amount of room air (21% oxygen). Commonly available masks deliver 24, 28, 35 or 40% oxygen. At concentrations above 24%, humidification may be required.

**Venturi nebulizer** a type of nebulizer used in AEROSOL therapy. The pressure drop of gas flowing through the nebulizer draws liquid from a capillary tube. As the liquid enters the gas stream it breaks up into a spray of small droplets.

**venule** ('venyool) a minute vein which collects blood from the capillaries.

**verapamil** (ve'rapə‚mil) a coronary dilator used in the treatment of supraventricular tachycardia and of angina pectoris.

**verbigeration** (‚vərbijə'rayshən) the monotonous repetition of phrases or meaningless words.

**vermicide** ('vərmi‚sied) an agent that destroys intestinal worms; an anthelmintic.

**vermiform** ('vərmi‚fawm) wormshaped. *V. appendix* the wormshaped structure attached to the caecum.

**vermifuge** ('vərmi‚fyooj) an agent that expels intestinal worms; an anthelmintic.

**verminous** ('vərminəs) infested with worms or other animal parasites, such as lice.

**vernix** ('vərniks) [L.] *varnish. V. caseosa* the fatty covering on the skin of the fetus during the last months of pregnancy. It consists of cells and sebaceous material.

**verruca** (və'rookə) a wart. Hypertrophy of the prickle cell layer of

the epidermis and thickening of the horny layer. A virus is the causative organism. *V. acuminata* a venereal wart that appears on the external genitalia. *V. plana* a small, smooth, usually skin-coloured or light-brown, slightly raised wart, sometimes occurring in great numbers; seen most often in children. *V. plantaris* a viral epidermal tumour on the sole of the foot.

**version** ('vərshən, -zhən) the turning of a part; applied particularly to the turning of a fetus in order to facilitate delivery. *External v.* manipulation of the uterus through the abdominal wall in order to change the position of the fetus. *Internal v.* rotation of the fetus by means of manipulation with one hand in the vagina. *Podalic v.* turning of the fetus so that the head is uppermost and the feet presenting. *Spontaneous v.* one that occurs naturally without the application of force.

**vertebra** ('vərtibrə) one of the 33 irregular bones forming the spinal column: 7 cervical, 12 thoracic, 5 lumbar, 5 sacral (sacrum) and 4 coccygeal (coccyx) vertebrae.

**vertebral** ('vərtibrəl) pertaining to a vertebra. *V. column* the spine or backbone.

**vertebrobasilar** (‚vərtibroh'basilə) pertaining to the vertebral and the basilar arteries. *V. disease* a condition affecting the flow of blood through the vertebral and basilar arteries which may cause recurrent attacks of blindness, diplopia, vertigo, dysarthria and hemiparesis.

**vertex** ('vərteks) the crown of the head. *V. presentation* position of the fetus such that the crown of the head appears in the vagina first.

**vertigo** ('vərti‚goh) a feeling of rotation or of going round, in either oneself or one's surroundings, particularly associated with disease of the cerebellum and the vestibular nerve of the ear. It may occur in diplopia or Menière's syndrome.

**vesicle** ('vesik'l) 1. in anatomy, a small bladder, usually containing fluid. 2. a very small blister, usually containing serum. *Seminal v.* one of a pair of sacs which arise from the vas deferens near the bladder and contain semen.

**vesicoureteric** (‚vesikoh.yoor'terik) relating to the urinary bladder and the ureters. *V. reflux* the passing of urine backwards up the ureter during micturition. A cause of pyelonephritis in children.

**vesicovaginal** (‚vesikohvə'jien'l) relating to the bladder and vagina. *See* FISTULA.

**vesicular** (ve'sikyuhlə) relating to or containing vesicles. *V. breathing* the soft murmur of normal respiration, as heard on auscultation. *V. mole* hydatidiform mole.

**vesiculitis** (ve‚sikyuh'lietis) inflammation of a vesicle, particularly the seminal vesicles.

**vessel** ('ves'l) a tube, duct or canal for conveying fluid, usually blood or lymph.

**vestibular** (ve'stibyuhlə) relating to a vestibule. *V. glands* those in the vestibule of the vagina, including Bartholin's glands. *V. nerve* a branch of the auditory nerve supplying the semicircular canals and concerned with balance and equilibrium.

**vestibule** ('vesti‚byool) a space or cavity at the entrance to another structure. *V. of the ear* the cavity at the entrance to the cochlea. *V. of the vagina* the space between the labia minora at the entrance to the vagina.

**vestibulocochlear** (ve‚stibyuhloh-'kokli.ə) pertaining to the vestibule of the ear and the cochlea. *V. nerve* the eighth cranial nerve. Also known as the auditory nerve.

**vestigial** (ve'stiji.əl) rudimentary. Referring to the remains of an anatomical structure which, being of no further use, has atrophied.

**viable** ('vieəb'l) capable of independent life.

**Viagra** (vie'agrə) a trade name for the oral drug sildenafil citrate, used for the treatment of erectile dysfunction. Viagra increases the man's ability to achieve and maintain a penile erection during sexual stimulation. It is given by mouth and is only available on medical prescription after appropriate assessment.

**Vibrio** ('vibrioh) a genus of Gram-negative bacteria, curved and motile by means of flagellae. *V. cholerae* that which causes cholera.

**vicarious** (vi'kairi.əs) 1. obtained or undergone at second hand through sympathetic participation in another's experiences. 2. substituted for another; used when one organ functions instead of another.

**villus** ('viləs) a small finger-like process projecting from a surface. *Chorionic v. see* CHORIONIC. *Intestinal villi* those of the mucous membrane of the small intestine, each of which contains a blood capillary and a lacteal.

**vinblastine** (vin'blasteen) a vinca alkaloid used as an antineoplastic in the treatment of Hodgkin's disease and testicular germinal cell cancer, usually in combination with other antineoplastic agents.

**Vincent's angina** ('vinsənts) *J.H. Vincent, French physician, 1862–1950. See* ANGINA.

**vincristine** (vin'kristeen) a vinca alkaloid used as an antineoplastic in the treatment of acute leukaemias, Hodgkin's disease, non-Hodgkin's lymphomas and some solid tumours, usually in combination with other antineoplastic agents.

**vinyl** ('vien'l) a plastic material now used extensively for medical equipment. *V. ether* a short-acting inhalation anaesthetic drug used mainly for inducing anaesthesia and for minor surgery.

**viraemia** (vie'reemi.ə) the presence of viruses in the blood.

**virilism** ('viri.lizəm) masculine traits exhibited by a female owing to the production of excessive amounts of androgenic hormone either in the adrenal cortex or from an ovarian tumour. *See* ARRHENOBLASTOMA.

**virion** (vie.riən) a fully developed complete infectious viral particle consisting of its nucleic acid and a surrounding coat of protein (capsid); the extracellular (cell-free) form of a virus.

**virology** (vie'roləjee) the scientific study of viruses, their growth and the diseases caused by them.

**virulence** ('virələns) the power of a microorganism to produce toxins or poisons. This depends on (a) the number and power of the invading organisms, and (b) the power of the microorganism to overcome host resistance.

**virulent** ('virələnt) dangerously poisonous.

**virus** ('vierəs) any member of a unique class of infectious agents, which were originally distinguished by their smallness and their inability to replicate outside a living host cell; because these properties are shared by certain other microorganisms (rickettsiae, chlamydiae), viruses are now characterized by their simple organization and their unique mode of replication. A virus consists of genetic material, which may be either DNA or RNA, and is surrounded by a protein coat and, in some viruses, by a membranous envelope. They cause many diseases, including chickenpox (varicella), herpes zoster (shingles), herpes infec-

tions, measles (rubeola), German measles (rubella), mumps, infectious mononucleosis, hepatitis A and B, yellow fever, the common cold, acquired immune deficiency syndrome (AIDS), influenza, certain types of pneumonia and croup and other respiratory infections, poliomyelitis, and several types of encephalitis. There is evidence that certain viruses may be capable of causing cancer.

**viscera** ('visə.rə) *pl.* of VISCUS.

**viscid** ('visid) sticky and glutinous.

**viscosity** (vi'skositee) resistance to flowing. A sticky and glutinous quality.

**viscus** ('viskəs) any of the organs contained in the body cavities, especially in the abdomen.

**vision** ('vizhən) the faculty of seeing. Sight.

**visual** ('vizhyooəl) relating to sight. *V. acuity* sharpness of vision. It is assessed by reading test types. *V. cells* the rods and cones of the retina. *V. field* the area within which objects can be seen when looking straight ahead. *V. purple* the pigment in the outer layers of the retina. Rhodopsin.

**visualization** (.vizhyooəlie-'zayshən) the technique of using the imagination and relaxation to create any desired changes in an individual's life.

**vital** ('viet'l) relating to life. *V. capacity* the amount of air that can be expelled from the lungs after a full inspiration. *V. signs* the signs of life, namely pulse, respiration and temperature. *V. statistics* the records kept of births and deaths among the population, including the causes of death, and the factors that seem to influence their rise and fall.

**vitallium** (vie'tali.əm) a metal alloy used in dentistry and for prostheses in bone surgery.

**vitamin** ('vitəmin) any of a group of accessory food factors which are contained in foodstuffs and are essential to life, growth and reproduction. *See* Appendices.

**vitiligo** (,viti'liegoh) a skin disease marked by an absence of pigment, producing white patches on the face and body. Leukoderma.

**vitrectomy** (vi'trektəmee) surgical extraction of the vitreous humour and its replacement by a physiological solution in the treatment of vitreous haemorrhage in diabetic retinopathy.

**vitreous** ('vitri.əs) glassy. *V. humour* the transparent jelly-like substance filling the posterior of the eye, from lens to retina.

**vocal** ('vohk'l) pertaining to the voice, or the organs that produce the voice. *V. cords* the two folds of tissue in the larynx, formed of fibrous tissue covered with squamous epithelium. *V. resonance* the normal sounds of speech heard through the chest wall by means of a stethoscope.

**volatile** ('volə,tiel) having a tendency to evaporate readily.

**volition** (və'lishən) the conscious adoption by the individual of a line of action.

**Volkmann's contracture** ('vohlk-mənz) *R. von Volkmann, German surgeon, 1830–1889.* Contraction of the fingers and sometimes of the wrist or of analogous parts of the foot, with loss of power, after severe injury or improper use of a tourniquet or cast.

**volume** ('volyoom) the space occupied by a substance. *Minute v.* the total volume of air breathed in or out in 1 min. *Packed cell v.* that occupied by the blood cells after centrifuging (about 45% of the blood sample). *Residual v.* the amount of air left in the lungs after breathing out fully.

**voluntary** ('voləntə.ree) under the control of the will. *See* INVOLUNTARY.

**volvulus** ('volvyuhləs) twisting of a loop of bowel causing obstruction. Most common in the sigmoid colon.

**vomer** ('vohmə) a thin plate of bone forming the posterior septum of the nose.

**vomit** ('vomit) 1. matter ejected from the stomach through the mouth (vomitus). 2. to eject material in this way. *Bilious v.* vomit mixed with bile. The vomit is stained yellow or green. *Coffee-ground v.* ejected matter that contains small quantities of altered blood, which has the appearance of coffee grounds. *Faecal* or *stercoraceous v.* vomit mixed with faeces. Occurs in intestinal obstruction when the contents of the upper intestine regurgitate back into the stomach. It is dark brown with an unpleasant odour.

**vomiting** ('vomiting) a reflex act of expulsion of the stomach contents via the oesophagus and mouth. It may be preceded by nausea and excess salivation if the cause is local irritation in the stomach. *Cyclical v.* recurrent attacks of vomiting often occurring in children and associated with acidosis. *Projectile v.* the forcible ejection of the gastric contents, usually without warning. Present in hypertrophic pyloric stenosis and in cerebral diseases. *V. of pregnancy* vomiting occurring in the months of pregnancy. Morning sickness.

**von Willebrand's disease** (von 'vili.brants) *E.A. von Willebrand, Finnish physician, 1870–1949.* A bleeding disorder inherited as an autosomal dominant trait (rarely recessive), characterized by a prolonged bleeding time, deficiency of coagulation factor VIII, and associated with epistaxis and increased bleeding after trauma or surgery, menorrhagia and postpartum bleeding.

**VSD** ventricular septal defect.

**vulnerability** (ˌvulnə.rə'bilitee) weakness. Susceptibility to injury or infection.

**vulva** ('vulvə) the external female genital organs.

**vulvectomy** (vul'vektəmee) excision of the vulva.

**vulvitis** (vul'vietis) inflammation of the vulva.

**vulvovaginitis** (ˌvulvohˌvaji'nietis) inflammation of the vulva and vagina.

# W

**Waldeyer's ring** ('valdieəz ˌring)
H.W.G. von Waldeyer-Hartz, German
anatomist, 1836–1921. The circle of
lymphoid tissue in the pharynx
formed by the lingual, faucial and
pharyngeal tonsils.

**Wangensteen tube** ('wangenˌsteen)
O.H. Wangensteen, American surgeon, 1898–1981. A gastrointestinal
aspiration tube with a tip that is
opaque to X-rays.

**warfarin** ('wawfə.rin) an oral anticoagulant drug that depresses the
prothrombin level. Used mainly in
the treatment of coronary and
venous thrombosis.

**wart** (wawt) an elevation of the
skin, often of a brownish colour,
caused by hypertrophy of papillae
in the dermis due to a virus infection. See VERRUCA and CONDYLOMA.

**Wassermann test (reaction)** ('vasə-
mən) A.P. von Wassermann, German
bacteriologist, 1866–1925. A
complement-fixation test used in
the diagnosis of syphilis.

**water** ('wawtə) a clear, colourless,
tasteless liquid composed of
hydrogen and oxygen ($H_2O$).
**W. balance** fluid balance. That
between the fluid taken in by all
routes and the fluid lost by all
routes. **W.-borne** descriptive of certain diseases that are spread by
contaminated water. **W.-brash** the
eructation of dilute acid from
the stomach to the pharynx, giving
a burning sensation. Pyrosis. Heart-

burn. **W.-seal drainage** a closed
method of drainage from the pleural space allowing the escape of
fluid and air but preventing air
entering because the drainage tube
discharges under water.

**Waterhouse–Friderichsen syndrome**
(ˌwawtəhows'freedriksən) R.
Waterhouse, British physician,
1873–1958; C. Friderichsen, Danish
physician, b. 1886. A rare disorder.
Meningococcal MENINGITIS, which
is marked by sudden onset and
short course, fever, coma, cyanosis,
haemorrhages from the skin and
mucous membranes, and haemorrhage into the adrenal glands.

**Watson–Crick helix** (ˌwotsən'krik)
J.D. Watson, American geneticist,
b.1928; F. Crick, British biochemist, b.
1916. Double helix; a representation
of the structure of DEOXYRIBO-
NUCLEIC ACID (DNA), consisting of
two coiled chains, each of which contains information completely speci-
fying the other chain.

**waxy flexibility** (ˌwaksi ˌfleksi'bilitee) a cataleptic state in which a
patient's limbs are held in-
definitely in any position in
which they have been placed. See
CATATONIA.

**weal** (weel) a raised stripe on the
skin, as is caused by the lash of a
whip. Typical of urticaria.

**wean** (ween) 1. to discontinue breast
or bottle-feeding and substitute
other feeding habits, e.g. solid

foods. This should be effected gradually at about the 4th–6th month. 2. in respiratory therapy, to gradually decrease dependence on assisted ventilation until the patient is able to breathe spontaneously.

**webbing** ('webing) the state of being connected by a membrane or a fold of skin. *W. of the hands* or *feet* congenital abnormality in which the digits are not separated from each other. Syndactyly. *W. of the neck* folds of skin in the neck, giving it a webbed appearance. Occurs in certain congenital conditions, e.g. Turner's syndrome.

**Weil's disease** ('vielz) *A. Weil, German physician, 1848–1916.* Spirochaetal jaundice. The organism, *Leptospira icterohaemorrhagiae*, is harboured and excreted by rats and enters through a bite or skin abrasion, or infected food or water.

**Weil–Felix reaction** (,viel'feliks) *E. Weil, Austrian physician, 1880–1922; A. Felix, Czech bacteriologist, 1887–1956.* An agglutination test of blood serum used in the diagnosis of typhus.

**well-baby clinic** (,wel) mothers are encouraged to bring their infants to these clinics for assessment and monitoring of the child's health. Immunization is available and there are opportunities for 'family' health promotion.

**well-man clinic** ('man) a health promotion clinic available for men to screen for health problems and to promote health, e.g. self-examination of the testicles. *See* TESTICULAR SELF-EXAMINATION.

**well-woman clinic** ('wumən) a health promotion clinic available to screen women for breast and cervical cancer, anaemia, diabetes and hypertension and to promote health, e.g. self-examination of the breasts. *See* BREAST.

**wellness** ('welnəs) the development of a personal lifestyle that promotes feelings of wellbeing, achieves the highest level of health within one's capability, and minimizes chances of becoming ill. It is guided by a developing sense of self-awareness and self-responsibility encompassing emotional, mental, physical, social, spiritual and environmental health.

**Welsh National Board for Nursing, Midwifery and Health Visiting** (welsh) *see* NATIONAL BOARDS.

**wen** (wen) a small sebaceous cyst; a steatoma.

**Werdnig–Hoffmann disease** (,vərdnig'hofmən) *G. Werdnig, Austrian neurologist, 1844–1919; J. E. Hoffmann, German neurologist, 1857–1919.* Disease characterized by progressive spinal muscular atrophy affecting the shoulder, neck, pelvis and eventually the respiratory muscles of infants.

**Werner's syndrome** ('vərnəz) *C.W.O. Werner, German physician, 1879–1936.* A hereditary condition characterized by cataracts, osteoporosis, stunted growth and premature greying of the hair.

**Wernicke–Korsakoff syndrome** (,vərnikə'kawsəkof) *K. Wernicke, German neurologist, 1848–1905; S.S. Korsakoff, Russian neurologist, 1854–1900.* A disorder of the central nervous system, usually associated with chronic alcoholism, nutritional deficiency and severe deficiency of vitamin $B_1$. It is characterized by a combination of motor and sensory disturbances and disordered memory function. One form is Wernicke's encephalopathy, a neurological condition due to vitamin $B_1$ deficiency. Untreated, it progresses from mental confusion and double vision to lethargy and coma.

**Wertheim's operation** ('vərt- .hiemz) *E. Wertheim, Austrian gynaecologist, 1864–1920. See* HYSTERECTOMY.

**wet nurse** ('wet) a lactating woman who breast feeds another woman's child.

**Wharton's jelly** ('wawtənz) *T. Wharton, British physician, 1614–1673.* The connective tissue of the umbilical cord.

**wheezing** ('weezing) breathing with a rasp or whistling sound. It results from constriction or obstruction of the throat, pharynx, trachea or bronchi.

**whiplash injury** ('wip,lash ,injəree) injury to the spinal cord, nerve roots, ligaments or vertebrae in the cervical region due to a sudden jerking back of the head and neck. Common in road traffic accidents where there is sudden acceleration or deceleration of the vehicle.

**whiplash shake syndrome** (shayk) a constellation of injuries to the brain and eye that may occur when a young child is shaken vigorously with the head unsupported. This causes stretching and tearing of the cerebral vessels and brain substance, commonly leading to subdural haematomas and retinal haemorrhages. It may result in paralysis, blindness and other visual disturbances, convulsions and death. *See* SHAKEN BABY SYNDROME.

**Whipple's operation** ('wip'lz) *A.O. Whipple, American surgeon, 1881–1963.* Radical pancreatoduodenectomy performed for carcinoma of the head of the pancreas.

**whipworm** ('wip,wərm) *see* TRICHURIS.

**white leg** (wiet) milk leg. *See* PHLEGMASIA.

**whitlow** ('witloh) a felon; a suppurating inflammation of a finger near the nail. *Melanotic w.* a malignant tumour of the nail bed characterized by formation of melanotic tissue. *Subperiosteal w.* one in which the infection involves the bone covering. *Superficial w.* a pustule between the true skin and cuticle. *See* PARONYCHIA.

**WHO** (hoo) World Health Organization.

**whole time equivalent** ('hohl,tiem ə'kwivələnt) total weekly contracted hours of full- and part-time staff expressed as a multiple of the standard working week.

**whooping cough** ('hooping) a notifiable infectious disease characterized by catarrh of the respiratory tract and paroxysms of coughing, ending in a prolonged whooping respiration; called also pertussis. The causative organism is *Bordetella pertussis*. Whooping cough is a serious disease; most cases occur in children. All babies should be immunized against whooping cough unless there is a sound medical objection.

**Widal reaction** (vee'dahl) *G.F.I. Widal, French physician, 1862–1929.* A blood agglutination test for typhoid fever.

**Wilms' tumour** ('vilmz) *M. Wilms, German surgeon, 1867–1918.* A highly malignant tumour of the kidney occurring in young children. A nephroblastoma.

**Wilson's disease** ('wilsənz) *S.A.K. Wilson, British neurologist, 1878–1937.* Hepatolenticular degeneration. A congenital abnormality in the metabolism of copper, leading to neurological degeneration.

**wiring** ('wieəring) the fixing together of a broken or split bone by the use of a wire. Commonly used for the jaw, the patella and the sternum.

**wisdom teeth** ('wizdəm) the back molar teeth, the eruption of which is often delayed until maturity.

**wish fulfilment** ('wish fuhl,filmənt) a desire, not always acknowledged consciously by the person, which is fulfilled through dreams or by day-dreaming.

**withdrawal** (widh'draw'l) 1. a pathological retreat from reality. 2.

abstention from drugs to which one is habituated or addicted; also denoting the symptoms occasioned by such withdrawal. *W. symptoms* symptoms brought about by abrupt withdrawal of a narcotic or other drug to which a person has become addicted; called also abstinence syndrome. The usual reactions to withdrawal may include anxiety, weakness, gastrointestinal symptoms, nausea and vomiting, tremor, fever, rapid heartbeat, convulsions and delirium.

**Wolff–Parkinson–White syndrome** (ˌwuhlfˌpahkinsənˈwiet) *L. Wolff, American cardiologist, 1898–1972; Sir J. Parkinson, British physician, 1885–1976; P. D. White, American cardiologist, 1886–1973.* Abnormal heart rhythm caused by an accessory bundle between the atria and ventricles. A congenital disorder.

**womb** (woom) the uterus.

**Wood's light** (ˈwuhdz) *R.W. Wood, American physicist, 1868–1953.* Ultraviolet light transmitted through a glass filter containing nickel oxide. It produces fluorescence of infected hairs when placed over a scalp affected with ringworm.

**woolsorter's disease** (ˈwuhlsawtəz) pulmonary anthrax.

**word blindness** (ˈwərd) *see* DYSLEXIA.

**word salad** (ˌsalad) rapid speech in which the words are strung together without meaning.

**World Health Organization** (ˌwərld ˈhelth ˌawgəniˌzayshən) abbreviated WHO. The specialized agency of the United Nations that is concerned with health at an international level. WHO organizes health compaigns against infectious diseases and sponsors research in medical laboratories. It also provides expert advice on all matters directly or indirectly concerned with physical or mental health to all member states.

**worm** (wərm) any one of a number of groups of long soft-bodied invertebrates, some of which are parasitic to humans.

**wound** (woond) a cut or break in continuity of any tissue, caused by injury or operation. It is classified according to its nature. *Abrased w.* the skin is scraped off, but there is no deeper injury. *Contused w.* with bruising of the surrounding tissue. *Incised w.* usually the result of operation, and produced by a knife or similar instrument. The edges of the wound can remain in apposition, and it should heal by first intention. *Lacerated w.* one with torn edges and tissues, usually the result of accident or injury. It is often septic and heals by second intention. *Open w.* a gaping wound on the body surface. *Penetrating w.* often made by gunshot, shrapnel, etc. There may be an inlet and outlet hole and vital organs are often penetrated by the missile. *Punctured w.* made by a pointed or spiked instrument. *Septic w.* any type into which infection has been introduced, causing suppurative inflammation. It heals by second intention. *W. healing* the restoration of integrity to injured tissues by replacement of dead tissue with viable tissue. The process starts immediately after an injury and may continue for months or years. *See* HEALING.

**wrist** (rist) the point of the carpus and bones of the forearm. *W. drop* loss of power in the muscles of the hand. It may be due to nerve or tendon injury, but can result from lack of sufficient support by splint or sling.

**writer's cramp** (ˌrietəz) a colloquial term for painful spasm of the hand and forearm, caused by excessive writing and poor posture.

**wryneck** ('rie͵nek) *see* TORTICOLLIS.
***Wuchereria*** (͵vookə'riə.ri.ə) a genus
of nematode worms which are the

principal vectors of filariasis. ***W. bancrofti*** the most common species in
tropical and subtropical areas.

# X

X chromosome the female sex chromosome, being present in all female gametes and only half the male gametes. When union takes place two X chromosomes result in a female child (XX) but one of each results in a male child (XY). *See* Y CHROMOSOME.

X-linked (ˌlinkt) pertaining to the genes, or the effect of these genes, situated on the X chromosome. X-linked disorders are those caused by the genes on the X chromosome.

X-rays (ˌrayz) electromagnetic waves of short length which are capable of penetrating many substances and of producing chemical changes and reactions in living matter. They are used both to aid diagnosis and to treat disease. Also called Röntgen rays.

xanthelasma (ˌzanthəˈlazmə) a disease marked by the formation of flat or slightly raised yellow cholesterol deposits on the eyelids.

xanthine ('zantheen) a compound found in plant and animal tissues; the forerunner of uric acid in nucleoprotein metabolism.

xanthochromia (ˌzanthohˈkrohmi.ə) 1. the presence of yellow patches on the skin. 2. the yellow colouring of cerebrospinal fluid seen in patients who have had a subarachnoid haemorrhage.

xanthoma (zanˈthohmə) the presence in the skin of flat areas of yellowish pigmentation due to deposits of lipids. There are several varieties. *X. palpebrarum* xanthelasma.

xanthopsia (zanˈthopsi.ə) a disturbance of vision in which all objects appear yellow.

xanthosis (zanˈthohsis) a yellow skin pigmentation, seen in some cases of diabetes and poliomyelitis.

*Xenopsylla* (ˌzenopˈsilə) a genus of fleas, some of which are vectors of plague. *X. cheopis* the rat flea, which transmits bubonic plague.

xeroderma (ˌziə.rohˈdərmə) a hereditary condition in which there is excessive dryness of the skin. A mild form of ichthyosis. *X. pigmentosum* a rare hereditary and often fatal disease in which there is extreme sensitivity of the skin and eyes to light. It begins in childhood and rapidly progresses. The formation of malignant neoplasms is common.

xerophthalmia (ˌzir.rofˈthalmi.ə) a condition in which the cornea and conjunctiva become horny and necrosed owing to a deficiency of vitamin A. Xeroma.

xerosis (ziˈrohsis) a condition of dryness, especially of the eyes, mouth, vagina or skin.

**xerostomia** (ˌziə.roh'stohmi.ə) dryness of the mouth due to a failure of salivary gland secretion.

**Xylocaine** ('zieloh͵kayn) a proprietary preparation of lignocaine used for local anaesthesia.

**xylose** ('zielohz) a pentose sugar, found in connective tissue and sometimes in urine, which is not metabolized in the body.

**XYY syndrome** an extremely rare condition in males in which there is an extra Y chromosome, making a total of 47 chromosomes in each body cell. *See* KLINEFELTER'S SYNDROME.

# Y

**Y chromosome** the male sex chromosome, being present in half the male gametes and none of the female. It carries few major genes. *See* X CHROMOSOME.

**yawning** ('yawning) an involuntary act in which the mouth is opened wide and air is drawn in and exhaled. It may accompany tiredness or boredom.

**yaws** (yorz) framboesia. A skin infection common in tropical countries. Caused by *Treponema pertenue*, it is common among people, especially children, who live under primitive conditions in equatorial Africa, South America, and the East and West Indies.

**yeast** (yeest) any of the fungi of the genus *Saccharomyces*. They produce fermentation in malt and in sweetened fruit juices, resulting in the formation of alcoholic solutions such as beer and wines.

**yellow fever** ('yeloh) an acute, notifiable, infectious disease of the tropics caused by a virus and transmitted by a mosquito (*Aëdes aegypti*). The virus attacks the liver and kidneys and the symptoms include rigor, headache, pain in the back and limbs, high fever and black vomit. Haemorrhage from the intestinal mucous membrane may occur. There is a high mortality rate.

**yin and yang** (,yin ənd 'yang) the two complementary principles of Chinese philosophy incorporated

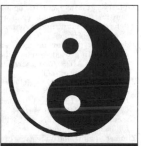

**THE CHINESE SYMBOL FOR YIN–YANG**

into traditional Chinese medicine. Yin is feminine, dark and negative; yang is masculine, bright and positive. Together, the Yin–Yang interaction and balance is believed to maintain the harmony of the body and, in a healthy person, maintain a state of dynamic balance (*see* Figure).

**yoga** ('yohgə) one of the six systems of Indian philosophy which emphasizes personal physical preparation using isometric exercises, relaxation, breathing techniques and the attainment of defined body positions to achieve relaxation, with physical and emotional harmony and wellbeing.

# Z

**Z-plasty** (ˌplastee) a plastic operation for removing and repairing deformity resulting from a contraction scar (*see* Figure).

**zidovudine** (zieˈdovyuhˌdeen) an antiviral drug used to retard the progress of AIDS. Also known as azidothymidine or AZT.

**Ziehl–Neelsen method** (ˌzielˈneelsən ˌmethəd) *F. Ziehl, German bacteriologist, 1857–1926; F.K.A. Neelsen, German pathologist, 1854–1894.* A method of staining tubercle bacilli for microscopic study.

**Zimmer** (ˈzimə) the trade name of a metal, light-weight walking aid, commonly applied to other products of similar design and weight. Predominantly used by the elderly to assist in rehabilitation.

**zinc** (zingk) *symbol* Zn. A trace element which is essential in the body for cell growth and multiplication. The recommended daily intake of zinc is 15 mg for an adult. A severe deficiency of zinc can retard growth in children, cause a low sperm count in adult males, and retard wound healing.

**Zn** symbol for *zinc*.

**Zollinger–Ellison syndrome** (ˌzolinjəˈelisən) *R.M. Zollinger, American physician, b. 1903; E.H. Ellison, American physician, 1918–1970.* A rare condition in which a pancreatic tumour causes excessive outpouring of gastric juice. Peptic ulcers may occur.

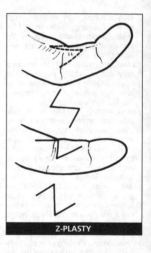

**Z-PLASTY**

**zona** (ˈzohnə) a zone. **Z. facialis** herpes of the face. **Z. pellucida** the membrane surrounding the ovum.

**zonula** (ˈzonyuhlə) a zonule. In anatomy, a small, usually circular, area. *Ciliary z.* the area surrounded by the suspensory ligaments of the eye.

**zonulysin** (ˌzonyuhˈliesin) a proteolytic enzyme that may be used in eye surgery to dissolve the suspensory ligament.

**zoonosis** (ˌzoh.əˈnohsis, ˌzooə-) a disease of animals that is transmissible to humans, e.g. anthrax, cat-scratch fever, etc.

**zoster** (ˈzostə) *see* HERPES.

**zygoma** (zieˈgohmə, zi-) the arch formed by the union of the temporal bone with the malar bone in front of the ear.

**zygote** (ˈziegoht, ˈzi-) a single fertilized cell formed from the union of a male and a female gamete.

**zymosis** (zieˈmohsis) fermentation.

# Appendices

# Appendix 1
# NUTRITION

## Artifical Nutritional Support
### HILARY PEAKE

### Indications

- Failure to meet nutritional requirements with food.

### Types

- Enteral nutrition, e.g. nutritional supplements (sip feeds) or tube feeding.
- Parenteral nutrition, including central and peripheral administration.

Enteral nutrition should be the first-line route for the provision of nutritional support. If the gut works, enteral feeding should be used.

## Enteral Nutrition
Refer to the dictionary for a definition.

### Indications for Enteral Tube Feeding
See Box 1.1.

| BOX 1.1 | INDICATIONS FOR ENTERAL TUBE FEEDING |
| --- | --- |

**Increased nutritional requirements**
- E.g. sepsis, burns, trauma, postoperative stress

**Inadequate oral intake**
- Anorexia
- Nil by mouth
- Swallowing difficulties, e.g. cerebrovascular accident, oesphageal carcinoma

### Contraindications

- Patients with a non-functioning gut (refer to parenteral nutrition section).

**Enteral Nutrition Routes**
- Oral diet.
- Nutritional supplements, e.g. sip feeds.
- Tube feeding, including:
—Pre-pyloric, e.g. nasogastric, gastrostomy (surgical or endoscopic).
—Post-pyloric, e.g. nasoduodenal/jejunal, jejunostomy, gastrostomy with an extension jejunostomy.
- N.B. A team decision is required to select the most appropriate route.

**Composition of Enteral Tube Feeds**
All enteral feeds contain protein, carbohydrate, fat, electrolytes, vitamins and minerals:

- Standard feeds: 1 kcal per ml.
- High-energy feeds: 1.5 kcal per ml.

A variety of specialist feeds are also available—for example, for the management of renal failure, malabsorption and inflammatory bowel disease.

**Tube Feeding Regimens**
Regimen depends on the route of tube feeding and the aims and objectives of nutritional support. Most regimens include a rest to allow for the stomach to re-acidify. This is not required for patients fed past the pylorus.

**Complications**

| TABLE 1.1 | COMPLICATIONS OF ENTERAL TUBE FEEDING |
|---|---|
| Complication | Recommendation |
| Diarrhoea, (listed below are possible causes) | Check medical history for bowel disease<br>Record stool output daily |
| • Infective diarrhoea | Send stool sample<br>Ensure a clean technique is used when handling enteral feeds and flushing feeding tubes |
| • Medication, e.g. motility agents, antibiotics, medication containing sorbitol | Review medication, especially antibiotics |
| • Bacterial overgrowth | Hydrogen breath test |
| • Malabsorption | Check for pancreatic, biliary or gastrointestinal disease |

| Complication | Recommendation |
|---|---|
| Diarrhoea (*contd.*) | |
| • Hypoalbuminaemia | Discuss with dietitian |
| • Hyperosmolar feeds | Discuss with dietitian |
| N.B. Most feeds are lactose- and gluten-free | |
| Constipation | Check fluid intake<br>Consider using a fibre feed, discuss with dietitian<br>Consider laxatives prescription, discuss with medical team |
| Mucosal erosion and oesophageal strictures | Use fine-bore feeding tubes instead of wide-bore PVC tubes, e.g. ryles |
| Regurgitation | Rate of feed must not exceed the patient's absorption<br>Tilt the head of the bed by 30 degrees when tube-feeding supine patients |
| Psychological problems, **e.g.** | Where possible involve patients in their care |
| • Altered body image | |
| • Hunger | |
| • Loss of autonomy | |
| • Loss of the pleasure of eating | |

### Monitoring

Effective monitoring can reduce the complications associated with enteral nutritional support (see Table 1.1). It is very important to:

- Check the tube is accurately positioned prior to commencing feed.
- Flush the tube regularly.
- Monitor gastrointestinal function, e.g.:
—Bowel movements.
—Nausea and vomiting.
—Bloating.
—Gastric distension.
—Gastric aspirate volume.

## Parenteral nutrition

Parenteral nutrition (PN) should be used to prevent or treat malnutrition when the intestine is unavailable or intestinal function is inadequate. N.B. Consider and discuss all enteral feeding access routes prior to commencing parenteral nutrition.

**Possible Indications for Parenteral Nutrition**

| BOX 1.2 | POSSIBLE INDICATIONS FOR PARENTERAL NUTRITION |
|---|---|

**Failure to tolerate enteral nutritional support**
- E.g. paralytic ileus, vomiting, profuse diarrhoea

**Intestinal failure**
- Intestinal atresia, short bowel syndrome, motility disorders

**Severe malabsorption**
- Cannot be managed by an elemental diet

**Severe pancreatitis**
- Unable to tolerate jejunal feeding

**Severe mucositis**
- Unable to pass enteral tube

**Bowel rest**
- Post-gastrointestinal surgery; cannot be achieved by an elemental diet

**Full nutritional requirements cannot be met via the enteral route**

**Parenteral Nutrition Routes**
The perceived length of feeding and nutritional requirements (energy, amino acid, electrolytes and fluid) will influence the route of nutritional support:

- Central access
—Short-term: multilumen lines.
—Long-term: e.g. Hickman line or Portacath.
- Peripheral access (at/below antecubital fossa)
—Peripherally inserted central catheter (PICC) >15 cm long; (> 5 days–4 weeks).
—Midline, e.g. a peripherally inserted catheter (PIC) approximately 15 cm long (5 days–2 weeks).

**Composition of Parenteral Nutrition Feeds**
PN is usually administered in an all-in-one bag which contains:

- 10%, 20%, 50% glucose.
- 10%, 20% , 30% lipid.
- Amino acids.
- Electrolytes.
- Water.
- Fat- and water-soluble vitamins.
- Trace elements.

A variety of standard bags are usually available to meet patients' requirements. If required special bags can be compounded by some units. Sequential, single-bottle or multiple-bottle regimens using a Y or W connector are now used less frequently.

## Parenteral Feeding Regimens

- In all cases the lumen used for PN should be dedicated.
- Strict flow control is essential using volumetric pumps fitted with occlusion and air-in-line alarms.
- PN is usually administered over 24 hours but can be administered over shorter periods of time.

## Complications
See Table 1.2.

| TABLE 1.2 | COMPLICATIONS OF PARENTERAL NUTRITION |
|---|---|
| **Complication** | **Comment** |
| **Catheter-related** | |
| Catheter-related infection | Meticulous care of the line and catheter site can prevent sepsis |
| Central venous thrombosis | Discuss with medical team |
| Catheter occlusion and damage | Discuss with medical team |
| **Nutritional and metabolic** | |
| Dehydration | Monitor abnormal losses, e.g. fistulae or diarrhoea<br>N.B. Additional IV fluids may be required |
| Over-hydration | Monitor all other IV fluids that are administered, e.g. antibiotics, chemotherapy |
| Hyperglycaemia | Discuss carbohydrate content of PN with dietitian<br>Discuss blood sugar management with medical team |
| Hypoglycaemia | Hypoglycaemia can occur if PN is stopped immediately<br>PN infusion rate should be decreased slowly; if this is not possible provide an IV glucose solution and monitor blood glucose 4-hourly for 24 hours |
| Lipaemia | At-risk patients include critically ill, septic or those with renal failure |
| Electrolyte imbalance | Over- or under-administration of electrolytes |
| **Effect on other organ systems** | |
| Hepatobiliary disease | Consider impact of underlying disease and PN composition |
| Metabolic bone disease | Consider poor nutritional status and exposure to corticosteriod therapy |

Careful monitoring detects most of the complications associated with nutritional support. Multidisciplinary team management is essential.

## Basic Monitoring for Enteral (Tube Feeding) and Parenteral Nutrition

N.B. The frequency of monitoring can be reduced for stable patients; refer to figures in brackets in Table 1.3.

| TABLE 1.3 | MONITORING OF ENTERAL AND PARENTERAL NUTRITION | | |
|---|---|---|---|
| Parameter | Assessment | Frequency Enteral | Parenteral |
| Clinical | Temperature, pulse, respiration and blood pressure | 4-hourly | 4-hourly |
| | Ward urine analysis | Daily | Daily |
| Fluid balance | Fluid balance | At each bottle change | Hourly |
| | Serum urea | Daily (2 x weekly) | Daily |
| | Body weight | 2 x weekly | Daily |
| Biochemistry | Full serum electrolyte profile | Daily (2 x weekly) | Daily |
| | Glucose | Daily (2 x weekly) | 4-hourly blood (urinalysis) |
| | Liver function chemistry | 2 x weekly | 2 x weekly |
| | Zinc, copper and selenium | Monthly | Every 2 weeks |
| Nutritional status | Nutrient intake | Daily | Daily |
| | Body weight | Weekly | Weekly |
| Haematology | Full blood count | 2 x weekly | Daily |
| | Prothrombin time | As indicated | Weekly |
| Lipaemia | Cholesterol and triacylglycerol | As indicated | On initiation and then weekly |

BIBLIOGRAPHY

American Gastroenterological Association 1999 American Gastroenterology Association technical review on tube feeding for enteral nutrition. Gastroenterology 108: 1282–301

Arrowsmith H, McWhirter J, Payne-James J, Silk D A B, Stanford J, Teahon K 1999 Current perspectives on enteral nutrition in adults. McAtear C A (ed). ADM, Biddenden, Kent

ASPEN board of directors 1986 Guidelines for use of total parenteral nutrition in the hospitalized adult patient. Journal of Parenteral and Enteral Nutrition 10: 441–5

Fawcett H, MacFie J, McWhirter J, Sizer T, Whitney S 1996 Current perspectives on parenteral nutrition in adults. Pennington C R (ed). ADM, Biddenden, Kent

Heimburger D C 1990 Diarrhea with enteral feeding: will the real cause please stand up? American Journal of Medicine 88: 89–90

Lipman T O 1998 Grains or veins: is enteral nutrition really better than parenteral nutrition? A look at the evidence. Journal of Enteral and Parenteral Nutrition 22: 167–82

# Nutritional Management of Coronary Heart Disease, Obesity and Diabetes
## GARY FROST

Coronary heart disease, obesity and diabetes account for a large percentage of mortality and morbidity within the UK. Nutritional advice plays a key role in the prevention and treatment of all three. It is important that the messages given to people regarding prevention and treatment of these diseases are consistent. The following sections are aimed at giving a consensus overview of dietetic advice.

## Healthy Eating

Over the past few years the publicity surrounding healthy eating has quite often been confusing. There is widespread agreement, however, about the principles of a healthy diet and a healthy lifestyle which have not changed over the past 15 years. We now have a better understanding than ever before of the relationship between diet and health.

### The Healthy Eating Message

Healthy eating is used as an approach to reducing the risks of some of the major diseases of later life. There is a clear relationship between too much saturated fat and heart disease. Breast cancer has also been associated with a higher-fat diet. Continuing research is showing that being overweight increases your chances of developing diabetes, heart disease or high blood pressure. High blood pressure causes kidney disease as well as strokes and heart disease. Low-fibre diets have also been associated with bowel cancers and bowel disease. By keeping your weight down and following a healthy diet you can reduce the risk of developing some of these diseases.

## What does the Healthy Eating Message Aim to Convey?

A healthy diet works by supplying the correct mix of nutrients, vitamins and minerals for the body to perform at optimum level. There are four major food groups: protein, fat, carbohydrate, and vitamins and minerals. The well-balanced diet provides enough energy for the body to function optimumly and includes a mixture of foods from all the food groups which is high in starchy food, fibre, fruit and vegetables but low in fat.

As well as considering the types of food to eat, we should remember that quantities are also important. Keeping body weight down goes a long way towards maintaining a healthy lifestyle.

Healthy eating does not have to be more expensive. Larger portions of starchy foods such as bread, potatoes, rice and pasta are recommended and these tend to be less expensive; meats, cheeses, dairy products and so on, which cost more, should be taken in smaller portions.

## What does a Healthy Diet Involve?

There are five main areas to focus on, as described below.

## Total Energy

One of the major aims of healthy eating advice is to reduce the incidence of obesity. To this end a healthy diet provides enough energy for the body to function to its maximum but avoids weight gain. This is called energy balance; the energy going into the body which is provided by food is equal to the energy which is expended through keeping the heart beating and the cells of the body functioning and allowing for exercise. Weight gain takes place when the amount of energy going in is greater than that which is being expended.

In terms of healthy eating, the foods that provide energy to the body, i.e. fat and carbohydrate, are described in terms of their percentage contribution to total energy intake.

As far as fat is concerned, the overall message is 'Eat less fat and fatty food'. Fat should provide 30% of total energy intake. The link between total fat and saturated fat intake and coronary heart disease (CHD) is well established. One of the main reasons why healthy eating guidelines were originally written was to combat the rise in CHD and target a reduction in fat. All types of fat are high in calories. Fat contains 9 kcal per gram, compared with 4 kcal per gram for protein and carbohydrate. There is some evidence that diets high in fat are likely to lead to over consumption of energy and could contribute to obesity. Therefore fat should be used in moderation. Saturated fat consumption should be reduced and unsaturated fats used where there is a need to add fat. Principles behind the standard advice are as follows:

- The following foods should be reduced: lard, butter, cheese, fat on meat, cream, suet, meat produce, e.g. sausages, pâté etc.
- Where fat is necessary in cooking use a mono- (olive oil or rapeseed oil) or polyunsaturated oil (corn, sunflower, etc.). The advice is to throw out the frying pan and grill, bake, microwave, poach or boil meals instead.
- Eat fish and chicken more often and red meats less often. Buy lean cuts of red meat. Limit portion sizes to 125–200 grams (4–6 oz). Roast poultry or meat on a rack to drain the fat. Remove the skin from poultry before cooking.
- Use skimmed or semi-skimmed milk instead of full-cream milk. Try low-fat yoghurt instead of cream.
- Use low-fat spreads rather than butter or margarine and spread them thinly.
- Buy low-fat cheese or edam, camembert, brie or cottage cheese, etc. Avoid high-fat cheeses like cheddar. Limit hard cheese to a matchbox-size portion. Grated cheese goes further.

With carbohydrates, the overall message is 'Starchy high-fibre food should be included regularly in the diet'. Carbohydrate should provide 50% of total energy intake. To balance the decrease in fat and to avoid CHD intake should be increased. At present there is no evidence that high-carbohydrate diets are linked to CHD or diabetes. Carbohydrates that are high in fibre should be encouraged.

Fibre is also sometimes called roughage or non-starch polysaccharide (NSP), the latter being the name for the cell wall or plant structure. To simplify things, fibre is divided into two categories: insoluble and soluble. Insoluble fibre, e.g. wholegrain and wholemeal breads and cereals, the stringy bits in celery, etc., is good for the bowels. It helps prevent constipation and some studies suggest it reduces the risk of bowel cancer. Soluble fibre is good for the heart and is found in foods such as beans, pulses, oats and bananas. Many studies show that this type of fibre lowers the cholesterol and also improves blood sugar control in diabetes. Many foods contain a mixture of the two.

*Increase Fruit and Vegetable Consumption*
The current targets are for people to eat at least five portions of fruit and vegetables (excluding potatoes) a day.

*Reduce Sugar Intake*
A high-sugar diet causes tooth decay. Teeth should be brushed at least twice a day. Sugar is a nutrient which has no other goodness (e.g. vitamins or minerals). The calories it provides are known as 'empty calories'.

*Reduce Salt Intake*
Research suggests that on average we consume ten times more salt than is required. In people at risk of blood pressure problems salty foods can adversely affect blood pressure. This in turn increases the risk of heart and kidney disease or stroke. The rule is 'Add salt at the table but not during cooking' or vice versa. Cut down on as many processed or packaged foods, e.g. cheese, crisps, bacon, sausages, as possible because they contain high amounts of salt and preservative. Instead use more herbs and spices to flavour food, such as chives with potatoes and mustard with roast beef.

*Enjoy Alcohol in Moderation*
Follow the government guidelines for safe limits of alcohol: 21 units per week for men, and 14 units per week for women. One unit is equivalent to half a pint of lager, a small glass of wine or a pub measure of spirits. Alcohol is another form of empty calories so beware if watching your weight. Drinking alcohol is not recommended during pregnancy.

Research suggests that red wine contains anti-oxidants that have a protective effect against heart disease; these anti-oxidants are also found in fruit, vegetables and wholegrain products. Alcohol is not recommended as a health benefit to the younger generation (because the main cause of death in this age group is from accidents). However, there is much discussion in the over-40s generation, where the risk of heart disease and stroke is much higher. It could be an advantage in this age group to have a modest medicinal drink before bed!

**Conclusion**
Diet is just one part of the equation. For a healthy lifestyle other factors such as smoking, stress and lack of exercise play a part. All of these risk factors are avoidable. People need encouragement and even getting over one simple message will help reduce the risk of them developing some of the many diseases and conditions that have been mentioned—and they can still enjoy their food!

# Coronary Heart Disease
The UK has one of the highest rates of CHD in the world. One risk factor for the development of heart disease is a raised level of cholesterol in the

blood, but it is becoming clear that risk factors are many and varied. It is important that the healthy eating messages above are put across to people who are at risk or who have developed CHD.

Discussed below are a number of issues relating specifically to the risk factor of a raised plasma cholesterol, which is common. There are many ways of assessing risk relating to cholesterol. The main aim for those who have diagnosed CHD or who have other risk factors such as diabetes is that levels should be maintained below 5.2 mmol/l.

## How Diet is Important to Lowering Cholesterol

A cholesterol-lowering diet is used to lower the level of 'blood cholesterol'. Blood cholesterol is made in the body from the saturated fat found in the diet. Cholesterol found in food (e.g. eggs, shellfish) is thought to make only a small contribution to actual blood cholesterol levels. The main focus of a cholesterol-lowering diet is (a) reducing all fat in the diet and (b) changing fat from saturated to unsaturated. Thus a cholesterol-lowering diet is different from a low-cholesterol diet. Blood cholesterol itself, in normal amounts, has many important body functions.

As with all diets, the change to a healthier diet needs to be permanent rather than a short-term crash diet. Other areas to consider are weight, exercise and smoking habits, as it is a healthy lifestyle and not just a low saturated fat diet which reduces the risk of heart disease.

## Solving Some Common Problems

*What about Fat?*
Reduce the total amount of fat, especially saturated fat, in your diet. Fat is found in two forms: saturated and unsaturated (see Box 1.3.) Saturated fat raises the blood cholesterol while polyunsaturated fat lowers blood cholesterol. Monounsaturated fat does not increase or

---

**BOX 1.3**                                    **TYPES OF FAT IN FOODS**

**Saturated fat**
- Lard, butter, cheese, fat on red meat, cream, suet, meat produce, e.g. sausages, pâté.

**Monounsaturated**
- Olive oil, rapeseed oil, avocado

**Polyunsaturated**
- Sunflower oil and spreads, soya oil, corn oil

**Marine oils**
- Fish oil

decrease it. All types of fat are high in calories; therefore use fat in small amounts if you are overweight. If oil is needed in cooking use a mono- or polyunsaturated fat. Grill, bake, microwave, poach or boil meals instead of frying them.

### Is Oily Fish High in Fat?

Oily fish include salmon, mackerel, herring and pilchards. They are high in fat but it is a good type of fat (polyunsaturated). They are also rich in omega-3 fatty acids. It has been proposed that these fatty acids reduce the risk of a second heart attack after a first. There is evidence that they make blood less likely to clot and less viscous. Oily fish should be included in the diet at least twice a week. Some tasty examples are tinned fish on sandwiches or in a baked potato or fresh fish (which is coming down in price) baked or grilled.

### Margarine or Butter?

Butter is high in saturated fat and calories. Margarine (poly-unsaturated, sunflower) has the same amount of calories but may contain a better type of fat. Encourage people to check the label and buy one that is high in mono/polyunsaturates. Low-fat spread contains half of the fat (and therefore half of the calories) of butter. Recommended for people aiming to lose weight. Remember— whichever one you use, spread it thinly!

### Vegetables and Fruit

It is even more important that people with risk factors for CHD such as raised cholesterol increase their fruit and vegetable consumption towards five portions per day.

### Is Fibre Good for Lowering Cholesterol?

There are two groups of fibre: insoluble and soluble. As we have seen, insoluble fibre is good for the bowels; it is found in foods such as wholegrain and wholemeal breads and cereals. Soluble fibre is good for lowering cholesterol and is found in foods such as beans, pulses, oats and bananas. Many foods contain a mixture of the two. Include five portions of fruit and vegetables daily for a well-balanced diet.

### Why Do the French Drink so much Red Wine and yet Have a Lower Incidence of Heart Disease?

Research suggests that red wine contains anti-oxidants that have a protective effect. Anti-oxidants are also found in fruit, vegetables and wholegrain products.

# Obesity

## What Is It?
Nearly one half of the UK population is overweight. In the last 10 years the number of people who are very overweight has doubled. There are more overweight men than women but more women fall into the very overweight category. In 1993 the Government published a report called 'Health of the Nation', stating that it aimed to reduce the levels of obesity in men by 25% and women by 33% by 2005. There is no doubt that the more overweight a person becomes, the greater the risk of many chronic diseases such as diabetes and heart disease. The real cost to the nation is through the increased morbidity suffered through conditions like back pain. The rapid rise in obesity is totally explained by changes in lifestyle over the past 30 years which have created an environment of energy excess and decreasing physical activity.

The slimming industry made £80 million in 1994 on meal replacement products. This suggests that many people are trying to lose weight but the ever-increasing numbers of overweight people indicate little success. Data also suggest that people are becoming less active through performing fewer manual tasks and having increased access to cars, mechanization, etc. Recent advice on slimming may have been confusing at times but all the experts do agree that the best way for maintained weight loss is to follow a healthy lifestyle.

## Prevention is Better than Cure
All the current reviews of obesity management agree that there should be a greater focus on the prevention of obesity. However, the best way of achieving this is still a topic of current research.

## Why Should the Overweight Lose Weight?
Weight loss is of benefit in many conditions. Two stones overweight does not sound much but if you think of it as equivalent to carrying a 2-year-old child around, all day, every day, the extra stress put on your heart and circulation and other organs becomes obvious. Weight loss is of particular benefit in diabetes, high blood pressure, shortness of breath, joint problems and raised cholesterol.

## Body Mass Index
This is used to calculate healthy weight (see Box 1.4). Measure weight in kilograms and height in metres. Then take your weight and divide it by the square of your height (i.e. your height x height).

| BOX 1.4 | BODY MASS INDEX |
|---|---|

**20–25**
- Ideal body weight

**25–30**
- Overweight; it would be a good idea to lose some weight

**30–40**
- Obese; you must try to lose some weight

**40+**
- Very obese; you are putting your health at serious risk and must lose weight

Rapid weight loss is associated with muscle loss.

### What does Losing Weight Involve?
There is no way to avoid eating less than energy requirements. This means both cutting down on the total amounts of food eaten, especially fatty foods, and increasing daily activity and exercise.

*Practical Guidelines (see also Total Energy, pp. 438–439)*

Enjoy regular fruit and vegetables:

- All fruit and vegetables are recommended. Enjoy up to five or six portions a day. (One portion is equal to one piece of fruit or a serving of vegetables.)
- Grab a piece of fruit rather than raiding the refrigerator or the biscuit barrel.

Fill up on high-fibre/high-carbohydrate choices:

- Bulky high-fibre foods such as wholemeal pasta, wholemeal rice, wholegrain bread, etc. are more filling and curb hunger for longer.
- Carbohydrate foods, e.g. potatoes and bread, are good for you and should fill up your plate along with vegetables, at the expense of fatty protein foods.

### How to Achieve Weight Loss
Weight loss is individual. A diet that one person finds easy to follow may not be easy for another. The key to long-term success is slow, steady weight loss. This is why the most successful diets are usually the ones making small permanent changes to your normal eating habits. Beware of 'gimmick' diets which may help to promote weight loss in the short term but after a few weeks become dull and repetitive, causing old habits to return. To keep weight off in the long term it is usually necessary to deal with the problems that caused the weight

gain in the first place. Thus, unfortunately for those who are looking for a miracle cure or a magic bullet, the best approach to weight loss is sensible, regular healthy eating with a calorie intake which is less than your requirements. (500 kcal a day less than requirements leads to a weight loss of $\frac{1}{3}$ kg (1 lb) a week.)

**Increasing the Risk**
Being overweight puts a person at greater risk of developing heart disease or diabetes. This is especially true if the weight is carried around the waist (known as apple shape or trunkal obesity) rather than around the hips (known as pear shape). Men should aim to maintain a waistline of less than or equal to 94 cm, and lose weight from a waistline of more than 102 cm. In women the ideal waistline is less than 80 cm. More than 88 cm indicates the need for weight loss.

# Nutritional Advice for People with Diabetes
There are two main categories of diabetes: type 1, which used to be called insulin-dependent or juvenile onset diabetes; and type 2 diabetes, which used to be called non-insulin-dependent diabetes. In both cases dietary advice forms the cornerstone of treatment. Without getting the diet right it would be impossible to meet the glycaemic control targets which are important in both cases. However, nutritional advice is not just about blood glucose; it is also about preventing long-term complications such as heart disease. The following sections are written in a patient-centred way to help in advising on some common problems relating to the diabetes mellitus diet.

**What does a Healthy Diabetic Diet Involve?**
We believe there are six important points to consider:

- Firstly, your weight. If you are overweight then losing even a few pounds can have dramatic effects in helping to control your blood sugar and overall health.
- Secondly, it is important to eat regularly. At a minimum this would mean breakfast, lunch and your evening meal. Some people may be encouraged to have snacks between meals. People who eat more frequently tend to have better blood sugar control.
- Thirdly, eat more fibre-rich foods. Some foods, such as oats, beans, dahl and pulses, can help control your blood sugar.
- Fourthly, try to include vegetables and fresh fruit at each of your meals. This is important in trying to protect your heart.
- Fifthly, cutting down the fat in your food will help protect your heart. Cutting down on the amount of sugar you eat will make

your blood sugar easier to control. Cutting down on your salt intake will help with your blood pressure.

- Lastly, do not cut down on starchy foods such as bread, chapattis, rice, pasta and potatoes. Many people believe that if you have diabetes, you should eat less of these foods, but that is not the case. You should carry on enjoying these foods in the amounts you currently eat.

These six points can be summarized by imagining a plate. At meal times most people's plates consist of large portions of meat, fish, eggs or cheese. These high-fat foods often cover half of the plate, leaving very little room for vegetables, fruit and starchy foods such as potatoes, rice, pasta, chapattis and yam. We recommend that the amount of potatoes, other starchy foods, vegetables and fruit is increased so that they cover most of your plate, and that the amount of meat, fish, eggs or cheese is reduced so that it makes up the smallest portion of food on your plate. In this way the fatty foods you eat are reduced.

## Some Common Questions

*Are There Foods you can Eat that will not Affect your Blood Sugar?*
Yes, there are many foods you can eat and enjoy that will not affect your blood sugar and some foods that can positively help control your blood sugar. The main groups of foods that you can eat without worrying are vegetables and fruit. In fact, the vitamins help protect your heart. Within this food group, the pulse vegetables, such as lentils, black-eyed beans, chick peas, moong beans, haricot beans, butter beans, red kidney beans and even baked beans, can actually reduce the amount of sugar in the blood if you eat them regularly. We encourage people to eat as much fruit as possible. Try to become used to having fruit for your snacks or when feeling hungry rather than nibbling on things like biscuits that have a high fat content.

Drinks such as water, soda water, tea and coffee without sugar, sugar-free squash and diet drinks are all fine. Feel free to use sweeteners, if you think it is necessary.

As we already said, you should not be afraid to eat starchy foods. Starchy foods such as bread, breakfast cereal, potatoes, rice, pasta, green banana, yam and chapatti should form the basis of your meals. Again, some of these starchy foods can help to control blood sugar. You should try to eat these foods as regularly as possible.

All fish is very good for you, and there is evidence to suggest that oily fish such as mackerel, sardines, pilchards, salmon and herring have a positive effect on the health of your heart.

*Why Cut Down on Fat?*

Probably the most important thing you should do is to try to cut down on your fat and oil intake. Two of the major aims of the diet are to reduce the risk of heart disease and reduce your weight. Fats and oils (no matter what kind) in large amounts are bad for your heart. The general message is to eat less of these. They are also very high in energy, so reducing your use of fats and oils will help you lose weight

*Which Foods are High in Fat?*

There are visible fats—the fat that you can see in or on foods, such as cooking oils, including all the vegetable oils, ghee, lard, butter, margarine, meat fat and dripping. There are also foods that have hidden fats, such as biscuits, where the high fat content is not obvious. In general you should try to cut down on fried foods, snacks such as samosas and high-fat foods that come from takeaways. You should remove the fat from your meat, and perhaps use less butter, margarine or ghee in your food. Try a low-fat spread instead. You should try to encourage your family to move from using full-fat milk to a lower-fat milk such as semi-skimmed or skimmed, and reduce the amount of cheese that you eat. Make yoghurt using skimmed milk or buy low-fat types. Obviously, cream and chocolate-covered biscuits and cakes should only be eaten on occasion, as should pies and pasties.

*Which Foods should you Avoid?*

There are no hard and fast rules. We do discourage you from eating certain foods on a regular basis but do not say you should never eat these. Certainly you should attempt to reduce the amount of sugar in your diet, particularly if you are overweight. If you are going to eat foods which are high in sugar, such as sugar itself, chocolates, sweets, jams and honey, cakes and puddings, tinned fruit in syrup, ordinary squashes and fizzy drinks such as cola or Lucozade, then you should try and have them with other foods. If they are taken as part of a meal the glycaemic response is blunted. In general it is better for your overall health and diabetic control if you can avoid these foods.

**What to Watch Out For**

Please try to remember that diabetes is not just a disease involving sugar and is not just about cutting out sugar from your diet. It is about adding foods to the diet that will help control your blood sugar, limiting the amount of fat, and increasing the amount of vegetables and fresh fruit that you eat. It is about finding a new way to enjoy a wide variety of foods and drinks.

## Useful Address
British Diabetes Association
10 Queen Anne Street
London
WIM 0BD

## Paediatrics
CAROLINE KING

Due to their rapid growth rates children have higher nutritional requirements per kilogram body weight. These requirements gradually decline with age (see Table 1.4).

| TABLE 1.4 | ESTIMATED AVERAGE REQUIREMENTS/KG BODY WEIGHT* | | |
|---|---|---|---|
| Age | Fluid (ml) | Energy (kcal) | Protein (g) |
| Preterm | 150–200 | 120 | 3.5 |
| 0–3 months | 150 | 115–100 | 2.1 |
| 4–6 months | 130 | 95 | 1.6 |
| 7–9 months | 120 | 95 | 1.5 |
| 10–12 months | 110 | 95 | 1.5 |
| 1–3 years | 95 | 95 | 1.1 |
| 4–6 years | 85 | 90 | 1.1 |
| 7–10 years | 75 | 85 | No COMA rec |
| 11–14 years | 55 | 65 | No COMA rec |
| 15–18 years | 35–50 | 40 | 0.6 |

Note: The higher fluid requirements result in an increased risk of dehydration during illness.
* Committee on Medical Aspects of Food (COMA) 1991 DOH Report on health and social subjects, no. 41. HMSO, ISBN 0–11–321397–2

## Infants
Breast milk is the preferred feed in the vast majority and can be expressed and administered via tube in those unable, or too ill, to breast-feed. The alternative is a formula milk for which there are usually nutritional guidelines from government bodies regarding nutrient composition. Specialized formulas include preterm, high-energy, thickened, soya-based, semi-elemental, elemental, lactose-free, low-calcium and many more, such as those catering for increased requirements, malabsorption, inborn errors of metabolism, etc.

## Pre-school Children

This is a vulnerable group, with socio-economically disadvantaged children and those from some ethnic groups being prone to nutritional deficiencies. Iron and vitamin D are the most common micronutrients at risk of deficiency in the UK. Low-energy intakes due to poverty, poor parenting skills or neglect occur in a significant number of pre-schoolers, leading to failure to thrive. Conversely, obesity can have its roots in early childhood and keeping weight gain within accepted centiles should be the aim.

## Adolescents

The pubertal growth spurt represents a time of accelerated growth, almost matching that of early infancy, resulting in high nutrient requirements. However, an increasingly sedentary lifestyle coupled with easily available energy-dense food has led to an increased risk of obesity in young people.

# Appendix 2
# Resuscitation*
LINDSAY CREEK

The act of resuscitation can be split into two component parts: basic life support and advanced life support. This appendix concentrates on basic life support, and is structured around the 1998 guidelines published by the European Resuscitation Council and the Resuscitation Council (UK).

## The Chain of Survival

The Chain of Survival consists of four links. If a patient is to have the optimum chance of survival, *all* aspects of this 'Chain' must be present. If only one link fails, then the patient's chances are severely reduced, to the point where survival may not be the outcome at all. The four links are as follows:

- Early access.
- Early basic life support.
- Early defibrillation.
- Early advanced life support.

Early access involves the concept of early recognition of a cardiac arrest, and as a result the prompt activation of the emergency services. Assistance is accessed via the 999 system, and more recently by dialling 112 (the standardized emergency number throughout Europe).

Early basic life support is essential in the prevention of brain damage. Statistics demonstrate that it takes 3–4 minutes for a patient to suffer irreversible brain damage after collapse, less if the patient was initially hypoxic (Handley et al 1998: 67). As well as preventing this damage, basic life support can buy time for the arrival of a defibrillator, research demonstrating that the patient stays in ventricular fibrillation for a longer period of time (cited in Cummins et al 1991: 1834). Unfortunately, the application of basic life support techniques by members of the public in the UK tends to be extremely rare. This is largely due to ignorance and fear, the majority of people never having received any form of training. This deficit is now being addressed, and gradually we are seeing the advent of Community

---

* The illustrations in this appendix are reproduced with kind permission of the Resuscitation Council.

Resuscitation Training Officers, who are responsible for coordinating training for members of the public, businesses and industry, GPs, dentists and schools. Community-based courses are run by a variety of other agencies as well, and include Heartstart sessions supported by the British Heart Foundation, and courses run by the British Red Cross, St John's Ambulance, St Andrew's Ambulance Association and the Royal Life Saving Society.

Defibrillation, if applied as soon as possible in a cardiac arrest, is often successful. Research has shown that the patient's chances of survival after collapse from cardiac arrest decrease by 7–10% for every minute without defibrillation (cited in Bossaert et al 1998: 91). Nowadays, the advent of automated external defibrillators has enabled the concept of defibrillation to be introduced within the community, initially within high-risk areas such as golf courses, shopping centres and leisure and fitness centres. A few Ambulance NHS Trusts are also experimenting with Community Responder Schemes, in which members of a community are trained in emergency life support techniques and defibrillation, and are activated within their village/ town when an appropriate call is received by ambulance control. Life saving interventions can therefore be provided as soon as is humanly possible, and in the majority of cases, prior to the arrival of an ambulance.

Early advanced life support is the application of techniques that attempt to stabilize the patient's condition. Practical skills, such as obtaining intravenous access, the administration of drugs and endotracheal intubation, are included. The standardization of advanced life support has occurred over the past few years with the advent of specific courses for health-care professionals, coordinated by the Resuscitation Council (UK).

## The 1998 Resuscitation Guidelines

These guidelines concern the adult patient and do not involve the use of any adjuncts. They are based on out-of-hospital scenarios, and can be adapted for in-hospital arrests, where defibrillators and assistance are generally more readily available.

*Ensure safety:*                 Approach any situation with extreme care, ensuring there is no further danger to yourself or the casualty. Hazards will very much depend on the situation you are in at the time, but can include traffic, electricity, chemical leaks, animals, kitchen implements, falling masonry, etc.

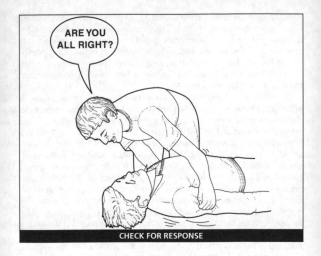

CHECK FOR RESPONSE

*Check for response*    As you approach the casualty shout at the person to obtain a response. If there is no response, then gently shake the casualty by the shoulders and shout again.

## The casualty responds to you

*Assess the situation:*    Assess the problem/situation and if required go for help. After obtaining assistance, return and remain with the casualty, providing first aid if necessary. Reassess at regular intervals.

## The casualty does not respond

*Shout for help*    It is possible that someone in the vicinity may hear your call and will respond.

*Open the airway:*    Look in the mouth for foreign bodies (dentures can be left in place if they fit well). If anything is seen, remove it carefully with a finger sweep. To open the airway you need to perform a head tilt/chin lift manoeuvre. To do this, place one hand on the

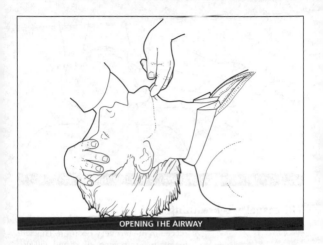

**OPENING THE AIRWAY**

forehead and tilt the head back; at the same time, with two fingers of your other hand, lift the chin. This action will lift the tongue from the back of the throat, thus opening the airway.

If you suspect that the casualty may have a cervical spine injury, attempt to open the airway by using jaw thrust, thus minimizing any movement to the neck. To perform a jaw thrust, place your fingers behind the angle of the jaw and apply a steady pressure to bring the jaw upwards and forwards.

*Check for breathing*   In order to check for breathing you must maintain the airway manoeuvre. Bring your cheek over the mouth and nose of the casualty and look along the line of the chest:

- Look for chest movement.
- Listen for breath sounds.
- Feel for breathing on your cheek.

You have 10 seconds in which to do this.

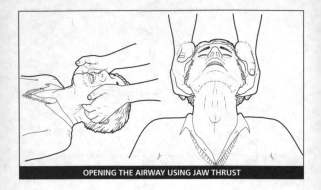

**OPENING THE AIRWAY USING JAW THRUST**

## The casualty is breathing

*Place in the recovery position* An unconscious casualty needs to be placed in the recovery position. This will maintain the airway position and will also ensure that if the patient vomits, stomach contents may drain out of the mouth rather than being aspirated into the lungs:

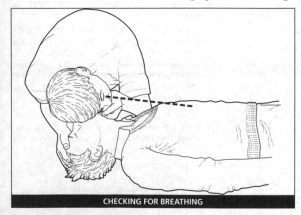

**CHECKING FOR BREATHING**

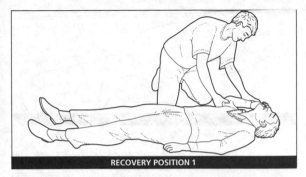

RECOVERY POSITION 1

RECOVERY POSITION 2

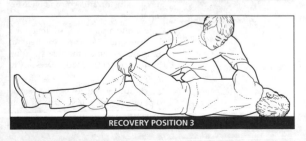

RECOVERY POSITION 3

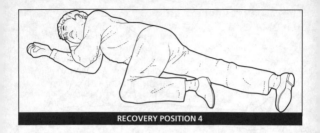

**RECOVERY POSITION 4**

- Before moving the casualty remove his or her glasses (if worn), and any keys or sharp objects from the pockets. To remove objects safely from pockets gently pull the linings out, thus avoiding personal injury from sharps, etc.

- Kneel beside the casualty. Place the arm nearest you at right angles to the casualty's body. Bend the elbow, keeping the palm uppermost.

- Bring the far arm across the casualty's chest and hold the back of the casualty's hand against the nearest cheek.

- With your other hand grasp the far thigh just above the knee. Pull it up, keeping the foot on the ground. Pull the casualty towards you and on to his or her side.

- Adjust the upper leg so that both the hip and the knee are bent at right angles. Open the airway, using the hand under the head if necessary to assist.

- If assistance is available send someone to phone for help. If you are on your own go for help, returning to check the casualty's breathing.

# The casualty is not breathing

*Go for help*

If someone responds to your shout for help send that person to phone for an ambulance. If you are on your own then leave the casualty at this point and make the phone call yourself. The only exceptions to this rule are if the person has collapsed as a result of trauma or drowning, or if the casualty is a child.

*Give two rescue breaths*

If the patient is not already on his or her back you will need to move the casualty. Hold the airway open and pinch the patient's nose closed. Seal your lips around the mouth and blow steadily for $1\frac{1}{2}$–2 seconds, looking for the chest rising. Bring your mouth away and allow the chest to fall completely before giving another breath. You have up to five attempts to give two effective ventilations. An adequate ventilation is one which causes the chest to rise (a volume of approximately 400–500 ml of air).

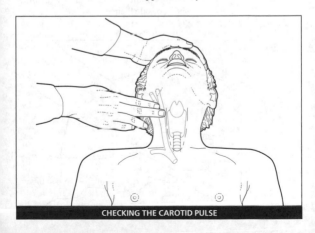

CHECKING THE CAROTID PULSE

*Check circulation*

Look for any signs of movement/signs of a circulation including swallowing, breathing or moving. At the same time check the carotid pulse for 10 seconds.

## Pulse is present
*Continue rescue breathing*

Rescue breathing should be continued for 1 minute before the circulation is checked again for 10 seconds. If the pulse remains present continue breathing, stopping only for pulse checks every minute. If you are ventilating a casualty at the correct rate, you should achieve 10–12 breaths in a minute.

## There is no pulse
*Start chest compressions*

To perform chest compressions effectively the casualty needs to be lying on his or her back on a firm surface. If possible, expose the chest to enable you to find the correct hand position. Run your fingers along the lowest ribs to the point where they join the sternum. Place two fingers on this point and the heel of your other hand beside them.

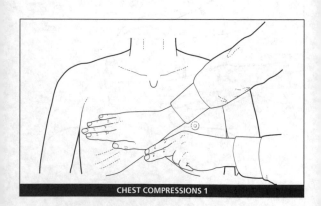

**CHEST COMPRESSIONS 1**

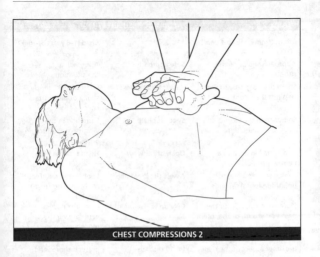

**CHEST COMPRESSIONS 2**

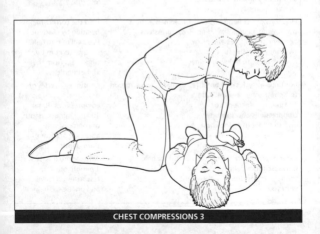

**CHEST COMPRESSIONS 3**

| TABLE 2.1 | PAEDIATRIC RESUSCITATION | |
| --- | --- | --- |
| **Infant (from birth to 1 year)** | | **Child (1–8 years of age)** |
| Approach and assess the situation | Safe approach | Approach and assess the situation |
| Shout at and gently shake or pinch the infant | Assess for response | Shout at and gently shake or pinch the child |
| Someone in the vicinity can call for an ambulance | Shout for help | Someone in the vicinity can call for an ambulance |
| Head tilt/chin lift into a neutral position | Open the airway | Head tilt/chin lift |
| Look, listen and feel for breathing for 10 seconds | Assess the breathing | Look, listen and feel for breathing for 10 seconds |
| Place your mouth over the nose and mouth of the infant | Give up to five breaths | Pinch the nose and ventilate via the mouth |
| Check the brachial pulse on the inner aspect of the upper arm. If pulse is 60 per minute or below, or is absent, commence chest compressions | Assess the circulation for 10 seconds | Check the carotid pulse. If there is no pulse commence chest compressions |
| Find the correct hand position by drawing an imaginary line between the nipples and place two fingers on the sternum one finger's breadth below this line | Commence chest compressions | Find the correct hand position by placing the heel of one hand on the sternum two fingers up from the xiphoid process |
| Continue in cycles of 1 breath to 5 chest compressions. Rate 100 per minute, depth of compressions approximately one-third depth of the chest | Continue resuscitation | Continue in cycles of one breath to five chest compressions. Rate 100 per minute, depth of compressions approximately one-third depth of the chest |
| After approximately 1 minute of resuscitation leave and phone for help. If possible take the infant with you | Go for help | After approximately 1 minute of resuscitation leave and phone for help |

Place the heel of your other hand over the first, and interlock your fingers pulling them clear of the chest. This will ensure that pressure is delivered purely by the heel of your hand.

Keep your elbows straight and bring your elbows over the casualty's chest. Commence 15 chest compressions, aiming to depress the sternum by 4–5 cm. The compressions should be delivered smoothly at a rate of 100 per minute. Continue to alternate 15 chest compressions with two ventilations, ensuring that each time you move back to the chest, you find the correct hand position again.

*Continue*

It is unlikely that basic life support alone will revive the casualty; therefore don't stop to check breathing or circulation unless the patient moves or takes a breath. Do *not* stop resuscitation because the patient does not respond, but continue until help arrives, or until you are too exhausted to keep going.

## When to Go for Help

This will depend upon the situation in which you may find yourself. In the majority of cases an adult will arrest as a result of a sudden cardiac event. In these patients, the lone rescuer should seek help as soon as it has been established that the patient is not breathing. If the cause of the collapse is thought to be trauma or drowning, or if the victim is an infant or a child, 1 minute of resuscitation should be performed by the lone rescuer before leaving to phone for help.

If there is more than one rescuer, one person should commence resuscitation while the other leaves to obtain help. If, however, you are a lone rescuer and someone responded to your shout for help, you can send that person to call an ambulance. If you do this, ensure that your helper knows your location, and request that the person returns and informs you that the telephone call has been made.

**In-hospital Resuscitation**

Many hospitals adapt the above guidelines subject to availability of defibrillators and experienced assistance. Ensure that you are aware of your hospital's resuscitation policy, including the number you need to call in order to activate the cardiac arrest team. The majority of hospitals now have a Resuscitation Training Officer in post, who is available for information and training issues relating to resuscitation.

# Paediatric Resuscitation

The priority, as far as children are concerned, is to prevent cardiac arrest in the first place. Thus, greater emphasis is placed upon recognition of the sick child and appropriate treatment to prevent decline. Children have a tendency to arrest as a result of respiratory difficulties rather than a primary cardiac dysfunction, and as a result they more commonly arrest into an asystolic or non-shockable rhythm.

There are a few fundamental differences within the paediatric basic life support algorithm, reflecting the varying sizes of child encountered. Of particular importance is the relative positioning of the airway. Infants require very little movement to achieve adequate airway position; often the head only needs to be placed in a neutral position. A child will require a slightly increased head tilt/chin lift from the infant, but not to the same extent as an adult. In all cases you should take particular care to obtain the chin lift by placing the fingers on the bony aspect of the chin, as pressing on the soft tissues can cause airway obstruction. The technique for rescue breathing also differs between age groups, the infant receiving mouth-to-mouth and nose ventilations, the older child receiving mouth-to-mouth. Up to five initial breaths should be given, as it may take a few attempts to achieve the correct airway position and therefore adequate ventilation.

The brachial pulse is recommended for the pulse check in infants, and the carotid pulse in a child over the age of 1 year. Chest compressions differ, in that infants require a two-finger technique (see Table 2.1) and the older child requires compression delivered with the heel of one hand. For children up to the age of 8, compressions and ventilation should be in continued cycles of 5:1. The child above 8 years of age will probably require a ratio of 15 compressions to 2 ventilations, and may need the two-handed compression technique. In all cases, resuscitation should be continued for 1 minute before leaving to phone for an ambulance if no one else has done so. The advantage with younger children is that it may be possible to take them to a phone with you.

REFERENCES

Bossaert L, Hanley A, Marsden A et al 1998 European Resuscitation Council guidelines for the use of automated external defibrillators by EMS providers and first responders. Resuscitation 37: 91–94

Cummins R, Ornato J, Thies W, Pepe P 1991 Improving survival from sudden cardiac arrest: the 'Chain of Survival' concept. Circulation May 83(5): 1832–47

Handley A, Bahr J, Baskett P et al 1998 The 1998 European Resuscitation Council guidelines for adult single rescuer basic life support. Resuscitation 37: 67–80

BIBLIOGRAPHY

American Heart Association 1997 Paediatric advanced life support, 3rd edn. American Heart Association

Colquhoun M, Handley A, Evans T 1995 ABC of resuscitation, 3rd edn. BMJ Publishing Group, London

Resuscitation Council (UK) 1998 Advanced life support course provider manual, 3rd edn. Resuscitation Council (UK), London

# Appendix 3
# Drugs and their Control*
CHRIS EVANS

The two acts that control the manufacture, supply and use of drugs are the Medicines Act 1968 and the Misuse of Drugs Act 1971.

## The Medicines Act

The Act defines 'medicinal products' as substances sold or supplied for administration to humans or animals for medicinal purposes. Part 3 of the Act, and order made under it, control the manufacture and sale or supply of medicines, and for this purpose broadly classify them into three classes:

1. Prescription-only medicines (PoM).
2. Pharmacy medicines (P).
3. General sales list medicines (GSL).

Different legal requirements apply to the sale, supply and labelling of each class.

In hospitals and other institutions, all medicines should be appropriately and securely stored in order to ensure that they remain safe and effective in use and to deter unauthorized access to them and hence possible misuse (see Department of Health 1988).

## The Misuse of Drugs Act

This Act designates and defines as Controlled Drugs a number of 'dangerous or otherwise harmful' substances. These substances are all also by definition prescription-only medicines under the Medicines Act. The controls imposed by the Misuse of Drugs Act are therefore additional to those under the Medicines Act. The main purpose of the Misuse of Drugs Act is to prevent abuse of Controlled Drugs by prohibiting their manufacture or supply except in accordance with various regulations made under the Act. Other regulations govern requirements for safe custody, destruction and supply to addicts.

For these purposes, under the current (1985) Regulations, Controlled Drugs are classified into five Schedules, each representing a different level of control. For practical purposes Schedule 2 is the most relevant to hospital and community nursing practice. It includes: cocaine; the major opioids such as diamorphine, methadone, morphine, papaveretum and pethidine, and the major stimulant amphetamine (and related drugs). (Amendments to this list and the list of drugs in the other Schedules may be made from time to time.)

Prescriptions for Schedule 2 drugs (and for those in Schedules 1 and 3) must:

1. Be handwritten, signed and dated by the prescriber.
2. Be in ink or be otherwise indelible.
3. Include the name and address of the patient.
4. State (in words and figures) the total quantity of the drug to be supplied.
5. State the dose to be taken.

(Some of these requirements may be relaxed for the prescription of some Controlled Drugs to addicts, for the treatment of their addiction, by doctors who hold a special Home Office licence.)

In hospitals, ordering, supply and storage of Controlled Drugs is subject to tight control:

1. They are stored separately in a locked cupboard (which may be within a second outer cupboard) to which access is restricted. The key to the cupboard is held by a first level nurse.
2. Supply from the pharmacy is made to a ward or department only on receipt of a written order signed by a responsible nurse.
3. A record is kept of stock held and details of doses given. A special register is used for this and no other purpose, and it is usually the case that each entry is countersigned by two nurses. The records should be regularly checked by the nurse in charge and by a pharmacist, according to health authority policy.

## Abbreviations Used in Prescriptions

Abbreviations of Latin are being replaced by English versions, which are considered safer; however, the nurse may still meet the Latin abbreviations given in Table 3.1.

## Self-administration of Drugs by Hospital Inpatients

For the inpatient approaching discharge, there are obvious benefits to be gained from the opportunity to assume responsibility for self-administration of prescribed medicines while access to professional support and advice is still readily available (UKCC 1992). Schemes to allow self-administration of their medicines by various groups of hospital inpatients have been established in several National Health Service (NHS) hospitals. Self-administration shifts the balance of

| TABLE 3.1 | ABBREVIATIONS USED IN PRESCRIPTIONS | |
|---|---|---|
| Abbreviation | Latin | English |
| a.c. | ante cibum | before food |
| ad lib. | ad libitum | to the desired amount |
| b.d. or b.i.d. | bis in die | twice a day |
| c. | cum | with |
| o.m. | omni mane | every morning |
| o.n. | omni nocte | every night |
| p.c. | post cibum | after food |
| p.r.n. | pro re nata | whenever necessary |
| q.d. | quaque die | every day |
| q.d.s. | quaque die sumendum | four times daily |
| q.i.d. | quater in die | four times a day |
| q.q.h. | quater quaque hora | every four hours |
| R | recipe | take |
| s.o.s. | si opus sit | if necessary |
| stat. | statim | at once |
| t.d.s. | ter die sumendum | three times a day |
| t.i.d. | ter in die | three times a day |

responsibility for this part of their care further towards patients. The nurse's fundamental professional duty of care is, however, undiminished and it is essential that local policies and procedures are adequate to ensure that this responsibility is, and can be shown to be, discharged.

## Administration of Medicines: UKCC Advisory Paper

The United Kingdom Central Council (UKCC), in an advisory paper on the administration of medicines, clearly states the role and responsibility of the nurse, midwife and health visitor in the administration of prescribed drugs. This paper is reproduced below.

1. This standards paper replaces the Council's advisory paper *Administration of medicines* (UKCC 1986) and the supplementary circular *The administration of medicines* (UKCC 1988). The Council has prepared this paper to assist practitioners to fulfil the expectations which it has of them, to serve more effectively the interests of patients and clients and to maintain and enhance standards of practice.

2. The administration of medicines is an important aspect of the professional practice of persons whose names are on the Council's

register. It is not solely a mechanistic task to be performed in strict compliance with the written prescription of a medical practitioner. It requires thought and the exercise of professional judgement which is directed to the following:

2.1 Confirming the correctness of the prescription.

2.2 Judging the suitability of administration at the scheduled time of administration.

2.3 Reinforcing the positive effect of the treatment.

2.4 Enhancing the understanding of patients in respect of their prescribed medication and the avoidance of misuse of these and other medicines.

2.5 Assisting in assessing the efficacy of medicines and the identification of side-effects and interactions.

3. To meet the standards set out in this paper is to honour, in this aspect of practice, the Council's expectation (set out in the Council's *Code of professional conduct* (UKCC 1992), that: As a registered nurse, midwife or health visitor you are personally accountable for your practice and, in the exercise of your professional accountability, must:

(a) Act always in such a manner as to promote and safeguard the interests and wellbeing of patients and clients.

(b) Ensure that no action or omission on your part, or within your sphere of responsibility, is detrimental to the interests, condition or safety of patients and clients.

(c) Maintain and improve your professional knowledge and competence.

(d) Acknowledge any limitations in your knowledge and competence and decline any duties or responsibilities unless able to perform them in a safe and skilled manner.

4. This extract from the *Code of professional conduct* applies to all persons on the Council's register irrespective of the part of the register on which their name appears. Although the content of pre-registration education programmes varies, dependent on the part or level of the register involved, the Council expects that, in this area of practice as in all others, all practitioners will have taken steps to develop their knowledge and competence and will have been assisted to this end. The word 'practitioner' is, therefore, used in the remainder of this paper to refer to all registered nurses, midwives and health visitors, each of whom must recognize the personal professional accountability which they bear for their actions. The Council therefore imposes no arbitrary boundaries between

the role of the first level and second level registered practitioner in this respect.

**Treatment with Medicines**

5. The treatment of a patient with medicines for therapeutic, diagnostic or preventative purposes is a process which involves prescribing, dispensing, administering, receiving and recording. The word 'patient' is used for convenience, but implies not only a patient in a hospital or nursing home, but also a resident of a residential home, a client in her or his own home or in a community home, a person attending a clinical or a general practitioner's surgery and an employee attending a workplace occupational health department. 'Patient' refers to the person receiving a prescribed medicine. Each medicine has a product licence, which means that authority has been given to a manufacturer to market a particular product for administration in a particular dosage range and by specified routes.

**Prescription**

6. The practitioner administering a medicine against a prescription written by a registered medical practitioner, like the pharmacist responsible for dispensing it, can reasonably expect that the prescription satisfies the following criteria:

6.1 It is based, whenever possible, on the patient's awareness of the purpose of the treatment and consent (commonly implicit).

6.2 The prescription is either clearly written, typed or computer-generated, and the entry is indelible and dated.

6.3 Where the new prescription replaces an earlier prescription, the latter has been cancelled clearly and the cancellation signed and dated by an authorized registered medical practitioner.

6.4 Where a prescribed substance (which replaces an earlier prescription) has been provided for a person residing at home or in a residential care home and who is dependent on others to assist with the administration, information about the change has been properly communicated.

6.5 The prescription provides clear and unequivocal identification of the patient for whom the medicine is intended.

6.6 The substance to be administered is clearly specified and, where appropriate, its form (for example, tablet, capsule, suppository) stated, together with the strength, dosage, timing and frequency of administration and route of administration.

6.7 Where the prescription is provided in an outpatient or community setting, it states the duration of the course before review.

6.8 In the case of controlled drugs, the dosage is written, together with the number of dosage units or total course if in an outpatient or community setting, the whole being in the prescriber's own handwriting.

6.9 All other prescriptions will, as a minimum, have been signed by the prescribing doctor and dated.

6.10 The registered medical practitioner understands that the administration of medicines on verbal instructions, whether she or he is present or absent, other than in exceptional circumstances, is not acceptable unless covered by the protocol method referred to in paragraph 6.11.

6.11 It is understood that, unless provided for in a specific protocol, instruction by telephone to a practitioner to administer a previously unprescribed substance is not acceptable, the use of facsimile transmission (fax) being the preferred method in exceptional circumstances or isolated locations.

6.12 Where it is the wish of the professional staff concerned that practitioners in a particular setting be authorized to administer, on their own authority, certain medicines, a local protocol has been agreed between medical practitioners, nurses and midwives and the pharmacist.

## Dispensing

7. The practitioner administering a medicine dispensed by a pharmacist in response to a medical prescription can reasonably expect that:

7.1 The pharmacist has checked that the prescription is written correctly so as to avoid misunderstanding or error and is signed by an authorized prescriber.

7.2 The pharmacist is satisfied that any newly prescribed medicines will not dangerously interact with or nullify each other.

7.3 The pharmacist has provided the medicine in a form relevant for administration to the particular patient, provided it in an appropriate container giving the relevant information and advised appropriately on storage and security conditions.

7.4  Where the substance is prescribed in a dose or to be administered by a route which falls outside its product licence, unless to be administered from a stock supply, the pharmacist will have taken steps to ensure that the prescriber is aware of and has chosen to exceed that licence.

7.5  Where the prescription for a specific item falls outside the terms of the product licence, whether as to its route of administration, the dosage or some other key factor, the pharmacist will have ensured that the prescriber is aware of this fact and, mindful of her or his accountability in the matter, has made a record on the prescription to this effect and has agreed to dispense the medicine ordered.

7.6  If the prescription bears any written amendments made and signed by the pharmacist, the prescriber has been consulted and advised and the amendments have been accepted.

7.7  The pharmacist, in pursuit of her or his role in monitoring the adverse side-effects of medicines, wishes to be sent any information that the administering practitioner deems relevant.

## Standards for the Administration of Medicines

8.  Notwithstanding the expected adherence by registered medical practitioners and pharmacists to the criteria set out in paragraphs 6 and 7 of this paper, the nurse, midwife or health visitor must, in administering any medicines, in assisting with administration or overseeing any self-administration of medicines, exercise professional judgement and apply knowledge and skill to the situation that pertains at the time.

9.  This means that, as a matter of basic principle, whether administering a medicine, assisting in its administration or overseeing self-administration, the practitioner will be satisfied that she or he:

9.1  Has an understanding of the substances used for therapeutic purposes.

9.2  Is able to justify any actions taken.

9.3  Is prepared to be accountable for the action taken.

10.  Against this background, the practitioner, acting in the interests of the patient, will:

10.1  Be certain of the identity of the patient to whom the medicine is to be administered.

10.2  Ensure that she or he is aware of the patient's current assessment and planned programme of care.

10.3  Pay due regard to the environment in which that care is being given.

10.4 Scrutinize carefully, in the interests of safety, the prescription, where available, and the information provided on the relevant containers.

10.5 Question the medical practitioner or pharmacist, as appropriate, if the prescription or container information is illegible, unclear, ambiguous or incomplete or where it is believed that the dosage or route of administration falls outside the product licence for the particular substance and, where believed necessary, refuse to administer the prescribed substance.

10.6 Refuse to prepare substances for injection in advance of their immediate use and refuse to administer a medicine not placed in a container or drawn into a syringe by her or him, in her or his presence, or prepared by a pharmacist, except in the specific circumstances described in paragraph 40 of this paper and others where similar issues arise.

10.7 Draw the attention of patients, as appropriate, to patient information leaflets concerning their prescribed medicines.

11. In addition, acting in the interests of the patient, the practitioner will:

11.1 Check the expiry data of any medicine, if on the container.

11.2 Carefully consider the dosage, method of administration, and route and timing of administration in the context of the condition of the specific patient at the operative time.

11.3 Carefully consider whether any of the prescribed medicines will or may dangerously interact with each other.

11.4 Determine whether it is necessary or advisable to withhold the medicine pending consultation with the prescribing medical practitioner, the pharmacist or a fellow professional colleague.

11.5 Contact the prescriber without delay where contraindications to the administration of any prescribed medicine are observed, first taking the advice of the pharmacist where considered appropriate.

11.6 Make clear, accurate and contemporaneous record of the administration of all medicines administered or deliberately withheld, ensuring that any written entries and the signature are clear and legible.

11.7 Where a medicine is refused by the patient, or the parent refuses to administer or allow administration of that medicine, make a clear and accurate record of the fact without delay, consider whether the refusal of that medicine compromises the patient's condition or the effect of other medicines, assess the situation and contact the prescriber.

11.8 Use the opportunity which administration of a medicine provides for emphasizing, to patients and their carers, the importance and implications of the prescribed treatment and for enhancing their understanding of its effects and side-effects.

11.9 Record the positive and negative effects of the medicine and make them known to the prescribing medical practitioner and the pharmacist.

11.10 Take all possible steps to ensure that replaced prescription entries are correctly deleted to avoid duplication of medicines.

## Applying the Standards in a Range of Settings

*Who can administer medicines?*

12. There is a wide spectrum of situations in which medicines are administered, ranging, at one extreme, from the patient in an intensive therapy unit who is totally dependent on registered professional staff for her or his care to, at the other extreme, the person in her or his own home administering her or his own medicines or being assisted in this respect by a relative or another person. The answer to the question of who can administer a medicine must largely depend on where within that spectrum the recipient of the medicines lies.

*Administration in the hospital setting*

13. It is the Council's position that, at or near the first stated end of that spectrum, assessment of response to treatment and speedy recognition of contraindications and side-effects are of great importance. Therefore prescribed medicines should only be administered by registered practitioners who are competent for the purpose and aware of their personal accountability.

14. In this context it is the Council's position that, in the majority of circumstances, a first level registered nurse, a midwife, or a second level nurse, each of whom has demonstrated the necessary knowledge and competence, should be able to administer medicines without involving a second person. Exceptions to this might be where:

14.1 The practitioner is instructing a student.

14.2 The patient's condition makes it necessary.

14.3 Local circumstances make the involvement of two persons desirable in the interests of the patients (for example, in areas of specialist care, such as a paediatric unit without sufficient specialist paediatric nurses or in other acute units dependent on temporary agency or other locum staff).

15. In respect of the administration of intravenous drugs by practitioners, it is the Council's position that this is acceptable, provided that, as in all other aspects of practice, the practitioner is satisfied with her or his competence and mindful of her or his personal accountability.

16. The Council is opposed to the involvement of persons who are not registered practitioners in the administration of medicines in acute care settings and with ill or dependent patients, since the requirements of paragraphs 8 to 11 inclusive of this paper cannot then be satisfied. It accepts, however, that the professional judgement of an individual practitioner should be used to identify those situations in which informal carers might be instructed and prepared to accept a delegated responsibility in this respect.

*Administration in the domestic or quasi-domestic setting*

17. It is evident that in this setting, on the majority of occasions, there is no involvement of registered practitioners. Where a practitioner engaged in community practice does become involved in assisting with or overseeing administration, then she or he must observe paragraphs 8 to 11 of this paper and apply them to the required degree. She or he must also recognize that, even if not employed in posts requiring registration with the Council, she or he remains accountable to the Council.

18. The same principles apply where prescribed medicines are being administered to residents in small community homes or in residential care homes. To the maximum degree possible, though related to their ability to manage the care and administration of their prescribed medicines and comprehend their significance, the residents should be regarded as if in their own home. Where assistance is required, the person providing it fills the role of an informal carer, family member or friend. However, as with the situation described in paragraph 17, where a professional practitioner is involved, a personal accountability is borne. The advice of a community pharmacist should be sought when necessary.

*Self-administration of medicines in hospitals or registered nursing homes*

19. The Council welcomes and supports the development of self-administration of medicines and administration by parents to children wherever it is appropriate and the necessary security and storage arrangements are available.

20. For the hospital patient approaching discharge, but who will continue on a prescribed medicines regimen following the return home, there are obvious benefits in adjusting to the responsibility of self-administration while still having access to professional support. It is accepted that, to facilitate this transition, practitioners may assist patients to administer their medicines safely by preparing a form of medication card containing information transcribed from other sources.

21. For the long-stay patient, whether in hospital or a nursing home, self-administration can help foster a feeling of independence and control in one aspect of life.

22. It is essential, however, that where self-administration is introduced for all or some patients, arrangements must be in place for the appropriate, safe and secure storage of the medicines, access to which is limited to the specific patient.

*The use of monitored dosage systems*

23. Monitored dosage systems, for the purpose of this paper, are systems which involve a community pharmacist, in response to the full prescription of medicines for a specific person, dispensing those medicines into a special container with sections for days of the week and times within those days and delivering the container, or supplying the medicines in a special container of blister packs, with appropriate additional information, to the nursing home, residential care home or domestic residence. The Council is aware of the development of such monitored dosage systems and accepts that, provided they are able to satisfy strict criteria established by the Royal Pharmaceutical Society of Great Britain and other official pharmaceutical organizations, that substances which react to each other are not supplied in this way and that they are suitable for the intended purpose as judged by the nursing profession, they have a valuable place in the administration of medicines.

24. While, to the present, their use has been primarily in registered nursing homes and some community or residential care homes, there seems no reason why, provided the systems can satisfy the standards referred to in paragraph 25, their use should not be extended.

25. In order to be acceptable for use in hospitals or registered nursing homes, the containers for the medicines must:

    25.1 Satisfy the requirements of the Royal Pharmaceutical Society of Great Britain for an original container.

25.2 Be filled by a pharmacist and sealed by her or him or under her or his control and delivered complete to the user.

25.3 Be accompanied by clear and comprehensive documentation which forms the medical practitioner's prescription.

25.4 Bear the means of identifying tablets of similar appearance so that, should it be necessary to withhold one tablet (for example, digoxin), it can be identified from those in the container space for the particular time and day.

25.5 Be able to be stored in a secure place.

25.6 Make it apparent if the containers (be they blister packs or spaces within a container) have been tampered with between the closure and sealing by the pharmacist at the time of administration.

26. While the introduction of a monitored dosage system transfers to the pharmacist the responsibility for being satisfied that the container is filled and sealed correctly so as to comply with the prescription, it does not alter the fact that the practitioner administering the medicines must still consider the appropriateness of each medicine at the time administration falls due. It is not the case, therefore, that the use of a monitored dosage system allows the administration of medicines to be undertaken by unqualified personnel.

27. It is not acceptable, in lieu of a pharmacist-filled monitored dosage system container, for a practitioner to transfer medicines from their original containers into an unsealed container for administration at a later stage by another person, whether or not that person is a registered practitioner. This is an unsafe practice which carries risks for both practitioner and patient. Similarly it is not acceptable to interfere with a sealed section at any time between its closure by the pharmacist and the scheduled time of administration.

*The role of nurses, midwives and health visitors in community*
*practice in the administration of medicines*

28. Any practitioner who, whether as a planned intervention or incidentally, becomes involved in administering a medicine, or assisting with or overseeing such administration, must apply paragraphs 8 to 11 of this paper to the degree to which they are relevant.

29. Where a practitioner working in the community becomes involved in obtaining prescribed medicines for patients, she or he

must recognize her or his responsibility for safe transit and correct delivery.

30. Community psychiatric nurses whose practice involves them in providing assistance to patients to reduce and eliminate their dependence on addictive drugs should ensure that they are aware of the potential value of short-term prescriptions and encourage their use where appropriate in the long-term interests of their clients. They must not resort to holding or carrying prescribed controlled drugs to avoid their misuse by those clients.

31. Special arrangements and certain exemptions apply to occupational health nurses. These are described in Information Document 11 and the appendices of *A guide to an occupational health nursing service: a handbook for employers and nurses* (Royal College of Nursing 1991).

32. Some practitioners employed in the community, including in particular community nurses, practice nurses and health visitors, in order to enhance disease prevention, will receive requests to participate in vaccination and immunization programmes. Normally these requests will be accompanied by specific named prescriptions or be covered by a protocol setting out the arrangements within which substances can be administered to certain categories of persons who meet the stated criteria. The facility provided by the Medicines Act 1968, for substances to be administered to a number of people in response to an advance 'direction', is valuable in this respect. Where preventive treatment has not been possible and there is no relevant protocol or advance direction, particularly in respect of patients about to travel abroad and requiring preventive treatment, a telephone conversation with a registered medical practitioner will suffice as authorization for a single administration. It is not, however, sufficient as a basis for supplying a quantity of medicines.

### Midwives and Midwifery Practice

33. Midwives should refer to the current editions of both the Council's *Midwives rules* (UKCC 1991a) and *A midwife's code of practice* (UKCC 1991b), and specifically to the sections concerning administration of medicines. At the time of publication of this paper, *Midwives rules* sets out the practising midwife's responsibility in respect of the administration of medicines and other forms of pain relief. *A midwife's code of*

*practice* refers to the authority provided by the Medicines Act 1968 and the Misuse of Drugs Act 1971, and regulations made as a result, for midwives to obtain and administer certain substances.

## What if the Council's Standards in Paragraphs 8 to 11 cannot be applied?

34. There are certain situations in which practitioners are involved in the administration of medicines where some of the criteria stated above either cannot be applied or, if applied, would introduce dangerous delay with consequent risk to patients. These will include occupational health settings in some industries, small hospitals with no resident medical staff and possibly some specialist units within larger hospitals and some community settings.

35. With the exception of the administration of substances for the purpose of vaccination or immunization described in paragraph 32 above, in any situation in which a practitioner may be expected or required to administer 'prescription-only medicines' which have not been directly prescribed for a named patient by a registered medical practitioner who has examined the patient and made a diagnosis, it is essential that a clear local policy be determined and made known to all practitioners involved with prescribing and administration. This will make it possible for action to be taken in patients' interests while protecting practitioners from the risk of complaint which might otherwise jeopardize their position.

36. Therefore, where such a situation will or may apply, a local policy should be agreed and documented which:

    36.1  States the circumstances in which particular 'prescription-only medicines' may be administered in advance of examination by a doctor.

    36.2  Ensures the relevant knowledge and skill of those to be involved in administration.

    36.3  Describes the form, route and dosage range of the medicines so authorized.

    36.4  Wherever possible, satisfies the requirements of Section 58 of the Medicines Act 1968 as a 'direction'.

## Substances for Topical Application

37. The standards set out in this paper apply, to the degree to which they are relevant, to substances used for wound dressing and

other topical applications. Where a practitioner uses a substance or product which has not been prescribed, she or he must have considered the matter sufficiently to be able to justify its use in the particular circumstances.

## The Administration of Homeopathic or Herbal Substances

38. Homeopathic and herbal medicines are subject to the licensing provisions of the Medicines Act 1968, although those on the market when that Act became operative (which means most of those now available) received product licences without any evaluation of their efficacy, safety or quality. Practitioners should, therefore, make themselves generally aware of common substances used in their particular area of practice. It is necessary to respect the right of individuals to administer to themselves, or to request a practitioner to assist in the administration of substances in these categories. If, when faced with a patient or client whose desire to receive medicines of this kind appears to create potential difficulties, or if it is felt that the substances might be either an inappropriate response to the presenting symptoms or likely to negate or enhance the effect of prescribed medicines, the practitioner, acting in the interests of the patient or client, should consider contacting the relevant registered medical practitioner, but must also be mindful of the need not to override the patient's rights.

## Complementary and Alternative Therapies

39. Some registered nurses, midwives and health visitors, having first undertaken successfully a training in complementary or alternative therapy which involves the use of substances such as essential oils, apply their specialist knowledge and skill in their practice. It is essential that practice in these respects, as in all others, is based upon sound principles, available knowledge and skill. The importance of consent to the use of such treatment must be recognized. So, too, must the practitioner's personal accountability for professional practice.

## Practitioners Assuming Responsibility for Care which includes Medicines being Administered which were previously checked by other Practitioners

40. Paragraph 10.6 of this paper referred to the unacceptability of a practitioner administering a substance drawn into a syringe or container by another practitioner when the practitioner

taking over responsibility for the patient was not present. An exception to this is an already established intravenous infusion, the use of a syringe pump or some other kind of continuous or intermittent infusion or injection apparatus, where a valid prescription exists, a responsible practitioner has signed for the container of fluid and any additives being administered and the container is clearly and indelibly labelled. The label must clearly show the contents and be signed and dated. The same measures must apply equally to other means of administration of such substances through, for example, central venous, arterial or epidural lines. Strict discipline must be applied to the recording of any substances being administered by any of the methods referred to in this paragraph and to reporting procedures between staff as they change and transfer responsibility for care.

## Management of Errors or Incidents in the Administration of Medicines

41. In a number of its annual reports, the Council has recorded its concern that practitioners who have made mistakes under pressure of work, and have been honest and open about those mistakes to their senior staff, appear often to have been made the subject of disciplinary action in a way which seems likely to discourage the reporting of incidents and therefore be to the potential detriment of patients and of standards.

42. When considering allegations of misconduct arising out of errors in the administration of medicines, the Council's Professional Conduct Committee takes great care to distinguish between those cases where the error was the result of reckless practice and was concealed and those which resulted from serious pressure of work and where there was immediate, honest disclosure in the patient's interest. The Council recognizes the prerogative of managers to take local disciplinary action where it is considered to be appropriate but urges that they also consider each incident in its particular context and similarly discriminate between the two categories described.

43. The Council's position is that all errors and incidents require a thorough and careful investigation which takes full account of the circumstances and context of the event and the position of the practitioner involved. Events of this kind call equally for

sensitive management and a comprehensive assessment of all of the circumstances before a professional and managerial decision is reached on the appropriate way to proceed.

## Arrangements for Prescribing Nurses

44. In March 1992 the Act of Parliament entitled the Medicinal Products: Prescription by Nurses, etc. Act 1992 became law. This legislation came into operation in October 1993. It permits nurses with a district nursing or health visiting qualification to prescribe certain products from a Nurse Prescriber's Formulary. The statutory rules specify the categories of nurses who can prescribe under this limited legislation.

45. A nurse prescriber can be defined as a community nurse or practice nurse who is identified as a nurse prescriber on the UKCC register, writing a prescription for an item in the Nurse Prescriber's Formulary using form FP10(CN) or FP10(PN), within a Nurse Prescribing Demonstration Scheme or within a health authority or trust that has implemented nurse prescribing. Nurse prescribing can therefore only be undertaken in community or primary care settings. All other schemes, e.g. in hospitals, whereby nurses are able to supply or administer medicines cannot accurately be termed 'nurse prescribing', and should be retitled if necessary.

46. Statutory Instrument 1994 No 2402 sets out the necessary training and qualifications for nurses to prescribe. It states that nurses who are able to prescribe must:

    46.1 Be registered on parts 1 to 12 of the UKCC register.

    46.2 Have a district nurse qualification and be employed by a health authority, trust or fundholding practice.

    46.3 Be registered in part 11 as a health visitor and be employed by a health authority, trust or fundholding practice.

    46.4 Be named on the professional register and marked as qualified to prescribe. Amendments to this Statutory Instrument have been made to allow eligible nurses employed in Primary Care Act pilots to prescribe.

47. Nurse prescribers may only prescribe from the items listed in the Nurse Prescriber's Formulary.

48. Useful address: Association for Nurse Prescribing, Porters South, 4 Crinan St, London N1 9SQ (tel 0207 843 4517).

49. Enquiries in respect of this Council paper should be directed to the Registrar and Chief Executive, United Kingdom Central Council for Nursing, Midwifery and Health Visiting, 23 Portland Place, London W1N 3AF.

REFERENCES

Department of Health 1988 Guidelines for the safe and secure handling of medicines: the Duthie Report. Department of Health, London

Department of Health 1999 Review of prescribing, supply and administration of medicines: final report. Department of Health, London

Medicinal Products: Prescription by Nurses, etc. Act 1992. HMSO, London

Medicines Act 1968 (reprinted 1986). HMSO, London

Misuse of Drugs Act 1971 (reprinted 1985). HMSO, London

National Health Service Executive 1998 Nurse prescribing—a guide for implementation. NHSE, Leeds

Nurse Prescriber's Formulary 1998 British Medical Association and Royal Pharmaceutical Society of Great Britain, London

Royal College of Nursing 1991 A guide to an occupational health nursing service: a handbook for employers and nurses, 2nd edn. RCN, London

UKCC 1986 Administration of medicines. A UKCC advisory paper: a framework to assist individual professional judgement and the development of local policies and guidelines. UKCC, London

UKCC 1988 The administration of medicines, PC88/05. UKCC, London

UKCC 1991a Midwives rules. UKCC, London

UKCC 1991b A midwife's code of practice. UKCC, London

UKCC 1992 Code of professional conduct for the nurse, midwife and health visitor, 3rd edn. UKCC, London

# Appendix 4
# RCN Fact Sheet 10 Extending Prescribing Powers to Nurses

For the past 20 years the Royal College of Nursing (RCN) has campaigned to extend prescribing powers to specialist nurses and midwives who have completed a prescribing course. The RCN believes that extending prescribing powers to nurses is beneficial for patients because it leads to the swift start of effective treatment. It is also cost-effective for the National Health Service because it saves both doctors' and nurses' time.

Extending prescribing powers is common sense when, in many cases, nurses are the lead specialists in the management of conditions such as diabetes and asthma. The vision of a health service with an emphasis on accessible health care in the community relies heavily on nurses' ability to prescribe.

## The Reality and the Vision

### Changes in Health Care

Changes in health care over the past two decades have led to widespread recognition that the rules for prescribing medicines need updating. The pressures for change include developments in nursing: for example, the introduction of new specialties with recognized training programmes including intensive care, practice nursing, community children's nursing, respiratory care, sexual health, diabetes and tissue viability.

Changes have occurred in patient expectations, with many patients, especially those with chronic health problems, and their carers becoming increasingly expert in the management of their own conditions and seeking advice from a wider range of health professionals.

The relationship between professionals has also changed, with treatment and care increasingly provided by multidisciplinary teams of health professionals. Individual team members act with a degree of autonomy in relation to their area of expertise.

### Nurses and Prescribing

After the successful piloting of nurse prescribing, Health Secretary Frank Dobson announced at the 1998 RCN Congress the extension of prescribing powers to all health visitors and district nurses in England. This process has now started, with training programmes under way for health visitors and district nurses who wish to prescribe.

Evaluation of eight nurse prescribing pilot schemes showed that patients saved time, felt less anxiety and often began treatment quicker when nurses had prescribing powers (National Health Service Executive 1998).

Health visitors and district nurses prescribe from a 'nurse formulary', a limited range of products based on the provision of nursing care involving treatment of wounds, minor injuries and some fungal infections, and the supply of stoma care products. The formulary is outdated, essentially representing community nursing practice of 10 to 15 years ago.

(Alongside these developments in nurse prescribing, group protocols have been introduced to allow the supply and administration of prescription-only medicines by nurses without the need for an individual prescription from a medical practitioner. Group protocols involve nurses and doctors agreeing a range of prescription-only medicines that nurses can use in their practice with written authorization from the medical practitioner to that effect. The national immunization programme relies on the use of such protocols.)

### The Review of Prescribing, Supply and Administration of Medicines (the Crown II Report—Department of Health 1999)

In March 1999 the final report of the Department of Health's review of prescribing, supply and administration of medicines was published. Chaired by Dr June Crown, the review opens the door to extending prescribing powers to a range of specialist nurses.

The Crown Report recommends the introduction of two new groups of prescribers—independent and dependent. Independent prescribers would take responsibility for the initial clinical assessment of a patient (usually making a diagnosis) and then prescribe as appropriate. Dependent prescribers would not make the original diagnosis but, once a diagnosis had been made by an independent prescriber—for example, by a specialist nurse or doctor—the dependent prescriber would be able to prescribe as appropriate, usually informed by clinical guidelines.

The review recommends the setting up of an independent body to consider proposals from professional organizations for the extension of prescribing rights. Organizations such as the RCN would make submissions to the New Prescribers Advisory Committee on behalf of groups of nurses within its membership.

**Issues raised by the Crown Report**

After the report's publication in March 1999, the Government announced a consultation period which lasted until June. Key points from the RCN's response are detailed below.

# Independent and Dependent Prescribers—RCN View

The report suggests family planning and tissue viability nurses as early candidates for independent prescribing rights, and diabetes, asthma and palliative care specialist nurses for dependent prescribing rights. The RCN agrees with the creation of independent and dependent prescribers but believes a wider range of specialist nurses should be considered for independent prescriber status. For example, though nurses working in the fields of diabetes, asthma and palliative care may become dependent prescribers, there will be nurse specialists in these areas eligible for independent prescriber status.

The RCN believes all nurses administering medicines as part of their practice should be fully versed in the nature of the drugs they use, irrespective of whether they have the legal right to prescribe them. The pharmacological knowledge of independent and dependent prescribers should therefore be similar; it is only the ability to make a thorough physical assessment and diagnostic decision which differentiates the two groups.

# Regulation and Formulary (Range of Drugs which can be Prescribed)—RCN View

Nurses already work within a regulatory framework which governs their practice. As with any nursing role, the ability to prescribe should be covered by the existing system of individual professional responsibility and accountability. The Crown Report seems to accept this argument but does not extend the logic to the issue of the range of medicines which can be prescribed—the formulary, concluding that prescribers should only be allowed to prescribe from a limited formulary relating to their specialist area. The RCN argues that such an imposed restriction is unnecessary and needlessly bureaucratic, given the regulatory nature of nursing practice. For example, nurse specialists in diabetes care would not be prescribing a pain control drug for a terminally ill child unless they were competent to do so, even if they were legally able. Similarly, pain control specialists might have access to a formulary containing insulin but would not prescribe for patients with diabetes, this not being their specialist area.

Major US studies indicate that the appropriateness and accuracy of nurse prescribers are at least equal to, and often exceed, that of medical practitioners (US Congress 1986).

## New Prescribers Advisory Committee

The RCN welcomes the report's recommendation to set up a New Prescribers Advisory Committee and wants the committee established before the end of 1999 at the latest. Seats should be available on the committee for representatives of key professional organizations like the RCN.

## Facts and Figures

- Cost–benefit analysis of nurse prescribing by Touche Ross identified savings in district nurse and health visitor time of £15.88 million and £3.45 million per year respectively (Department of Health and Touche Ross 1991).
- The Touche Ross analysis also estimated a potential £7.34 million annual saving in general practitioner time.
- The Department of Health has always stressed the need for nurse prescribing to be 'cost neutral'; evaluation undertaken by the Universities of York and Manchester of the first eight pilot nurse prescribing sites revealed no significant increase in the drugs bill (Luker 1997).
- Nurse prescribing has the potential to cut costs; for example, as a result of bulk purchasing initiatives for nurse formulary items, the pilot site in Bolton identified savings in its drugs bill (Community Healthcare Bolton NHS Trust and Wigan Health Authority 1997).
- Nurse prescribing is soon to be extensively piloted in Australia and New Zealand and is commonplace in Sweden and the USA; in April 1998, Illinois became the last US state to introduce nurse prescribing.

The RCN calls for:

- The setting up by the end of 1999 of the New Prescribers Advisory Committee.
- An RCN representative on the New Prescribers Advisory Committee.
- The eventual extension of prescribing rights from the full formulary (i.e. not a restricted range of products) to all specialist nurses who have been properly trained.
- Any extension of prescribing rights, including those already extended to health visitors and district nurses, to apply to nurses throughout the UK.

REFERENCES

Community Healthcare Bolton NHS Trust and Wigan Health
　　Authority 1997 Evaluation of nurse prescribing in Bolton. Bolton,
　　Community Healthcare Bolton NHS Trust and Wigan Health
　　Authority
Department of Health 1999 Review of prescribing, supply and
　　administration of medicines. Final report (Chair Dr June Crown).
　　Department of Health, London
Department of Health and Touche Ross 1991 Nurse prescribing final
　　report: a cost–benefit study. Department of Health, London
Luker K A 1997 Evaluation of nurse prescribing. Final report
　　executive summary. University of Liverpool, Liverpool
National Health Service Executive 1998 HSC 1998/232 Nurse
　　prescribing. National Health Service Executive, Leeds
US Congress 1986 Nurse practitioners, physician assistants, and
　　certified nurse-midwives: a policy analysis. Health technology case
　　study 37, OTA-HCS-37. Office of Technological Assessment
　　Washington DC, US Government Printing Office

*Reproduced with kind permission of the Royal College of Nursing.*

# Appendix 5
# The Legal and Professional
# Framework of Nursing
HELEN CAULFIELD

## Types of Regulation

Health care is regulated in many ways and influenced to varying degrees by several types of rule or 'law'. These can be broadly divided as follows:

- Objective rules
  —'Law' as commonly identified (i.e. civil law and criminal law).
  —Nursing legislation.
  —Code of Professional Conduct.

- Subjective rules
  —Social standards.
  —Cultural standards.
  —Moral standards.
  —Personal standards.

Objective rules are characterised by being imposed, enforced and obligatory, and are frequently applied to areas of professional work where a clear statement of guidance and control is required for reasons of safety and public policy.

Subjective rules are naturally embodied in the standards, personally adopted by the nurse, and represent his or her unique contribution to the care given.

Nurses are subject to strict control by both types of rule, but here particular attention is given to those categorized as objective.

## Law (Young 1994)

The laws of the land bind nurses as citizens and professionals, comprising both criminal and civil law. Criminal law is contained in statutes (acts of parliament); violation of these is achieved by either performing a prohibited action or omitting to perform a required act, and constitutes a criminal offence against the State. Successful prosecution results in a variety of penalties, from fines to imprisonment.

| TABLE 5.1 MEDICAL STATUTES | |
|---|---|
| **Statute** | **Year** |
| Offences against the Person Act | 1861 |
| Perjury Act | 1911 |
| Venereal Diseases Act | 1917 |
| Infant Life (Preservation) Act | 1929 |
| Children and Young Persons Act | 1933 |
| National Assistance Act | 1948 |
| Sexual Offences Act | 1956 |
| Mental Health Act | 1959 |
| Human Tissue Act | 1961 |
| Suicide Act | 1961 |
| Abortion Act | 1967 |
| Medicines Act | 1968 |
| Family Law Reform Act | 1969 |
| Misuse of Drugs Act | 1971 |
| Congenital Disabilities (Civil Liability) Act | 1976 |
| National Health Service Act | 1977 |
| Unfair Contract Terms Act | 1977 |
| Vaccine Damage Payments Act | 1979 |
| Mental Health Act | 1983 |
| Medical Act | 1983 |
| Public Health (Control of Disease) Act | 1984 |
| Data Protection Act | 1984 |
| Enduring Powers of Attorney Act | 1985 |
| Prohibition of Female Circumcision Act | 1985 |
| Hospital Complaints Procedure Act | 1985 |
| Surrogacy Arrangements Act | 1985 |
| Family Law Reform Act | 1987 |
| Access to Medical Records Act | 1988 |
| Human Organ Transplant Act | 1989 |
| Children Act | 1989 |
| Access to Health Records Act | 1990 |
| NHS and Community Care Act | 1990 |
| Human Fertilization and Embryology Act | 1990 |
| Medicinal Products: Prescription by Nurses Act | 1992 |
| Nurses, Midwives and Health Visitors Act | 1997 |
| Data Protection Act | 1998 |
| Health Act | 1999 |
| Care Standards Act | 2000 |

Source: Kennedy & Grubb (1994), updated

Table 5.1 lists the statutes which relate directly to the clinical and health-care environment. They dictate clearly what is acceptable and what is not, within an extensive sphere of clinical and related activities, and represent control exerted directly by Parliament in response to the social and cultural demands of society.

## Professional Negligence

Perhaps the most commonly identified laws in the sphere of nursing relate to the potential for an allegation of professional negligence. 'Negligence' is a tort (a civil wrong), evolving under the civil law which regulates the behaviour (in terms of rights and duties) of one individual towards another.

A serious but often misunderstood legal issue, negligence is developed around the concept of a 'duty of care' or 'responsibility', and the subsequent harm that can be caused to an individual if this duty or responsibility fails. If an allegation is made, liability for negligence will only be proven if three key concepts can be satisfied, as follows:

1. Did a duty of care (responsibility) exist?
2. Was that breached?
3. Was the subsequent harm caused by the breach?

A critical part of the test for negligence is to show that harm or loss has been inflicted, and that it was caused directly by the negligent or careless act (or omission) undertaken by the accused. It is a legal requirement that the resulting loss is directly related to the negligent event, although it does not have to be the sole or main cause. If all the criteria are satisfied, the victim of the wrongful act will be financially compensated, the amount awarded being decided by the court.

When an assessment of negligence is made, judgement is directed at evaluating the level of professional behaviour shown by the individual when the alleged negligent event occurred. The assessment is made by comparison with two standards:

1. The professional person must deliver the standard of care expected from a reasonably competent person exercising that professional skill.
2. The professional person must act in accordance with practice accepted by a body of responsible and skilled professional opinion.

If either of the above is inapplicable then negligence can be inferred. It is essential to recognize here the importance of adherence to the Code of Professional Conduct and all local policies relating to the clinical environment because both will offer legal protection. Proof of professional negligence is generally difficult if accepted and up-to-date practice is followed.

## Legal Issues Affecting Clinical Practice

An objective of this appendix is to present a concise guide to legal controls on commonly encountered nursing procedures and situations. In so doing, it is essential to bear in mind, firstly, any relevant statutes (see Table 5.1) and, secondly, the Code of Professional Conduct (see Appendix 6). Where there is no specific statute to cover any particular area, compliance with professional regulations and local hospital policies will contribute to a defence in the face of any legal claims under civil law, specifically negligence.

## Consent

This issue embodies the fundamental principle that every person has a right to choose what happens to him or her. Broadly, this can encompass both physical and psychological treatment, but is generally related to the giving of consent for physical invasive procedures.

This subject is covered by both criminal law (Offences against the Person Act 1861) and precedent set by the courts in civil cases. It is a basic rule of law that no one has a right to touch another physically without consent. To do so would create the possibility of a claim for assault (an attempt to apply force to another, such as to put him or her in fear of physical violence) or battery (the actual application of physical force). The physical force does not have to be substantial and damage does not have to be caused, but intent to carry out the non-consensual contact must be present.

As the major legal defence against assault and battery is consent, the agreement of the patient must be sought before any physical treatment can be given by doctor or nurse. In practice, this often amounts to an informal verbal agreement between the patient and health-care professionals, but in certain situations, e.g. when surgery is required, written consent to a specific treatment has to be obtained.

Consequently, the giving of consent is of paramount importance, and the law relating to this is strict. It is a legal requirement that an effective consent must satisfy the following criteria to ensure that it is a true consent (Carson & Montgomery 1991):

1. The patient must be able to understand the choices he or she is required to make.
2. Consent must be free and voluntary.

3. The procedure for which consent is sought must have been explained to the patient. It may be negligent to withhold important information.
4. Consent must not be procured by deceit.

To take account of the nature of medical and nursing practice, three exceptions to giving consent as above are acceptable but should be used with caution.

Firstly, as outlined previously, an informal explanation and verbal agreement between patient and nurses are often sufficient to allow routine clinical care and treatment to be performed. This mainly involves care that the patient would normally carry out personally and excludes any medical intervention.

Secondly, the principle of 'necessity' will justify treatment of a patient where consent cannot be given, primarily in an emergency situation. As such, this exception permits life-saving treatment but should be applied in extreme situations only. The subsequent risk of a claim of assault and battery may be high if the patient would, in retrospect, have declined the treatment, or had previously expressed such a preference.

Thirdly, and similarly to the above, an 'implied consent' can be relied upon if there is sufficient certainty that the patient would have requested or acceded to the treatment had it been offered in more controlled circumstances. Again, this applies to emergency events where either an initiation of a new treatment or an extension of an existing one is needed. In such events, it is ethically correct to consider that the treatment should be of obvious benefit to the patient, that it would be unreasonable to withhold it, and that no express objection has previously been given.

Children under 16 years of age can legally give their own consent if it is recognized that they have the capacity to understand what is involved and the consent is valid.

Relatives and close friends are frequently involved in care and consultation about patients, although they cannot in any situation legally give consent on behalf of the patient. This is governed by the legal rule that one adult does not have the authority to give consent for another adult.

## Confidentiality

In the course of their duties, nurses are in a position to collect a large quantity of confidential information about patients. The control of such sensitive details is regulated by statute, specifically the Access to

---

> **BOX 5.1    PRINCIPLES OF HOLDING PERSONAL DATA (DATA PROTECTION ACT 1984 AND 1998)**
>
> 1. Data are obtained fairly and lawfully
> 2. Data are held for one or more lawful purpose only (specified in the Data User's register entry—a legal requirement)
> 3. Data are used or disclosed only in accordance with the Data User's register entry
> 4. Data are adequate, relevant and not excessive for the purpose
> 5. Data are accurate and up to date
> 6. Data are not kept longer than necessary for a specific purpose
> 7. Data are made available to data subjects upon request
> 8. Data are properly protected against loss or disclosure

---

Health Records Act 1990 and the Access to Medical Records Act 1988, and also by the Code of Professional Conduct (clause 10). These statutes ensure that written information is accessible to those it concerns, but also that access to it can be restricted if necessary. Professionally, nurses are required to prioritize the protection of all confidential information and only to disclose it under specific conditions.

Information entered and stored on a computer is controlled by the two Data Protection Acts 1984 and 1998. Box 5.1 lists the principles concerning the collection and storing of all confidential patient data.

Breach of confidentiality can lead to three substantial penalties. Firstly, failing to secure confidential information could lead to prosecution under the Data Protection Act 1984 and 1998. Secondly, the United Kingdom Central Council For Nurses, Midwives and Health Visitors (UKCC) has power to consider whether a charge of professional misconduct applies, therefore risking removal from the register. Thirdly, an employer can issue a dismissal for breach of contract. (It is intended that the UKCC will be replaced with a new body, probably to be known as The Nurses and Midwives Council, during 2001.)

Four clear exceptions to maintaining confidentiality are recognized (UKCC 1992), as follows:

1. Where the patient consents to disclosure.
2. Where the information is required to continue a patient's care.
3. Where the law requires disclosure, e.g. accidents, firearm incidents, drug-related activities, reporting of notifiable diseases.
4. Where the public interest is deemed of greater importance than confidentiality, e.g. child abuse, drug-related offences.

Nurses should abide strictly by the rules of confidentiality unless one of these exceptions clearly applies.

## Drug Administration

The responsibility of the nurse for storage and administration of medicines is discussed in Appendix 3.

## Safety

Nurses have a comprehensive responsibility for the safety of patients in their care, some of which is shared clinically with doctors and environmentally with employers.

Nurses are legally bound by the civil law 'duty of care' doctrine, which formalizes the responsibility that nurses have to their patients, the violation of which entitles the sufferer of any ensuing harm to make a claim of negligence. Nurses are also professionally instructed in the Code of Professional Conduct (clause 2) to be aware of this duty.

In the general ward environment, safety is maintained by attention to three main areas. Firstly, by formal identification of the patient and the implementation of a system, which could include the use of personal photographs or the wearing of non-removable identity bands. The personal details recorded on the bands should be consistent with all documents. Secondly, the careful compilation of admission, inpatient and discharge charts and documents ensures that all plans and information are current and safety is not compromised by unnecessary loss or duplication. Thirdly, the conscientious dissemination of information between the patient and all members of the medical multidisciplinary team is essential. This allows the patient to have an understanding of the plan of care and also enables clinical treatment to proceed as safely as possible.

Application of these safety principles will be enhanced in certain acute and specialist environments. In these areas, identification of the patient and the passing on of accurate and detailed information is critical. Nurses trained in these areas will also be likely to have particular routines and procedures for which they may incur additional accountability. Nurses should also be aware of their own practical and experiential limitations, as encouraged in the Code of Professional Conduct (clause 4), to exert caution and not undertake to enter situations that compromise their clinical ability and the patient's safety.

The responsibility for safety within the physical environment of care and the facilities therein is allocated to health-care management and ultimately the health authority. Since the removal of Crown immunity from many statutes by the National Health Service and Community Care Act 1990, many facilities are now subject to quality controls as defined by individual statutes, e.g. incineration (Environment Protection Act 1990) and waste disposal (Control of Pollution Act 1974).

Within the ward, management has specific responsibility for providing adequate basic safety measures, e.g. fire precautions.

Nurses are instructed in the Code of Professional Conduct (clause 11) to evaluate the safety of the environment and to take action if this is jeopardized. Nursing staff are also required to be professionally aware of other factors affecting safety, particularly quality and availability of resources. This applies specifically to potentially unsafe staffing levels, skill mix or a demanding combination of patients and clinical conditions.

## Documentation

The range of documentation requiring nursing attention is plentiful, wide-ranging and detailed, much of it not directly related to nursing activities. As a result some documents will have a legal significance while others will not. The purpose of documentation is fourfold, as follows:

1. Legal or non-legal record-keeping.
2. Ease of administration.
3. Maintaining standards.
4. Ensuring continuity and safety.

Legal record-keeping infiltrates the nursing environment in several areas, e.g. administration of medicines, recording usage of controlled drugs, and contracts of employment between nurses and employing authorities. Nursing records are potentially legal documents, their main function being to evidence the care planned, treatment received and outcomes of a patient's stay. As a comprehensive record of the patient's visit, they form an important defence against allegations of misconduct or negligence. The time within which potential legal actions can be initiated under the Limitations Act 1939–75 (until a child reaches 21 years or 3 years from the date of damage) makes the necessity for accurate documentation of actions obvious.

The principle that a strong defence is much more likely from the basis of clear, precise documentation written at the time of the incident is an important supplementary reason for much clinical record-keeping. Difficulty is often encountered in achieving a balance in the detail to be given in nursing records and the frequency at which entries should be made, although there is no legal direction given for this. Maximum responsibility can be achieved by recording events, decisions and evaluations at the time they are undertaken, and experience should guide us as to the amount of detail which is appropriate.

Of equivalent importance to patient records are documents affecting staff, visitors and members of the public that could subsequently acquire a legal significance, e.g. accident reporting forces. Employers are legally required to report accidents, injuries and dangerous incidents to the Health and Safety Executive, and are required to act under the Reporting of Injuries, Diseases and Dangerous Occurrences Regulations 1985 and the Occupiers Liability Act 1957 and 1984.

## Decisions made by Patients

Protection of doctors and nurses from potential legal repercussions is required in situations where patients choose to make a decision contrary to professional advice. This occurs mainly in two areas. Firstly, where the patient refuses recommended treatment. Under the law governing consent (see above) the patient must have been given a suitably detailed explanation of the proposed treatment. Not to do so invalidates any subsequent consent and also presents the possibility of negligent action by the nurse. A consequence of a full description of proposed treatment may be refusal by the patient to undertake this recommended course of action. The individual patient has an absolute and inviolable right under civil law to accept treatment or to decline it. Doctors and nurses must ensure that these decisions are recorded, as an ultimate defence against possible resulting negligence actions if the outcome of declining treatment is unfavourable.

Secondly, patients may choose to discharge themselves from medical care against the advice of doctors and nurses. Patients cannot be legally detained (unless subject to various sections of the Mental Health Act 1983) and are free to leave at their will. A 'discharge against medical advice' form is valuable as a record of a discussion with a patient and as a place to note that the unplanned and unadvised discharge is of the patient's choice. The form should be witnessed by clinical staff involved, although the patient cannot be legally compelled to sign it.

## Complaints Procedure

This procedure is governed by the Hospital Complaints Procedure Act 1985. This legislation imposes a duty on each health authority to

| BOX 5.2 | PRINCIPLES OF COMPLAINTS PROCEDURES (HOSPITAL COMPLAINTS PROCEDURE ACT 1985) |
|---|---|

1. The complaints procedure must be adequately publicized and accessible
2. Complaints must be made in writing within 6 months of the incident
3. Complaints can be made by a personal representative of a deceased patient or one who is unable to act personally
4. A designated officer sufficiently senior to command staff cooperation and patient confidence should receive the complaint
5. Complaints are to be investigated thoroughly, fairly and speedily
6. All involved are to be kept informed of the progress of the investigation
7. Staff implicated should have the opportunity to reply

institute a complaints procedure that incorporates all the features listed in Box 5.2.

The Act covers hospital situations involving inpatients, outpatients and accident and emergency admissions only. If a complaint is not satisfactorily resolved at health authority level a legal case may ensue or the problem can be referred to the Health Service Commissioner.

## Patients' Property

Patients' property requires careful attention from nurses at all stages during a patient's hospitalization—from admission, while an inpatient, during any transfers between clinical areas, and on discharge.

The actions taken to safeguard property are to protect the patient from incurring a loss and to provide the nursing staff with an adequate defence against an allegation of theft.

If conscious and capable, the patient will automatically retain control of any property although some facilities for the safekeeping of valuables may be offered. In many cases the patient will be required to sign a disclaimer form, which will absolve the hospital during the patient's stay. If any items are retained for security by the hospital a patient will receive a signed receipt.

If the patient is unable to take responsibility for personal property while unconscious, confused or mentally incapacitated, the nurse will be required to take charge of it. The nurse's legal responsibility in this position assumes that of an 'involuntary bailee' (technically a person to whom goods are entrusted with no intention of transferring ownership). This demands that the nurse takes care of the property to the same degree that the patient would have done had he or she been able.

The well-established procedure of written documentation, double-checking and witnessing with another member of staff, and finally signing in duplicate for property received, is vital to ensure protection against accusations of theft. Accurate and careful description of all property held is prudent. On discharge all property must be returned to the patient, and on death to authorized receivers, in both cases in exchange for a signed receipt.

The penalties for inadequate or careless control of a patient's property are individual prosecutions for theft or activation of the health authority's liability for negligence. A nurse may also potentially face dismissal and be reported to the UKCC for professional misconduct.

REFERENCES

Carson D, Montgomery J 1991 Nursing and the law. Macmillan, London
Kennedy I, Grubb A 1994 Medical law. Butterworth, London
UKCC 1992 Guidelines for professional practice. UKCC, London
Young A P 1994 Law and professional conduct in nursing. Scutari, London


FURTHER READING

Brazier M 1992 Medicine, patients and the law. Penguin, London
Dyer C (ed) 1992 Doctors, patients and the law. Blackwell, Oxford
McCall Smith A, Mason J K 1994 Law and medical ethics. Butterworth, London
Rumbold G 1999 Ethics in nursing practice, 3rd edn. Baillière Tindall, London
Tingle J, Cribb A (eds) 1995 Nursing law and ethics. Blackwell Scientific, Oxford
Tschudin V 1991 Ethics in nursing. Heinemann, London

# Appendix 6
# United Kingdom Central Council for Nursing, Midwifery and Health Visiting Code of Professional Conduct

Each registered nurse, midwife and health visitor shall act, at all times, in such a manner as to:

- Safeguard and promote the interests of individual patients and clients.
- Serve the interests of society.
- Justify public trust and confidence.
- Uphold and enhance the good standing and reputation of the professions.

As a registered nurse, midwife or health visitor, you are personally accountable for your practice and, in the exercise of your professional accountability, must:

1. Act always in such a manner as to promote and safeguard the interests and wellbeing of patients and clients.
2. Ensure that no action or omission on your part, or within your sphere of responsibility, is detrimental to the interests, condition or safety of patients and clients.
3. Maintain and improve your professional knowledge and competence.
4. Acknowledge any limitations in your knowledge and competence and decline any duties or responsibilities unless able to perform them in a safe and skilled manner.
5. Work in an open and cooperative manner with patients, clients and their families, foster their independence and recognise and respect their involvement in the planning and delivery of care.
6. Work in a collaborative and cooperative manner with health care professionals and others involved in providing care, and recognise and respect their particular contributions within the care team.
7. Recognise and respect the uniqueness and dignity of each patient and client, and respond to their need for care, irrespective of their ethnic origin, religious beliefs, personal attributes, the nature of their health problems or any other factor.

8.  Report to an appropriate person or authority, at the earliest possible time, any conscientious objection which may be relevant to your professional practice.

9.  Avoid any abuse of your privileged relationship with patients and clients and of the privileged access allowed to their person, property, residence or workplace.

10. Protect all confidential information concerning patients and clients obtained in the course of professional practice and make disclosures only with consent, where required by the order of a court or where you can justify disclosure in the wider public interest.

11. Report to an appropriate person or authority, having regard to the physical, psychological and social effects on patients and clients, any circumstances in the environment of care which could jeopardise standards of practice.

12. Report to an appropriate person or authority any circumstances in which safe and appropriate care for patients and clients cannot be provided.

13. Report to an appropriate person or authority where it appears that the health or safety of colleagues is at risk, as such circumstances may compromise standards of practice and care.

14. Assist professional colleagues, in the context of your own knowledge, experience and sphere of responsibility, to develop their professional competence, and assist others in the care team, including informal carers, to contribute safely and to a degree appropriate to their roles.

15. Refuse any gift, favour or hospitality from patients or clients currently in your care which might be interpreted as seeking to exert influence to obtain preferential consideration.

16. Ensure that your registration status is not used in the promotion of commercial products or services, declare any financial or other interests in relevant organisations providing such goods or services and ensure that your professional judgement is not influenced by any commercial considerations.

## Notice to all Registered Nurses, Midwives and Health Visitors

This Code of Professional Conduct for the Nurse, Midwife and Health Visitor is issued to all registered nurses, midwives and health visitors by the United Kingdom Central Council for Nursing, Midwifery and Health Visiting. The Council is the regulatory body responsible for the standards of these professions to practise and conduct themselves within the standards and framework provided by the Code.

The Council's Code is kept under review and any recommendations for change and improvement would be welcomed and should be addressed to the Registrar and Chief Executive, United Kingdom Central Council for Nursing, Midwifery and Health Visiting, 23 Portland Place, London W1N 4JT.

# Appendix 7
# Professional Organizations and Trade Unions

## Community and District Nursing Association (CDNA)

The CDNA is a specialist professional association and trade union affiliated to the Trades Union Congress (TUC) and Scottish Trades Union Congress (STUC). For 30 years the Community and District Nursing Association has taken an active role in campaigning on issues affecting its membership.

For nearly 35 years the CDNA (formerly the DNA) has been the only professional body which solely represents the interests of community and district nurses. The CDNA is run by people who have worked in primary health care and nursing education so they are well aware of the issues facing their members.

The Association recognizes that, with all the changes and development taking place within health care in the community, a body which represents the sole interests of nurses who practise in the community is needed now more than ever.

For further information: http://www.cdna.tvu.ac.uk.


## UNISON

UNISON is the UK's biggest trade union with over 1.3 million members.

UNISON members are people working in the public services, for private contractors providing public services, and in the essential utilities. They include manual and white collar staff working full- or part time in local authorities, the National Health Service (NHS), colleges and schools, the electricity, gas and water industries, transport and the voluntary sector.

Every member of UNISON belongs to a branch which is made up of people working for the same employer.

Local stewards represent members at work and help find the answers to any problems. They are volunteers and play a vital role in recruiting new members and organizing the branches.

**The Organization**

UNISON has a clear structure to make sure that all members can have their say. The union is divided into 13 regions, each with its own regional council made up of delegates elected from branches in the area.

The governing body of UNISON is the annual national delegate conference, where the union's policy is decided by delegates elected from branches, regions and self-organized groups (see below). Policies decided at conference are carried out by the National Executive Council (NEC) which is elected from the regions and service groups.

Alongside this local structure, UNISON has six service groups which bring together members working in similar areas. These are: local government, health care, higher education, energy, water and transport.

Women make up two-thirds of UNISON's members so care is taken to ensure that their voices are heard through the union. At every level of the union, when people are elected to committees or delegations, women must be elected in fair proportion to their membership. Even the NEC has to elect 44 women out of its 67 seats and 13 are held by low-paid women. UNISON calls this 'proportionality'.

UNISON also has 'self-organized groups' to represent people who are likely to face particular discrimination at work—women, black members, disabled members and lesbians and gay men.

UNISON is the largest union in the TUC and plays an important role in developing policy. It has a big voice too in the Scottish, Welsh and Irish trades union congresses.

For further information: http://www.unison.org.uk.

# Royal College of Nursing (RCN)

**What is the RCN?**

With more than 310 000 members, the RCN is the world's largest professional union of nurses. The RCN is run by nurses for nurses, it campaigns on the part of the profession, and is a leading player in the development of nursing practice and standards of care. It is a provider of higher education and promotes research, quality and practice development through the RCN Institute. It is also a registered charity.

The RCN promotes the interests of nurses and patients by working with government, MPs, other unions, professional bodies and voluntary organizations. It is the voice of British nursing both at home and abroad, with representatives on a number of European, Commonwealth and international bodies. The RCN also represents the United Kingdom on the International Council for Nurses.

## The RCN's Royal Charter

The Royal Charter sets out the purposes of the RCN:

- To promote the science and art of nursing and the better education and training of nurses and their efficiency in the profession of nursing.
- To promote the advance of nursing as a profession in all or any of its branches.
- To promote the professional standing and interests of members of the nursing profession.
- To promote the above aims in both the UK and other countries through the medium of international agencies and other means.
- To assist nurses who, by reason of ill health or other adversity, are in need of assistance of any nature.
- To institute and conduct examinations, and to grant certificates and diplomas to those who satisfy the requirements laid down by the Council of the College.

## Working for Nurses

For busy professionals and nursing students, the RCN offers its members a wide range of services including:

- Advice and support with problems at work.
- Legal representation.
- A range of education and continuing professional development activities.
- Professional advice.
- A counselling and personal advice service.
- Immigration advice.
- Support and activities for nursing students.
- Free publications on nursing, health-care and employment issues.
- The largest nursing library in Europe.

## RCN Council

This is the RCN's ruling body, democratically elected by the members. Its 25 representatives include 14 from England and two each from

Northern Ireland, Scotland and Wales. Students have two elected representatives. The other three members are the RCN president, deputy president and chair of the RCN Congress. The RCN Council is responsible for the policies of the RCN and the general secretary is responsible for implementing policy. Council takes account of resolutions carried by the RCN Congress and recommendations from its standing committees.

### RCN Congress

Congress is the RCN's main annual debating forum. It plays a major part in shaping policy and initiating activity through resolutions and matters of discussion. Congress voters are drawn from branches and national forums but members may also attend as non-voting delegates.

RCN branches, national forums, Council and its standing committees, the RCN National Boards, the UK Stewards Committee and the UK Safety Representatives' Committee submit resolutions and matters for discussion on a wide range of issues. These are submitted to the Congress Agenda Committee who develop and manage the Congress agenda.

At local level the RCN has board offices in Northern Ireland, Scotland and Wales and offices throughout England. It has over 274 branches throughout the UK, over 70 professional groups covering a wide range of nursing specialisms and special interests, and a network of stewards and safety representatives in the workplace.

For further information: http://www.rcn.org.uk.

## International Council of Nurses (ICN)

The ICN's mission is: to represent nursing worldwide, advancing the profession and influencing health policy.

It is a federation of national nurses' associations (NNAs) representing nurses in more than 120 countries. Founded in 1899, the ICN is the world's first and widest-reaching international organization for health professionals. Operated by nurses for nurses, the ICN works to ensure quality nursing care for all, sound health policies globally, the advancement of nursing knowledge, and the presence worldwide of a respected nursing profession and a competent and satisfied nursing workforce.

The ICN Code for Nurses is the foundation of ethical nursing practice throughout the world. ICN standards, guidelines and policies for nursing practice, education, management, research and socio-economic welfare are accepted globally as the basis of nursing policy.

The ICN advances nursing, nurses and health through its policies, partnerships, advocacy, leadership development, networks, congresses and special projects, and by its work in the arenas of professional practice, regulation and socio-economic welfare. It is particularly active in:

- Professional nursing practice
  —International classification of nursing practice.
  —Advanced nursing practice and entrepreneurship.
  —HIV/AIDS.
  —Women's health.
  —Primary health care.

- Nursing regulation
  —Continuing education.
  —Ethics and human rights.
  —Credentialing.

- Socio-economic welfare for nurses
  —Occupational health and safety.
  —Remuneration.
  —Human resources planning.

- Career development.

Partnerships and strategic alliances include links with governmental and non-governmental agencies, foundations, regional groups, national associations and individuals assisting the ICN in advancing nursing worldwide.

### ICN Goals and Values

Three goals and five core values guide and motivate all ICN activities.

The goals are:

- To bring nursing together worldwide.
- To advance nurses and nursing worldwide.
- To influence health policy.

The five core values are:

- Visionary leadership.
- Inclusiveness.
- Flexibility.
- Partnership.
- Achievement.

The ICN is based in Geneva, Switzerland. For further information on ICN structure, publications and activities: http://www.icn.ch.

# Royal College of Midwives (RCM)

The RCM represents over 96% of the UK's practising midwives and is the world's largest and oldest professional midwifery organization. It works to advance the interests of midwives and the midwifery profession—and, by doing so, enhances the wellbeing of women, babies and families.

The RCM is governed by an elected Council of practising midwives. Each of the four UK countries—Scotland, Northern Ireland, England and Wales—has its own RCM Board, which provides services to midwives in those countries and advises the Council on strategic issues. In addition, the London-based headquarters provide a range of UK-wide functions and services.

Over 200 RCM branches hold regular meetings where members can give and receive support and discuss professional and workplace issues.

### Working for midwifery, working for midwives

The vast majority of UK midwives belong to the RCM because of the combined professional, trade union and educational benefits that only the RCM can offer. These include:

- Education and research
  —A range of training and professional development courses, to promote clinical excellence and to develop the midwifery leaders of tomorrow.
  —Active promotion of research, evidence-based practice and the development of midwifery as a learning profession.
  —The largest midwifery library in the world. The RCM collection, which reflects more than a century of change for midwifery and women, includes journals, theses and over 5000 books.

- Professional affairs
  —An extensive range of publications and policy papers, providing guidance and comment on the challenges facing mothers and midwives.
  —The *RCM Midwives' Journal*, devoted exclusively to midwifery matters, delivered direct to each member every month.
  —A voice for midwifery in national policy forums.

- Industrial relations
  - —Regional officers through the UK, who are all practising midwives. Only the RCM provides field-based staff who combine expertise in both midwifery and industrial relations.
  - —Over 600 workplace-based stewards and health and safety representatives, themselves midwives working in the NHS.
  - —Medical malpractice insurance, giving cover against legal liability to the sum of £3 million.

## Working for women

The RCM is committed to developing a maternity service that truly meets women's and babies' physical, psychological and emotional needs throughout pregnancy, labour and the postnatal period. The RCM sees this as a vital contribution to public health and an essential investment in the wellbeing of tomorrow's citizens. In partnership with service users themselves, the RCM has fought for a maternity service which treats women as partners in their own care, which respects the power of normal childbirth, and which puts both research evidence and the women's own wishes centre stage.

The RCM also uses its expertise to help improve the wider issues affecting women's and infants' health. It has campaigned for better support for women who are pregnant in prison, or suffering domestic violence or female genital mutilation (FGM). It works to promote breastfeeding, to improve neonatal care, and to help new parents feel confident and supported. It advises the Government, the NHS and others on how maternity care can help women enjoy not just a healthy pregnancy but increased quality of family life and wellbeing.

## Working internationally

As the only World Health Organization (WHO) Collaborating Centre for Midwifery, the RCM works with the Safe Motherhood Initiative (SMI) to promote maternal and infant health across the globe. It also works with a range of partners overseas, providing support and resources to help improve midwifery education and practice and maternal and infant health. The College is a founder member of the International Confederation of Midwives (ICM) and works with midwives worldwide, assisting with midwifery development by providing advice on legislation, research, education and practice.

For further information see RCM addresses in Appendix 8, Useful Addresses.

# Community Practitioners' and Health Visitors' Association (CPHVA)

The Community Practitioners' and Health Visitors' Association (CPHVA) is the UK professional body that represents registered nurses and health visitors who work in primary or community health settings. The CPHVA is an autonomous professional section of Manufacturing Science and Finance (MSF). MSF represents 65 000 professionals working in the NHS and altogether represents 400 000 members employed in the manufacturing, science and finance sectors.

With 18 000 members, the CPHVA is the third largest professional nursing union and is the only union which has public health at the centre of its activities and parliamentary lobbying. It campaigns to protect the status of community practitioners and the services they deliver, and influences policy decisions by the production of reports and consultation documents as well as the staging of conferences and seminars.

Membership includes:

- Access to expert advice on professional and clinical issues.
- Expert advice and representation on pay, contracts, and terms and conditions of employment.
- A comprehensive annual programme of specialist and professional development, education and training courses, conferences and seminars.
- An information resources centre.
- The award-winning *Community Practitioner* journal free every month and the *Opportunities* job supplement free every fortnight.
- Indemnity insurance cover against claims of up to £3 million.
- Access to the CPHVA's networks of special interest groups and databases.

As an autonomous section of MSF, CPHVA entitles its members to the range of updated benefits available to all MSF members. These include the MSF First CD-Rom with free Internet access direct to the home as well as the most competitive offers on items ranging from mobile phones to holidays, pensions and financial services.

# Appendix 8
# Useful addresses

Compiled By JOAN DATSUN

**Action for Sick Children** (formerly National Association for the
Welfare of Children in Hospital)
Argyle House
29–31 Euston Road
London
NW1 2SP

**Action for Smoking and Health (ASH)**
109 Gloucester Place
London
W1H 4EJ

**Age Concern England**
60 Pitcairn Road
Mitcham
Surrey
CR4 3LL

**Alcohol Concern** (National Agency of Alcohol
Misuse)
305 Gray's Inn Road
London
WC1X 8QF

**Alcoholics Anonymous**
P.O. Box 1
Stonebow House
Stonebow
York
Y01 2NJ

**Alzheimer's Disease Society**
3rd Floor Bank Building
Fulham Broadway
London
SW6 1EP

**APEX Partnership**
22–24 Worple Road
Wimbledon
London
SW19 4DD

**Arthritis and Rheumatism Council (ARC)**
41 Eagle Street
London
WC1R 4AR

**Association for Improvements in the Maternity Services (AIMS)**
163 Liverpool Road
London
N1 0RF

**Association of British Paediatric Nurses (ABPN)**
P.O. Box 14
Ashton-under-Lyne
Lancashire
OL5 9WW

**Association of Carers**
20–25 Glasshouse Yard
London
EC1A 4JS

**Association of Community Health Councils** (England and Wales)
30 Drayton Park
London
N5 1PB

**Association of Radical Midwives**
c/o Haringay Women's Centre
40 Turnpike Lane
London
N8 0PS

**Asthma Society** (merged with Asthma Research Council to become
National Asthma Campaign)
Providence House
Providence Place
London
N1 0NT

**Back Pain Association**
31–33 Park Road
Teddington
Middlesex
TW11 0AB

**Breast Care and Mastectomy Association**
15–19 Britton Street
London
SW3 3TZ

**British Association for Cancer United Patients (BACUP)**
3 Bath Place
Rivington Street
London
EC2A 3JR

**British Colostomy Association**
15 Station Road
Reading
RG1 1LG

**British Deaf Association**
38 Victoria Place
Carlisle
Cumbria
CA1 1HU

**British Diabetic Association**
10 Queen Anne Street
London
W1M 0BD

**British Dietetic Association**
Daimler House
Paradise Circus
Queensway
Birmingham
B1 2BJ

**British Epilepsy Association**
Anstey House
40 Hanover Square
Leeds
LS3 1BE

**British Geriatric Society (BGS)**
1 St Andrew's Place
London
NW1 4LB

**British Heart Foundation**
102 Gloucester Place
London
W1H 4DH

**British Nutrition Foundation**
High Holborn House
52–54 High Holborn
London
WCIV 6RQ

**British Pregnancy Advisory Service**
Austry Manor
Wooten
Waven
Solihull
West Midlands
BG5 6DA

**British Red Cross Society (BRCS)**
9 Grosvenor Crescent
London
SW1X 7EJ

**Cancer Link**
17 Britannia Street
London
WC1X 9JN

**Capability** (formerly Spastics Society)
12 Park Crescent
London
W1N 4EQ

**Carers' National Association**
20–25 Glasshouse Yard
London
EC1A 4JT

**Childline**
Royal Mail Building
Studd Street
London
N1 0QW

**Coeliac Society**
P.O. Box 220
High Wycombe
Buckinghamshire
HP11 2HY

**Commission for Racial Equality**
Elliot House
10–12 Allington Street
London
SW1E 5EH

**Commonwealth Nurses Association**
c/o International Department Royal College of Nursing
20 Cavendish Square
London
W1M 0AB

**Community Practitioners' and Health
  Visitors' Association**
40 Bermondsey Street
London
SE1 3UD

**Coronary Prevention Group**
Central Middlesex Hospital
Acton Lane
London
NW10 7NS

**CRUSE** (National Association for the Widowed and their
Children)
Cruse House
126 Sheen Road
Richmond
Surrey
TW9 1UR

**Department of Health** (England)
Richmond House
79 Whitehall
London
SW1A 2NS

**Department of Health** (Northern Ireland)
Dundonald House
Upper Newtonwards Road
Belfast
BT4 3SB

**Disabled Living Foundation**
380–384 Harrow Road
London
W9 2HU

**English National Board for Nursing, Midwifery and Health
Visiting (ENB)**
Victory House
170 Tottenham Court Road
London
W1T 0HA

**Equal Opportunities Commission**
Overseas House
Quay Street
Manchester
M3 3HN

**Family Planning Association (FPA)**
Margaret Pyke House
27–35 Mortimer Street
London
W1N 7RJ

**Foresight** (Association for the Promotion of Preconceptual Care)
The Old Vicarage
Church Lane
Witley
Godalming
Surrey
GU8 5PN

**Gamblers Anonymous and GAM-ANON**
17–23 Blantyre Street
Cheyne Walk
London
SW10 0DT

**General Medical Council (GMC)**
178 Great Portland Street
London
W1N 6JE

**Gerontology Nutrition Unit**
Royal Free Hospital
School of Medicine
21 Pond Street
London
NW3 2PN

**Haemophilia Society**
123 Westminster Bridge Road
London
SE1 7HR

**Health Education Authority**
Hamilton House
Mabledon Place
London
WC1H 9TX

**Health and Safety Executive**
2 Southwark Bridge
London
SE1 9HS

**Health Service Ombudsman**
Church House
Great Smith Street
London
SW1P 3BW

**Health Visitors Association**
50 Southwark Street
London
SE1 1UN

**Help the Aged**
16–18 St James's Walk
London
EC1R 0BE

**Hospice Information Service**
St Christopher's Hospice
51–59 Lawrie Park Road
Sydenham
London
SE26 6DZ

**Ileostomy Association** (now Ileostomy and Internal Pouch
Support Group)
Amblehurst House
P.O. Box 23
Mansfield
Nottinghamshire
NG18 4TT

**Infection Control Nurses Association (ICNA)**
c/o Janet Roberts
Clatterbridge Hospital
Bebington
Wirral
Merseyside
L63 4JY

**Institute of Complementary Medicine**
P.O. Box 194
London
SE15 1QZ

**International Confederation of Midwives**
10 Barley Mow Passage
Chiswick
London
W4 4PH

**International Council of Nurses**
37 rue Vermont
Geneva
Switzerland

**Invalids at Home**
23 Farm Avenue
London
NW2 2BJ

**King's Fund**
11–13 Cavendish Square
London
W1M 0AN

**Lady Hoare Trust for Physically Disabled Children**
(Associated with Arthritis Care)
7 North Street
Midhurst, West Sussex
GU29 9DJ

**Leukaemia Society**
14 Kingfisher Court
Venny Bridge
Pinhoe, Exeter
EX4 8JN

**Macmillan Cancer Relief**
Anchor House
15–19 Britten Street
London
SW3 3TZ

**Malcolm Sargent Cancer Fund for Children**
14 Abingdon Road
London
W8 6AF

**Marie Curie Memorial Foundation**
28 Belgrave Square
London
SW1X 8QG

**Medic-Alert Foundation**
11–13 Afton Terrace
London
N4 3JP

**Medicines Control Agency**
Market Towers
1 Nine Elms Lane
London
SW8 5NQ

**MIND** (National Association for Mental Health)
15–19 Broadway
London
E15 4BQ

**Multiple Sclerosis Society**
25 Effie Road
Fulham
London
SW6 1EE

**Narcotics Anonymous**
P.O. Box 246
London
SW12 8DL

**National Association of Theatre Nurses**
22 Mount Parade
Harrogate
HG1 1BX

**National Board for Nursing, Midwifery and Health Visiting for Northern Ireland**
RAC House
70 Chichester Street
Belfast
BT1 4JE

**National Board for Nursing, Midwifery and Health Visiting for Scotland**
  22 Queen Street
  Edinburgh
  EH2 1JZ

**National Childbirth Trust (NCT)**
  Alexandra House
  Oldham Terrace
  London
  Q3 6NH

**National Council for One Parent Families**
  255 Kentish Town Road
  London
  NW5 6NH

**National Council for Vocational Qualifications**
  222 Euston Road
  London
  NW1

**National Federation of Kidney Patients' Associations**
  Acorn Lodge
  Woodsets
  Nr Worksop
  Nottinghamshire
  S81 8AT

**National Institute of Clinical Excellence (NICE)**
  90 Long Acre
  London
  W3 6NH

**National Schizophrenia Fellowship**
  79 Victoria Road
  Surbiton, Surrey
  KT6 4NS

**National Society for Epilepsy**
Chalfont Centre for Epilepsy
Chalfont St Peter
Gerrards Cross, Buckinghamshire
SL9 0RJ

**National Society for the Prevention of Cruelty to Children**
(NSPCC)
67 Curtain Road
London
EC2A 3NH

**Neonatal Nurses Association (NNA)**
7 Milton Chambers
19 Milton Street
Nottingham
NG1 3EN

**NHS Management Executive**
Quarry House
Quarry Hill
Leeds
L52 7EU

**Nurses Welfare Service**
Victoria Chambers
16–18 Strutton Ground
London
SW1P 2HP

**Nursing and Hospital Carers Information Centre**
121 Edgware Road
London
W2 2HX

**Nursing and Midwifery Staffs Negotiating Council**
20 Cavendish Square
London
W1M 0AB

**Parent's Friend**
  c/o Voluntary Action
  Leeds Stringer House
  34 Lupton Street
  Hunslet; Leeds
  LS10 2QW

**Parkinson Disease Society**
  36 Portland Place
  London
  W1N 3DG

**Pregnancy Advisory Service**
  13 Charlotte Street
  London
  W1P 1HD

**Primary Nursing Network Nursing Developments**
  King's Fund Centre
  126 Albert Street
  London
  NW1 7NF

**Renal Society**
  64 South Hill Park
  London
  NW3 3SJ

**Royal Association in Aid of the Deaf and Dumb**
  27 Old Oak Road
  London
  W3 7SL

**Royal Association for Disability and Rehabilitation**
  Unit 12, City Forum
  250 City Road
  London
  EC1V 8AF

**Royal College of Midwives (RCM)**
  15 Mansfield Street
  London
  W1M 0BE

**RCM English Board**
  Kings House
  2nd Floor
  Kings Street
  Leeds LS1 2HH

**RCM Northern Ireland Board**
  Friends Provident Building
  58 Howard Street
  Belfast
  BT1 6PH

**RCM Scottish Board**
  37 Frederick Street
  Edinburgh
  EH2 1EP

**RCM Welsh Board**
  4 Cathedral Road
  Cardiff
  CF1 9LJ

**Royal College of Nursing of the United Kingdom (RCN)**
  20 Cavendish Square
  London
  W1M 0AB

**Royal College of Nursing (Northern Ireland)**
  17 Windsor Avenue
  Belfast
  BT9 6EE

**Royal College of Nursing (Scottish Board)**
  42 South Oswald Road
  Edinburgh
  EH9 2HH

**Royal College of Nursing (Welsh Board)**
  Ty Maeth
  King George V Drive
  East Cardiff
  CF4 4XZ

**Royal Commonwealth Society**
New Zealand House
Haymarket
London
SW1Y 4TQ

**Royal Institute of Public Health and Hygiene**
28 Portland Place
London
W1N 4DE

**Royal National Institute for the Blind (RNIB)**
224 Great Portland Place
London
W1N 6AA

**Royal National Institute for the Deaf (RNID)**
19–23 Featherstone Street
London
EC1Y 8SL

**Royal National Pension Fund for Nurses**
Burdett House
15 Buckingham Street
London
W2N 6ED

**Royal Society of Health**
38a St George's Drive
London
SW1Y 4BH

**Royal Society of Medicine**
1 Wimpole Street
London
W1M 8RE

**Royal Society for the Prevention of Accidents (ROSPA)**
Cannon House
The Priory
Queensway
Birmingham
B4 6BS

**St John Ambulance Association and Brigade**
1 Grosvenor Crescent
London
SW1X 7ES

**Samaritans Incorporated**
17 Uxbridge Road
Slough
Berkshire
SL1 1SN

**SCOPE**
12 Park Crescent
London
W1N 4EQ

**Scottish Home and Health Department**
St Andrew's House
Regent Road, Edinburgh
EH1 3DE

**Sickle Cell Society**
54 Station Road
London
NW10 4UA

**Society and College of Radiographers**
2 Carriage Row
183 Eversholt Green, London
NW1 1BU

**Standing Conference on Drug Abuse**
1–4 Hatton Place
Hatton Garden
London
EC1N 8ND

**Stillbirth and Neonatal Death Society (SANDS)**
28 Portland Place
London
W1N 4DE

**Stress Syndrome Foundation**
  Cedar House
  Yalding
  Kent
  ME18 6JD

**Sue Ryder Foundation**
  Cavendish
  Sudbury
  Suffolk
  CO10 8AY

**Terrence Higgins Trust**
  52–54 Gray's Inn Road
  London
  WC1X 8JU

**Twins and Multiple Birth Association**
  54 Broad Lane
  Hampton
  Middlesex
  TW12 3BG

**UNISON (Head Office)**
  1 Mabledon Place
  London
  WC1H 9HA

**United Kingdom Central Council for Nursing, Midwifery and Health Visiting (UKCC)**
  23 Portland Place
  London
  W1N 3AF

**Vegan Society**
  47 Highlands Road
  Leatherhead
  Surrey
  KT22 8NQ

**Welsh National Board for Nursing, Midwifery and Health Visiting**
13th Floor
Pearl Assurance House
Greyfriars Road
Cardiff
CF1 3AG

**Welsh Office**
Crown Buildings
Cathays Park
Cardiff
CG10 1DX

**Women's Health Concern (WHC)**
17 Earls Terrace
London
W8 6LP

**Women's Royal Voluntary Services (WRVS)**
17 Old Park Lane
London
W1Y 4AJ

**World Health Organization**
Avenue Appia 1211
Geneva 27
Switzerland

# Appendix 9
# Degrees, Diplomas and Organizations: Abbreviations in Nursing and Health Care

| | |
|---|---|
| AA | Alcoholics Anonymous |
| ABPN | Association of British Paediatric Nurses |
| AIMSW | Association of the Institute of Medical Social Workers |
| AOC | Aromatherapy Organizations Council |
| APEX | Association of Professional and Executive Staffs |
| ASH | Action on Smoking and Health |
| BA | Bachelor of Arts |
| BACUP | British Association of Cancer United Patients |
| BAON | British Association of Orthopaedic Nurses |
| BDA | British Dental Association |
| BDSc | Bachelor of Dental Science |
| BEd | Bachelor of Education |
| BITA | British Intravenous Therapy Association |
| BMAS | British Medical Acupuncture Society |
| BN | Bachelor of Nursing |
| BPOG | British Psychosocial Oncology Group |
| BRA | British Reflexology Association |
| BRCS | British Red Cross Society |
| BSc (Soc SC-Nurs) | Bachelor of Science (Nursing) |
| BSMDH | British Society of Medical and Dental Hypnosis |
| CATS | Credit Accumulation Transfer Scheme |
| CCETSW | Central Council for Educational Training in Social Work |
| CCHE | Central Council for Health Education |
| CMT | Clinical Midwife Teacher |
| CNAA | Council for National Academic Awards |
| CNF | Commonwealth Nurses Federation |
| CNN | Certificated Nursery Nurse |
| COSHH | Control of Substances Hazardous to Health |
| CSP | Chartered Society of Physiotherapists |
| DCH | Diploma in Child Health |

| | |
|---|---|
| DDA | Dangerous Drugs Act |
| DipAr | Diploma in Aromatherapy |
| DipEd | Diploma in Education |
| DipHyp | Diploma in Hypnotherapy |
| DipMedAc | Diploma in Medical Acupuncture |
| Dip NEd | Diploma in Nursing Education |
| DipPhyto | Diploma in Phytotherapy |
| DN | Diploma in Nursing |
| DNA | District Nursing Association |
| DNE | Diploma in Nursing Education |
| DoH | Department of Health |
| DPH | Diploma in Public Health |
| DPhil | Doctor of Philosophy |
| DPM | Diploma in Psychological Medicine |
| DSc | Doctor of Science |
| DTM&H | Diploma in Tropical Medicine and Hygiene |
| EN | Enrolled Nurse |
| ENB | English National Board for Nursing, Midwifery and Health Visiting |
| FCSP | Fellow of the Chartered Society of Physiotherapists |
| FETC | Further Education Teaching Certificate |
| FNIF | Florence Nightingale International Foundation |
| FNIMH | Fellow of National Institute of Medical Herbalists |
| FPA | Family Planning Association |
| FRcn | Fellow of the Royal College of Nursing |
| FRS | Fellow of the Royal Society |
| FRSH | Fellow of the Royal Society of Health |
| GMC | General Medical Council |
| GNVQ | General National Vocational Qualification |
| HEA | Health Education Authority |
| HFEA | Human Fertilization and Embryology Authority |
| HSA | Hospital Savings Association |
| HV | Health Visitor |
| HVA | Health Visitors' Association |
| ICN | International Council of Nurses |
| ICNA | Infection Control Nurses Association |
| ICW | International Council of Women |
| IFA | International Federation of Aromatherapists |

| | |
|---|---|
| IHF | International Hospital Federation |
| INR | Index of Nursing Research |
| LFHom | Licensed Associate of the Faculty of Homeopathy |
| MA | Master of Arts |
| MAACP | Member of Acupuncture Association of Chartered Physiotherapists |
| MAO | Master of the Art of Obstetrics |
| MAOT | Member of the Association of Occupational Therapists |
| MBA | Master of Business Administration |
| MBAC | Member of British Acupuncture Council |
| MBIM | Member of the British Institute of Management |
| MCSP | Member of the Chartered Society of Physiotherapists |
| MFHom | Member of Faculty of Homeopathy |
| MIND | National Association for Mental Health |
| MMAA | Member of Modern Acupuncture Association |
| MPhil | Master of Philosophy |
| MRC | Medical Research Council |
| MRSH | Member of the Royal Society of Health |
| MRSHom | Member of Royal Society of Homeopaths |
| MRSS | Member of Register of Shiatsu Society |
| MSc | Master of Science |
| MSF | Manufacturing Science and Finance |
| MSRG | Member of the Society of Remedial Gymnasts |
| MSR(R) | Member of the Society of Radiographers (Radiography) |
| MSR(T) | Member of the Society of Radiographers (Radiotherapy) |
| MTD | Midwife Teachers' Diploma |
| NAMCW | National Association for Maternal and Child Welfare |
| NAMH | National Association for Mental Health |
| NATN | National Association of Theatre Nurses |
| NAWCH | National Association for the Welfare of Children in Hospital |
| NHS | National Health Service |
| NIB | Northern Ireland Board for Nursing, Midwifery and Health Visiting |
| NIMH | National Institute of Medical Herbalists |

| | |
|---|---|
| NNA | Neonatal Nurses Association |
| NNEB | National Nursery Education Board |
| NUMINE | Network of Users of Microcomputers in Nurse Education |
| NUS | National Union of Students |
| NVQ | National Vocational Qualification |
| OHNC | Occupational Health Nursing Certificate |
| ONC | Orthopaedic Nurses' Certificate |
| OND | Ophthalmic Nursing Diploma |
| OT | Occupational Therapist |
| PhD | Doctor of Philosophy |
| PMRAFNS | Princess Mary's Royal Air Force Nursing Service |
| PNA | Psychiatric Nurses' Association |
| ProfDipAr | Professional Diploma in Aromatherapy |
| QARANC | Queen Alexandra's Royal Army Nursing Corps |
| QARNNS | Queen Alexandra's Royal Naval Nursing Service |
| QIDN | Queen's Institute of District Nursing |
| QNI | Queen's Nursing Institute |
| RCM | Royal College of Midwives |
| Rcn | Royal College of Nursing |
| RGN | Registered General Nurse |
| RHV | Regional Health Visitor |
| RM | Registered Midwife |
| RMN | Registered Mental Nurse |
| RN | Registered Nurse |
| RNMH | Registered Nurse for the Mentally Handicapped |
| RNT | Registered Nurse Tutor |
| RSCN | Registered Sick Children's Nurse |
| StAAA | St Andrew's Ambulance Association |
| StJAA | St John Ambulance Association |
| StJAB | St John Ambulance Brigade |
| SCM | State Certified Midwife |
| SHHD | Scottish Home and Health Department |
| SNB | Scottish National Board for Nursing, Midwifery and Health Visiting |
| SNNEB | Scottish National Nursing Examination Board |
| SRN | State Registered Nurse |

| | |
|---|---|
| SSStJ | Serving Sister of the Order of St John of Jerusalem |
| ST | Speech Therapist |
| UKCC | United Kingdom Central Council for Nursing, Midwifery and Health Visiting |
| VSO | Voluntary Service Overseas |
| WFH | Word Federation of Hypnotherapists |
| WHO | World Health Organization |
| WNB | Welsh National Board for Nursing, Midwifery and Health Visiting |
| WRVS | Women's Royal Voluntary Service |

# Appendix 10
## Units of Measurement and Tables of Normal Values

## SI Units (Système International d'Unités)

**Base Units**

| Physical quantity | Name of unit | Symbol |
|---|---|---|
| Mass | kilogram | kg |
| Length | metre | m |
| Time | second | s |
| Electric current | ampere | A |
| Temperature | kelvin | K |
| Luminous intensity | candela | cd |
| Amount of substance | mole | mol |

**Derived Units**
Derived units to measure other quantities are obtained by multiplying or dividing any two or more of the seven base units. Some of these have their own names and symbols. For example:

| Physical quantity | Name of unit | Symbol | Base or derived units |
|---|---|---|---|
| Force | newton | N | $kg.m.s^{-2}$ |
| Pressure | pascal | Pa | $N.m^{-2}$ |
| Energy, work, heat | joule | J | $N.m$ |
| Power | watt | W | $J.s^{-1}$ |

### Prefixes used for Multiples

| Factor | Prefix | Symbol |
|--------|--------|--------|
| $10^{-12}$ | pico | p |
| $10^{-9}$ | nano | n |
| $10^{-6}$ | micro | μ |
| $10^{-3}$ | milli | m |
| $10^{-2}$ | centi | c |
| $10^{-1}$ | deci | d |
| $10$ | deca | da |
| $10^{2}$ | hecto | h |
| $10^{3}$ | kilo | k |
| $10^{6}$ | mega | M |
| $10^{9}$ | giga | G |
| $10^{12}$ | tera | T |

### Capacity

The SI unit of *volume* is the cubic metre ($m^3$), but the litre (l) is more commonly used and accepted (it is equivalent to 1 $dm^3$).

| | | |
|---|---|---|
| 1000 microlitres (μl) | = 1 millilitre (ml) | |
| 10 millilitres | = 1 centilitre (cl) | |
| 100 millilitres | = 10 centilitres | |
| 1000 millilitres | = 100 centilitres | = 1 decilitre(dl) |
| | | = 10 decilitres = 1 litre (l) |

1 cubic centimetre ($cm^3$ or cc) = 1 millilitre
1 cubic decimetre ($dm^3$) = 1 litre

### Domestic Equivalents (approximate)

| | | |
|---|---|---|
| 1 teaspoon | = | 5 ml |
| 1 dessertspoon | = | 10 ml |
| 1 tablespoon | = | 20 ml |
| 1 sherry glass | = | 60 ml |
| 1 teacup | = | 142 ml |
| 1 breakfast cup | = | 230 ml |
| 1 tumbler | = | 285 ml |

### Weights

| | |
|---|---|
| 1000 micrograms (μg) | = 1 milligram (mg) |
| 1000 milligrams | = 1 gram (g) |
| 1000 grams | = 1 kilogram (kg) |
| 1000 kilograms | = 1 metric tonne |

**Energy**

A dietetic calorie is the amount of heat required to raise the temperature of 1 litre of water by 1°C and is equal to 4.184 kilojoules.

1 g fat will produce 38 kilojoules or 9 calories.

1 g protein will produce 17 kilojoules or 4 calories.

1 g carbohydrate will produce 17 kilojoules or 4 calories.

**Comparative Temperatures**

| Celsius (°C) | Fahrenheit (°F) | Celsius (°C) | Fahrenheit (°F) |
|---|---|---|---|
| 100 (boiling point) | 212 | 38.5 | 101.3 |
| 95 | 203 | 38 | 100.4 |
| 90 | 194 | 37.5 | 99.5 |
| 85 | 185 | 37 | 98.6 |
| 80 | 176 | 36.5 | 97.7 |
| 75 | 167 | 36 | 96.8 |
| 70 | 158 | 35.5 | 95.9 |
| 65 | 149 | 35 | 95 |
| 60 | 140 | 34 | 93.2 |
| 55 | 131 | 33 | 91.4 |
| 50 | 122 | 32 | 89.6 |
| 45 | 113 | 31 | 87.8 |
| 44 | 112.2 | 30 | 86 |
| 43 | 109.4 | 25 | 77 |
| 42 | 107.6 | 20 | 68 |
| 41 | 105.8 | 15 | 59 |
| 40 | 104 | 10 | 50 |
| 39.5 | 103.1 | 5 | 41 |
| 39 | 102.2 | 0 (freezing point) | 32 |

To convert readings of the Fahrenheit scale into Celsius degrees subtract 32, multiply by 5, and divide by 9, for example:

$98 - 32 = 66 \times 5 = 330 \div 9 = 36.6$
Therefore $98°F = 36.6°C$

To convert readings of the Celsius scale into Fahrenheit degrees multiply by 9, divide by 5, and add 32, for example:

$36.6 \times 9 = 330 \div 5 = 66 + 32 = 98$
Therefore $36.6°C = 98°F$

The term 'Celsius' (from the name of the Swede who invented the scale in 1742) is now being internationally used instead of 'centigrade', which term is employed in some countries to denote fractions of an angle.

# Normal Values

| Analysis | Reference range |
|---|---|
| **Haematology** | |
| Haemoglobin | |
| Male | 14.0–17.7 g dL$^{-1}$ |
| Female | 12.0–16.0 g dL$^{-1}$ |
| Mean corpuscular volume (MCV) | 80–96 fl |
| White cell count | 4–11 ×10$^9$/litre |
| Platelet count | 150–400 × 10$^9$/litre |
| Serum B$_{12}$ | 160–925 ng L$^{-1}$ |
| | (150–675 pmol L$^{-1}$) |
| Serum folate | 4–18 µg L$^{-1}$ |
| | (5–63 nmol L$^{-1}$) |
| Erythrocyte sedimentation rate (ESR) | < 20 mm in 1 hour |
| **Coagulation** | |
| Partial thromboplastin time (PTTK) | 24–31 s |
| Prothrombin time | 12–16 s |
| **Serum biochemistry** | |
| Alanine aminotransferase (ALT) | 5–40 U L$^{-1}$ |
| Albumin | 36–53 g L$^{-1}$ |
| Alkaline phosphatase | 25–115 U L$^{-1}$ |
| Amylase | < 220 U L$^{-1}$ |
| Aspartate aminotransferase (AST) | 7–40 U L$^{-1}$ |
| Bicarbonate | 22–30 mmol L$^{-1}$ |
| Bilirubin | < 17 µmol L$^{-1}$ |
| | (0.3–1.5 mg dL$^{-1}$) |
| Calcium | 2.20–2.67 mmol L$^{-1}$ |
| | (8.5–10.5 mg dL$^{-1}$) |
| Chloride | 95–106 mmol L$^{-1}$ |
| Creatinine | 0.06–0.12 mmol L$^{-1}$ |
| | (0.6–1.5 mg dL$^{-1}$) |
| Ferritin | |
| Female | 6–110 µg L$^{-1}$ |
| Male | 20–260 µg L$^{-1}$ |
| Post-menopausal | 12–230 µg L$^{-1}$ |
| Glucose | 4.5–5.6 mmol L$^{-1}$ |
| | (70–110 mg dL$^{-1}$) |
| Potassium | 3.5–5.0 mmol L$^{-1}$ |
| Sodium | 135–146 mmol L$^{-1}$ |
| Urea | 2.5–6.7 mmol L$^{-1}$ |
| | (8–25 mg dL$^{-1}$) |

Source: Saunders' Pocket Essentials of Clinical Medicine (2nd edn). Anne Ballinger and Stephen Patchett. WB Saunders 1999.

# Appendix 11
# Immunization

Table 11.1 represents an example of a standard childhood immunization programme. Please note, however, that individual considerations always need to be borne in mind regarding childhood immunization—both in terms of possible contraindications and adverse reactions.

## Immunization Aftercare and Side-effects

### BCG
BCG immunization should not cause any pyrexia.

Between 2 and 6 weeks after the injection, there may be a small swelling at the injection site with scaling, crusting and bruising. The injection site should be kept exposed to air. Avoid covering it with a plaster. Eventually it will heal on its own and leave a small scar.

### Diphtheria, Tetanus, Whooping cough, Polio, Hib and Meningitis C vaccine
Some children become irritable and may develop a slight fever between 6 and 24 hours after immunization. This is not serious. A patch of redness around the injection site is also common.

| TABLE 11.1 | EXAMPLE OF CHILD IMMUNIZATION SCHEDULE |
|---|---|
| **Age Due** | **Immunization** |
| At 2 months | Polio |
| | Hib |
| | Diphtheria |
| | Tetanus |
| | Whooping cough |
| | Meningitis C |
| At 3 months | Polio |
| | Hib |
| | Diphtheria |
| | Tetanus |
| | Whooping cough |
| | Meningitis C |
| At 4 months | Polio |
| | Hib |
| | Diphtheria |
| | Tetanus |
| | Whooping cough |
| | Meningitis C |
| At 12–15 months | Measles |
| | Mumps |
| | Rubella |
| 3–5 years (usually before the child starts school) | Measles |
| | Mumps |
| | Rubella |
| | Diphtheria |
| | Tetanus |
| | Polio |
| 10–14 years (sometimes shortly after birth) | BCG (against tuberculosis) |
| School leavers (13–18 years) | Diphtheria |
| | Tetanus |
| | Polio |

## Measles, Mumps and Rubella (MMR)

A week to 10 days after the injection the child may become pyrexial for 1–2 days. There may also be a rash. Swollen lymph glands in the neck may occur 2–3 weeks after immunization. These reactions are not serious or contagious.

# Appendix 12
# Community Care
PAUL THACKER

A simple definition of community care might be: 'the help and support that people need so that they can live as independently as possible in their own home or in homely surroundings in the community'.

The NHS and Community Care Act 1990 has enabled restructuring of the way in which care is delivered, placing the emphasis on the above definition. Care in the community is not alien to the National Health Service (NHS) or to the nurses who work within it. The Act reconfigures some of the funding, gearing it more towards local needs, and formalizes what we all know to be true about working together to enable the best outcome for the patient/client/user. Initially, the main groups affected by the reforms were elderly and disabled people, people with mental illness or mental handicap, people with acquired immune deficiency syndrome (AIDS), and those with drug and alcohol problems. As time has gone on, however, the need to define parameters of health and social care has brought about the introduction of 'eligibility criteria'. These are matrices designed to offer a testing-ground for making decisions about whose budget shall carry responsibility for care provision. The health element of care in the community is known as 'NHS continuing care' and might be described as 'the provision of NHS-funded health care and support on a short- or long-term basis to meet the needs of patients who could not—or would not—respond to intensive treatment'.

The NHS and Community Care Act itself is divided into two parts.

Part One, implemented in 1991, created a new structure in the NHS and introduced the internal market and the purchaser/provider split. In simple terms, those of us controlling funds that used to be in the hands of the old health authorities are now more accountable for how that money is spent. It is a question of learning the art of good housekeeping, as part of our professional role, and not abdicating responsibility for budgetary control. In broader terms, each Trust acts as a business in the 'marketplace'; it invests, spends, advances, retreats, expands and contracts as market forces dictate, in order to stay, quite literally, in 'credit'.

Part Two of the Act, implemented in April 1993, deals with the provision of community care. It is this that affects the majority of ward/field staff. The 'key components' are:

- Services that respond flexibly and sensitively to the needs of individuals and their carers.
- Services that allow a range of options for consumers.
- Services that intervene—no more than is necessary—to foster independence.
- Services that concentrate on those with the greatest need.

Such key elements focus on patient-centred care, which nurses have advocated for many years. All nurses strive to help their patients to be independent and self-reliant.

Nor has dependence ever been fostered in social care provision. After years of providing their own caring services in local areas, however, social services are changing from being solely a 'provider' to encompassing a 'purchaser' role. They have, in effect, become the enabler of the entire service. The main provisions relating to social services in the Act are as follows:

- The transfer of responsibility and resources from the DSS to local authorities.
- Lead responsibility for the assessment of needs.
- The preparation of Community Care Plans (on an annual basis).
- A duty to consult not only with other agencies but also with users and carers.
- Establishment of a complaints procedure and independent inspection units.
- Application of registration standards for residential homes.

The fundamental aim is to provide acceptable, high-quality care within a community setting. This places responsibilities upon all the agencies and individuals involved. It is a process of cooperation designed to deliver a unified approach to meeting the needs of the people who are our customers.

Also in 1993, as part of the implementation of the Act, health and social service authorities all over the UK were required to reach agreement on their respective responsibilities for care services. They undertook to review and reconfirm their agreements annually. Most authorities now identify and share information on levels of care services and undertake not to make unilateral changes in resources. Social service eligibility criteria are, however, different in form from continuing health care eligibility criteria. They do not define, for example, the dependency level of people for whom the social services provide care, as opposed to continuing health care. This has meant that 'working together' has become increasingly more important if customers are not to fall through 'gaps' in care provision.

The eligibility criteria for NHS-funded continuing care are set out by each purchaser area in the UK but, typically, would include care provision to various dependency levels of:

- Frail elderly.
- Elderly people with mental health problems.
- People with dementia.
- Children and young people.
- Adults with a learning disability.
- People with a physical and/or sensory disability.

Such categories might also be subdivided in terms of respite care, palliative care, specialist equipment and specialist transport.

## Roles
Everyone has a role in making the Act a reality.

### The Role of the Local Authorities
The local authorities have lead responsibility. Their main tasks are as follows:

- Making information about the service easily available to potential customers and their carers. This includes the range of services, how they are provided and assessed, and how to complain.
- Assessing community care needs—in *consultation* with other agencies.
- Telling the customer the outcome of these assessments.
- Undertaking regular reviews of individual care needs.
- Providing feedback of information into the overall planning system.

### The Role of the Health Authorities and NHS Trusts
Health Authorities and NHS Trusts must play a full and active part in the cooperative process, both in assessing needs and in responding to them. Their key responsibilities are as follows:

- To identify which health-care professionals will take part in the assessment of care needs (with local authorities).
- To set up systems for the feeding back of health-care needs information to the NHS.
- To agree necessary arrangements for the appointment of health-care professionals as named assessors (where appropriate).
- To be certain that the right health care (as assessed) is being provided.

- To have in place the necessary arrangements to review health-care needs and revise provision of care.
- To develop improved lines of communication with local authorities.

**The Role of the General Practitioner**

This is very important. The general practitioner is often the first contact for potential customers. The role of the general practitioner is to:

- Advise patients on the range and availability of local social services.
- Refer patients to social services through a locally agreed system.
- Advise social services (with the consent of the patient) of clinical information relevant to the patient's current health and ability to cope at home.
- Become involved in complex cases where professional medical advice is requested.

For agencies to cooperate effectively, a mechanism—based on local circumstances and concerns—needs to be agreed. This is the process called *assessment and care management*. If there is no agreed mechanism, ignorance will very quickly lead to chaos! It simply involves the members of the different agencies—along with the user and carers—working in partnership.

A referral to any of the agencies will prompt an assessment of need which may lead to the involvement of a further agency. The different *assessments* make up the whole picture of *need*. Managing that need is the responsibility of one named person (the named assessor, usually from the social services department), who is *independent* of service provision and helps to prevent conflict of interest or 'tramlining' into particular services. This system also promotes a flexibility of response to individual need and customer choice. The named assessor is accountable to the customer or client, and this has the practical advantage of reducing the number of contacts the customer has to make in order to alter the level of help required.

## Hospital Discharge Arrangements

There is little doubt that advancements in both medical and nursing science over the years have increased the rate at which patients flow through the acute hospital system. Shorter stays following surgery—and even day surgery—are now commonplace.

It is all the more important, then, to ensure that agencies work together. That is why hospital discharge arrangements are so important. How various agencies interact with regard to individual discharge arrangements may be seen as a key indicator of performance. The 'Hospital discharge workbook' (produced by the Department of Health (1994) and available free of charge from The Health Publications Unit, Storage and Distribution Centre, Heywood Stores, Manchester Road, Heywood, Lancs OL10 2PZ) sets out a framework for good practice in this field which addresses the major issues identified in recent findings. In particular, it is designed to:

- Address both quality *and* efficiency issues.
- Be outcome-orientated, both in relation to individual service users, and to the service overall.
- Provide practical help based on experience that has been proved to work (examples of innovative practice are included throughout the workbook).
- Recognise and address *all* the various stakeholders, from service users and their carers, to health and social services staff responsible for purchasing and providing services.

The robust application of multi-agency working in 'discharge' or 'transfer of care' is as much a useful model for overall working practice in the community environment as in the acute setting. Using a three-cornered approach—acute health, community health, local authority—the different agencies can set joint agreements in place that will help cement the best of working relationships.

To summarize:

- Keep the customer at the centre.
- Assess needs professionally.
- Refer to others where necessary, allowing them make their assessments.
- Work as a team.
- Talk to customer, carers and each other.
- Keep customer, carers and each other involved and informed at all stages of planning.
- Do not take away independence in hospital (e.g. encourage patients to give their own insulin if that is what they normally do).
- Set appropriate and individual care packages.
- Only give what is yours to give.
- Do not spend other people's money.

- Check everything is in place *before* setting your plans in motion.
- In short, be sensitive, selective and systematic in and with the care situation.

REFERENCES AND BIBLIOGRAPHY

Caring for people: community care in the next decade and beyond. 1989 HMSO, London
Community care in the next decade and beyond: policy guidance. 1990 HMSO, London
Getting better: inspection of hospital discharge (care management) arrangements for older people. 1998 HMSO, London
Partnership in action: a discussion document. 1998 HMSO, London
HC(89)5 and LAC(89)7 Discharge of patients from hospital. 1989 HMSO, London
Hospital discharge workbook. HMSO, London
National Health Service and Community Care Act 1990. HMSO, London
Neill J, Williams J 1992 Leaving hospital: elderly people and their discharge to community care (briefing paper). National Institute for Social Work, Research Unit, HMSO, London
The patient's charter. 1991 HMSO, London

# Appendix 13
# Occupational Health and Safety
JUDY RIVETT

The Health and Safety at Work etc. Act 1974 provided the structure
for all modern health and safety legislation. The foundation Act
placed duties on employers for the health, safety and welfare of
their employees while at work as far as is reasonably predictable. It
also placed a duty on the employees to cooperate with their
employers in adhering to the safe systems of work implemented by
the employers and not to interfere or misuse anything provided for
this purpose.

## Health and Safety Commission and Health and Safety Executive
The Act also established the Health and Safety Commission and the
Health and Safety Executive. The role of the Commission is to advise
the appropriate ministers on the need for new health and safety
regulations. It is a tripartite body comprising representatives from the
Confederation of British Industry (CBI), the Trades Union Congress
(TUC), local authorities and the Health and Safety Executive (HSE),
and invited representatives from independent and local authorities.
The HSE is a separate statutory body appointed by the Commission
and undertakes the work required by the Commission. The Executive
is the enforcing body for health and safety law and provides an
advisory service to both sides of industry and commerce.

Since 1974 an enormous tranche of regulations controlling more
specific aspects of industry and commerce have become law. The
Control of Substances Hazardous to Health Regulations 1988
(amended 1998) and the 'Six Pack' of 1992 (see below), driven by the
European Parliament, have had a tremendous impact on improving
conditions at work for the nation's workforce.

## The Control of Substances Hazardous to Health Regulations 1988 (amended 1998)
These regulations introduced the idea of risk assessment in the
workplace. Employers are required to assess the substances used in
their workplace for their potential as health hazards under the
categories 'very toxic', 'toxic', 'harmful', 'corrosive' or 'irritant'.
The assessment should also include the measures required to
control the risks, whether by eliminating the substances from the work

process; containing the substance in an enclosed system thus preventing exposure; or safeguarding the individual with protective equipment or workwear. Whichever control measure is introduced, the system must be monitored and reviewed continuously.

## Health Surveillance

As part of the monitoring system, health surveillance should be undertaken if appropriate. The health of employees exposed to hazardous substances can be affected through absorption into the body. The absorption route can be by inhalation, by ingestion, through the skin or a combination of these. When inside the body the substances are metabolized. Metabolites can target various organs of the body which can be harmful. A classic example of this is exposure to asbestos. The small fibres are breathed in and lodge in the lungs and pleura. Asbestosis, mesothelioma and lung cancer can be fatal outcomes. Health surveillance therefore requires biological monitoring. At its simplest this could be a skin inspection ensuring no dermatitic changes have occurred as a result of exposure to an irritant, through to lung function tests and urine, breath or blood analyses. The criteria used to decide which type of surveillance is appropriate depend on whether a test is available. Tributyl tin oxide was once used as a timber preservation treatment; however, it was not known how it was metabolized in the body and therefore no appropriate test existed. The potential for it to cause harm could not be eradicated and, as many occupational diseases have a long latency period—up to 40 years for asbestosis, for example, tributyl tin oxide was withdrawn from use.

## Environmental Monitoring

Monitoring the work environment is imperative to ensure that all control measures are effective. This may include checking that local exhaust ventilation systems are functioning properly; checking that noise levels are not above legal limits; or asking people to wear passive air samplers to ensure they are not inhaling possible contaminants.

## Records

Results of all monitoring must be recorded. Health surveillance records must be treated in confidence although a 'fitness to work' certificate should be given to the employer. As health surveillance records have to be kept for 40 years, the appropriate place for storing these documents is with an occupational health service. Records for environmental monitoring should be designed so that data can be read alongside data from fitness certificates. This will help to identify any failing control measures at a glance.

## The Reporting of Injuries, Disease and Dangerous Substances Regulations 1985

Employers are required to report to the HSE (or local authority for retail premises) certain injuries, diseases or dangerous occurrences that have stemmed from work activities. The aim of the regulations is to provide information to the HSE for epidemiological purposes. Analysis of the information may suggest a pattern of disease or injury associated with a particular industry. Action can be taken to establish the cause of the risk and its prevention.

## The 'Six Pack' 1992

Six new sets of regulations were produced in 1992 in response to the European Parliament Framework Directive. These are:

- Management of Health and Safety at Work.
- Manual Handling Operations.
- Personal Protective Equipment at Work.
- Health and Safety (Display Screen Equipment).
- Provision and Use of Work Equipment.
- Workplace (Health, Safety and Welfare).

While each set of regulations focuses on specific aspects of the workplace, they all have a common theme. They reinforce the need for risk assessments, introducing control measures and follow-up monitoring and review systems. However, for the first time the idea of

---

**BOX 13.1**          **A STEP-BY-STEP GUIDE**

- The employer has duty for assessing risks in the workplace
- Is anyone at work knowledgeable about health and safety?
- Appoint a person to carry out health risk assessment
- Refer to the Health and Safety Regulations and HSE guidance for help in health risk identification
- Could employees be harmed?
- What can be done about the risks?
- Has the appointed person sufficient specialist knowledge about controlling the risks?
- Is expert help needed?

a 'competent person' is introduced. The employer is required to appoint one or more competent persons to assist in undertaking the measures needed to comply with the relevant statutory provisions. In small businesses this may be the employer in person or a colleague. In larger organizations it is likely to be a full occupational health and safety service. Whoever it is, the person must be knowledgeable about the risks to health and safety within that workplace.

Another important aspect of the 'Six Pack' is the need to provide information, instruction and training for employees. In practice this means providing factual information about the risks and the measures used to control them, telling people what they must do for their protection and training them how to do it (see Box 13.1).

### Hazard and Risk

Frequently, there is confusion about the terms 'hazard' and 'risk'. 'Hazard' is something which will cause harm if not controlled. 'Risk' is the potential for harm when control measures are in place. An unguarded guillotine, for example, poses a tremendous hazard to health — certainly it did for many French aristocrats! Guarded industrial guillotine machines, which can only be operated from a safe distance, pose little risk.

### Failing to Safety as Opposed to Failing to Danger

It is a fact of life that things break down. All systems introduced to protect the health, safety and welfare of employees need to be assessed for their potential to fail to safety—not to danger. A simple example of this is hand-washing. Where there is a risk of employees ingesting a toxic residue on their hands, one of the control measures associated with the work process would be to ask them to wash their hands before eating. People in general will not go out of their way to find washing facilities so it is imperative to ensure there are adequate facilities adjacent to the area in which they will be eating. On a building site, construction workers burning lead paint from girders were absorbing high levels of lead. They had been provided with protective air-fed helmets, gloves and overalls. Their work site was opposite the Portakabin used as a canteen. The lavatory and washing facilities were on the opposite side of the site. Clearly, they just removed their helmets and gloves before going into the canteen. Not only did they remove their helmets and gloves but they stored the dust-laden gloves neatly tucked into the breathing zone of their helmets—a natural act for the many bikers among them! The obvious solution to this problem was to install a second Portakabin with washing facilities and storage for the gloves and the helmets in front of the canteen. Their lead levels subsequently reduced.

## Safe Systems of Work and Human Factors

Safe systems of work are not achieved by writing a policy document and putting it in a manual in a cupboard. They involve understanding how people go about their work and incorporating their natural behaviour into the system. In the hand-washing example given previously, guiding the construction workers through the washing facilities to gain access to the canteen made it quite natural for them to wash their hands. Yes, even bikers!

# Appendix 14
# Nursing on the Internet

CHRISTINE BISHOP

**For the health-care professional, the Internet provides a veritable treasure chest of information, but mixed in with the nuggets of gold is a vast amount of irrelevant or useless data. Many hours can be wasted searching for the precise information you require, so the trick is to learn to navigate the Net without too much frustration.**

The various types of information accessible via the Web include:

- Information about professional organizations, academic institutions and hospitals, e.g. the Royal College of Nursing.
- Full text or abstracts of many published articles—available through Medline. In addition many journals are now accessible online, either free of charge or on a subscription basis.
- Information about disease states, e.g. AIDS Insite (http://hivinsite.ucsf.edu/).
- Information about drugs.
- Support groups for parents, e.g. Web sites for parents of premature infants (http://www2.medsch.wisc.edu/ childrenshosp/parents_of_preemies/toc.html).
- Details of conferences.

In fact, information on almost any topic is probably now available electronically if you know where to find it.

If you don't know the URL or 'address' of the Web page you want to access, then you need to use one of the search engines such as Yahoo or AltaVista, which should be easily accessible via your browser (e.g. Netscape Navigator or Microsoft Internet Explorer).

When you type in a keyword for the site you want to access, the search engine will bring up a list of all the sites on the Web containing that particular keyword. Obviously if it is a common word, such as 'nurse' you can end up with several thousand sites, which can be very tedious to go through. So if possible restrict the list by being more precise—for example, 'nurse and education' or 'nurse and journals'.

Once you have found a site which interests you make sure you bookmark it so that you can find it again. Many sites include links to related Web sites and these are a good source of high-quality information.

To help you find your way around the World Wide Web, listed below are some nursing sites which you may find useful, but do bear in mind that sites are constantly being added and deleted, so you will need to do your own research.

# Medisearch

To focus on the large amount of useful health information there is on the Internet, the UK search engine Mirago has launched a special service called Medisearch (www.medisearch.co.uk), which offers search services for 'authoritative' medical information.

The documents categorized by the Mirago robots as containing medical resources have been compiled in conjunction with UK health professionals, who have classified sites considered to be repositories of 'authoritative' medical information. These resources include UK and international professional, research, administrative, charitable, support and commercial sites in both the private and public sectors. The Medisearch index encompasses hundreds of thousands of pages on health-related topics with the index completely refreshed every 2–3 weeks.

Apart from a free searchable service for health professionals and patients, Medisearch offers news and topic-oriented Web guides linking to thousands of useful health-related sites.

### American Association of Colleges of Nursing (AACN)
(http://www.aacn.nche.edu/index.html)
Web homepage of the AACN, the national voice of America's university and higher-degree nursing education programmes. For members only there is an interactive issues forum.

### Community Practitioners' and Health Visitors' Association (CPHVA)
http://www.msfcphva.org.uk)
The UK professional body that represents registered nurses and health visitors who work in primary or community health settings.

### English National Board for Nursing, Midwifery and Health Visiting (ENB) Link Home Page
(http://www.enb.org.uk/)
This site aims to disseminate Board information to nurses, midwives and health visitors in England and includes details of current circulars, courses and contact information. There are links to Research Digest listing, the commissioned research and the ENB Health Care Database of nursing literature abstracts.

**Health Education Authority (HEA)**
(http://www.hea.org.uk)
Web homepage of the UK Health Education Authority. It contains news, press releases and publications produced by the HEA, as well as details of conferences and events relating to health promotion and research programmes currently under the aegis of the HEA. A new Web site on immunization has proved very successful.
(http://www.immunisation.org.uk).

**Index Medicus**
(http://www.medscape.com/Home/Search/Index Medicus)
A full listing of journal abbreviations used for Index Medicus.

**Medscape**
(http://www.medscape.com)
Permits free access to full text of a selection of peer-reviewed journals as well as the latest news in different specialities. Registration is required. Also gives free access to Medline.

**Medscape—Drug Information**
(http://www.medscape.com/misc/formdrugs.html)
Information on more than 200 000 prescription and over-the-counter drugs including indications, interactions and precautions. The site also enables you to find drugs to treat a disease and includes an online medical dictionary.

**Mining Co Guide to Nursing**
(http://nursing.miningco.com/)
A useful resource for nurses offering Net links, features, bulletin boards, chat and a free newsletter. There are also further links to an evolving index of Net resources on nursing divided by specialty.

**National Board for Nursing, Midwifery and Health Visiting for Northern Ireland**
(http://www.n-i.nhs.uk/NBNI/index.htm)
Provides advice and information on training for nurses, midwives and health visitors in Northern Ireland.

**National Board for Nursing, Midwifery and Health Visiting for Scotland**
(http://www.nbs.org.uk/)

Responsible for standards of education and training for nurses, midwives and health visitors in Scotland. Provides career information for these professions.

## National League for Nursing (NLN)
(http://www.nln.org/)
The NLN aims to promote quality nursing education in the US. Information is provided on membership, accreditation programme, career and education opportunities, as well as news and events.

## Nurses on the Web
(http://www.cp-tel.net/pamnorth/webnurse.htm)
A nursing site designed to bring both students and professional nurses together to offer support, communication and assistance. The pages are frequently updated and include information on nursing journals, nursing practice and further nursing links.

## Nursing Around the World
(http://www.nurse-dk.com/)
A free access site offering online chat, the Nursing Forums, the Nursing Connection and reviews. A world-nurse listserv allows members to read or debate global nursing issues with nurses internationally.

## Nursing Connection
(http://www.nursecon.htm)
This provides a free listing service for nurses around the world. Each listing includes an e-mail link as well as a description of the individual's interests, location and specialty.

## Nursing (Medicine)
(http://galaxy.tradewave.com/galaxy/Medicine/Health-Occupations/nursing.html)
A directory of nursing resources with links to nursing research, theory and specialities. Further links to US organisations and nursing directories.

## PubMed
(http://www.ncbi.nlminih.gov/PubMed/)
The National Library of Medicine's free search service with access to 9 million citations in Medline with links to participating online journals.

**Raven's Child—Nursing Links**
(http://home.att.net/~ravenschild/)
Homepage linking to sites on community health nursing, ICU nursing and trauma. This site is designed as a resource for students, nurses and other medical personnel.

**Royal College of Nursing, Australia (RCNA)**
(http://www.rcna.org.au)
Web pages for this organisation for nurses from all practice areas throughout Australia.

**Royal College of Nursing Conference and Exhibition Unit**
(http://www.nursing-standard.co.uk/confs.htm)
A listing of conferences organised by the RCN in the UK and Europe.

**Royal College of Nursing UK**
(http://www.rcn.org.uk)
The RCN is the world's largest professional union for registered nurses, midwives and health visitors. The site provides information about the organisation and a service for members who require professional, legal and educational advice.

**Royal Windsor Society for Nursing Research** ('For Your Information')
(http://www.windsor.igs.net/~nhodgins/)
A useful new resource designed to promote nursing research at a global level. It includes online workshops, a nursing journals database and newsgroup. There is also a listing of professional services and opportunities and recent publications. There are plans to include an online workshop on database design/software choice as well as a basic nursing research study Web site design.

**UK Central Council (UKCC)**
(http://www.healthworks.co.uk/hw/orgs/UKCC.html)
Information on the organisation, structure, funding and membership of the UKCC plus contact details.

**Welsh National Board for Nursing, Midwifery and Health Visiting**
(http://www.wnb.org.uk/)

Provides information relevant to nurses, midwives and health visitors working in Wales and also those wishing to enter the profession.

**Worldwide Nurse**
(http://www.wwnurse.com)
A valuable site with an extensive compilation of links to online nursing sites and journals, colleges and universities, lists of employment vacancies and nursing humour.

# Appendix 15
# Universal Precautions/Infection Control Guidelines

Health-care workers who come into contact with blood, secretions and excreta may be exposed to pathogens, including blood-borne viruses such as human immunodeficiency virus (HIV) and hepatitis B and C. It is impossible to identify all those with infection, blood-borne or otherwise. Therefore it is recommended that all body fluids be regarded as potentially infectious and universal precautions be used.

The most common means of transmission is direct contact, particularly via hands. Blood-borne infections are most likely to be transmitted by direct sharps injury. Blood contact with broken skin or mucous membranes also provides a route of transmission whenever contact with blood or other body fluids is anticipated (UK Health Departments 1998).

Staff should ensure that they are familiar with local infection control policies which will provide explicit guidance.

## Handwashing
Handwashing must be carried out after removal of protective clothing, between patient contacts, after contact with blood and body fluids, before invasive procedures and before handling food (Infection Control Nurses Association 1997).

## Skin
Cuts and abrasions in any area of exposed skin should be covered with a dressing which is waterproof, breathable and is an effective viral and bacterial barrier.

## Gloves
Seamless, non-powdered gloves should be worn whenever contact with body fluids is anticipated. Potential contact with blood or blood-stained body fluids requires powder-free natural rubber latex gloves to minimize risks relating to virus permeability. Sterile gloves are required for invasive procedures (Infection Control Nurses Association 1999).

## Aprons

Disposable plastic aprons or water-impermeable gowns should be worn whenever splashing with body fluids is anticipated.

## Eye Protection

Visors, goggles or safety spectacles should be worn whenever splashing with body fluids or flying contaminated debris/tissue is anticipated.

## Masks

Water-repellent masks are worn when there is a risk of blood splash to the face. For the care of patients with smear-positive respiratory tuberculosis, high-efficiency filter masks are worn during cough induction, bronchoscopy and for prolonged contact (Department of Health 1996).

## Sharps

Take care during the use and disposal of sharps. Do not resheathe sharps. Dispose of all sharps at the point of use into an approved sharps container (Medical Devices Agency 1993). Do not overfill containers.

## Needlestick Injury

In the event of a sharps or needlestick injury:

1. Encourage bleeding from the wound. Do not suck or rub.
2. Wash area thoroughly with soap and water.
3. Cover with a waterproof dressing.
4. If known, note the name of the patient.
5. Report to occupational health.
6. Notify line manager and document incident.
7. If the patient is thought to be HIV-positive post-exposure prophylaxis (PEP) may be required. This should be given as soon as possible after injury. Staff must be familiar with local PEP guidance (Department of Health 1997).

## Conjunctivae/mucous membranes

If splashed with blood/blood-stained body fluids irrigate with copious amounts of saline and follow steps 4–7 above.

## Spillages

Wear an apron and non-powdered latex gloves. Absorb liquid using paper towels. For blood spills either apply 10 000 ppm (1%)

hypochlorite solution or sprinkle with NaDCC granules and leave for several minutes. Clean area with detergent and water and dry. In the absence of disinfectants, and for spillage of all other body fluids, clean area thoroughly with detergent and water wearing protective clothing. Discard all equipment into yellow clinical waste bags.

## Waste

All waste contaminated with blood or body fluids must be discarded into yellow clinical waste sacks, labelled and sent for incineration according to local policy. For further details and local requirements, refer to your local infection control policy or infection control nurse.

REFERENCES

Department of Health–Interdepartmental Working Group on Tuberculosis 1996 The prevention and control of tuberculosis in the United Kingdom: recommendations for the prevention and control of tuberculosis at a local level, Department of Health and the Welsh Office. HMSO, London
Department of Health 1997 Guidelines on post-exposure prophylaxis for health care workers occupationally exposed to HIV PL/CO(97)1. HMSO, London (This guidance is due for update Spring 2000)
Infection Control Nurses Association 1997 Guidelines for hand hygiene. ICNA
Infection Control Nurses Association 1999 Glove usage guidelines. ICNA
Medical Devices Agency 1993 Use and management of sharps containers. Safety Action Bulletin no. 102, MDA
UK Health Departments 1998 Guidance for clinical health care workers: protection against infection with blood-borne viruses. HMSO, London

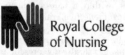 Royal College of Nursing

The above is available as a poster from RCN Direct on 0345 726 1000 quoting publication code 264.

*Reproduced with kind permission of the Royal College of Nursing, March 2000.*

# Appendix 16
# Clinical Supervision
JOHN DRISCOLL

The need to formalize opportunities for talking to each another during worktime, in order to learn as well as to support each other in practice, is legitimized by the Chief Nursing Officers of the UK. *A Vision for the Future* (Department of Health 1993) sought to provide a blueprint for nursing, midwifery and health visiting activities into the new millennium. It emphasized the development of clinical supervision as a key target for registered nurses in order to maintain clinical competence and to become more personally responsible in practice. Some of these ideas have now been given an added impetus with the demand to modernize the NHS (Department of Health 1998a, 1998b) and the expected nursing, midwifery and health visiting contribution in enhancing the quality of UK health-care provision (Department of Health 1999).

The concept of clinical supervision evolved throughout the 1990s. Its key themes are:

- A formal (contractual) process of professional support and learning.
- A way of enabling practitioners to share and learn from experience.
- A way of enhancing consumer protection and safety of care.
- A formal arrangement enabling nurses to discuss their work, at work, as regards sustaining and developing professional practice.
- The development of professional skills and competence.
- Formalized reflective practice in practice contributing to quality patient services (Driscoll 2000).

In helping practitioners implement clinical supervision, Bishop (1998) offers a useful definition for clinical practice that encompasses many of the previous ideas: 'Clinical supervision is a designated interaction between two or more practitioners, within a safe/supportive environment, which enables a continuum of reflective, critical analysis of care, to ensure quality patient services.'

While clinical supervision might be a new concept to many practitioners, its three main components are already present in everyday practice:

- Supervised clinical practice and learning.
- Organizational supervision.
- Supportive supervision.

## Supervised Clinical Practice and Learning

This type of supervision is well known to practitioners. Both parties in this relationship operate in well-defined roles in which success is identified in the form of learning outcomes. The supervisory role is usually one of assessor or mentor. This is achieved by giving regular feedback on the student's ability to meet designated learning outcomes and by making judgements about the learner's clinical competence.

## Organizational Supervision

Not unlike supervised practice, organizational or managerial supervision focuses on employee performance in the health-care setting, e.g. risk management, maintaining quality care, operationalizing human resources, financial planning or associated activities, and can be either formal or informal. Perhaps it is not surprising that the introduction of badly-thought-out clinical 'supervision' in practice can evoke suspicion, or feelings on the part of practitioners that they are being 'watched' or 'controlled' in some way by those responsible for the overall management of service delivery. The UKCC (1996), however, unequivocally states that clinical supervision is not:

- The exercise of overt managerial responsibility or managerial supervision.
- A system of formal individual performance review.
- Hierarchical in nature.

The more traditional aims and goals of management supervision, which tend to constitute a formal, monitoring process that insists on good practice, differ from clinical supervision, which is intended to be a more enabling process, focused on supporting effective practice.

## Supportive Supervision

Support systems have always been a feature of nursing practice. Some emerge from working with and knowing that you can trust particular people, that they will not laugh at you, and that they are prepared to listen to your practice concerns. Butterworth et al (1998) describe these well-known ad hoc and unplanned forms of supportive supervision as 'tear breaks', in which caring for oneself forms an important way of surviving the business of caring for others. Clinical supervision is not intended to replace such episodes in practice, but is an additional source of formalized help available to all practitioners.

Formalizing clinical supervision ensures that it becomes a legitimate part of everyday practice. Whether sessions are held one to one or in groups, the participants together negotiate and agree a written contract which identifies ground rules governing the supervision process to be undertaken. One of the fundamental differences between clinical supervision and other types of supervision already in place is the adoption of 'the qualified nurse also as a lifelong learner in practice' concept. This can be extremely challenging, whereas the previous norms of supervision in practice have tended to be more hierarchical in nature. Therefore the sorts of issue to consider in any clinical supervision contract are likely to be:

- The purpose of clinical supervision and knowing what it is not.
- Obtaining agreement on how often sessions will occur and be organized.
- How participants will know if clinical supervision is working or not.

The functions of clinical supervision in social work practice have also formed the basis of supervisory functions within much of the UK nursing literature on clinical supervision. Brigid Proctor's (1986) Interactive Model of Clinical Supervision describes three supervisory components that are not dissimilar to those previously described (supervised practice, organizational supervision and supportive supervision):

- Normative (managerial/organizational function).
- Formative (learning/educational function).
- Restorative (supportive function).

Being aware of the different functions and possibilities of supervision is not only useful for the clinical supervisor in finding a structure and establishing criteria for supervision, but also for the supervisee to maximize the use of the session time available (Driscoll 1999). The three functions can also remind practitioners of the different 'supervisory hats' or approaches among the more traditional supervision activities in practice outlined previously. Proctor's (1986) supervisory components have also formed the basis for evidencing clinical supervision outcomes in UK nursing (Bowles & Young 1999, Rafferty et al 1998).

For clinical supervision to be sustained in clinical practice in the face of all the other demands for practitioners' time, its effectiveness needs to be evaluated. For the most part, UK health employers have invested in clinical supervision largely on the assumption that it will be advantageous in clinical practice but will need to be convinced that further investment is warranted. Research is now beginning to surface about the benefits and outcomes of implementing clinical supervision in practice (Butterworth et al 1997, WMCSLS 1998).

Breaking down clinical supervision into its different component parts is easier than thinking of the topic as a whole and of how it can be monitored for effectiveness. One of the obvious things to do is to keep some record or documentation of what happens in clinical supervision rather than having to remember a specific detail when asked. Any monitoring of the effectiveness of clinical supervision should ideally rest with the supervisees' personal experience, as it is they who understand what effective and ineffective clinical supervision really are. This means taking into account qualititative not just quantitative research methods. Butterworth & Bishop (1994: 42–4) suggest it is possible to audit clinical supervision through existing reporting mechanisms.

Clinical supervision, in addition to more traditional forms of supervision in UK practice, offers many possibilities for nurse practitioners, for the organizations in which they work and, most importantly, for the persons that they care for. While the work ethic of clinical practice continues, from within modern health care there is emerging a genuine concern for the personal health of a work force increasingly faced with more complex practice challenges. Clinical supervision is about caring for oneself enough to continue to deliver effective care for others. The vehicle of clinical supervision is formalized reflective practice in practice for already qualified practitioners. Accepting the importance of being able formally to stop and intentionally reflect with others about practice, in practice, and putting back that learning for the benefit of others are fundamental principles of the remodernization of state-run health-care provision in the UK.

## References

Bishop V 1998 (ed) Clinical supervision in practice – some questions, answers and guidelines. Macmillan/Nursing Times Research, London

Bowles N, Young C 1999 An evaluative study of clinical supervision based on Proctor's three function interactive model. Journal of Advanced Nursing 30(4): 958–64

Butterworth T, Bishop V (eds) 1994 Proceedings of the Clinical Supervision Conference held on 29th November at the National Motorcycle Museum, Birmingham. NHS Executive, London

Butterworth T, Carson J, White E, Jeacock A, Clements A, Bishop V 1997 It is good to talk. An evaluation study in England and Scotland. The School of Nursing, Midwifery and Health Visiting, University of Manchester, Manchester

Butterworth T, Faugier J, Burnard P 1998 (eds) Clinical supervision and mentorship in nursing, 2nd edn. Stanley Thornes, Cheltenham, pp 1–18

Department of Health 1993 A vision for the future: the nursing, midwifery and health visiting contribution to health and health care. HMSO, London

Department of Health 1998a A first class service – quality in the new NHS. Department of Health, Leeds

Department of Health 1998b The new NHS – working together: securing a quality workforce for the NHS. Department of Health, London

Department of Health 1999 Making a difference. Strengthening the nursing, midwifery and health visiting contribution to health and healthcare. Department of Health, London

Driscoll J J 1999 Getting the most from clinical supervision: part one. The supervisee. Mental Health Practice 2(6): 28–35

Driscoll J J 2000 Practising clinical supervision: a reflective approach. Baillière Tindall (in association with the RCN), London

Proctor B 1986 Supervision: a co-operative exercise in accountability. In: Marken M, Payne M (eds) Enabling and ensuring – supervision in practice. National Youth Bureau, Council for Education and Training in Youth and Community Work, Leicester

Rafferty M, Jenkins E, Parke S 1998 Clinical supervision: what's happening in practice? A report submitted to the Clinical Effectiveness Support Unit (Wales), University of Wales, Swansea

United Kingdom Central Council for Nursing, Midwifery and Health Visiting 1996 Position statement on clinical supervision for nursing and health visiting. UKCC, London

West Midlands Clinical Supervision Learning Set (WMCSLS) 1998 Clinical supervision: getting it right in your organisation. A critical guide to good practice. West Midlands Clinical Supervision Learning Set, University of Birmingham, Birmingham

# Appendix 17
# Clinical Governance
JOHN DRISCOLL

Clinical governance has been introduced throughout the UK in order to tackle the wide differences in the quality of health care and also to address public concerns about well-publicized cases of poor professional performance (King's Fund 1999). It is one of a number of Quality NHS Reforms (Department of Health 1998a, 1998b, 1999a, 1999b) that set out to help practitioners of all professional groups maintain and improve high standards of patient care.

Other reforms being implemented alongside clinical governance as part of the remodernization of the NHS include the development of:

- National Institute for Clinical Excellence (NICE): this new special health authority has been established with responsibility for assessing the clinical and cost effectiveness of new and existing health technologies and providing guidance to the NHS on their adoption.
- National Service Frameworks (NSFs): these are templates or blueprints for care in major service areas, developed nationally by NICE, which will be used locally by the NHS Executive and other health-care organizations to review and reshape local service provision. The first two NSFs on coronary heart disease and mental health were due to be published early in 2000.
- A National Framework for Assessing Performance: a new set of performance measures or indicators is being developed, to include 41 indicators looking at the work of the NHS across six broad dimensions of performance within health care: health improvement, fair access, effective delivery of appropriate health care, patient and carer experience, health outcomes of NHS care, and efficiency (National Health Service Executive 1999a). Using these criteria the performance of health authorities and trusts will be compared and reviewed. Each health-care organization will be required to produce an annual public clinical governance report, the first of which was to be published in April 2000. The data will be collated and used by the Department of Health in the form of published 'league tables' for monitoring the different elements of quality in health-care provision.

- A Commission for Health Improvement (CHI): this new statutory body will report directly to the Secretary of State for Health and will ensure that all NHS trusts have adequate systems of clinical governance in place and are implementing national policies and guidelines issued by NICE and the NHS Executive. The Inspectorate will visit each trust periodically and have extensive powers to access information, interview staff and recommend changes where necessary.

Although quality is not a new idea in care provision, many people would agree that the use and application of quality systems in the NHS are extremely variable, producing marked differences between actual and expected levels of care. Clinical governance is aimed at coordinating the quality of clinical care delivered and ensuring that existing quality assurance initiatives within health-care organizations meet national standards. It is by far the most ambitious quality initiative that has ever been implemented in the NHS (Scally & Donaldson 1998), bringing together existing quality assurance and audit processes within health care under one national umbrella.

The UK Government expects the principles of clinical governance to apply to all those who provide or manage patient care services in the NHS (Department of Health 1998a). Every hospital, community and ambulance trust, and GP service will appoint a named lead clinician, who will ensure on behalf of the chief executive that the clinical governance framework is sufficiently robust to coordinate and monitor new and existing quality initiatives in the organization. NHS trust chief executives will be accountable for clinical governance and report regularly to publicly held trust board meetings in much the same way as for financial and resourcing matters. Health authorities and regional NHS Executive offices will ensure that the providers of health care are developing systems of clinical governance.

Clinical governance is an organization-wide initiative that requires the commitment and support of all staff for significant sustained improvement to occur. A shift in the organizational culture away from blame and punitive action towards an open, questioning, participative environment which promotes multidisciplinary activities such as team working, learning and research is necessary to create an environment conducive to clinical excellence. The chief executive and clinical directors will encourage their staff to learn from past mistakes and will be active in demonstrating the behaviours and standards required to deliver a quality service.

At a more local level, familiar quality improvement activities that directly link to clinical governance are:

- Clinical audit.
- Clinical effectiveness.
- Standard setting and monitoring.
- Evidence-based practice.
- Critical incident reporting.
- Complaints procedures.
- Clinical supervision and reflective practice.
- Risk management.

Risk management has been extended and developed in the context of controls assurance (NHS Executive 1999b) to provide a system of management to inform the trust board about significant risks within its organization.

All provide feedback and data to practitioners to enable them to assess performance, identify areas of concern, implement plans for improvement, anticipate potential problems and prevent them from developing (United Kingdom Central Council for Nursing, Midwifery and Health Visiting 1999). Obtaining regular and formalized feedback on practice such as in clinical supervision is a clear demonstration of an individual nurse or health visitor exercising responsibility under clinical governance (Butterworth & Woods 1999). In addition clinical governance in nursing, midwifery and health visiting in the UK is linked with and supported by professional self-regulation and continuing professional development activities (United Kingdom Central Council for Nursing, Midwifery and Health Visiting 1999). In many respects related health disciplines may look towards local leads and initiatives already being taken by many nurses in practice.

The Royal College of Nursing (1998) advocates a number of key principles to underpin the implementation of clinical governance:

- It must be focused on improving the quality of patient care.
- It should apply to all health care, whether in hospitals, health centres or in the community.
- It demands partnerships between clinicians and managers and between clinicians and patients.
- It should directly involve users of the health services and the wider public.
- It must recognize the key role of nursing skills and expertise around improving quality.
- It will develop in an enabling culture which celebrates success as well as learning from mistakes, rather than attributing blame.

- It applies to all NHS staff and must be clearly defined and communicated.
- It does not replace professional self-regulation or individual clinical judgement but provides a framework in which practitioners can operate.

Nursing has no need to reinvent the wheel when examining its contribution to the clinical governance agenda. What is needed is the will to adopt and capitalize on existing nursing quality initiatives. The recent publication *Making a Difference* (Department of Health 1999b) reinforces the value and importance the Government places on nursing, midwifery and health visiting and their contribution to quality improvement in UK health care.

For perhaps the first time clinical governance provides a formal link between the individual nurse, at whatever level, and the organization itself. The challenge for nursing is not only to demonstrate concern for nurses' own individual autonomy and accountability but also to join forces with its peers in demonstrating a collective interest in the quality and standard of the nursing service that is to be delivered by the organization (Castledine 1999). Such changes will not happen overnight, but should be seen as part of an overall strategy to modernize and shape the NHS well into the 21st century. Clinical governance builds on quality practices that already exist, but with a more coherent and systematic approach than has previously been seen in state-run health provision within the UK. In essence, quality has now become every health-care practitioner's responsibility.

REFERENCES

Butterworth T, Woods D 1999 Clinical governance and clinical supervision: working together to ensure safe and accountable practice (a briefing paper). School of Nursing, Midwifery and Health Visiting, University of Manchester, Manchester
Castledine G 1999 Clinical governance and self regulation in nursing. British Journal of Nursing 8(7): 4
Department of Health 1998a A first class service—quality in the new NHS. Department of Health, Leeds
Department of Health 1998b The new NHS—working together: securing a quality workforce for the NHS. Department of Health, London

Department of Health 1999a Clinical governance: quality in the new NHS. Department of Health, Leeds

Department of Health 1999b Making a difference: strengthening the nursing, midwifery and health visiting contribution to health and healthcare. Department of Health, London

King's Fund 1999 What is clinical governance? a briefing paper, February. King's Fund, London

National Health Service Executive 1999a The NHS performance assessment and network. National Health Service Executive, Leeds

National Health Service Executive 1999b Guidelines for implementing controls assurance in the NHS. National Health Service Executive, Leeds

Royal College of Nursing 1998 Guidance for nurses on clinical governance. Royal College of Nursing, London

Scally G, Donaldson L 1998 Clinical governance and the drive for quality improvement in the new NHS in England. British Medical Journal 317: 61–5

United Kingdom Central Council for Nursing, Midwifery and Health Visiting 1999 Professional self-regulation and clinical governance. UKCC, London

FURTHER READING

Brocklehurst N, Walshe K 1999 Quality and the NHS, Nursing Standard 13(51):46–53

Crinson I 1999 Clinical governance: the new NHS, new responsibilities?'. British Journal of Nursing 8(7): 449–53

Dewar S 1999 Clinical governance under construction. Harcourt Brace, London

Fatchett A 1998 Nursing in the new NHS: modern, dependable? Baillière Tindall, London

Hale C 1999 Providing support for nurses in general practice through clinical supervision: a key element of the clinical governance framework'. Journal of Clinical Governance 7: 162–5

Lilley R 1999 Making sense of clinical governance: a workbook for NHS doctors, nurses and managers (includes a CD-ROM with clinical governance planning and information system). Radcliffe Medical, Abingdon

Royal College of Nursing Institute (open learning pack) 1999 Realising clinical effectiveness and clinical governance through clinical supervision. Radcliffe Medical, Abingdon

ONLINE RESOURCES

- The Department of Health (UK) website: www.doh.gov.uk/ dhhome.htm
- The NHS Performance Assessment Framework (NHSE 1999): www.doh.gov.uk/nhsexec/nhspaf.htm
- A very detailed website resource for practitioners involved in clinical governance, whether in hospitals or the community by Wisdom–Trent NHSE: The Wisdom Centre—A Resource Pack for Clinical Governance: www.wisdom.org.uk/clingov.html
- A Model of Clinical Governance in Bradford and detailed Discussion Paper provided by Northern and Yorkshire NHS Executive Regional Office: www.doh.gov.uk/nyro/clingov/ cgbrad.htm
- The NHS Executive Regional Offices and Clinical Governance Resources: www.doh.gov.uk/nhsexec/nhseros.htm